国际经典内科学教科书

第10版
Cecil Essentials of Medicine
希氏内科学精要
中英双语版

原　著　**Edward J. Wing, MD, FACP, FIDSA**
Former Dean of Medicine and Biological Sciences
Professor of Medicine
Warren Alpert Medical School of Brown University, Providence, Rhode Island

Fred J. Schiffman, MD, MACP
Sigal Family Professor of Humanistic Medicine
Vice Chair, Department of Medicine
Warren Alpert Medical School of Brown University, Providence, Rhode Island

中英双语版　编辑委员会　主任委员　王　辰

── 第9分册 ──

感染性疾病

主　译　刘海鹰　张福杰　曹　彬

北京大学医学出版社

XISHI NEIKEXUE JINGYAO（DI 10 BAN） DI 9 FENCE　GANRANXING JIBING（ZHONGYING SHUANGYU BAN）

图书在版编目（CIP）数据

希氏内科学精要 ：第 10 版 . 第 9 分册，感染性疾病 ：汉、英 ／（美）爱德华·温（Edward J. Wing），（美）弗雷德·谢夫曼（Fred J. Schiffman）原著；刘海鹰，张福杰，曹彬主译 . -- 北京 ：北京大学医学出版社，2024. 11. -- ISBN 978-7-5659-3275-5

Ⅰ. R5

中国国家版本馆 CIP 数据核字第 20248FN453 号

北京市版权局著作权合同登记号：图字：01-2024-4518

Elsevier (Singapore) Pte Ltd.
3 Killiney Road, #08-01 Winsland House I, Singapore 239519
Tel: (65) 6349-0200; Fax: (65) 6733-1817

Cecil Essentials of Medicine, Tenth Edition
Copyright © 2022 by Elsevier, Inc. All rights are reserved, including those for text and data mining, AI training, and similar technologies.
Publisher's note: Elsevier takes a neutral position with respect to territorial disputes or jurisdictional claims in its published content, including in maps and institutional affiliations.
Previous editions copyrighted 2016, 2010, 2007, 2004, 2001, 1997, 1993, 1990, and 1986.
ISBN-13: 978-0-323-72271-1

This translation of Cecil Essentials of Medicine, Tenth Edition by Edward J. Wing and Fred J. Schiffman was undertaken by Peking University Medical Press and is published by arrangement with Elsevier (Singapore) Pte Ltd.

Cecil Essentials of Medicine, Tenth Edition by Edward J. Wing and Fred J. Schiffman 由北京大学医学出版社进行翻译，并根据北京大学医学出版社与爱思唯尔（新加坡）私人有限公司的协议约定出版。

《希氏内科学精要（第 10 版） 第 9 分册　感染性疾病（中英双语版）》（刘海鹰　张福杰　曹 彬　主译）
ISBN: 978-7-5659-3275-5
Copyright © 2024 by Elsevier (Singapore) Pte Ltd. and Peking University Medical Press.
All rights reserved. No part of this publication may be reproduced or transmitted in any form or by any means, electronic or mechanical, including photocopying, recording, or any information storage and retrieval system, without permission in writing from Elsevier (Singapore) Pte Ltd. and Peking University Medical Press.

注　意

本译本由北京大学医学出版社独立完成。相关从业及研究人员必须凭借其自身经验和知识对文中描述的信息数据、方法策略、搭配组合、实验操作进行评估和使用。由于医学科学发展迅速，临床诊断和给药剂量尤其需要经过独立验证。在法律允许的最大范围内，爱思唯尔、译文的原文作者、原文编辑及原文内容提供者均不对译文或因产品责任、疏忽或其他操作造成的人身及（或）财产伤害及（或）损失承担责任，亦不对由于使用文中提到的方法、产品、说明或思想而导致的人身及（或）财产伤害及（或）损失承担责任。

Published in China by Peking University Medical Press under special arrangement with Elsevier (Singapore) Pte Ltd. This edition is authorized for sale in the People's Republic of China only, excluding Hong Kong SAR, Macau SAR and Taiwan. Unauthorized export of this edition is a violation of the contract.

希氏内科学精要（第 10 版）　第 9 分册　感染性疾病（中英双语版）

主　　译：刘海鹰　张福杰　曹　彬

出版发行：北京大学医学出版社

地　　址：（100191）北京市海淀区学院路 38 号　北京大学医学部院内

电　　话：发行部 010-82802230；图书邮购 010-82802495

网　　址：http://www.pumpress.com.cn

E - m a i l：booksale@bjmu.edu.cn

印　　刷：北京信彩瑞禾印刷厂

经　　销：新华书店

策划编辑：高　瑾

责任编辑：董　梁　　责任校对：靳新强　　责任印制：李　啸

开　　本：889 mm×1194 mm　1/16　　印张：22.75　　字数：850 千字

版　　次：2024 年 11 月第 1 版　2024 年 11 月第 1 次印刷

书　　号：ISBN 978-7-5659-3275-5

定　　价：150.00 元

版权所有，违者必究

（凡属质量问题请与本社发行部联系退换）

中英双语版 编辑委员会

主任委员

王　辰

委　　员（按姓氏笔画排序）

王　洁	王伊龙	王建祥	巴　一	代华平	宁　光	宁晓红	朱　兰
任景怡	刘海鹰	李小鹰	李梦涛	李雪梅	杨爱明	张福杰	郑金刚
房静远	赵　晶	赵明辉	郝　伟	姜　辉	栗占国	贾继东	夏维波
黄　慧	黄晓军	曹　彬	彭　斌	潘　慧

第 1 分册　内科学概论·呼吸与危重症医学·术前和术后照护
　　　　　　主译　王　辰　代华平　赵　晶　黄　慧

第 2 分册　心血管疾病
　　　　　　主译　郑金刚　任景怡

第 3 分册　肾脏疾病
　　　　　　主译　李雪梅　赵明辉

第 4 分册　胃肠疾病·肝脏与胆道系统疾病
　　　　　　主译　房静远　杨爱明　贾继东

第 5 分册　血液疾病
　　　　　　主译　黄晓军　王建祥

第 6 分册　肿瘤疾病
　　　　　　主译　王　洁　巴　一

第 7 分册　内分泌疾病与代谢疾病·女性健康·男性健康·骨与骨矿物质代谢疾病
　　　　　　主译　宁　光　朱　兰　姜　辉　夏维波　潘　慧

第 8 分册　肌肉骨骼与结缔组织疾病
　　　　　　主译　栗占国　李梦涛

第 9 分册　感染性疾病
　　　　　　主译　刘海鹰　张福杰　曹　彬

第 10 分册　神经疾病·老年医学·缓和医疗·酒精和物质使用
　　　　　　主译　彭　斌　王伊龙　李小鹰　宁晓红　郝　伟

医学名词审定指导

任慧玲　李晓瑛　冀玉静　张燕舞　李军莲

中英双语版 序言

让我国医学生与国际医学生站在同一起跑线上的首要之事,是为其提供具有世界先进水平的标准教材。我们应争取使每一位医学生都能接触到内容经典、充分代表现代医学水平的国际权威原文教材并力求准确翻译,提供原文与中文双语对照版本,使医学生和医生在学习中形成双语医学词语、概念、概念间逻辑及由此构成的医学知识体系。在这样的思想驱动下,国际经典内科学教科书《希氏内科学精要(第10版)》中英双语版应运而生。

《希氏内科学》原著以其论述严谨准确、系统全面,被誉为"标准的内科学参考书"。自1927年首次出版以来,在内科学领域渐享世界级声誉,成为全球众多优秀医学院校,包括哈佛医学院、斯坦福大学医学院、约翰斯·霍普金斯大学医学院、牛津大学医学部、剑桥大学医学院、墨尔本大学医学院、新加坡国立大学医学院及多伦多大学医学院等普遍采用的内科学参考书。首版《希氏内科学精要》则诞生于1986年,旨在凝炼其全本的精华和要点,以最为简洁明确的方式向以医学生为主体的医学界精辟传达《希氏内科学》的核心信息,包括书中所体现出的人文精神。此后,每版精要本都力求凝炼地反映当时最新医学成果和医疗实践指南,愈来愈成为各国医学生、住院医师、专培医师及教师学习和传授内科学的主要教本,在世界医学教材体系中居引领地位。《希氏内科学》和《希氏内科学精要》两个版本不仅在英语国家被广泛使用,更被翻译为葡萄牙语、西班牙语、希腊语、意大利语、日语、简体中文版,为全球医学界广泛采用。

中国的医学生、住院医师、专培医师需要培养国际专业信息获取能力。将精要本原文引进并准确翻译,以中英文对照的形式呈现,便于读者进行双语对照阅读和学习,使之在学习理解国际标准医学内容的同时,学习好中英文医学词语,为国际医学交流打好基础。相信此举对于提高我国的医学教育水平,培养国际型医学人才至为有益。

《希氏内科学精要》精练地涵盖了内科学的所有主要领域,包括心血管疾病、呼吸疾病与危重症、消化疾病、肾脏疾病、内分泌和代谢疾病、风湿疾病、血液疾病、肿瘤、感染性疾病、神经与老年疾病等,构建了较为系统的知识体系。在翻译引进过程中,我们遵循将相关内容集中的原则,将原书按系统器官拆分为十个分册,使其更具有专科阅读的对应性,以更加灵活轻便的形式为读者提供多样化的阅读选择。

为确保译文质量，我们在译者遴选上采取了严谨的标准。从《希氏内科学（第26版）》翻译团队中择优选取责任心强、译文优质的译者，同时吸纳了临床医学专业"101"计划核心教材的编者团队。每个分册均由主译专家带领各自译者团队完成翻译、审校、交叉互审、通审四级审校工作。这些译者具备扎实的英语与专业能力，他们在翻译过程中，深入理解原文，准确阐述作者思想，并多角度审视译文的准确性、流畅性与风格一致性，确保译文的忠实性、规范性与可读性，在不同的语言和文化间架起坚实的桥梁。尤其值得称赞的是，对原著中疏漏或不够完善之处，译文中以"译者注"的形式加以适当解释和说明，使译文内容在忠实于原著的基础上更为准确。

本书读者定位于具有一定学习能力和基础的高等医学院校医学专业 8 年制、5 年制学生以及相关医学专业人员，可作为医务人员的内科学参考书、住院医师规范化培训和专科医师规范化培训辅导教材、研究生入学考试辅导教材、内科学教师参考书、内科学各专科医师复习回顾其他专科知识的重要读本。

呼吸与危重症医学教授
中国医学科学院院长
北京协和医学院校长
2024 年 11 月

对学习者教科书重要。
对学医者内科学重要。
世界上的内科学教科书，
首推《希氏内科学精要》。

中文是中国医生主要执业用语。
英文是国际医学交流的主要文字。
学习医学，当以双语对应阅读为好。
如此，可获纵横国际之效。

本书力求有助于此。

In Memoriam

Thomas E. Andreoli, MD

Dr. Thomas Andreoli, along with Drs. Lloyd Hollingsworth (Holly) Smith, Jr., Fred Plum, and Charles C.J. Carpenter, was one of the four founding editors of *Cecil Essentials of Medicine*. He served as editor for editions one through eight before he passed away on April 14, 2009. Dr. Andreoli was born in the Bronx, New York, in 1935, attended Catholic primary and high schools, and graduated from St. Vincent College and the Georgetown School of Medicine. He trained as a resident at Duke University under legendary Chair of Medicine Dr. Eugene Stead, who recognized him as a brilliant physician and scientist and encouraged his research career. Dr. Andreoli received his research training at the NIH and then in the laboratory of Dr. Tosteson at Duke. His research focused on the biochemical and biophysical properties of renal tubular cell membranes and their role in water and electrolyte transport. He made fundamental discoveries on the normal renal physiology, illuminating the way to subsequent work by many others on renal health and disease. His research was recognized with numerous awards and election to honorific societies both in the United States and in Europe. Dr. Andreoli also served as editor of *The American Journal of Physiology: Renal Physiology* and Editor in Chief of *Kidney International*.

Tom's national prominence and leadership qualities were recognized early in his career when he became head of Nephrology at the University of Alabama in Birmingham. There he helped faculty and trainees develop outstanding research, organized clinical services, and created a hemodialysis program to build one of the outstanding Divisions of Nephrology in the country. In 1979, Dr. Andreoli was appointed Chair of the Department of Internal Medicine at the University of Texas, Houston, where he assembled an outstanding faculty focused on research, clinical care, and teaching. In 1988, he accepted the position as Chairman of Internal Medicine at the University of Arkansas School of Medicine, a position he held until his death. There he again assembled a distinguished faculty who were outstanding researchers but also dedicated to outstanding clinical care and teaching. Morning report and clinical rounds with Dr. Andreoli were rigorous and riveting, focusing on the individual patient, not only their diagnoses and treatment but also on each patient's personal concerns and well-being. Dr. Andreoli was revered by medical students, his house staff, faculty, and colleagues, and I (EJW) personally can attest to what he regarded as his most cherished role—the mentorship and education of the next generation of physicians.

One of Dr. Andreoli's great interests was *Cecil Essentials of Medicine*, for which he was the editor/chief editor for eight of its ten editions, an interest that reflected his commitment to the education of students, house staff, and other physicians in the "essentials" of Internal Medicine.

Dr. Andreoli was devoted to his family. He was married to Elizabeth Berglund Andreoli from 1987 until his death. He was previously married to Dr. Kathleen Gainor Andreoli, mother of his three children and their ten grandchildren. Being of Italian ancestry and from Bronx, New York, it is not surprising that Dr. Andreoli was a passionate fan of the New York Yankees, Italian opera, which he could sing in Italian, and Frank Sinatra.

Dr. Andreoli's legacy lives on in his numerous previous students, house staff, colleagues, and in this book.

缅 怀

托马斯·安德里奥利博士

托马斯·安德里奥利（Thomas E. Andreoli）博士携手李奥德·霍灵斯沃斯·史密斯［Lloyd Hollingsworth（Holly）Smith］博士、弗雷德·普拉姆（Fred Plum）博士和查尔斯·卡彭特（Charles C.J. Carpenter）博士同为《希氏内科学精要》的创始编者。他在2009年4月14日去世前，曾担任该书第1至第8版的编者。安德里奥利博士于1935年出生于美国纽约布朗克斯区，就读于天主教小学和中学，后毕业于圣文森特学院和乔治城大学医学院。他在杜克大学医学院接受住院医师培训期间师从著名内科主任尤金·斯特德（Eugene Stead）博士，后者将其视为杰出的医生和科学家，并鼓励他投身科研事业。安德里奥利博士在美国国立卫生研究院接受科研训练后，前往杜克大学托斯特森（Tosteson）博士的实验室继续深造。他重点研究肾小管细胞膜的生化和生物物理特性及其在水和电解质转运中所发挥的作用。他在正常肾脏生理学方面的重要发现为后续关于肾脏健康和疾病的研究铺平了道路。安德里奥利博士的研究工作荣获多个学术奖项，并入选美国和欧洲的多个荣誉学会。他还担任《美国生理学杂志：肾脏生理学篇》（*The American Journal of Physiology: Renal Physiology*）的编辑以及《国际肾脏杂志》（*Kidney International*）的主编。

安德里奥利博士担任阿拉巴马大学伯明翰分校肾脏病学系主任后不久，即因其杰出领导力而赢得全美业内声誉。他帮助本校师生们取得科研突破，负责临床业务的组织实施，并因开创血液透析业务而使该科跻身全美顶级肾脏内科之列。1979年，安德里奥利博士被任命为得克萨斯大学休斯敦分校内科学系主任，他在该系组建了一支科研、临床诊疗和教学并重的优秀教职团队。自1988年起，他担任阿肯色大学医学院内科学系主任，直至辞世。在这里他再次组建了一支卓越的教职团队，他们不仅科研工作出色，临床诊疗和教学工作也出类拔萃。安德里奥利博士带领的晨会报告和查房非常严谨而引人入胜，不仅尽心竭力于每位患者的诊断和治疗，还关注到他们每个人的个体情况和福祉。安德里奥利博士深受医学生、住院医师、教职人员和同事的崇敬，我（EJW）可以证明，他最珍视的角色当属培养和教育下一代医生。

安德里奥利博士对《希氏内科学精要》倾注了满腔热忱，先后担任了该书10版中8版的编者/主编，践行他为医学生、住院医师和其他各科医生们传授内科学"精要"的承诺。

安德里奥利博士高度重视家庭。他与第二任妻子伊丽莎白·伯格兰德·安德里奥利（Elizabeth Berglund Andreoli）的婚姻从1987年延续到辞世。他与第一任妻子凯瑟琳·盖娜·安德里奥利（Kathleen Gainor Andreoli）博士育有三个子女和十个孙辈。作为意大利裔和纽约布朗克斯人，安德里奥利博士是纽约洋基队、意大利歌剧（他能用意大利语演唱）和美国著名歌手、演员、主持人弗兰克·辛纳屈（Frank Sinatra）的忠实拥趸。安德里奥利博士将永远被他的众多学生、住院医师和同事怀念，并因本书而流芳百世。

In Memoriam

Charles C.J. Carpenter, MD

Dr. Charles C.J. Carpenter joined Drs. Thomas Andreoli, Lloyd Hollingsworth Smith, Jr., and Fred Plum as a founder of *Cecil Essentials of Medicine*. He served as editor for seven editions and was followed in that role by Dr. Ivor Benjamin and then Dr. Edward Wing. Sadly, Chuck passed away on March 19, 2020, surrounded by his wife and children. He was Professor Emeritus of Medicine at The Warren Alpert Medical School of Brown University and Physician-in-Chief Emeritus at The Miriam Hospital.

Chuck was born in Savannah, Georgia, on January 5, 1931. He attended college at Princeton and medical school at Johns Hopkins where he also did his house staff training, including chief residency, and then joined the Johns Hopkins faculty. With his young family, he travelled to Calcutta, India, where he carried out landmark studies for the treatment of cholera.

Before coming to Brown in 1986, he was Chair of Medicine at Baltimore City Hospital and Case Western Reserve University.

His contributions to medical science and clinical care were many. While in Calcutta, using basic scientific evidence coupled with practical approaches, Dr. Carpenter developed "oral rehydration therapy" to address the cholera epidemic there. This treatment has saved millions of lives. While at Case, one of his innovations was to develop the nation's first Division of Geographic Medicine because of his strong belief that all physicians should be medical citizens of the world. In 1987, as he became deeply involved in the clinical management of persons living with HIV, he initiated a unique program in which Brown University faculty and trainees assumed responsibility for all HIV care in the Rhode Island State prison system.

Dr. Carpenter served as Chairman of the American Board of Internal Medicine and President of the Association of American Physicians. He has been a member of the NIH AIDS Executive Committee, the National Advisory Allergy and Infectious Diseases Council, and the USPHS AIDS Task Force. He was Chair of the Antiretroviral Treatment Panel of the International AIDS Society-USA and authored their recommendations on antiretroviral treatment. He also served as Chair of the Treatment Committee to evaluate the President's Emergency Plan for HIV/AIDS Relief. He became the director of the Brown University International Health Institute and the director of the Lifespan/Brown Center for AIDS Research with several Boston hospitals.

Throughout his career, Dr. Carpenter was the recipient of many international, national, and regional awards, accepting each with characteristic humility. With both small and large groups of learners, Chuck made certain that every member of his team was well educated, and each felt that they contributed to the well-being of their patients. His ability to sit calmly at the bedside, hold the patient's hand, comfort them, and listen in a genuinely focused way, influenced so many physicians. He was truly grateful for the opportunity to care for those less fortunate than he, and the feeling of being privileged to do so was clearly transmitted to all. Dr. Carpenter was a wonderful blend of profound compassion combined with the adherence to scholarship and teaching. Sir William Osler wrote that physicians should "Do the kind thing and do it first." Chuck lived by this precept. Vigor and insight characterized his approach to clinical and ethical challenges, always with younger colleagues at his side. In a recent tribute to him, many emphasized that Dr. Carpenter dedicated his life to his patients, many of whom were the most vulnerable members of society. We hope that we will have some of his strength and use his example as our compass as we are challenged to reduce suffering and improve the health of all for whom we are responsible.

He is survived by his wife of 61 years, Sally; three sons, Charles, Murray, and Andrew; and seven grandchildren.

缅 怀

查尔斯·卡彭特博士

查尔斯·卡彭特（Charles C.J. Carpenter）博士与托马斯·安德里奥利（Thomas E. Andreoli）博士、李奥德·霍灵斯沃斯·史密斯（Lloyd Hollingsworth Smith）博士和弗雷德·普拉姆（Fred Plum）博士共同开创了《希氏内科学精要》。他共担任了7版的编者，嗣后由艾弗·本杰明（Ivor Benjamin）博士和爱德华·温（Edward Wing）博士接任。查尔斯·卡彭特博士于2020年3月19日在妻子和子女们的陪伴下辞世。他曾担任布朗大学沃伦·阿尔珀特医学院的内科学系名誉教授和米里亚姆医院的名誉主任医师。

查尔斯·卡彭特博士于1931年1月5日出生于美国佐治亚州萨凡纳市。他在普林斯顿大学获得学士学位后进入约翰斯·霍普金斯大学医学院，并完成了包括住院总医师在内的住院医师培训，随后加入了约翰斯·霍普金斯大学的教职团队。他曾携妻子和年幼的孩子前往印度加尔各答，在当地对霍乱的治疗进行了具有里程碑意义的研究工作。

在1986年入职布朗大学之前，他曾担任巴尔的摩市医院和凯斯西储大学医学院的内科学主任。

他在医学科学研究和临床诊疗领域建树颇多。在加尔各答期间，基于基础科学证据及临床实践，查尔斯·卡彭特博士开创了"口服补液疗法"以遏制当地的霍乱疫情。这一疗法拯救了数百万人的生命。秉承医生无国界的世界公民理念，他在凯斯西储大学做了一项开创性工作，建立了美国首个地缘医学部（研究地理环境因素对人体健康和疾病影响的学科）。1987年，他深度参与人类免疫缺陷病毒（HIV）携带者的临床管理，并发起了一个独特的项目——由布朗大学教职团队和医学生们承担罗德岛州监狱系统内所有艾滋病相关诊疗工作。

查尔斯·卡彭特博士曾担任美国内科医师委员会主席和美国医师协会主席。他曾是美国国立卫生研究院艾滋病行政委员会、美国国家过敏与传染病咨询委员会以及公共卫生服务部艾滋病工作组的成员。他还曾担任国际艾滋病学会-美国分会抗逆转录病毒治疗组主席，并撰写了抗逆转录病毒治疗建议。他还担任过艾滋病治疗委员会主席，该委员会负责评估美国总统防治艾滋病紧急救援计划；曾担任布朗大学国际健康研究所所长，以及大学与多家波士顿当地医院合办的生命周期/布朗大学艾滋病研究中心主任。

查尔斯·卡彭特博士在职业生涯中获得过诸多国际性、全美和地区性奖项，同时展现其谦逊品格。无论学员人数多寡，查尔斯·卡彭特博士都会确保人人都能受到良好教育，并让他们感到自己也对患者的健康做出了贡献。他能够安静地坐在病床边，握住患者的手，安慰他们，并全神贯注地听取患者倾诉，这一举动深深地感染了许多医生。他十分珍视诊治不幸染病者的机会，并且能够将这种殊荣感传递给所有人。查尔斯·卡彭特博士完美地融汇了对患者的宅心仁厚与对学术和教学的坚守。威廉·奥斯勒（William Osler）爵士曾写道，医生应该"行善事，为人先"，而这正是查尔斯·卡彭特博士一生奉行的信条。他在面对临床和伦理挑战时充满活力和洞察力，始终重视提携年轻同事。许多人的悼词中都重点指出，查尔斯·卡彭特博士将毕生致力于患者福祉，其中许多人属于社会上最弱势群体。我们希望，在我们面临减少患者痛苦及改善其健康状况的挑战时，能够拥有他的力量，并以他为榜样获得指引。

查尔斯·卡彭特博士与妻子萨丽（Sally）共度了61年的婚姻时光，育有查尔斯（Charles）、穆雷（Murray）和安德鲁（Andrew）三子以及七个孙辈。

ABOUT THE EDITORS

Dr. Edward J. Wing was an editor of *Cecil Essentials of Medicine,* editions 8 and 9, and is the lead editor of edition 10. He graduated from Williams College in 1967 and from the Harvard Medical School in 1971. He was a resident in Internal Medicine at the Peter Bent Brigham and completed an Infectious Diseases Fellowship at Stanford University. Joining the faculty at the University of Pittsburgh in 1975, he focused his NIH-funded research on mechanisms of cell-mediated immunity as well as various clinical aspects of Infectious Diseases. From 1990 to 1998, the University and UPMC appointed him as Physician-in-Chief at Montefiore Hospital, then Chief of Infectious Diseases, and finally Interim Chair of Medicine.

In 1998, Dr. Wing became Chair of Medicine at Brown University (1998–2008) where he consolidated the department across hospitals, practice plans, and training programs. As Dean of Medicine and Biological Sciences at Brown University (2008–2013) he strengthened ties with affiliated hospitals (Lifespan and Care New England), increased research, and oversaw the construction of a new medical school building. International exchange programs with medical schools in Kenya, the Dominican Republic, and Haiti were established during his years as chairman and dean. Dr. Wing has cared for patients with HIV since the beginning of the epidemic in outpatient clinics. He continues to be active in research, clinical care, and teaching.

Dr. Fred J. Schiffman, who along with Dr. Edward Wing is editor of *Cecil Essentials of Medicine,* 10th edition, attended Wagner College and then the New York University School of Medicine, from which he graduated in 1973. He performed his early house staff training at Yale-New Haven Hospital and then spent two years at the National Cancer Institute. He returned to Yale as Chief Medical Resident followed by a hematology fellowship. He became Medical Director of Yale's Primary Care Center before coming to Brown University in 1983, where he has been a leader in the medical residency program as well as Associate Physician-in-Chief at The Miriam Hospital.

Dr. Schiffman holds The Sigal Family Professorship in Humanistic Medicine at The Warren Alpert Medical School of Brown University. His scholarly interests include the structure and function of the human spleen and the intersection of the arts and medical care. He has directed or championed many projects and programs, including those that encourage and reinforce wellness and resilience in patients, families, and caregivers. He began a novel program that places medical students and physicians with other nonmedical professionals as they share in the viewing of works of art in the Museum of the Rhode Island School of Design. Dr. Schiffman recently led a Brown University edX course entitled, "Artful Medicine: Art's Power to Enrich Patient Care," with worldwide participation. Dr. Schiffman has also edited texts on hematologic pathophysiology, consultative hematology, and the anemias.

原著主编

爱德华·温（Edward J. Wing）博士是《希氏内科学精要》第 8 版和第 9 版的编者，以及第 10 版的主编。他先后于 1967 年和 1971 年毕业于威廉姆斯学院和哈佛医学院。他曾在彼得·本特·布里格姆医院任内科住院医师，后在斯坦福大学完成了传染病学的专科医师（Fellowship）课程。自 1975 年加入匹兹堡大学医学院以来，他通过美国国立卫生研究院资助的研究项目，探索细胞介导免疫的机制以及传染病学各领域的临床诊疗工作。1990—1998 年期间，他先后被匹兹堡大学及其医学中心任命为蒙特菲奥里医院的主任医师、传染病科主任，后担任内科临聘主任。

1998 年起，温博士担任布朗大学医学院的内科主任（1998—2008 年）。在此期间，他在不同医院、实践计划和培训项目间对内科进行整合。在担任布朗大学医学与生物科学院院长（2008—2013 年）期间，他加强了与各附属医院（Lifespan 医院和 Care New England 医院）间的联系，提升了科研工作的水准，并为医学院建成了一座新楼。在担任主任和院长期间，他还建立了与肯尼亚、多米尼加共和国和海地的医学院的国际交流项目。温博士自艾滋病流行初期便在门诊诊治艾滋病患者，并始终工作在科研、临床和教学一线。

弗雷德·谢夫曼（Fred J. Schiffman）博士与爱德华·温（Edward Wing）博士共同担任《希氏内科学精要》第 10 版的主编。他就读于瓦格纳学院，随后进入纽约大学医学院，并于 1973 年毕业。他在耶鲁大学附属纽黑文医院接受早期住院医师培训，随后在美国国家癌症研究所工作了两年。回到耶鲁大学后，他担任住院总医师，然后完成了血液学专科医师课程，随后成为耶鲁初级保健中心医学主任。他于 1983 年入职布朗大学，领导医学住院医师项目并担任米里亚姆医院的副主任医师。

谢夫曼博士担任布朗大学沃伦·阿尔珀特医学院人文医学系的西格尔家庭医学教授。他的学术兴趣涵盖人体脾脏的结构和功能，以及艺术与医疗的交叉融合。他主持或参与了许多项目和计划，其中包括许多旨在鼓励和加强患者、家人和医护人员的福祉与康复能力的项目。他所创办的一个新项目可以让医学生和医生与其他非医学专业人士一起，共同欣赏罗德岛设计学院博物馆的艺术作品。谢夫曼博士近期还主持了布朗大学名为"艺术与医学：艺术赋能患者照护"的 edX 课程，此课程的参与者来自全球多个国家。谢夫曼博士还出版了有关血液病理生理学、血液科会诊和贫血的著作。

原著者名单

Jinnette Dawn Abbott, MD
Rajiv Agarwal, MD
Marwa Al-Badri, MD
Hyeon-Ju Ryoo Ali, MD
Jason M. Aliotta, MD
Khaldoun Almhanna, MD, MPH
Mohanad T. Al-Qaisi, MD
Zuhal Arzomand, MD
Akwi W. Asombang, MD, MPH
Su N. Aung, MD, MPH
Christopher G. Azzoli, MD
Christina Bandera, MD
Debasree Banerjee, MD
Mashal Batheja, MD
Jeffrey J. Bazarian, MD, MPH
Selim R. Benbadis, MD
Ivor J. Benjamin, MD, FAHA, FACC
Eric Benoit, MD
Marcie G. Berger, MD
Clemens Bergwitz, MD
Nancy Berliner, MD
Jeffrey S. Berns, MD
Pooja Bhadbhade, DO
Ratna Bhavaraju-Sanka, MD
Tanmayee Bichile, MD
Ariel E. Birnbaum, MD
Charles M. Bliss, Jr., MD
Andrew S. Blum, MD, PhD
Bryan J. Bonder, MD
Russell Bratman, MD
Glenn D. Braunstein, MD
Alma M. Guerrero Bready, MD
Richard Bungiro, PhD
Anna Marie Burgner, MD, MEHP
Jonathan Cahill, MD
Andrew Canakis, DO
Benedito A. Carneiro, MD, MS
Brian Casserly, MD
Abdullah Chahin, MD, MA, MSc
Philip A. Chan, MD
Kimberle Chapin, MD
William P. Cheshire, Jr., MD
Waihong Chung, MD, PhD
Emma Ciafaloni, MD

Joaquin E. Cigarroa, MD
Michael P. Cinquegrani, MD
Andreea Coca, MD, MPH
Harvey Jay Cohen, MD
Scott Cohen, MD, MPH
Beatrice P. Concepcion, MD, MS
Nathan T. Connell, MD, MPH
Maria Constantinou, MD
Roberto Cortez, MD
Timothy J. Counihan, MD, FRCPI
Anne Haney Cross, MD
Cheston B. Cunha, MD, FACP
Joanne S. Cunha, MD
Susan Cu-Uvin, MD
Noura M. Dabbouseh, MD
Kwame Dapaah-Afriyie, MD, MBA
Erin M. Denney-Koelsch, MD
Andre De Souza, MD
An S. De Vriese, MD, PhD
Neal D. Dharmadhikari, MD
Leah Dickstein, MD
Don Dizon, MD, FACP, FASCO
Robyn T. Domsic, MD, MPH
Kim A. Eagle, MD
Michael G. Earing, MD
Pamela Egan, MD
Wafik S. El-Deiry, MD, PhD, FACP
Mitchell S. V. Elkind, MD, MS
Tarra B. Evans, MD
Michael B. Fallon, MD
Dimitrios Farmakiotis, MD
Francis A. Farraye, MD
Ronan Farrell, MD
Panayotis Fasseas, MD, FACC
Mary Anne Fenton, MD
Fernando C. Fervenza, MD, PhD
Sean Fine, MD
Arkadiy Finn, MD
Timothy Flanigan, MD
Brisas M. Flores, MD
Andrew E. Foderaro, MD
Theodore C. Friedman, MD, PhD
Joseph Metmowlee Garland, MD, AAHIVM

Eric J. Gartman, MD
Abdallah Geara, MD
Raul Macias Gil, MD
Timothy Gilligan, MD, FASCO
Michael Raymond Goggins, MB BCh BAO, MRCPI
Geetha Gopalakrishnan, MD
Vidya Gopinath, MD
Susan L. Greenspan, MD, FACP
Osama Hamdy, MD, PhD
Johanna Hamel, MD
Sajeev Handa, MD, SFHM
Mitchell T. Heflin, MD, MHS
Robert G. Holloway, MD, MPH
Christopher S. Huang, MD
Zilla Hussain, MD
T. Alp Ikizler, MD
Iris Isufi, MD
Carlayne E. Jackson, MD
Paul G. Jacob, MD, MPH
Matthew D. Jankowich, MD
Niels V. Johnsen, MD, MPH
Jessica E. Johnson, MD
Rayford R. June, MD
Tareq Kheirbek, MD, ScM, FACS
Alok A. Khorana, MD, FACP, FASCO
Sena Kilic, MD
David Kim, MD
James Kleczka, MD
James R. Klinger, MD
Patrick Koo, MD, ScM
Pooja Koolwal, MD
Mary P. Kotlarczyk, PhD
Nicole M. Kuderer, MD
Awewura Kwara, MD
Jennifer M. Kwon, MD, MPH
Richard A. Lange, MD, MBA
Jerome Larkin, MD
Alfred I. Lee, MD, PhD
Daniel J. Levine, MD
David E. Lewandowski, MD
Kelly V. Liang, MD, MS
Kimberly P. Liang, MD, MS
David R. Lichtenstein, MD

扫描二维码了解更多信息

Douglas W. Lienesch, MD
Geoffrey S.F. Ling, MD, PhD
Ester Little, MD, FACP
Yi Liu, MD
Nicole L. Lohr, MD, PhD
John R. Lonks, MD, FACP, FIDSA, FSHEA
Gary H. Lyman, MD, MPH
Jeffrey M. Lyness, MD
Shane Lyons, MD, MRCPI, MRCP(UK)
Diana Maas, MD
Talha A. Malik, MD, MSPH
Sonia Manocha, MD
Susan Manzi, MD, MPH
Frederick J. Marshall, MD
F. Dennis McCool, MD
Russell J. McCulloh, MD
Kelly McGarry, MD, FACP
Eavan Mc Govern, MD, PhD
Robin L. McKinney, MD
Anthony Mega, MD
Shivang Mehta, MD
Douglas F. Milam, MD
Maria D. Mileno, MD
Abhinav Kumar Misra, MBBS, MD
Orson W. Moe, MD
Niveditha Mohan, MBBS
Larry W. Moreland, MD
Alan R. Morrison, MD, PhD
Steven F. Moss, MD
Christopher J. Mullin, MD, MHS
Sinéad M. Murphy, MB, BCh, MD, FRCPI
Sagarika Nallu, MD, FAAP, FAAN, FAASM
Javier A. Neyra, MD, MSCS
Ghaith Noaiseh, MD
Thomas A. Ollila, MD
Steven M. Opal, MD
Biff F. Palmer, MD
Jen Jung Pan, MD, PhD
Anna Papazoglou, MD
Aric Parnes, MD
Nayan M. Patel, DO, MPH
Ari Pelcovits, MD
Mark A. Perazella, MD
Michael F. Picco, MD, PhD
Kate E. Powers, DO
Laura A. Previll, MD, MPH
Nilum Rajora, MD
Adolfo Ramirez-Zamora, MD
John Reagan, MD
Rebecca Reece, MD
Harlan Rich, MD, AGAF, FACP
Jennifer H. Richman, MD
Lisa R. Rogers, DO
Ralph Rogers, MD
Michal G. Rose, MD
James A. Roth, MD
Sharon Rounds, MD
Jason C. Rubenstein, MD
Abbas Rupawala, MD
Jenna Sarvaideo, DO
Ramesh Saxena, MD, PhD
Fred J. Schiffman, MD, MACP
Ruth B. Schneider, MD
Kristin A. Seaborg, MD
Anil Seetharam, MD
Stuart Seropian, MD
Jigme Michael Sethi, MD
Sanjeev Sethi, MD, PhD
Elizabeth Shane, MD
Esseim Sharma, MD
Shani Shastri, MD, MPH
Barry S. Shea, MD
Lauren Shevell, MD, MPH
Joseph A. Smith, Jr., MD
Robert J. Smith, MD
Davendra P.S. Sohal, MD, MPH
Christopher Song, MD, FACC
Thomas Sperry, MD
Jeffrey M. Statland, MD
Emily M. Stein, MD
Jennifer L. Strande, MD, PhD
Rochelle Strenger, MD
Thomas R. Talbot, MD, MPH
Christopher G. Tarolli, MD, MSEd
Yael Tarshish, MD
Pushpak Taunk, MD
Philip Tsoukas, MD
Allan R. Tunkel, MD, PhD
Jeffrey M. Turner, MD
Zoe G.S. Vazquez, MD
Stacie A. F. Vela, MD
Paul M. Vespa, MD, FCCM, FAAN, FANA, FNCS
Wanpen Vongpatanasin, MD
Marcella D. Walker, MD
Eunice S. Wang, MD
Sharmeel K. Wasan, MD
Thomas J. Weber, MD
Brandon J. Wilcoxson, MD
Edward J. Wing, MD, FACP, FIDSA
Ellice Wong, MD
John J. Wysolmerski, MD
Rayan Yousefzai, MD
Thomas R. Ziegler, MD
Rebecca Zon, MD

ACKNOWLEDGMENTS

Dr. Schiffman and I wish to thank first of all, the authors of the 128 chapters that make up the tenth edition of *Cecil Essentials of Medicine.* They have worked diligently to compose the material for each chapter and apply their mastery as they added the newest information, in clear language, to the text. Their efforts are apparent in the excellence of the book, and we are immensely grateful for their work. We wish to also thank Marybeth Thiel, Jennifer Ehlers, and Dan Fitzgerald from Elsevier who guided and supported our work as editors and whose expertise has made this volume possible. Finally, we are always thankful to our wives, Dr. Rena Wing and Ms. Gerri Schiffman, without whose love, support, and especially humor, this book would not have happened.

致 谢

　　谢夫曼博士和我首先要致谢《希氏内科学精要》第10版全书128章的各位作者。感谢他们精益求精地撰写每一章节，并运用其专业知识，以简明的语言将前沿资讯呈现在书中。正是他们的辛勤努力确保了本书的卓越地位，对他们唯有由衷的感激。我们还要感谢爱思唯尔出版集团的玛丽贝丝·蒂尔（Marybeth Thiel）、詹妮弗·埃勒斯（Jennifer Ehlers）和丹·菲茨杰拉德（Dan Fitzgerald），他们对本书的编辑工作给予了指导和支持，其专业水准保障了本书的完稿。最后，要特别感谢我们的妻子——蕾娜·温（Rena Wing）博士和盖瑞·谢夫曼（Gerri Schiffman）女士，对她们的爱和支持，特别是积极乐观的心态始终心存感激，她们为本书的圆满完成发挥了不可或缺的作用。

总目录

第 1 分册

第 1 篇　内科学概论　Introduction to Medicine
第 2 篇　呼吸与危重症医学　Pulmonary and Critical Care Medicine
第 3 篇　术前和术后照护　Preoperative and Postoperative Care

第 2 分册

心血管疾病　Cardiovascular Disease

第 3 分册

肾脏疾病　Renal Disease

第 4 分册

第 1 篇　胃肠疾病　Gastrointestinal Disease
第 2 篇　肝脏与胆道系统疾病　Diseases of the Liver and Biliary System

第 5 分册

血液疾病　Hematologic Disease

第 6 分册

肿瘤疾病　Oncologic Disease

第 7 分册

第 1 篇　内分泌疾病与代谢疾病　Endocrine Disease and Metabolic Disease
第 2 篇　女性健康　Women's Health
第 3 篇　男性健康　Men's Health
第 4 篇　骨与骨矿物质代谢疾病　Diseases of Bone and Bone Mineral Metabolism

第 8 分册

肌肉骨骼与结缔组织疾病　Musculoskeletal and Connective Tissue Disease

第 9 分册

感染性疾病　Infectious Disease

第 10 分册

第 1 篇　神经疾病　Neurologic Disease
第 2 篇　老年医学　Geriatrics
第 3 篇　缓和医疗　Palliative Care
第 4 篇　酒精和物质使用　Alcohol and Substance Use

第 9 分册

感染性疾病

第9分册译者名单

主 译

刘海鹰　张福杰　曹　彬

译 者（按姓氏笔画排序）

王　芳	首都医科大学附属北京地坛医院	张福杰	首都医科大学附属北京地坛医院
田　地	首都医科大学附属北京地坛医院	张碧莹	北京大学第三医院
代丽丽	首都医科大学附属北京佑安医院	郑和义	中国医学科学院北京协和医院
宁永忠	北京市垂杨柳医院	黄　磊	中国人民解放军总医院第五医学中心
朱华栋	中国医学科学院北京协和医院	曹　玮	中国医学科学院北京协和医院
刘明娟	中国医学科学院北京协和医院	曹　彬	中日友好医院
刘海鹰	中国医学科学院病原生物学研究所	崔晓敬	中日友好医院
刘智博	中日友好医院	康　梅	四川大学华西医院
阮巧玲	复旦大学附属华山医院	彭俊平	中国医学科学院病原生物学研究所
李　军	中国医学科学院北京协和医院	葛　瑛	中国医学科学院北京协和医院
李太生	中国医学科学院北京协和医院	韩　宁	首都医科大学附属北京地坛医院
杨　帆	中国医学科学院病原生物学研究所	韩　红	中国医学科学院北京协和医院
杨雯婷	中日友好医院	舒跃龙	中国医学科学院病原生物学研究所
肖　江	首都医科大学附属北京地坛医院	鲁炳怀	中日友好医院
张文宏	复旦大学附属华山医院	路　明	北京大学第三医院
张利军	重庆医科大学附属第二医院		

第9分册目录

感染性疾病　Infectious Disease

1. Host Defenses Against Infection, 4
   宿主对感染的防御，5

2. Laboratory Diagnosis of Infectious Diseases, 28
   感染性疾病的实验室诊断，29

3. Fever and Febrile Syndromes, 40
   发热和发热性综合征，41

4. Bacteremia and Sepsis, 60
   菌血症和感染中毒症，61

5. Infections of the Central Nervous System, 74
   中枢神经系统感染，75

6. Infections of the Head and Neck, 108
   头颈部感染，109

7. Infections of the Lower Respiratory Tract, 118
   下呼吸道感染，119

8. Infections of the Heart and Blood Vessels, 134
   心脏和血管的感染，135

9. Acute Bacterial Skin and Skin Structure Infections, 150
   急性细菌性皮肤和皮肤结构感染，151

10. Intraabdominal Infections, 164
    腹腔内感染，165

11. Infectious Diarrhea, 176
    感染性腹泻，177

12. Infections Involving Bone and Joints, 188
    累及骨和关节的感染，189

13. Urinary Tract Infections, 194
    尿路感染，195

14. Health Care-Associated Infections, 202
    医疗照护相关感染，203

15. Sexually Transmitted Infections, 214
    性传播感染，215

16 Human Immunodeficiency Virus Infection, 232
人类免疫缺陷病毒感染，233

17 Infections in the Immunocompromised Host, 270
免疫妥协宿主的感染，271

18 Infectious Diseases of Travelers: Protozoal and Helminthic Infections, 290
旅行者感染性疾病：原虫和蠕虫感染，291

附录 Coronavirus Disease 2019 (COVID-19), 304
2019 冠状病毒病（COVID-19），305

索引 Index，320

CECIL ESSENTIALS OF MEDICINE

Infectious Disease

Infectious Disease

1. Host Defenses Against Infection, 4
2. Laboratory Diagnosis of Infectious Diseases, 28
3. Fever and Febrile Syndromes, 40
4. Bacteremia and Sepsis, 60
5. Infections of the Central Nervous System, 74
6. Infections of the Head and Neck, 108
7. Infections of the Lower Respiratory Tract, 118
8. Infections of the Heart and Blood Vessels, 134
9. Acute Bacterial Skin and Skin Structure Infections, 150
10. Intraabdominal Infections, 164
11. Infectious Diarrhea, 176
12. Infections Involving Bone and Joints, 188
13. Urinary Tract Infections, 194
14. Health Care-Associated Infections, 202
15. Sexually Transmitted Infections, 214
16. Human Immunodeficiency Virus Infection, 232
17. Infections in the Immunocompromised Host, 270
18. Infectious Diseases of Travelers: Protozoal and Helminthic Infections, 290

APPENDIX   Coronavirus Disease 2019 (COVID-19), 304

感染性疾病

1 宿主对感染的防御，5

2 感染性疾病的实验室诊断，29

3 发热和发热性综合征，41

4 菌血症和感染中毒症，61

5 中枢神经系统感染，75

6 头颈部感染，109

7 下呼吸道感染，119

8 心脏和血管的感染，135

9 急性细菌性皮肤和皮肤结构感染，151

10 腹腔内感染，165

11 感染性腹泻，177

12 累及骨和关节的感染，189

13 尿路感染，195

14 医疗照护相关感染，203

15 性传播感染，215

16 人类免疫缺陷病毒感染，233

17 免疫妥协宿主的感染，271

18 旅行者感染性疾病：原虫和蠕虫感染，291

附录 2019 冠状病毒病（COVID-19），305

1

Host Defenses Against Infection

Richard Bungiro, Edward J. Wing

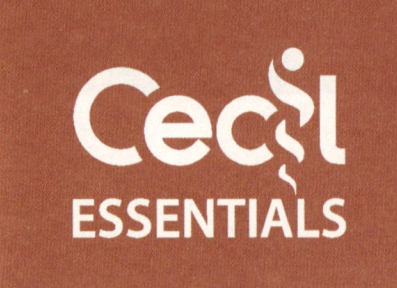

HOST VERSUS PATHOGEN: VICTORY, DEATH, OR COEXISTENCE

Many factors determine whether we coexist peacefully with our normal microbial flora and also whether we live or die in an environment filled with a wide spectrum of potentially pathogenic microbes. Factors such as age, nutritional status, underlying medical conditions (e.g., diabetes mellitus, chronic pulmonary disease), and the nature of the exposure (e.g., microbial virulence, inoculum size) may affect our response to infectious disease, with the outcome ultimately determined by our host defenses, which include anatomic (e.g., skin) and physiologic barriers (e.g., stomach acid), innate immune responses (e.g., phagocytes, microbial pattern receptors), and adaptive responses that include specific antibodies and cell–mediated immunity.

Humans are equipped with a multilayered host defense system to counter infectious organisms, and the interaction between a potential pathogen and a human can lead to one of three basic outcomes: death of the human host, elimination of the pathogen (with or without clinical symptoms), or an ongoing symbiotic relationship whose nature may change with time and under additional biologic pressures. For example, while some healthy humans are colonized by *Streptococcus pneumoniae*, pneumonia or meningitis may be caused by virulent strains, leading to death if the host's defenses cannot eliminate the pathogen in time. Most individuals exposed to *Mycobacterium tuberculosis* are asymptomatic because the adaptive immune response contains the organism in a live but nonreplicating (latent) state. Almost one third of the world's population is so infected, but only about 10% progress to active disease. Immunologic impairment (e.g., as a result of human immunodeficiency virus [HIV] infection) and factors such as age-associated immune senescence increase the risk of progressing from latent to active disease.

The asymptomatic nature of an infection should not automatically be equated with latency or dormancy of the pathogen. For example, chronic HIV infection was initially incorrectly characterized as having a prolonged latent or silent stage before the host developed immunodeficiency and opportunistic infections. However, most untreated HIV-infected individuals harbor actively replicating virus that kill $CD4^+$ T lymphocytes on a daily basis, although the aggregate effects are not appreciated until $CD4^+$ T lymphocyte levels are reduced to below 200 cells/mL, typically after 8 to 10 years of infection without antiretroviral treatment. Infected individuals are contagious to others despite their relatively asymptomatic state, thus treatment (when available) is recommended regardless of $CD4^+$ T lymphocyte levels. Treatment halts viral immune destruction and reduces viral burden in blood and genital secretions, thus decreasing an infected individual's risk of transmitting HIV.

CATEGORIES OF HOST DEFENSES AND RISKS OF INFECTION

The relative importance of the innate and adaptive immune defenses is best illustrated by individuals who are deficient in a particular immunological component. For example, cancer chemotherapy may lead to the depletion of innate cells such as neutrophils, rendering the host more susceptible to bacterial and fungal infections. Congenital deficiency of immunoglobulins increases the risk of infections that are usually thwarted by antibody responses such as those associated with *Streptococcus pneumoniae* and *Haemophilus influenzae*. Pharmacologic inhibition of tumor necrosis factor-α (TNF-α) for the treatment of chronic inflammatory disease such as Crohn's or psoriasis increases the risk of developing active tuberculosis among those with latent infection. In 1981 astute clinicians, recognizing the increased incidence of an atypical pneumonia caused by *Pneumocystis jirovecii* (formerly *P. carinii*) among young men, sounded the alarm that a novel acquired immunodeficiency syndrome (eventually shown to primarily affect $CD4^+$ T lymphocytes) had appeared that was later ascribed to HIV.

Host defenses to infection can be classified as nonimmunologic barriers, innate immunity, and specific or adaptive immunity. Immune defenses against microbial pathogens are composed of cells and molecules located in the blood, peripheral sites such as the skin and submucosal regions, and in secondary lymphoid tissues such as the lymph nodes, tonsils, spleen, and Peyer patches.

For a deeper discussion of these topics, please see Chapters 39 through 44 in Section VII, "Principles of Immunology and Inflammation," in *Goldman-Cecil Medicine*, 26th Edition.

Nonimmunologic Host Defenses

Nonimmunologic host defenses include anatomic and physiologic barriers that prevent the entry of pathogens into the body. Injuries or devices that damage or bypass anatomic barriers frequently lead to infection. Examples include burns, intravenous catheters, intubation, urinary tract catheters, surgery, and trauma.

The respiratory tract defenses depend on mucus that entraps pathogens and on ciliary action and cough that continuously clear the mucus and organisms from the lungs and upper airways. Respiratory viruses, including influenza, may inhibit ciliary action or denude the mucous membrane completely, allowing bacteria to colonize and cause secondary infection. Stroke, medications, or other causes of reduced cough reflex may lead to poor clearance of secretions, mucus, and pathogens, leading to lung infection. Smoking and exposure to industrial toxins such as silica may similarly reduce lung host defenses, such as by reducing ciliary action and inhibiting alveolar macrophage function respectively. Alveolar macrophages located in the lung parenchyma play an essential role in the initial clearance and killing of pathogens.

宿主对感染的防御

刘海鹰 译 舒跃龙 李太生 审校 刘海鹰 通审

宿主 vs. 病原体：胜利，死亡或共存

众多因素决定了我们是否能与正常的微生物菌群和平共处，以及我们是否能在充满各种潜在致病微生物的环境中生存或死亡。年龄、营养状况、基础疾病（如糖尿病、慢性肺病）和暴露的性质（如微生物毒力、接种量）等因素可能会影响我们对感染性疾病的反应，其结果最终取决于我们的宿主防御系统，包括解剖屏障（如皮肤）和生理屏障（如胃酸）、先天免疫应答（如吞噬细胞、微生物模式受体）以及包括特异性抗体和细胞介导的适应性免疫应答。

人类拥有多个层次的宿主防御系统来对抗感染性生物体，潜在病原体与人类之间的相互作用可能导致三种基本结果之一：人类宿主死亡、病原体被消除（可能伴有或不伴有临床症状），或者形成持续的共生关系，其性质可能会随着时间的推移和生物压力的增加而发生变化。例如，虽然肺炎链球菌可以定植于一些健康人体内，但感染其毒力株可导致肺炎或脑膜炎，如果宿主的防御不能及时消除病原体，就会导致死亡。大多数个体感染结核分枝杆菌后都是无症状的，因为适应性免疫应答可使这一生物体处于存活但非复制（潜伏）状态。世界上近 1/3 的人口感染了结核分枝杆菌，但只有约 10% 发展为活动性疾病。免疫损伤［如，由于感染人类免疫缺陷病毒（HIV）］和年龄相关的免疫衰老等因素增加了从潜伏状态发展为活动性疾病的风险。

无症状感染并不意味着病原体处于潜伏期或休眠状态。例如，慢性 HIV 感染最初被错误地描述为在宿主出现免疫缺陷和机会性感染之前有一个长期的潜伏或沉默阶段。然而，大多数未经治疗的 HIV 感染者体内都有活跃复制的病毒，每天都在杀死 $CD4^+$ T 细胞，尽管在 $CD4^+$ T 细胞水平降低到 200/ml 以下（通常是感染 8～10 年后且未经抗逆转录病毒治疗）时，这种综合效应才会显现出来。尽管感染者相对无症状，但仍会传染给其他人，因此无论 $CD4^+$ T 细胞水平如何，都建议进行治疗（如果有条件）。治疗可阻止病毒破坏免疫系统，减少血液和生殖道分泌物中的病毒载量，从而降低感染者传播 HIV 的风险。

宿主防御的分类和感染风险

先天性和适应性免疫防御的相对重要性可以通过缺乏特定免疫成分的人得到最好的说明。例如，癌症化疗可能导致中性粒细胞等先天免疫细胞耗竭，使宿主更容易感染细菌和真菌。先天性缺乏免疫球蛋白会增加感染的风险，而这些感染通常被抗体反应（例如与肺炎链球菌和流感嗜血杆菌相关的抗体反应）阻断。使用抑制肿瘤坏死因子 -α（TNF-α）的药物来治疗慢性炎症性疾病（如克罗恩病或银屑病）会增加结核分枝杆菌潜伏感染患者发展为活动性结核病的风险。1981 年，敏锐的临床医生发现年轻男性中由耶氏肺孢子虫（以前称为卡氏肺孢子虫）引起的非典型肺炎发病率增加，于是敲响了一种新型获得性免疫缺陷综合征出现的警钟，最终证明其主要影响 $CD4^+$ T 细胞，后来被归因于 HIV。

宿主对感染的防御可分为非免疫屏障、先天免疫和特异性或适应性免疫。针对微生物病原体的免疫防御系统由位于血液、皮肤和黏膜下区域等外周部位以及淋巴结、扁桃体、脾和派尔集合淋巴结等次级淋巴组织中的细胞和分子组成。

有关此专题的深入讨论，请参阅 *Goldman-Cecil Medicine* 第 26 版第 7 篇"免疫学和炎症原理"中的第 39～44 章。

非免疫性宿主防御

非免疫性宿主防御包括防止病原体进入体内的解剖学和生理学屏障。损伤或破坏或绕过解剖屏障的装置经常导致感染，包括烧伤、静脉导管、气管插管、尿路导管、手术和创伤。

呼吸道的防御功能依赖于捕获病原体的黏液，以及不断清除肺部和上呼吸道黏液和病原体的纤毛运动和咳嗽。呼吸道病毒感染，包括流感，可能会抑制纤毛运动或使黏膜完全脱落，从而使细菌定植并引起继发感染。卒中、药物或其他导致咳嗽反射减弱的原因可能导致分泌物、黏液和病原体清除不畅，导致肺部感染。吸烟和暴露于工业毒素（如二氧化硅）分别通过减少纤毛运动和抑制肺泡巨噬细胞功能，也同样能降低肺部宿主防御能力。位于肺实质中的肺泡巨噬细胞在最初清除和杀死病原体方面发挥着重要作用。

Nonimmune gastrointestinal defenses include gastric acidity, which kills many microorganisms, and vomiting and diarrhea, which help to clear pathogens from the gut. Bacteria vary greatly in their susceptibility to gastrointestinal host defenses. For example, as few as 10 *Shigella* sp bacteria can cause infection, whereas 10^5 to 10^8 *Vibrio cholera* bacteria are required for infection.

The urinary tract is protected physically by regular urine flow, the acidity of the urine, and antimicrobial peptides. Conditions that interfere with these factors (e.g., prostatic hypertrophy, renal stones) may lead to stasis and infection. Mechanical injection of bacteria through the urethra into the bladder, as may occur in women during sexual intercourse, can lead to colonization of the bladder and infection. Urinary tract catheters bypass normal mechanical barriers allowing bacteria to enter the bladder retrograde resulting in urinary tract infections.

The normal microbiologic flora on the skin and in the respiratory and gastrointestinal tracts is an important component of host defenses. Normal florae compete with pathogens for nutrients and have antimicrobial activity of their own. To illustrate, certain commensal bacteria of the skin secrete acid that prevents colonization by species more likely to cause disease. Disruption of the normal flora, such as by antibiotic treatment, allows opportunistic organisms such as *Clostridioides difficile* in the gut and *Candida* sp in the mouth or vagina to colonize and cause disease.

Organs that clear organisms from the bloodstream and lymph, including the liver, spleen, and lymph nodes, play an essential role after a pathogen has breached the primary anatomic barriers. Lack of a spleen increases a person's susceptibility to overwhelming sepsis caused by encapsulated bacteria including *S. pneumoniae*, *Neisseria meningitidis*, and *H. influenzae*. Cirrhosis of the liver allows portal vein blood to bypass the liver, increasing susceptibility to infection by gut flora.

Innate Immunity

Innate immunity refers to inborn resistance mechanisms that rapidly recognize pathogens and promote inflammation at the site of infection, thus comprising a critical first line of defense against pathogens. Fig. 1.1 compares the major features of innate and adaptive immunity.

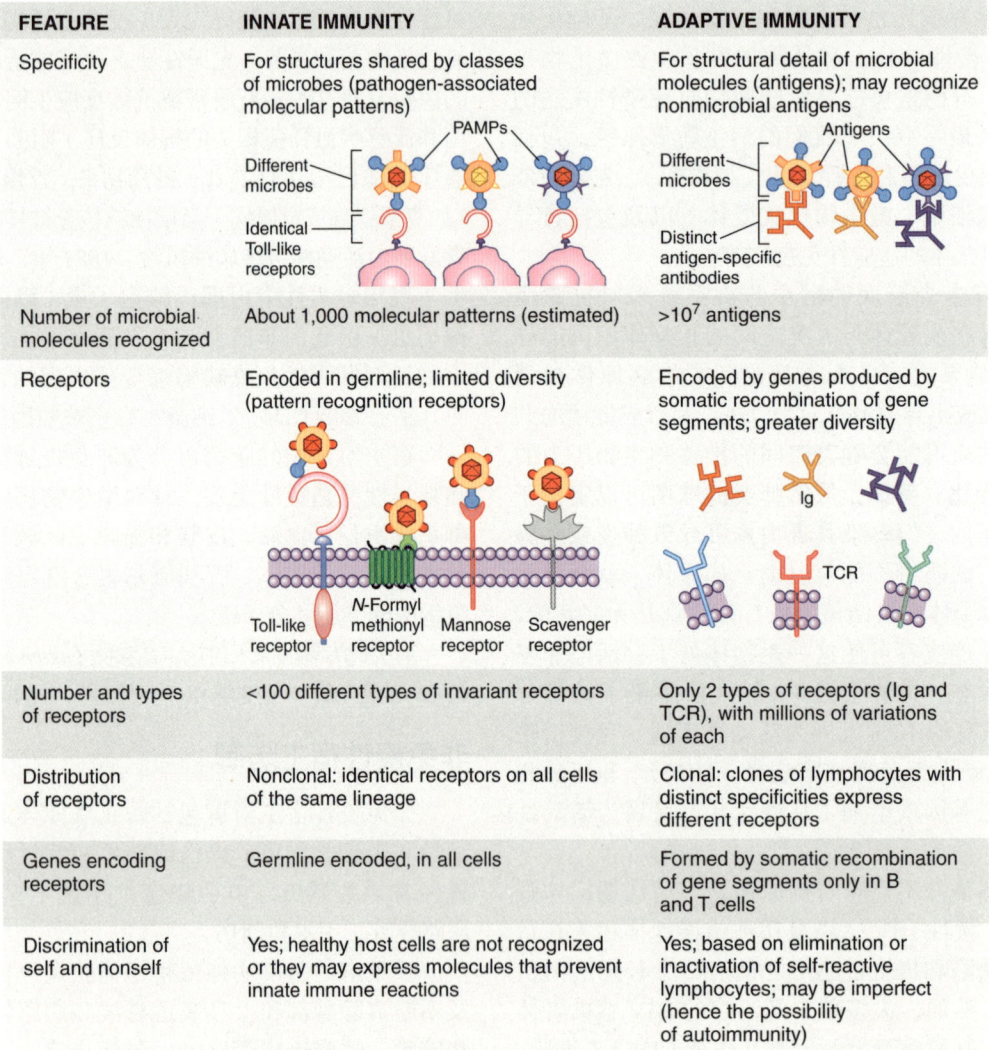

Fig. 1.1 Specificity and receptors of innate immunity and adaptive immunity. This summarizes the important features of the specificity and receptors of innate and adaptive immunity, with select examples illustrated. *Ig*, Immunoglobulin (antibody); *TCR*, T cell receptor. (From Abbas A K, Lichtman A H, Pillai S: Basic immunology: functions and disorders of the immune system, 6th ed. Philadelphia, Elsevier, 2018.)

非免疫性胃肠道防御功能包括胃酸，它可以杀死许多微生物，导致呕吐和腹泻，这有助于清除肠道中的病原体。细菌对胃肠道宿主防御系统的敏感性差异很大。例如，只要 10 个志贺菌就能引起感染，而 $10^5 \sim 10^8$ 个霍乱弧菌才能导致感染。

尿路受到有规律的尿液流动、尿液酸度和抗菌肽的物理保护。影响这些因素的情况（如前列腺增生、肾结石）可能会导致尿流淤积和感染。女性在性交过程中可能机械性地将细菌通过尿道注入膀胱而导致膀胱细菌定植和感染。尿路导管绕过正常的机械屏障，使细菌逆行进入膀胱，导致尿路感染。

皮肤、呼吸道和胃肠道中的正常微生物群是宿主防御系统的重要组成部分。正常菌群与病原体竞争营养，并具有自己的抗微生物活性。例如，皮肤上的某些共生菌分泌酸性物质，防止更有可能致病的菌种定植。通过抗生素治疗等方式破坏正常菌群，使肠道中的艰难梭菌和口腔或阴道中的念珠菌等机会性病原体定植并致病。

清除血液和淋巴中微生物的器官包括肝、脾和淋巴结等，它们在病原体突破初步解剖屏障后发挥着重要作用。缺乏脾会增加患者对可引起感染中毒症的肺炎链球菌、脑膜炎奈瑟球菌和流感嗜血杆菌等荚膜细菌的易感性。肝硬化使门静脉血液绕过肝，增加了肠道菌群感染的易感性。

先天免疫

先天免疫是指与生俱来的抵抗机制，它能迅速识别病原体并促进感染部位的炎症反应，从而构成抵御病原体的第一道关键防线。图 1.1 比较了先天免疫和适应性免疫的主要特征。先天免疫应答是相对非特异性的、不变

特征	先天免疫	适应性免疫
特异性	用于各类微生物共用的结构（病原体相关分子模式） 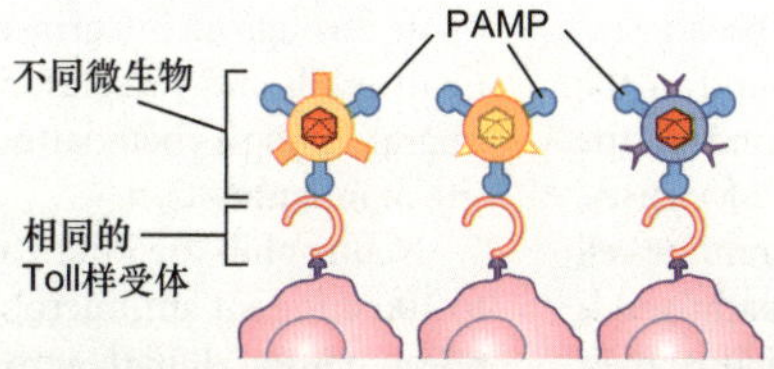	了解微生物分子（抗原）的结构细节；可识别非微生物抗原 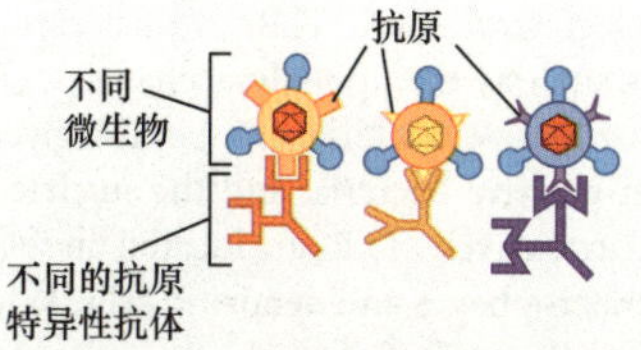
识别的微生物分子数量	约1000种分子模式（估计）	>10^7 抗原
受体	在种系中编码；有限的多样性（模式识别受体） 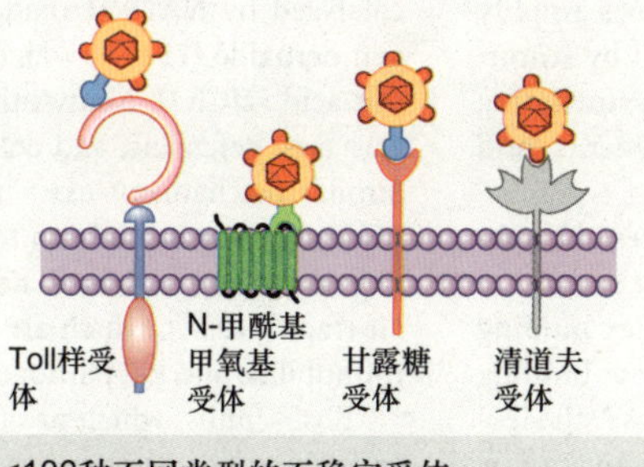	由基因片段体细胞重组产生的基因编码；具有更大的多样性 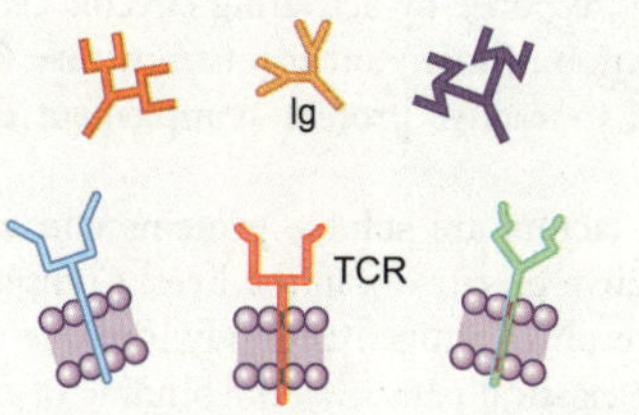
受体的数量和类型	<100种不同类型的不稳定受体	只有两种受体（Ig和TCR），每种受体的变异数以百万计
受体的分布	非克隆：在同一谱系的所有细胞上都具有相同的受体	克隆：具有独特特异性的淋巴细胞克隆表达不同的受体
编码受体的基因	种系编码，在所有细胞中	仅在B细胞和T细胞中通过基因片段的体细胞重组而形成
自体与非体的区分	能够；健康宿主细胞不能被识别，或者它们可能表达阻止先天免疫反应的分子	能够；基于自我反应淋巴细胞的消灭或失活；可能不完善（因此有自身免疫的可能性）

图 1.1 先天免疫和适应性免疫的特异性和受体。本图总结了先天免疫和适应性免疫的特异性和受体的重要特征，并举例说明。Ig，免疫球蛋白（抗体）；TCR，T细胞受体（引自 Abbas A K, Lichtman A H, Pillai S：Basic immunology：functions and disorders of the immune system，6th ed. Philadelphia，Elsevier，2018.）

The response of innate immunity is relatively nonspecific, invariant, rapid, and largely without memory. By contrast, adaptive immunity is highly specific and diverse but relatively slow during a primary infection, typically requiring days or even weeks to reach maximal activation. However, adaptive responses typically lead to the formation of durable memory that can be recalled upon secondary infection with a more rapid, robust response.

The molecules involved in innate immune responses include cytokines, chemokines, integrins, and pattern receptors. Cytokines are soluble proteins that have numerous functions, including promoting cellular growth and activation as well as regulating adaptive immune responses (Table 1.1). Their functions range from stimulating the production of and activating inflammatory cells, including neutrophils, macrophages, and eosinophils, to the direct antiviral action of interferons. Some activate endothelial cells and cause fever, whereas others regulate the inflammatory response.

Concentration gradients of chemokines in tissue attract leukocytes to areas of inflammation. Integrins on the surface of leukocytes allow adhesion to receptors on other types of cells such as vascular endothelium. This is the first step in recruiting and localizing leukocytes to areas of inflammation.

Pathogen pattern recognition receptors on phagocytes include toll-like receptors (TLRs), named for their homology to the toll molecule which was originally identified in the fruit fly, *Drosophila*; nucleotide oligomerization domain–like receptors (often abbreviated as Nod-like receptors, or NLRs); C-type lectin-like receptors (CLRs); and retinoic acid-inducible gene-I-like receptors (RLRs), which are intracellular receptors that detect viral RNA. TLRs, which recognize broad features of microbes such as the lipopolysaccharide (LPS) found in the cell wall of gram-negative bacteria, the peptidoglycan found in the cell walls of gram-positive bacteria, and the nucleic acids of viruses, have been studied extensively. TLRs are located on several immune cell types, including macrophages and dendritic cells. When a pathogen is detected by TLRs on the surface of a cell or associated with endosomes, signaling cascades are initiated that lead to the activation of nuclear transcription factors such as nuclear factor-κB (NF-κB). This stimulates the production of numerous cytokines important in the inflammatory response, including interleukin-1 (IL-1), IL-6, IL-10, IL-15, TNF-α, and growth factors (see Table 1.1). These cytokines amplify the inflammatory response by activating effector cells and by stimulating the production of many other inflammatory factors, including IL-2, interferons, C-reactive protein, complement components, and growth factors.

Complement factors are soluble proteins and enzymes that are produced as inactive precursors in the liver. Complement activation may occur as a result of antigen-antibody immune complex binding by factor C1 (the classical pathway), the binding of mannose-binding lectin (MBL) to microbial glycoproteins containing mannose (the lectin pathway), or the alternative pathway, which can be activated by bacterial cell wall components.

Regardless of how the complement system is activated, the cascade results in the production of C3 convertase, a protein that cleaves C3 into C3a and C3b fragments. This is followed by the production of a C5 convertase, which cleaves C5 into C5a and C5b. C3a and C5a, also known as anaphylatoxins, stimulate histamine release from mast cells leading to vasodilatation, increase vascular permeability and attract activated macrophages. C3b binds to the microbial surface and in conjunction with pathogen-specific immunoglobulin G (IgG) may stimulate phagocytosis. C5b serves as a nucleation point for the assembly of the membrane attack complex (MAC) that consists of C5b, C6, C7, C8 and multiple molecules of C9. MAC assembly results in pore formation that leads to bacterial lysis. Patients deficient in any of the MAC components C5 to C9 appear to be particularly susceptible to organisms such as *Neisseria meningitides* and *N. gonorrhoeae*. The complement system is regulated by numerous factors including soluble C1 inhibitor, which causes breakdown of the C1 complex, as well as the membrane-bound proteins decay-acceleration factor (DAF), which breaks down C3 convertases, and protectin, which inhibits MAC formation. These regulatory factors help to ensure that the complement system is not activated inappropriately against host cells.

The inflammatory response results in the classic clinical signs of inflammation, including erythema, pain, warmth, swelling, and loss of function. It can be initiated by microorganisms in tissue, tissue injury, or dysfunctional adaptive immunity (e.g., autoantibodies). The response includes inflammatory molecules as previously described and tissue and migrating leukocytes. Neutrophils are central to the clinical manifestations of inflammation in tissue, and patients with neutropenia or functional deficits in neutrophil function often lack the signs of inflammation at the site of serious infection.

Neutrophils are bone marrow–derived phagocytes whose production is greatly stimulated by infection through the action of macrophage-produced growth factors, including granulocyte colony-stimulating factor (G-CSF) and granulocyte-macrophage colony-stimulating factor (GM-CSF). Neutrophils circulate in blood (where they are the most abundant white blood cell), are attracted to sites of inflammation, and are activated by chemotactic factors, including formyl peptides derived from bacteria, complement factors C3a and C5a, IL-8, interferon, and leukotrienes, particularly leukotriene B_4. Neutrophils migrate from the endovascular space into inflammatory tissue through an integrin-regulated process that includes receptors on neutrophils and vascular endothelial cells. Activated neutrophils then migrate using a chemoattractive (i.e., chemokine) gradient toward the site of inflammation.

Neutrophils are killing machines containing granules that have up to 100 different antimicrobial molecules. The contents of granules are released intracellularly into phagosomes after phagocytosis of a pathogen or released extracellularly in the vicinity of pathogens. Phagocytosis is greatly enhanced by opsonization (i.e., antibody and complement binding) of pathogens. The major microbicidal mechanism of neutrophils is the superoxide burst (i.e., production of superoxide anion catalyzed by NADPH oxidase) and then the dismutation to hydrogen peroxide (H_2O_2), which may in turn be converted to hypochlorous acid (HClO). Many other granule molecules, such as cathepsins, elastases, defensins, and collagenase contribute to the killing process. Similar mechanisms exist in other phagocytes such as macrophages. More recently it has been found that in addition to phagocytosis and degranulation, activated neutrophils produce neutrophil extracellular traps (NETs), which are webs of chromatin and proteases that can immobilize and kill pathogenic microbes.

Eosinophils, which are found more in tissue than the circulation, are primarily important in host defenses against multicellular parasites such as parasitic worms. Growth and differentiation of eosinophils is promoted by IL-5. Eosinophils are activated and recruited by a variety of mediators, including complement factors and leukotrienes. Eosinophil granules contain specific cationic proteins that are toxic to parasites. Eosinophils also play key roles in the pathogenesis of allergic reactions and diseases such as asthma.

Basophils in blood and mast cells in tissue contain granules with high concentrations of histamine and other inflammatory mediators. Basophils and mast cells express receptors for complement factors and others that bind immunoglobulin E (IgE) produced by B cells. They can be activated by complement factors C3a and C5a and by cross-linking of IgE by antigen on the surface of mast cells. Histamine is a short-acting, low-molecular-weight amine that acts through four

的、快速的，而且基本上没有记忆。相比之下，适应性免疫具有高度特异性和多样性，但在原发性感染期间启动相对较慢，通常需要数天甚至数周才能达到最大激活。然而，适应性免疫应答通常会形成持久记忆，这种记忆可以在继发感染时以更快速、更强大的反应被唤起。

参与先天免疫应答的分子包括细胞因子、趋化因子、整合素和模式受体。细胞因子是具有多种功能的可溶性蛋白质，包括促进细胞生长和活化以及调节适应性免疫应答（表1.1）。细胞因子的功能包括刺激中性粒细胞、巨噬细胞和嗜酸性粒细胞等炎症细胞的产生和活化，也包括干扰素的直接抗病毒作用。有些能激活内皮细胞并引起发热，而另一些则能调节炎症反应。

组织中趋化因子的浓度梯度将白细胞吸引到炎症区域。白细胞表面的整合素使其黏附到其他类型的细胞（如血管内皮）上的受体。这是募集白细胞并将其定位到炎症部位的第一步。

吞噬细胞上的病原体模式识别受体包括Toll样受体（TLR），因其与最初在果蝇中发现的Toll受体的同源性而得名；核苷酸寡聚化结构域样受体（通常缩写为Nod样受体，或NLR）；C型凝集素样受体（CLR）；以及视黄酸诱导基因I样受体（RLR），后者是识别病毒RNA的细胞内受体。TLR已被广泛研究，其可以识别微生物的多种特征，例如革兰氏阴性菌细胞壁中的脂多糖（LPS）、革兰氏阳性菌细胞壁中的肽聚糖和病毒的核酸。TLR位于几种类型的免疫细胞上，包括巨噬细胞和树突状细胞。当病原体被细胞表面或与内质体相关的TLR检测到时，会启动信号级联反应，从而激活核转录因子，如核因子-κB（NF-κB）。这会刺激产生多种对炎症反应很重要的细胞因子，包括白细胞介素-1（IL-1）、IL-6、IL-10、L-15、TNF-a和生长因子（表1.1）。这些细胞因子通过激活效应细胞和刺激其产生其他炎症因子（包括IL-2、干扰素、C反应蛋白、补体成分和生长因子）来放大炎症反应。

补体因子是在肝中以非活性前体形式产生的可溶性蛋白质和酶。补体激活可能是由于因子C1与抗原-抗体免疫复合物结合（经典途径）、甘露糖结合凝集素（MBL）与含甘露糖的微生物糖蛋白结合（凝集素途径）或可由细菌细胞壁成分激活的替代途径。

无论补体系统如何被激活，级联反应都会导致产生C3转化酶，这是一种将C3分解成C3a和C3b片段的蛋白质。随后产生C5转化酶，将C5转化为C5a和C5b。C3a和C5a，也称为过敏毒素，可刺激肥大细胞释放组胺导致血管舒张，增加血管通透性并吸引活化的巨噬细胞。C3b与微生物表面结合，并与病原体特异性免疫球蛋白G（IgG）结合可刺激吞噬作用。C5b是由C5b、C6、C7、C8和多个C9分子组成的膜攻击复合体（MAC）组装的成核点。膜攻击复合体组装后形成孔隙，导致细菌裂解。缺乏任何MAC组分C5至C9的患者似乎特别容易感染如脑膜炎奈瑟球菌和淋病奈瑟球菌等微生物。该复合系统受多种因素的调节，其中包括导致C1复合物分解的可溶性C1抑制剂，以及能分解C3转化酶的膜结合蛋白衰变加速因子（DAF）和能抑制MAC生成的保护蛋白。这些调节因子有助于确保补体系统不会对宿主细胞不适当地激活。

炎症反应会导致典型的临床表现，包括红斑、疼痛、发热、肿胀和功能丧失。它可能是由组织中的微生物、组织损伤或适应性免疫失调（如自身抗体）引起的。这种反应包括前文所述的炎症分子以及组织内和迁移的白细胞。中性粒细胞是组织炎症临床表现的核心，患有中性粒细胞缺乏症或中性粒细胞功能障碍的患者往往缺乏严重感染部位的炎症征象。

中性粒细胞来源于骨髓的吞噬细胞，感染时巨噬细胞产生的生长因子，包括粒细胞集落刺激因子（G-CSF）和粒细胞-巨噬细胞集落刺激因子（GM-CSF）会极大地刺激中性粒细胞的生成。中性粒细胞在血液中循环（它们是血液中含量最高的白细胞），被吸引到炎症部位，并被趋化因子激活，这些趋化因子包括来自细菌的甲酰肽、补体因子C3a和C5a、IL-8、干扰素和白三烯，尤其是白三烯B4。中性粒细胞通过整合素调控从血管内腔迁移到炎症组织中，该过程包括中性粒细胞和血管内皮细胞上的受体。然后，活化的中性粒细胞利用趋化诱导因子（即趋化因子）梯度向炎症部位迁移。

中性粒细胞是含有多达100种不同抗菌分子颗粒的杀伤机器。颗粒的内容物在病原吞噬作用后在细胞内释放到吞噬体中，或在病原体附近细胞外释放。病原体的调理作用（即抗体和补体结合）大大增强了吞噬作用。中性粒细胞的主要杀菌机制是超氧化物爆发（即由NADPH氧化酶催化的超氧阴离子的产生），然后突变为过氧化氢（H_2O_2），而过氧化氢又可能转化为次氯酸（HClO）。许多其他颗粒分子，如组织蛋白酶、弹性蛋白酶、防御素和胶原酶，都参与杀伤过程。其他吞噬细胞（如巨噬细胞）也存在类似的机制。最近发现，除了吞噬作用和脱颗粒作用外，活化的中性粒细胞还会产生中性粒细胞胞外陷阱（NET），NET是染色质和蛋白酶的网，可以固定和杀死病原微生物。

嗜酸性粒细胞在组织中分布多于外周循环，在宿主防御多细胞寄生虫（如蠕虫）方面尤为重要。IL-5促进嗜酸性粒细胞的生长和分化。嗜酸性粒细胞被多种介质激活和募集，包括补体因子和白三烯。嗜酸性粒细胞颗粒含有对寄生虫有毒的特定阳离子蛋白。嗜酸性粒细胞在过敏反应和哮喘等疾病的发病机制中也起着关键作用。

血液中的嗜碱性粒细胞和组织中的肥大细胞含有高浓度组胺和其他炎症介质的颗粒。嗜碱性粒细胞和肥大细胞表达补体因子和其他结合B细胞产生的免疫球蛋白E（IgE）的受体。它们可以被补体因子C3a和C5a以及肥大细胞表面的抗原和IgE交联激活。组胺是一种短效、低分子量的胺，通过四种不同的组胺受体发挥作用。其作用包括诱导支气管收缩和支气管平

TABLE 1.1 Cytokines

Cytokine and Subunits	Principal Cell Source	Cytokine Receptor and Subunits[a]	Principal Cellular Targets and Biologic Effects
Type I Cytokine Family Members			
Interleukin-2 (IL-2)	T cells	CD25 (IL-2Rα) CD122 (IL-2Rβ) CD132 (γc)	T cells: proliferation and differentiation into effector and memory cells; promotes regulatory T cell development, survival, and function NK cells: proliferation, activation B cells: proliferation, antibody synthesis (in vitro)
Interleukin-3 (IL-3)	T cells	CD123 (IL-3Rα) CD131 (βc)	Immature hematopoietic progenitors: induced maturation of all hematopoietic lineages
Interleukin-4 (IL-4)	CD4+ T cells (Th2, Tfh), mast cells	CD124 (IL-4Rα) CD132 (γc)	B cells: isotype switching to IgE T cells: Th2 differentiation, proliferation Macrophages: alternative activation and inhibition of IFN-γ–mediated classical activation
Interleukin-5 (IL-5)	CD4+ T cells (Th2), group 2 ILCs	CD125 (IL-5Rα) CD131 (βc)	Eosinophils: activation, increased generation
Interleukin-6 (IL-6)	Macrophages, endothelial cells, T cells	CD126 (IL-6Rα) CD130 (gp130)	Liver: synthesis of acute-phase protein B cells: proliferation of antibody-producing cells T cells: Th17 differentiation
Interleukin-7 (IL-7)	Fibroblasts, bone marrow stromal cells	CD127 (IL-7R) CD132 (γc)	Immature lymphoid progenitors: proliferation of early T and B cell progenitors T lymphocytes: survival of naïve and memory cells
Interleukin-9 (IL-9)	CD4+ T cells	CD129 (IL-9R) CD132 (γc)	Mast cells, B cells, T cells, and tissue cells: survival and activation
Interleukin-11 (IL-11)	Bone marrow stromal cells	IL-11Rα CD130 (gp130)	Production of platelets
Interleukin-12 (IL-12): IL-12A (p35) IL-12B (p40)	Macrophages, dendritic cells	CD212 (IL-12Rβ1) IL-12Rβ2	T cells: Th1 differentiation NK cells and T cells: IFN-γ synthesis, increased cytotoxic activity
Interleukin-13 (IL-13)	CD4+ T cells (Th2), NKT cells, group 2 ILCs, mast cells	CD213a1 (IL-13Rα1) CD213a2 (IL-13Rα2) CD132 (γc)	B cells: isotype switching to IgE Epithelial cells: increased mucus production Macrophages: alternative activation
Interleukin-15 (IL-15)	Macrophages, other cell types	IL-15Rα CD122 (IL-2Rβ) CD132 (γc)	NK cells: proliferation T cells: survival and proliferation of memory CD8+ cells
Interleukin-17A (IL-17A) Interleukin-17F (IL-17F)	CD4+ T cells (Th17), group 3 ILCs	CD217 (IL-17RA) IL-17RC	Epithelial cells, macrophages and other cell types: increased chemokine and cytokine production; GM-CSF and G-CSF production
Interleukin-21 (IL-21)	Th2 cells, Th17 cells, Tfh cells	CD360 (IL-21R) CD132 (γc)	B cells: activation, proliferation, differentiation Tfh cells: development Th17 cells: increased generation
Interleukin-23 (IL-23): IL-23A (p19) IL-12B (p40)	Macrophages, dendritic cells	IL-23R CD212 (IL-12Rβ1)	T cells: differentiation and expansion of Th17 cells
Interleukin-25 (IL-25; IL-17E)	T cells, mast cells, eosinophils, macrophages, mucosal epithelial cells	IL-17RB	T cells and various other cell types: expression of IL-4, IL-5, IL-13
Interleukin-27 (IL-27): IL-27 (p28) EBI3 (IL-27B)	Macrophages, dendritic cells	IL-27Rα CD130 (gp130)	T cells: enhancement of Th1 differentiation; inhibition of Th17 differentiation NK cells: IFN-γ synthesis?

Continued

表 1.1 细胞因子

细胞因子和亚单位	主要细胞来源	细胞因子受体和亚单位 [a]	主要细胞靶点和生物学效应
I 型细胞因子家族成员			
白细胞介素 -2（IL-2）	T 细胞	CD25（IL-2Rα） CD122（IL-2Rβ） CD132（γc）	T 细胞：增殖和分化为效应细胞和记忆细胞；促进调节 T 细胞的发育、存活和功能 NK 细胞：增殖、活化 B 细胞：增殖、抗体合成（体外）
白细胞介素 -3（IL-3）	T 细胞	CD123（IL-3Rα） CD131（βc）	未成熟造血干细胞：所有造血谱系的诱导成熟
白细胞介素 -4（IL-4）	CD4+ T 细胞（Th2，Tfh），肥大细胞	CD124（IL-4Rα） CD132（γc）	B 细胞：同型转化为 IgE T 细胞：Th2 分化、增殖 巨噬细胞：替代活化和抑制 IFN-γ 介导的经典激活
白细胞介素 -5（IL-5）	CD4+ T 细胞（Th2），II 型先天淋巴细胞	CD125（IL-5Rα） CD131（βc）	嗜酸性粒细胞：激活，增加生成
白细胞介素 -6（IL-6）	巨噬细胞、内皮细胞、T 细胞	CD126（IL-6Rα） CD130（gp130）	肝：合成急性期蛋白 B 细胞：产生抗体的细胞增殖 T 细胞：Th17 分化
白细胞介素 -7（IL-7）	成纤维细胞，骨髓基质细胞	CD127（IL-7R） CD132（γc）	未成熟淋巴样祖细胞：早期 T 和 B 细胞祖细胞的增殖 T 淋巴细胞：幼稚细胞和记忆细胞的存活
白细胞介素 -9（IL-9）	CD4+ T 细胞	CD129（IL-9R） CD132（γc）	肥大细胞、B 细胞、T 细胞和组织细胞：存活和激活
白细胞介素 -11（IL-11）	骨髓基质细胞	IL-11Rα CD130（gp130）	血小板的产生
白细胞介素 -12（IL-12） IL-12A（p35） IL-12B（p40）	巨噬细胞、树突状细胞	CD212（IL-12Rβ1） IL-12Rβ2	T 细胞：Th1 分化 NK 细胞和 T 细胞：IFN-γ 合成，细胞毒活性增加
白细胞介素 -13（IL-13）	CD4+ T 细胞（Th2），NKT 细胞，II 型先天淋巴细胞，肥大细胞	CD213a1（IL-13Rα1） CD213a2（IL-13Rα2） CD132（γc）	B 细胞：同型转换为 IgE 上皮细胞：黏液生成增加 巨噬细胞：替代活化
白细胞介素 -15（IL-15）	巨噬细胞，其他细胞类型	IL-15Rα CD122（IL-2Rβ） CD132（γc）	NK 细胞：增殖 T 细胞：记忆 CD8+ 细胞的存活和增殖
白细胞介素 -17A（IL-17A） 白细胞介素 -17F（IL-17F）	CD4+ T 细胞（Th17），III 型先天淋巴细胞	CD217（IL-17RA） IL-17RC	上皮细胞、巨噬细胞及其他细胞类型：趋化因子和细胞因子的产生增加；GM-CSF 和 G-CSF 的产生
白细胞介素 -21（IL-21）	Th2 细胞，Th17 细胞，Tfh 细胞	CD360（IL-21R） CD132（γc）	B 细胞：活化、增殖、分化 Tfh 细胞：发育 Th17：增殖
白细胞介素 -23（IL-23） IL-23A（p19） IL-12B（p40）	巨噬细胞、树突状细胞	IL-23R CD212（IL-12Rβ1）	T 细胞：Th17 细胞的分化和扩增
白细胞介素 -25（IL-25，IL-17E）	T 细胞、肥大细胞、嗜酸性粒细胞、巨噬细胞、黏膜上皮细胞	IL-17RB	T 细胞和各种其他细胞类型：IL-4、IL-5、IL-13 的表达
白细胞介素 -27（IL-27） IL-27（p28） EBI3（IL-27B）	巨噬细胞、树突状细胞	IL-27Rα CD130（gp130）	T 细胞：促进 Th1 分化；抑制 Th17 分化 NK 细胞：IFN-γ 合成？

TABLE 1.1 Cytokines—cont'd

Cytokine and Subunits	Principal Cell Source	Cytokine Receptor and Subunits[a]	Principal Cellular Targets and Biologic Effects
Stem cell factor (c-Kit ligand)	Bone marrow stromal cells	CD117 (KIT)	Pluripotent hematopoietic stem cells: induced maturation of all hematopoietic lineages
Granulocyte-monocyte CSF (GM-CSF)	T cells, macrophages, endothelial cells, fibroblasts	CD116 (GM-CSFRα) CD131 (βc)	Immature and committed progenitors, mature macrophages: induced maturation of granulocytes and monocytes, macrophage activation
Monocyte CSF (M-CSF, CSF1)	Macrophages, endothelial cells, bone marrow cells, fibroblasts	CD115 (CSF1R)	Committed hematopoietic progenitors: induced maturation of monocytes
Granulocyte CSF (G-CSF, CSF3)	Macrophages, fibroblasts, endothelial cells	CD114 (CSF3R)	Committed hematopoietic progenitors: induced maturation of granulocytes
Thymic stromal lymphopoietin (TSLP)	Keratinocytes, bronchial epithelial cells, fibroblasts, smooth muscle cells, endothelial cells, mast cells, macrophages, granulocytes and dendritic cells	TSLP-receptor CD127 (IL-7R)	Dendritic cells: activation Eosinophils: activation Mast cells: cytokine production T cells: Th2 differentiation
Type II Cytokine Family Members			
IFN-α (multiple proteins)	Plasmacytoid dendritic cells, macrophages	IFNAR1 CD118 (IFNAR2)	All cells: antiviral state, increased class I MHC expression NK cells: activation
IFN-β	Fibroblasts, plasmacytoid dendritic cells	IFNAR1 CD118 (IFNAR2)	All cells: antiviral state, increased class I MHC expression NK cells: activation
Interferon-γ (IFN-γ)	T cells (Th1, CD8+ T cells), NK cells	CD119 (IFNGR1) IFNGR2	Macrophages: classical activation (increased microbicidal functions) B cells: isotype switching to opsonizing and complement-fixing IgG subclasses (established in mice) T cells: Th1 differentiation Various cells: increased expression of class I and class II MHC molecules, increased antigen processing and presentation to T cells
Interleukin-10 (IL-10)	Macrophages, T cells (mainly regulatory T cells)	CD210 (IL-10Rα) IL-10Rβ	Macrophages, dendritic cells: inhibition of expression of IL-12, co-stimulators, and class II MHC
Interleukin-22 (IL-22)	Th17 cells	IL-22Rα1 or IL-22Rα2 IL-10Rβ2	Epithelial cells: production of defensins, increased barrier function Hepatocytes: survival
Interleukin-26 (IL-26)	T cells, monocytes	IL-20R1IL-10R2	Not established
Interferon-λs (type III interferons)	Dendritic cells	IFNLR1 (IL-28Rα) CD210B (IL-10Rβ2)	Epithelial cells: antiviral state
Leukemia inhibitory factor (LIF)	Embryonic trophectoderm, bone marrow stromal cells	CD118 (LIFR) CD130 (gp130)	Stem cells: block in differentiation
Oncostatin M	Bone marrow stromal cells	OSMR CD130 (gp130)	Endothelial cells: regulation of hematopoietic cytokine production Cancer cells: inhibition of proliferation
TNF Superfamily Cytokines[b]			
Tumor necrosis factor (TNF, TNFSF1)	Macrophages, NK cells, T cells	CD120a (TNFRSF1) or CD120b (TNFRSF2)	Endothelial cells: activation (inflammation, coagulation) Neutrophils: activation Hypothalamus: fever Muscle, fat: catabolism (cachexia)
Lymphotoxin-α (LTα, TNFSF1)	T cells, B cells	CD120a (TNFRSF1) or CD120b (TNFRSF2)	Same as TNF

表 1.1 细胞因子（续表）

细胞因子和亚单位	主要细胞来源	细胞因子受体和亚单位 [a]	主要细胞靶点和生物学效应
干细胞因子（c-Kit 配体）	骨髓基质细胞	CD117（KIT）	多能造血干细胞；所有造血谱系的诱导成熟
粒细胞-巨噬细胞 CSF（GM-CSF）	T 细胞、巨噬细胞、内皮细胞、成纤维细胞	CD116（GM-CSFRα） CD131（βc）	未成熟和成熟的前体，成熟巨噬细胞：诱导粒细胞和单核细胞成熟，巨噬细胞活化
巨噬细胞 CSF（M-CSF，CSF1）	巨噬细胞、内皮细胞、骨髓细胞、成纤维细胞	CD115（CSF1R）	定向造血祖细胞：诱导单核细胞成熟
粒细胞 CSF（G-CSF，CSF3）	巨噬细胞、成纤维细胞、内皮细胞	CD114（CSF3R）	定向造血祖细胞：诱导粒细胞成熟
胸腺基质淋巴细胞生成素（TSLP）	角质细胞、支气管上皮细胞、成纤维细胞、平滑肌细胞、内皮细胞、肥大细胞、巨噬细胞、粒细胞和树突状细胞	TSLP-受体 CD127（IL-7R）	树突状细胞：激活 嗜酸性粒细胞：激活 肥大细胞：细胞因子的产生 T 细胞：Th2 细胞分化
II 型细胞因子家族成员			
IFN-α（多种蛋白质）	浆细胞样树突状细胞、巨噬细胞	IFNAR1 CD118（IFNAR2）	所有细胞：抗病毒状态，增强 I 型 MHC 表达，NK 细胞激活
IFN-β	成纤维细胞、浆细胞样树突状细胞	IFNAR1 CD118（IFNAR2）	所有细胞：抗病毒状态，增强 I 型 MHC 表达 NK 细胞激活
IFN-γ	T 细胞（Th1、CD8[+] T 细胞）、NK 细胞	CD119（IFNGR1） IFNGR2	巨噬细胞：典型激活（增加杀微生物功能） B 细胞：同型转换为调理型和补体结合型 IgG 亚类（在小鼠中建立） T 细胞：Th1 分化 各种细胞：I 类和 II 类 MHC 分子表达增加，抗原处理和向 T 细胞提呈增加
白细胞介素 10（IL-10）	巨噬细胞、T 细胞（主要是调节性 T 细胞）	CD210（IL-10Rα） IL-10Rβ	巨噬细胞、树突状细胞：抑制 IL-12、共刺激因子和 II 类 MHC 的表达
白细胞介素 22（IL-22）	Th17 细胞	IL-22Rα1 或 IL-22Rα2 IL-10Rβ2	上皮细胞：产生防御素，屏障功能增强 肝细胞：存活
白细胞介素 26（IL-26）	T 细胞、单核细胞	IL-20R1、IL-10R2	尚未确定
IFN-λs（III 型 IFN）	树突状细胞	IFNLR1（IL-28Rα） CD210B（IL-10Rβ2）	上皮细胞：抗病毒状态
白血病抑制因子（LIF）	胚胎滋养外胚层，骨髓基质细胞	CD118（LIFR） CD130（gp130）	干细胞：分化受阻
抑瘤素 M	骨髓基质细胞	OSMR CD130（gp130）	内皮细胞：调节造血细胞因子的产生 癌细胞：抑制增殖
TNF 超家族细胞因子 [b]			
肿瘤坏死因子（TNF，TNFSF1）	巨噬细胞、NK 细胞、T 细胞	CD120a（TNFRSF1）或 CD120b（TNFRSF2）	内皮细胞：活化（炎症、凝血） 中性粒细胞：活化 下丘脑：发热 肌肉、脂肪：分解代谢（坏死）
淋巴毒素-α（LTα，TNFSF1）	T 细胞、B 细胞	CD120a（TNFRSF1） CD120b（TNFRSF2）	与 TNF 相同

TABLE 1.1 Cytokines—cont'd

Cytokine and Subunits	Principal Cell Source	Cytokine Receptor and Subunits[a]	Principal Cellular Targets and Biologic Effects
Lymphotoxin-αβ (LTαβ)	T cells, NK cells, follicular B cells, lymphoid inducer cells	LTβR	Lymphoid tissue stromal cells and follicular dendritic cells: chemokine expression and lymphoid organogenesis
BAFF (CD257, TNFSF13B)	Dendritic cells, monocytes, follicular dendritic cells, B cells	BAFF-R (TNFRSF13C) or TACI (TNFRSF13B) or BCMA (TNFRSF17)	B cells: survival, proliferation
APRIL (CD256, TNFSF13)	T cells, dendritic cells, monocytes, follicular dendritic cells	TACI (TNFRSF13B) or BCMA (TNFRSF17)	B cells: survival, proliferation
Osteoprotegerin (OPG, TNFRSF11B)	Osteoblasts	RANKL	Osteoclast precursor cells: inhibits osteoclast differentiation
IL-1 Family Cytokines			
Interleukin-1α (IL-1α)	Macrophages, dendritic cells, fibroblasts, endothelial cells, keratinocytes, hepatocytes	CD121a (IL-1R1) IL-1RAP or CD121b (IL-1R2)	Endothelial cells: activation (inflammation, coagulation) Hypothalamus: fever
Interleukin-1β (IL-1β)	Macrophages, dendritic cells, fibroblasts, endothelial cells, keratinocyte	CD121a (IL-1R1) IL-1RAP or CD121b (IL-1R2)	Endothelial cells: activation (inflammation, coagulation) Hypothalamus: fever Liver: synthesis of acute-phase proteins T cells: Th17 differentiation
Interleukin-1 receptor antagonist (IL-1RA)	Macrophages	CD121a (IL-1R1) IL-1RAP	Various cells: competitive antagonist of IL-1
Interleukin-18 (IL-18)	Monocytes, macrophages, dendritic cells, Kupffer cells, keratinocytes, chondrocytes, synovial fibroblasts, osteoblasts	CD218a (IL-18Rα) CD218b (IL-18Rβ)	NK cells and T cells: IFN-γ synthesis Monocytes: expression of GM-CSF, TNF, IL-1β Neutrophils: activation, cytokine release
Interleukin-33 (IL-33)	Endothelial cells, smooth muscle cells, keratinocytes, fibroblasts	ST2 (IL1RL1) IL-1 Receptor Accessory Protein (IL1RAP)	T cells: Th2 development ILCs: activation of group 2 ILCs
Other Cytokines			
Transforming growth factor-β (TGF-β)	T cells (mainly Tregs), macrophages, other cell types	TGF-β R1 TGF-β R2 TGF-β R3	T cells: inhibition of proliferation and effector functions; differentiation of Th17 and Treg B cells: inhibition of proliferation; IgA production Macrophages: inhibition of activation; stimulation of angiogenic factors Fibroblasts: increased collagen synthesis

APRIL, A proliferation-inducing ligand; *BAFF*, B cell–activating factor belonging to the TNF family; *BCMA*, B cell maturation protein; *CSF*, colony-stimulating factor; *IFN*, interferon; *IgE*, immunoglobulin E; *ILCs*, innate lymphoid cells; *MHC*, major histocompatibility complex; *NK cell*, natural killer cell; *NKT cell*, natural killer T cell; *OSMR*, oncostatin M receptor; *RANK*, receptor activator for nuclear factor κB ligand; *RANKL*, RANK ligand; *TACI*, transmembrane activator and calcium modulator and cyclophilin ligand interactor; *Th*, T helper; *Tfh*, T follicular helper; *TNF*, tumor necrosis factor; *TNFSF*, TNF superfamily; *TNFRSF*, TNF receptor superfamily; *Treg*, regulatory T cell.

[a]Most cytokine receptors are dimers or trimers composed of different polypeptide chains, some of which are shared between receptors for different cytokines. The set of polypeptides that compose a functional receptor (cytokine binding plus signaling) for each cytokine is listed. The functions of each subunit polypeptide are not listed.

[b]All TNF superfamily (TNFSF) members are expressed as cell surface transmembrane proteins, but only the subsets that are predominantly active as proteolytically released soluble cytokines are listed in the table. Other TNFSF members that function predominantly in the membrane-bound form and are not, strictly speaking, cytokines are not listed in the table. These membrane-bound proteins and the TNFRSF receptors they bind to include OX40L (CD252, TNFSF4):OX40 (CD134, TNFRSF4); CD40L (CD154, TNFSF5):CD40 (TNFRSF5); FasL (CD178, TNFSF6):Fas (CD95, TNFRSF6); CD70 (TNFSF7):CD27 (TNFRSF27); CD153 (TNFSF8):CD30 (TNFRSF8); TRAIL (CD253, TNFSF10):TRAIL-R (TNFRSF10A-D); RANKL (TNFSF11):RANK (TNFRSF11); TWEAK (CD257, TNFSF12):TWEAKR (CD266, TNFRSF12); LIGHT (CD258, TNFSF14):HVEM (TNFRSF14); GITRL (TNFSF18):GITR (CD357 TNFRSF18); and 4-IBBL:4-IBB (CD137).

From Abbas A K, Lichtman A H, Pillai S: Basic immunology: functions and disorders of the immune system, 6th ed. Philadelphia, Elsevier, 2018.

表 1.1 细胞因子（续表）

细胞因子和亚单位	主要细胞来源	细胞因子受体和亚单位 [a]	主要细胞靶点和生物学效应
淋巴毒素-αβ（LTαβ）	T细胞、NK细胞、滤泡性B细胞、淋巴样诱导细胞	LTβR	淋巴组织基质细胞和滤泡树突状细胞：趋化因子表达与淋巴器官发生
BAFF（CD257，TNFSF13B）	树突状细胞、单核细胞、滤泡树突状细胞、B细胞	BAFF-R（TNFRSF13C）或 TACI（TNFRSF13B）或 BCMA（TNFRSF17）	B细胞：存活、增殖
APRIL（CD256，TNFSF13）	T细胞、树突状细胞、单核细胞、滤泡树突状细胞	TACI（TNFRSF13B）或 BCMA（TNFRSF17）	B细胞：存活、增殖
骨保护素（OPG，TNFRSF11B）	成骨细胞	RANKL	破骨细胞前体细胞：抑制破骨细胞分化
IL-1家族细胞因子			
白细胞介素-1α（IL-1α）	巨噬细胞、树突状细胞、成纤维细胞、内皮细胞、角质细胞、肝细胞	CD121a（IL-1R1）IL-1RAP CD121b（IL-1R2）	内皮细胞：活化（炎症、凝血）下丘脑：发烧
白细胞介素-1β（IL-1β）	巨噬细胞、树突状核细胞、成纤维细胞、内皮细胞、角质细胞	CD121a（IL-1R1）IL-1RAP CD121b（IL-1R2）	内皮细胞：活化（炎症、凝血）下丘脑：发烧 肝：急性期蛋白质的合成 T细胞：Th17分化
白细胞介素-1受体拮抗剂（IL-1RA）	巨噬细胞	CD121a（IL-1R1）IL-1RAP	各种细胞：IL-1竞争性拮抗剂
白细胞介素-18（IL-18）	单核细胞、巨噬细胞、树突状细胞、Kupffer细胞、角质细胞、软骨细胞、滑膜成纤维细胞、成骨细胞	CD218a（IL-18Rα）CD218b（IL-18Rβ）	NK细胞和T细胞：IFN-γ合成 单核细胞：GM-CSF、TNF、IL-1β的表达 中性粒细胞：激活、细胞因子释放
白细胞介素-33（IL-33）	内皮细胞、平滑肌细胞、角质细胞、成纤维细胞	ST2（IL1RL1）IL-1受体辅助蛋白（IL1RAP）	T细胞：Th2发育 ILC：Ⅱ型ILC的激活
其他细胞因子			
转化生长因子-β（TGF-β）	T细胞（主要是Treg）、巨噬细胞、其他类型的细胞	TGF-β R1 TGF-β R2 TGF-β R3	T细胞：抑制增殖和效应功能；Th17和Treg的分化 B细胞：抑制增殖；IgA生产 巨噬细胞：抑制活化；刺激血管生成因子 成纤维细胞：胶原蛋白合成增加

APRIL，增殖诱导配体；BAFF，属于TNF家族的B细胞激活因子；BCMA，B细胞成熟蛋白；CSF，集落刺激因子；IFN，干扰素；IgE，免疫球蛋白E；ILC，先天淋巴细胞；MHC，主要组织相容性复合体；NK细胞，自然杀伤细胞；NKT细胞，自然杀伤T细胞；Th，T辅助细胞；Tfh，T滤泡辅助细胞；TNF，肿瘤坏死因子；TNFSF，TNF超家族；TNFRSF，TNF受体超家族；Treg，调节性T细胞。

[a] 大多数细胞因子受体是由不同多肽链组成的二聚体或三聚体，其中一些多肽链在不同细胞因子受体之间共享。表中列出了组成每种细胞因子功能受体（细胞因子结合加信号传导）的一组多肽。未列出每个亚基多肽的功能。

[b] 所有TNF超家族（TNFSF）成员都以细胞表面跨膜蛋白形式表达，但表中只列出了主要以蛋白水解释放的可溶性细胞因子形式发挥活性的亚群。表中未列出其他主要以膜结合形式起作用且严格来说不是细胞因子的TNFSF成员。这些膜结合蛋白及其结合的TNFRSF受体包括OX40L（CD252，TNFSF4）：OX40（CD134，TNFRSF4）；CD40L（CD154，TNFSF5）：CD40（TNFRSF5）；FasL（CD178，TNFSF6）：Fas（CD95，TNFRSF6）；CD70（TNFSF7）：CD27（TNFRSF27）；CD153（TNFSF8）：CD30（TNFRSF8）；trail（CD253，TNFSF10）：trail-R（TNFRSF10A-D）；rankl（TNFSF11）：rank（TNFRSF11）；tweak（CD257，TNFSF12）：TWEAKR（CD266，TNFRSF12）；LIGHT（CD258，TNFSF14）：HVEM（TNFRSF14）；GITRL（TNFSF18）：GITR（CD357 TNFRSF18）；4-IBBL：4-IBB（CD137）。

引自 Abbas A K，Lichtman A H，Pillai S：Basic immunology：functions and disorders of the immune system，6th ed. Philadelphia，Elsevier，2018.

different histamine receptors. Its actions include bronchoconstriction and bronchial smooth muscle contraction, itching, pain, vasodilation, and increased vascular permeability. Histamine also plays a role in gastric acid secretion, motion sickness, and sleep suppression. Commonly used antihistamines counter these effects.

Blood monocytes are produced in the bone marrow and circulate for several days in the blood. Some may migrate into tissues, where they may develop into macrophages that phagocytize pathogens and debris and kill microorganisms when activated by bacterial products such as lipopolysaccharide (LPS), interferon-γ, and other cytokines.

The properties and function of macrophages depend on the tissue. Alveolar macrophages in the lung are continuously exposed to airborne particles and pathogens, whereas microglia in the brain have a very different environment and function. Macrophages clear cellular debris after acute inflammation and thus are the custodians of peripheral tissue. Macrophages produce a variety of cytokines important in the inflammatory process, including IL-1, TNF-α, IL-6, IL-15, and leukocyte growth factors.

Fever during inflammation and infection results from cytokines such as IL-1 and TNF-α that are released by macrophages into the circulation. These molecules increase the level of prostaglandins in the hypothalamus, which elevates the normal temperature set point. This stimulates thermoregulatory mechanisms to elevate the core body temperature, which has antimicrobial effects.

Macrophages play a central role in granuloma formation. For example, macrophages are critical in controlling difficult-to-kill acid-fast mycobacteria such as *M. tuberculosis* or fungi by walling off viable organisms in granulomas. Macrophages also present antigen derived from microbial pathogens to T cells, helping to initiate the adaptive immune response.

Dendritic cells (DCs) are derived from myeloid or lymphocytic precursors. Dendritic cells of the myeloid lineage (also known as conventional DCs or cDCs) are found primarily in tissues where pathogens are likely to enter the body, such as the skin, gastrointestinal tract, spleen, and respiratory tract. These cells have branchlike cytoplasmic extensions (for which they are named), and they phagocytize pathogens in a manner similar to macrophages, then migrate to lymphoid organs where they interact with T cells. They are the major antigen-presenting cells (APCs) in the body and are critical for the initial activation of adaptive immune responses. Dendritic cells of the lymphoid lineage are known as plasmacytoid dendritic cells (pDCs). Like cDCs, pDCs may also present antigen to T cells; however, their major role is to produce copious amounts of interferon-α upon viral infection, providing a critical first line of defense.

Natural killer (NK) cells are large granular lymphocytes that kill abnormal cells, including virus-infected cells and certain tumor cells. NKs do not express immunoglobulins or T-cell receptors but rather employ a system of activating and inhibitory receptors to detect features of stressed cells such as reduction in the expression of major histocompatibility complex (MHC) molecules. Upon activation, NKs kill their targets by releasing granule contents that include the pore-forming protein perforin and various proteases known as granzymes, which may induce target cell death via lysis or apoptosis. NKs are part of the first line of defense against viral infections while adaptive immunity is developing. Patients with NK deficiencies have been shown to be highly susceptible to herpesvirus infection such as varicella-zoster virus.

Adaptive Immunity

The adaptive immune response is capable of producing exquisitely specific protective mechanisms against microbial pathogens (see Fig. 1.1). Adaptive responses to most protein-containing antigens produced by pathogens during a primary exposure leads to the

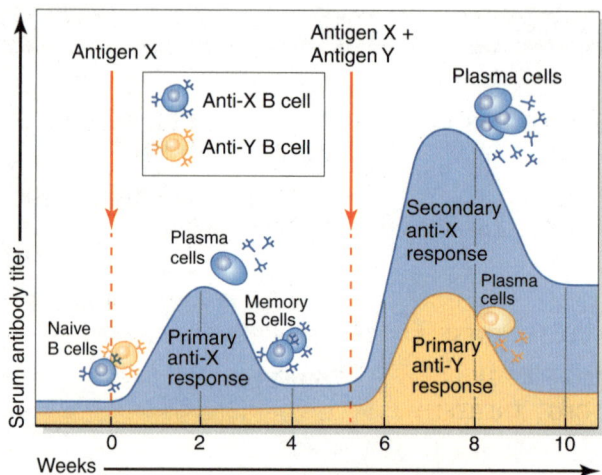

Fig. 1.2 Primary and secondary immune responses. The properties of memory and specificity can be demonstrated by repeated immunizations with defined antigens in animal experiments. Antigens X and Y induce the production of different antibodies (a reflection of specificity). The secondary response to antigen X is more rapid and larger than the primary response (illustrating memory) and is different from the primary response to antigen Y (again reflecting specificity). Antibody levels decline with time after each immunization. The level of antibody produced is shown as arbitrary values and varies with the type of antigen exposure. Only B cells are shown, but the same features are seen with T cell responses to antigens. The time after immunization may be 1 to 3 weeks for a primary response and 2 to 7 days for a secondary response, but the kinetics vary, depending on the antigen and the nature of immunization. (From Abbas A K, Lichtman A H, Pillai S: Basic immunology: functions and disorders of the immune system, 6th ed. Philadelphia, Elsevier, 2018.)

formation of memory B and T cells; secondary exposure to that antigen may recall the memory, leading to adaptive responses that are more rapid, of much greater magnitude, and of higher affinity than before (Fig. 1.2). The capacity of the adaptive immune system to protect against different pathogens is truly astounding. Through a process known as gene rearrangement it has been estimated that B cells can produce 10^{12} different immunoglobulin molecules and that T cells can have up to 10^{18} different T-cell receptors (TCRs) for specific antigens.

Antibodies and B Lymphocytes

Antibodies, also known as immunoglobulins (Igs), are variable glycoproteins produced by B cells that recognize specific structural motifs (epitopes) on the molecules (antigens) produced by microbial pathogens. In antimicrobial defense, binding of an antibody to a pathogen may inhibit (neutralize) the ability of the pathogen to infect a cell (e.g., influenza virus) or the ability of a toxin (e.g., tetanus toxin) to be effective; prompt phagocytosis by phagocytic cells such as neutrophils and macrophages (i.e., opsonization); activate the complement cascade; or kill an infected cell through the process known as antibody-dependent cellular cytotoxicity (ADCC), in which otherwise nonspecific immune cells such as neutrophils or macrophages are able to recognize antibodies bound to target cell surfaces and release cytolytic factors.

Antibody-mediated host defense occurs mainly in the extracellular space, as opposed to T cell–mediated host defenses that act primarily on intracellular pathogens (i.e., those that enter cells and survive intracellularly). The five major isotypes (also known as classes) of antibodies are summarized in Fig. 1.3 (note that IgG and IgA are further divided into subtypes). Effector functions mediated by antibodies include complement activation (IgM and IgG1/2/3),

滑肌收缩、瘙痒、疼痛、血管舒张和血管通透性增加。组胺还对胃酸分泌、晕动病和抑制睡眠方面发挥作用。常用的抗组胺药可以抵消这些作用。

血液单核细胞在骨髓中产生，并在血液中循环数天。有些可能迁移到组织中，在那里它们可能发育成巨噬细胞，当被脂多糖（LPS）、干扰素-γ 和其他细胞因子等细菌产物激活时，它们会吞噬病原体和碎片并杀死微生物。

巨噬细胞的性质和功能取决于它们所在的组织。例如，肺泡巨噬细胞持续暴露于空气中的颗粒和病原体，而大脑中的小胶质细胞则在非常不同的环境中发挥不同的功能。巨噬细胞清理急性炎症后的细胞碎片，因此是外周组织的监管员。巨噬细胞产生多种在炎症过程中重要的细胞因子，包括IL-1、TNF-α、IL-6、IL-15和白细胞生长因子。

炎症和感染期间的发热是由巨噬细胞释放到循环中的细胞因子（如IL-1和TNF-α）引起的。这些分子增加了下丘脑中前列腺素的水平，从而提高了正常温度调定点。这刺激了体温调节机制，提高了核心体温，从而起到抗菌作用。

巨噬细胞在肉芽肿形成过程中发挥着核心作用。例如，巨噬细胞在控制难以杀死的抗酸分枝杆菌（如结核杆菌）或真菌方面起着关键作用，它能在肉芽肿中为有活性的生物体筑墙。巨噬细胞还能将来自微生物病原体的抗原传递给T细胞，有助于启动适应性免疫应答。

树突状细胞（DC）来源于髓系或淋巴细胞前体。髓系的树突状细胞（也称为经典树突状细胞或cDC）主要存在于病原体可能进入的人体组织中，例如皮肤、胃肠道、脾和呼吸道。这些细胞具有树枝状细胞质突起（因此得名），它们以类似于巨噬细胞的方式吞噬病原体，然后迁移到淋巴器官，在那里它们与T细胞相互作用。它们是体内主要的抗原提呈细胞（APC），对适应性免疫应答的初始激活至关重要。淋巴系的树突状细胞被称为浆细胞样树突状细胞（pDC）。与cDC一样，pDC也可能向T细胞提呈抗原；不过，它们的主要作用是在病毒感染时产生大量的干扰素-α，提供关键的第一道防线。

自然杀伤（NK）细胞是杀死异常细胞、病毒感染细胞和某些肿瘤细胞的大颗粒淋巴细胞。NK不表达免疫球蛋白或T细胞受体，而是利用激活和抑制受体系统来检测应激细胞的特征，例如降低主要组织相容性复合物（MHC）分子的表达。激活后，NK通过释放颗粒内容物来杀死其靶标，这些颗粒内容物包括成孔蛋白穿孔素和各种称为颗粒酶的蛋白酶，这些蛋白酶可能通过裂解或凋亡诱导靶细胞死亡。当适应性免疫发展时，NK细胞是抵御病毒感染第一道防线的一部分。NK缺乏症患者已被证明对疱疹病毒（如水痘-带状疱疹病毒）感染高度易感。

适应性免疫

适应性免疫应答能够产生针对微生物病原体的精细的特异性保护机制（见图1.1）。在初次暴露期间，对病原体产生的大多数含蛋白质抗原的适应性免疫应

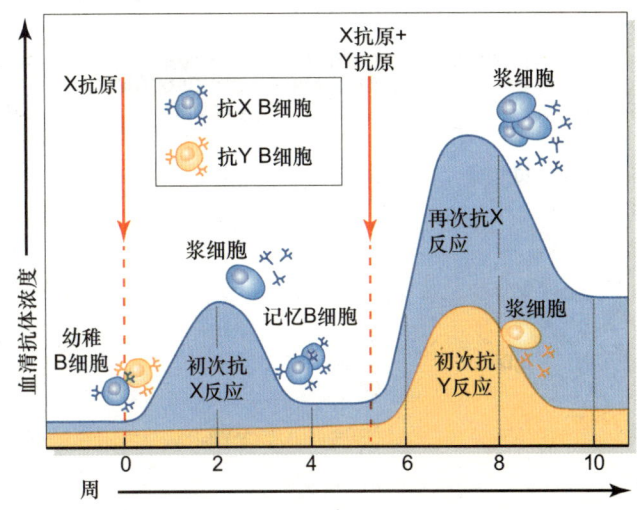

图1.2 初次和再次免疫应答。记忆和特异的特性可以通过在动物实验中用确定的抗原重复免疫来证明。抗原X和Y会诱导产生不同的抗体（反映了特异性）。对抗原X的再次应答比初次应答更快、更大（反映了记忆性），与对抗原Y的初次反应不同（再次反映了特异性）。每次免疫后，抗体水平都会随着时间的推移而下降。产生的抗体水平以任意值显示，并随抗原暴露类型的不同而变化。图中只显示了B细胞，但T细胞对抗原的反应也有同样的特征。初次应答的免疫时间可能为1～3周，再次反应的免疫时间可能为2～7天，但其动力学因抗原和免疫性质而异（引自 Abbas A K, Lichtman A H, Pillai S: Basic immunology: functions and disorders of the immune system, 6th ed. Philadelphia, Elsevier, 2018.）

答导致记忆B细胞和T细胞的形成；二次暴露于该抗原可能会唤起记忆，导致适应性免疫应答比以前更快、幅度更大、亲和力更高（图1.2）。适应性免疫系统抵御不同病原体的能力确实令人震惊。通过一种称为基因重排的过程，据估计，B细胞可以产生10^{12}种不同的免疫球蛋白分子，而T细胞可以产生多达10^{18}种不同的T细胞受体（TCR）来对抗特定的抗原。

抗体和B淋巴细胞

抗体，也称为免疫球蛋白（Ig），是由B细胞产生的可变糖蛋白，可识别微生物病原产生的分子（抗原）上的特定结构基序（表位）。在抗微生物防御中，抗体与病原体的结合可能会抑制（中和）病原体感染细胞的能力（例如流感病毒）或毒素（例如破伤风毒素）的有效能力；吞噬细胞（如中性粒细胞和巨噬细胞）的快速吞噬作用（即调理作用）；激活补体级联；或通过称为抗体依赖性细胞毒性（ADCC）的过程杀死受感染的细胞，其中非特异性免疫细胞（如中性粒细胞或巨噬细胞）能够识别与靶细胞表面结合的抗体并释放细胞溶解因子。

抗体介导的宿主防御主要发生在细胞外空间，而T细胞介导的宿主防御主要作用于细胞内病原体（即进入细胞并在细胞内存活的病原体）。图1.3总结了抗体的五种主要同种型（也称为类别）（请注意，IgG和IgA进一步分为亚型）。抗体介导的效应功能包括补体激活（IgM和IgG1/2/3）、调理作用（IgG）、中和作用

ISOTYPE OF ANTIBODY	SUBTYPES (H CHAIN)	PLASMA CONCENTRATION (mg/ml)	PLASMA HALF-LIFE (DAYS)	SECRETED FORM	FUNCTIONS
IgA	IgA 1,2 (α1 or α2)	3.5	6	Mainly dimer, also monomer, trimer	Mucosal immunity
IgD	None (δ)	Trace	3	Monomer	Naive B cell antigen receptor
IgE	None (ϵ)	0.05	2	Monomer	Defense against helminthic parasites, immediate hypersensitivity
IgG	IgG 1-4 (γ1, γ2, γ3 or γ4)	13.5	23	Monomer	Opsonization, complement activation, antibody-dependent cell-mediated cytotoxicity, neonatal immunity, feedback inhibition of B cells
IgM	None (μ)	1.5	5	Pentamer 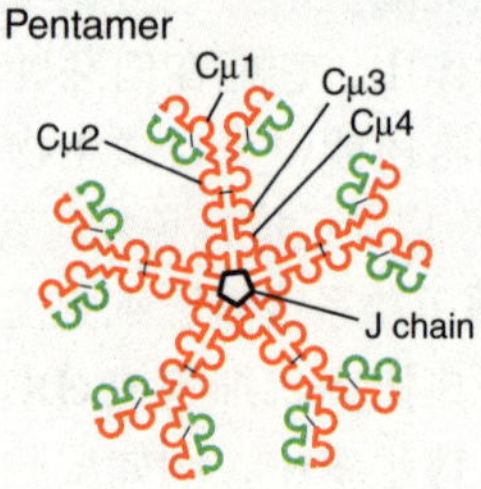	Naive B cell antigen receptor (monomeric form), complement activation

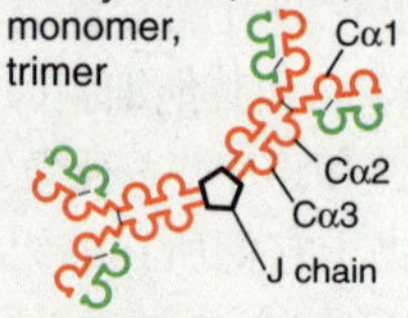

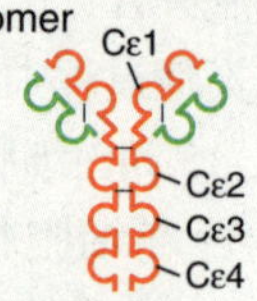

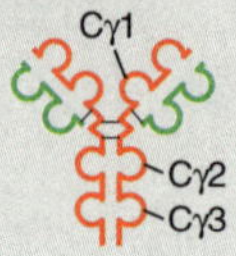

Fig. 1.3 Features of the major isotypes (classes) of antibodies. This figure summarizes some important features of the major antibody isotypes of humans. Isotypes are classified on the basis of their heavy (H) chains; each isotype may contain either κ or λ light chain. The schematic diagrams illustrate the distinct shapes of the secreted forms of these antibodies. Note that IgA consists of two subclasses, called IgA1 and IgA2, and IgG consists of four subclasses, called IgG1, IgG2, IgG3, and IgG4. Most of the opsonizing and complement fixation functions of IgG are attributable to IgG1 and IgG3. The domains of the heavy chains in each isotype are labeled. The plasma concentrations and half-lives are average values in normal individuals. *Ig*, Immunoglobulin. (From Abbas A K, Lichtman A H, Pillai S: Basic immunology: functions and disorders of the immune system, 6th ed. Philadelphia, Elsevier, 2018.)

opsonization (IgG), neutralization (IgM, IgG, and IgA) and mast cell degranulation (IgE) which mediates type I hypersensitivity. IgG antibodies cross the placenta, providing protective immunity to newborns for months after birth. IgA molecules are secretory antibodies that act at mucosal surfaces and are the predominant antibody in external secretions such as mucus, saliva, and breast milk. IgE is responsible for allergic responses and host defenses against parasites. IgM (in monomeric form) and IgD are found on the surface of naïve B cells and function in the initial antigen-mediated activation of these cells.

The basic structural unit of an antibody is composed of two identical "heavy" (H) chains and two identical "light" (L) chains (Fig. 1.4). Each heavy and light chain has constant and variable regions, the latter mediating antigen specificity. The five major types of heavy chains are designated mu, delta, gamma, epsilon and alpha (μ, δ, γ, ϵ, and α) and define the antibody isotype (IgM, IgD, IgG, IgE and IgA). There are two types of light chains, kappa and lambda (κ and λ), that may associate with any of the heavy chains. The antigen-binding site of each molecule is composed partly of the variable region of a heavy chain and partly of the variable region of a light chain. There are two such binding sites for each antibody monomer, although secreted antibodies may contain 2, 4, or 10 identical antigen binding sites depending on if they are secreted as a monomer (IgG, IgD, IgE), a dimer (IgA) or a pentamer (IgM) (see Fig. 1.3).

The B-cell receptor (BCR) is composed of the specific immunoglobulin produced by that B cell associated with signaling molecules on the cell surface. Naïve B cells simultaneously express BCRs that contain monomeric IgM or IgD, each with identical antigen specificity. When initially stimulated, B cells typically secrete pentameric IgM antibodies. Later in the immune response, a B cell may undergo a process that allows the isotype of immunoglobulin produced to switch (e.g., from IgM to IgG; see later).

同种型抗体	亚型（H链）	血浆浓度（mg/ml）	血浆半衰期（天）	分泌型	功能
IgA	IgA 1,2 (α1或α2)	3.5	6	主要是二聚体，也有单体，三聚体 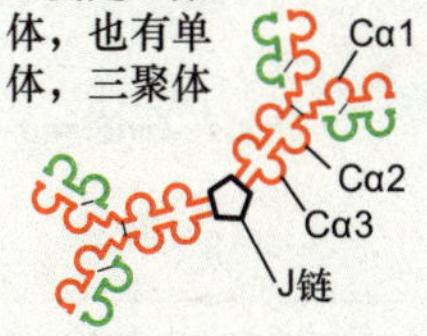	黏膜免疫
IgD	无 (δ)	痕量	3	单体	初始B细胞抗原受体
IgE	无 (ε)	0.05	2	单体 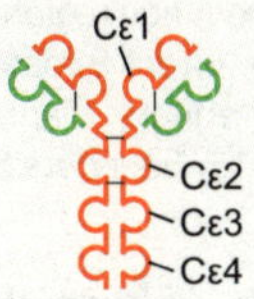	对蠕虫寄生虫的防御，即时超敏反应
IgG	IgG 1-4 (γ1,γ2,γ3或γ4)	13.5	23	单体 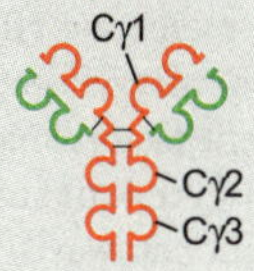	调理作用，补体激活，抗体依赖性细胞介导的细胞毒性，新生儿免疫，B细胞的反馈抑制
IgM	无 (μ)	1.5	5	五聚体 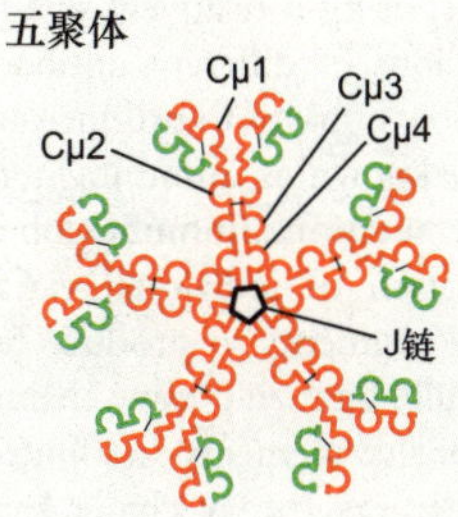	初始B细胞抗原受体（单体形式），补体激活

图 1.3 主要抗体类型的特征。本图总结了人类主要抗体类型的一些重要特征。抗体类型根据其重（H）链进行分类；每种类型可能包含 κ 或 λ 轻链。示意图说明了抗体分泌型的不同形状。请注意，IgA 由两个亚型组成，称为 IgA1 和 IgA2，IgG 由四个亚类组成，分别是 IgG1、gG2、lgG3 和 IgG4。IgG 的大部分调理作用和补体固定功能都归功于 IgG1 和 IgG3。每种类型的重链结构域都有标记。血浆浓度和半衰期是正常个体的平均值。Ig，免疫球蛋白（引自 Abbas A K, Lichtman A H, Pillai S: Basic immunology: functions and disorders of the immune system, 6th ed. Philadelphia, Elsevier, 2018.）

（IgM、IgG 和 IgA）和肥大细胞脱颗粒（IgE）介导的 I 型超敏反应。IgG 抗体穿过胎盘，在出生后数月内为新生儿提供保护性免疫。IgA 分子是作用于黏膜表面的分泌抗体，是黏液、唾液和母乳等外分泌物中的主要抗体。IgE 负责过敏反应和宿主对寄生虫的防御。IgM（单体形式）和 IgD 存在于初始 B 细胞的表面，并在这些细胞的初始抗原介导的激活中起作用。

抗体的基本结构单元由两条相同的"重"（H）链和两条相同的"轻"（L）链组成（图 1.4）。重链和轻链各有恒定和可变区域，后者介导抗原特异性。五种主要类型的重链被命名为 μ、δ、γ、ε 和 α，并定义了抗体同种型（IgM、IgD、IgG、IgE 和 IgA）。有两种类型的轻链，kappa 和 lambda（κ 和 λ），它们可以与任何重链相关联。每个分子的抗原结合位点部分由重链的可变区组成，部分由轻链的可变区组成。每个抗体单体都有两个这样的结合位点，但分泌的抗体可能含有 2、4 或 10 个相同的抗原结合位点，具体取决于它们是以单体（IgG、IgD、IgE）、二聚体（IgA）或五聚体（IgM）的形式分泌的（见图 1.3）。

B 细胞受体（BCR）由 B 细胞产生的特异性免疫球蛋白组成，与细胞表面的信号分子相关。新生 B 细胞同时表达含有单体 IgM 或 IgD 的 BCR，每种细胞都具有相同的抗原特异性。最初刺激时，B 细胞通常分泌五聚体 IgM 抗体。在免疫应答的后期，B 细胞可能会经历一个过程，该过程使产生的免疫球蛋白发生同型转换（例如，从 IgM 到 IgG；见下文）。

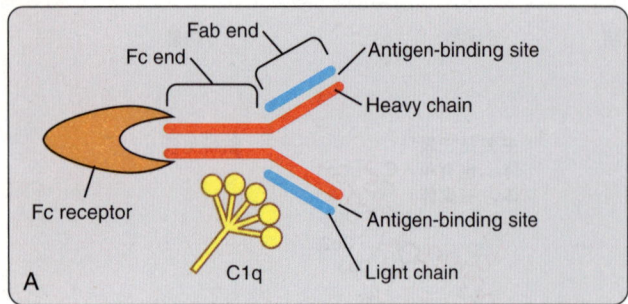
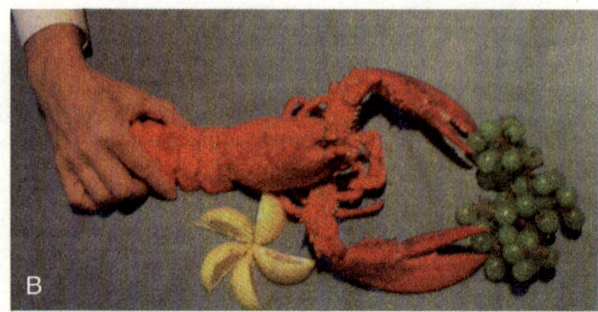

Fig. 1.4 Structure of antibodies. Antibody molecules are composed of two heavy chains *(red lines)* and two light chains *(blue lines)* held together by disulfide bonds. The two heavy chains join to form a tail (Fc end), which can interact with receptors (FcR) on a variety of cells. The heavy and light chains contribute to the Fab end. At the 5′ or amino-terminal end, these chains form two identical antigen-binding sites, much like two lobster claws. Near the hinge region of the antibody, there is a binding site for C1q, the first component of the complement cascade. (From Birdsall H: Adaptive immunity: antibodies and immunodeficiencies. In Bennett JE, Dolin R, Blaser M, editors: Mandell, Douglas, and Bennett's principles and practice of infectious diseases, ed 8, Philadelphia, 2015, Saunders.)

The constant region of the two antibody heavy chains comprises the Fc portion, which can be bound by various Fc receptors (FcRs) on the surface of immune cells (Fig. 1.4), mediating effector functions such as opsonization, ADCC, and degranulation, depending on the isotype and cell type. Soluble complement factors may also bind the Fc portion of antibodies that have bound soluble or surface-associated antigens, activating the classic complement pathway.

Much as a child might produce a large number of unique structures from a small set of building blocks, using a relatively small amount of DNA humans can generate billions of different antibodies. The two major genetic strategies that allow humans to produce antibodies specific to virtually any antigen are known as immunoglobulin gene rearrangement and somatic hypermutation. Immunoglobulin gene rearrangement involves recombination of individual variable (V), diversity (D), and joining (J) gene segments to produce functional genes that encode the immunoglobulin light and heavy chains.

Humans have about 130 functional V segments distributed among the three immunoglobulin gene clusters (heavy chain, kappa light chain, and lambda light chain); each cluster contains four to six functional J segments, with the heavy chain cluster also containing about 25 functional D segments. During B-cell development proteins known as recombination activating genes 1 and 2 (RAG-1/2) mediate random recombination of V, D, and J segments on heavy chain alleles and V and J segments on light chain alleles in a stepwise process. The combinational diversity of V(D)J rearrangement is greatly augmented by flexible joining events that can lead to insertion or deletion of nucleotides at each junction. In this manner, an enormously diverse set of variable chains—perhaps as many as 10^{12}—may be assembled. Further genetic variation arises through a process known as somatic hypermutation, which occurs in proliferating B cells following activation by foreign antigen in lymphoid tissues.

The adaptive humoral response begins with recognition of foreign antigen by specific B cells in secondary lymphoid organs. Before activation, B cells express IgM and IgD with a particular specificity on their membranes; following binding of a protein antigen the B cells internalize and process the antigen, then present peptides derived from it to CD4$^+$ helper T (Th) cells. Interaction with a Th that expresses a TCR specific for peptide derived from the foreign antigen allows a B cell to become activated, proliferate, and differentiate into antibody-secreting plasma cells or memory B cells. Proliferating B cells may begin to express antibody isotypes other than IgM and IgD (e.g., IgG, IgA, IgE) through a process known as isotype switching that is driven by cytokines such as IL-4, IL-10, IL-5 and others produced by T cells. Isotype switching, which does not affect the specificity of the antibody, allows the host to take advantage of the various effector functions mediated by the different isotypes (e.g., complement fixation for IgM, opsonic activity for IgG). As mentioned previously, proliferating B cells may also undergo somatic hypermutation, a process by which point mutations are randomly inserted into the immunoglobulin DNA. While most such mutations are deleterious, those B cells bearing mutations that enhance antigen binding activity (affinity) are selected and expanded, leading to an overall increase in the quality of the antibody response over time—this is known as affinity maturation. Furthermore, T-cell interaction typically drives the generation of a pool of memory B cells that persist for the life of the individual. Such memory cells have the capacity to be reactivated upon subsequent exposure to foreign antigen, leading to secondary antibody responses that are faster, of greater magnitude, and of higher affinity than the primary response (see Fig. 1.2).

Although most protein antigens are said to be T-dependent (i.e., require Th cells for optimal B-cell activation), some antigens can stimulate B cells to proliferate and produce antibody directly without the presence of Th cells (T-independent). T-independent antigens include microbial-derived molecules such as LPS, which bind pattern receptors (e.g., TLRs) on B cells and may stimulate them without regard to antigen specificity. Others, such as microbial-derived polysaccharides that contain repeating epitopes, specifically engage B cells with sufficient strength to bypass the requirement for Th cell interaction. More commonly, however, B cells are stimulated through synergistic action with Th cells. Specific antigen is bound to the surface immunoglobulin of the B cell, triggering endocytosis, degradation of the antigen, and presentation of peptide fragments in association with MHC class II molecules on the cell surface. Th cells with TCRs specific for the MHC-peptide complex interact with the B cell; this interaction is stabilized and strengthened through cell adhesion molecules and costimulatory activation molecules such as CD28 on the T cell and B7-1/2 (also known as CD80/86) on the B cell. Th cells then produce costimulatory molecules such as CD40L (which engages CD40 on the B cell) and cytokines such as IL-4 that drive activation and antibody production by the B cells.

T Lymphocytes

T cell precursors are produced in the bone marrow and migrate to the thymus where they undergo development and selection. At the conclusion of their development most T lymphocytes express either

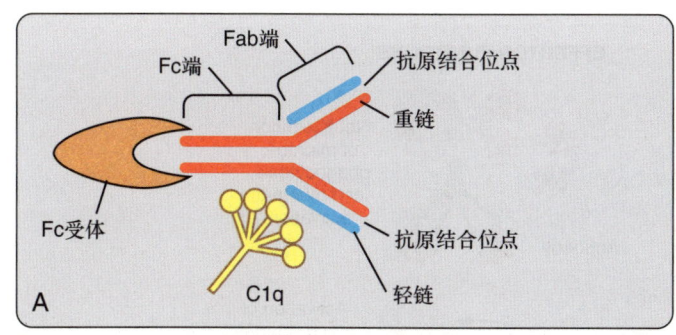 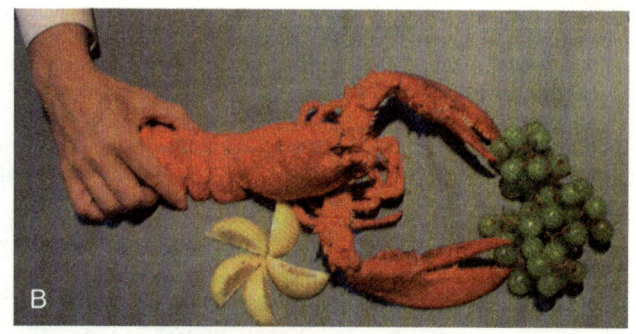

图 1.4 抗体结构。抗体分子由两条重链（红线）和两条轻链（蓝线）通过二硫键连接而成。两条重链连接形成尾部（Fc端），可以与多种细胞上的受体（FcR）相互作用。重链和轻链形成 Fab 端。在 5′ 或氨基末端，这些链形成两个相同的抗原结合位点，就像两个龙虾爪一样。在抗体的铰链区附近，有一个与补体级联的第一个成分，即 C1q 的结合位点（引自 Birdsall H: Adaptive immunity: antibodies and immunodeficiencies. In Bennett JE, Dolin R, Blaser M, editors: Mandell, Douglas, and Bennett's principles and practice of infectious diseases, ed 8, Philadelphia, 2015, Saunders.）

两条抗体重链的恒定区包括 Fc 部分，该部分可与免疫细胞表面的各种 Fc 受体（FcR）结合（图 1.4），介导调理、ADCC 和脱颗粒等效应功能，具体取决于同种型和细胞类型。可溶性补体因子还可以结合可溶性或表面相关抗原的抗体的 Fc 部分，激活经典的补体途径。

就像孩子可以用一小套积木制作出大量独特的结构一样，使用相对少量的 DNA，人类可以产生数十亿种不同的抗体。使人类产生对几乎任何抗原具有特异性抗体的两种主要遗传策略被称为免疫球蛋白基因重排和体细胞超突变。免疫球蛋白基因重排涉及个体变量（V）、多样性（D）和连接（J）基因片段的重组，以产生编码免疫球蛋白轻链和重链的功能基因。

人类约有 130 个功能 V 片段分布在 3 个免疫球蛋白基因簇（重链、κ 轻链和 λ 轻链）中；每个簇包含 4～6 个功能 J 段，重链簇还包含约 25 个功能 D 段。在 B 细胞发育过程中，称为重组激活基因 1 和 2（RAG-1/2）的蛋白质循序介导重链等位基因上 V、D 和 J 片段以及轻链等位基因上的 V 和 J 片段的随机重组。V(D)J 重排的复合多样性通过可导致每个连接处的核苷酸插入或缺失的灵活连接而大大增强。以这种方式，可以组装出一组非常多样化的可变链（可能多达 10^{12}）。进一步的遗传变异是通过一种称为体细胞过度突变的过程产生的，该过程发生在淋巴组织中被外来抗原激活后增殖的 B 细胞中。

适应性体液应答始于次级淋巴器官中特异性 B 细胞对外来抗原的识别。在激活之前，B 细胞在其膜上表达具有特异性的 IgM 和 IgD；与蛋白抗原结合后，B 细胞内化并处理抗原，然后将源自抗原的肽提呈给 $CD4^+$ 辅助性 T（Th）细胞。与表达源自外来抗原的肽特异性 TCR 的 Th 相互作用，使 B 细胞被激活、增殖并分化为分泌抗体的浆细胞或记忆 B 细胞。增殖的 B 细胞可能开始表达 IgM 和 IgD 以外的抗体同种型（例如 IgG、IgA、IgE），该过程称为同种型转换，该过程由 IL-4、IL-10、IL-5 等细胞因子和 T 细胞产生的其他细胞因子驱动。同种型转换不影响抗体的特异性，使宿主能够利用不同同种型介导的各种效应功能（例如，IgM 的补体结合、IgG 的调理活性）。如前所述，增殖的 B 细胞也可能经历体细胞超突变，这是一个将突变随机插入免疫球蛋白 DNA 的过程。虽然大多数此类突变是有害的，但那些携带增强抗原结合活性（亲和力）的突变的 B 细胞被选择和扩增，导致抗体反应质量随时间推移的整体提高——这被称为亲和力成熟。此外，T 细胞相互作用通常会驱动记忆 B 细胞池的产生，这些细胞会持续存在于个体的一生。这种记忆细胞具有在随后暴露于外来抗原时被重新激活的能力，导致比初次应答更快、幅度更大、亲和力更高的再次抗体应答（见图 1.2）。

尽管大多数蛋白质抗原被认为是 T 细胞依赖性的（即需要 Th 细胞才能实现最佳 B 细胞活化），但一些抗原可以直接刺激 B 细胞增殖并产生抗体，而不需要 Th 细胞（T 细胞非依赖性）。T 细胞非依赖性抗原包括微生物衍生的分子，如 LPS，它们与 B 细胞上的模式受体（如 TLR）结合，并可在不考虑抗原特异性的情况下刺激它们。其他抗原，如含有重复表位的微生物衍生多糖，以足够的强度特异性地与 B 细胞结合，以绕过 Th 细胞相互作用的要求。然而，更常见的是，B 细胞通过与 Th 细胞的协同作用受到刺激。特异性抗原与 B 细胞表面免疫球蛋白结合，触发内吞作用、抗原降解，及与细胞表面 MHC Ⅱ类分子结合提呈肽片段。具有 MHC-肽复合物特异性 TCR 的 Th 细胞与 B 细胞相互作用；这种相互作用通过细胞黏附分子和共刺激驱动分子［如 T 细胞上的 CD28 和 B 细胞上的 B7-1/2（也称为 CD80/86）］得到稳定和加强。然后，Th 细胞产生共刺激分子，如 CD40L（与 B 细胞上的 CD40 结合）和细胞因子，如 IL-4，驱动 B 细胞的活化和抗体产生。

T 淋巴细胞

T 细胞前体在骨髓中产生，并迁移到胸腺，在那里进行发育和选择。在其发育结束时，大多数 T 淋巴细胞在其表面表达 CD4 或 CD8 分子，以及对抗原肽和自

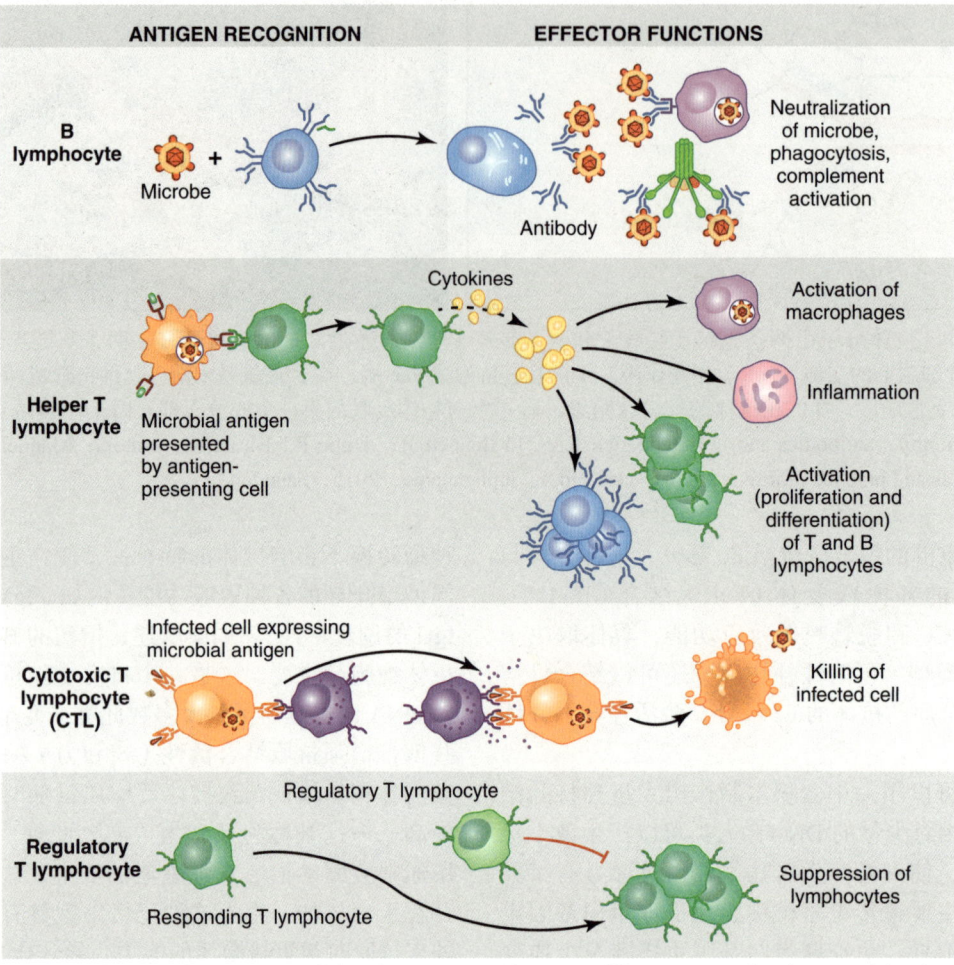

Fig. 1.5 Classes of lymphocytes. B lymphocytes recognize many different types of antigens and develop into antibody-secreting cells. Helper T lymphocytes recognize antigens on the surfaces of antigen-presenting cells and secrete cytokines, which stimulate different mechanisms of immunity and inflammation. Cytotoxic T lymphocytes recognize antigens on infected cells and kill these cells. Regulatory T cells suppress immune responses (e.g., to self antigens). (From Abbas A K, Lichtman A H, Pillai S: Basic immunology: functions and disorders of the immune system, 6th ed. Philadelphia, Elsevier, 2018.)

CD4 or CD8 molecules on their surface along with TCRs specific for a particular combination of antigenic peptide and self MHC. During development, the TCR is produced in a process involving V(D)J gene rearrangement mediated by RAG-1/2 in a manner broadly analogous to that of B cells. Most conventional T cells express TCRs that are a combination of alpha and beta TCR chains, each with constant and variable regions; others express TCRs consisting of gamma and delta TCR chains.

As maturation takes place in the thymus, T cells undergo selection processes that eliminate those whose TCRs have low affinity for self MHC (positive selection) or too high an affinity for self molecules (negative selection). The combination of positive and negative selection thus ensures that T-cell activation requires a combination of self MHC and foreign antigen. Naïve T cells, usually in regional lymph nodes or similar tissues such as Peyer patches in the gut, are sensitized by interaction with an APC such as a dendritic cell or memory B cell. The APC internalizes and processes microbial antigen and then presents peptides derived from that antigen to the associated T cell. Presentation of antigen occurs in association with MHC (also known as human leukocyte antigens, or HLA) class II molecules for CD4+ cells or MHC class I molecules for CD8+ cells. CD4+ cells are called helper T cells (Th) and develop into Th1, Th2, and Th17 subsets. CD8+ cells are cytotoxic T cells (CTLs; see Fig. 1.5).

CD4+ T cells play a central role in the activation of B lymphocytes, other CD4+ T cells, CD8+ T cells, and phagocytic cells such as macrophages. CD4+ T cells orchestrate host defenses against pathogens that are initially acquired by phagocytic cells during phagocytosis or pinocytosis. Dendritic cells, for example, take up pathogens or antigens by phagocytosis or pinocytosis and then degrade them within phagosomes.

Antigenic peptides, which are produced by proteolytic degradation of protein antigens in phagolysosomes, bind noncovalently to a grove in MHC class II molecules. The complex is then transported to the cell surface for presentation to T cells expressing CD4 molecules on their surface. CD4+ T cells with specificity for the antigen then bind via their TCRs to the MHC class II/antigen complex on the surface of the APC. CD4 also associates with MHC II, stabilizing the interaction between T cell and APC. Accessory molecules, such as the adhesion molecule lymphocyte function–associated antigen 1 (LFA-1) on T cells, which interacts with intercellular adhesion molecule 1 (ICAM-1)

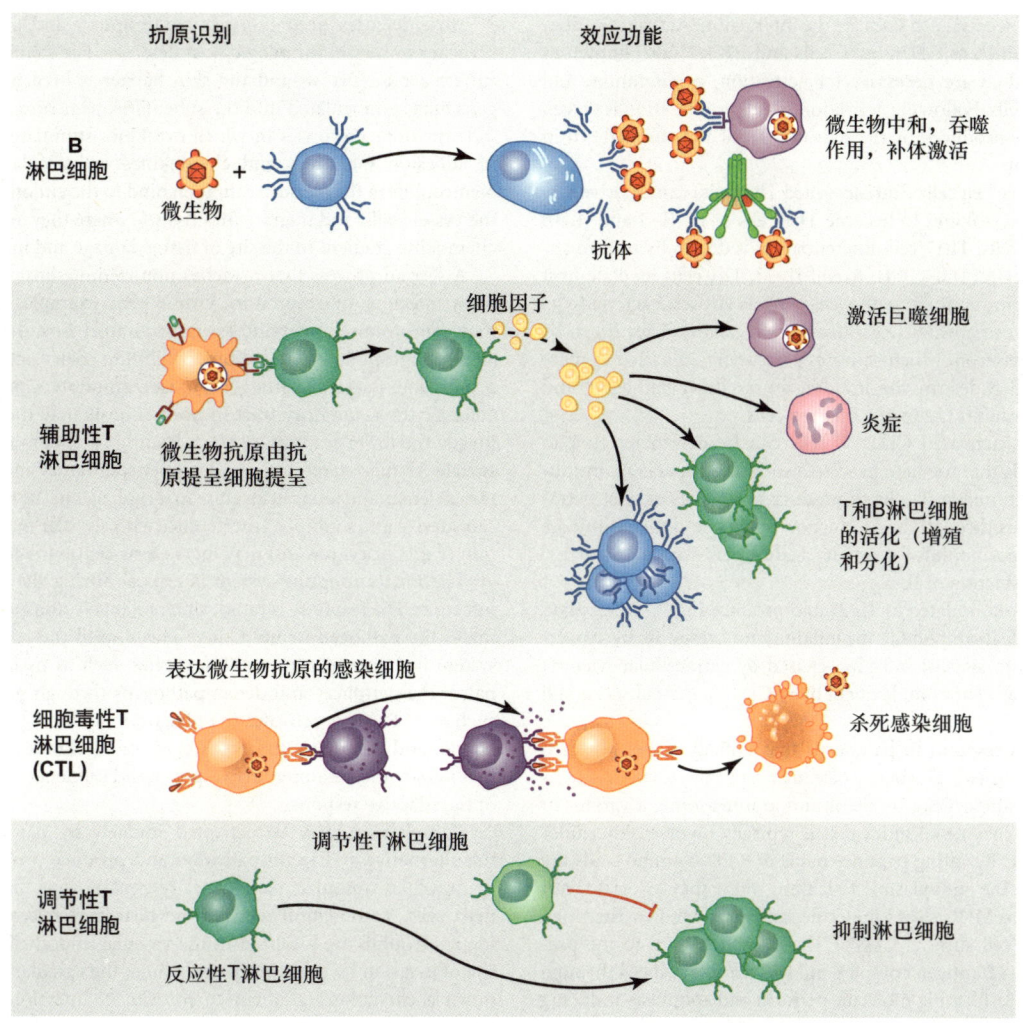

图1.5 淋巴细胞类别。B淋巴细胞能识别多种不同类型的抗原，并发育成分泌抗体的细胞。辅助性T淋巴细胞能识别抗原递呈细胞表面的抗原，并分泌细胞因子，刺激不同的免疫和炎症机制。细胞毒性T淋巴细胞能识别感染细胞上的抗原并杀死这些细胞。调节性T淋巴细胞抑制免疫应答（如对自身抗原的反应）（引自Abbas A K, Lichtman A H, Pillai S: Basic immunology: functions and disorders of the immune system, 6th ed. Philadelphia, Elsevier, 2018.）

身MHC的特定组合特异的TCR。在发育过程中，TCR是在由RAG-1/2介导的V（D）J基因重排的过程中产生的，其方式大致类似于B细胞。大多数经典T细胞表达的TCR是由α和β链组成的，每个TCR都具有恒定区和可变区；少部分表达由γ和δ链组成的TCR。

当T细胞在胸腺中成熟时，会经历选择过程，从而淘汰那些TCR对自身MHC的亲和力低（阳性选择）或对自身分子亲和力过高（阴性选择）的T细胞。因此，阳性和阴性选择的结合确保了T细胞活化需要自身MHC和外源抗原的组合。幼稚T细胞通常位于区域淋巴结或类似组织（如肠道中的派尔集合淋巴结）中，通过与树突状细胞或记忆B细胞等抗原提呈细胞（APC）相互作用而被致敏。APC对微生物抗原进行内化和处理，然后将源自该抗原的肽提呈给相关的T细胞。抗原提呈与$CD4^+$细胞的MHC（也称为人类白细胞抗原或HLA）Ⅱ类分子或$CD8^+$细胞的MHCⅠ类分子相关。$CD4^+$细胞称为辅助性T细胞（Th），可发育成Th1、Th2和Th17亚群。$CD8^+$细胞是细胞毒性T细胞（CTL；见图1.5）。

$CD4^+$ T细胞在B淋巴细胞、其他$CD4^+$ T细胞、$CD8^+$ T细胞和吞噬细胞（如巨噬细胞）的活化中起核心作用。$CD4^+$ T细胞协调宿主防御病原体，这些病原体最初由吞噬细胞在吞噬作用或胞饮作用期间获得。例如，树突状细胞通过吞噬作用或胞饮作用摄入病原体或抗原，然后在吞噬体内降解它们。

抗原肽是蛋白质抗原在吞噬溶酶体中被蛋白水解后产生的，与MHCⅡ类分子中的沟槽非共价结合。然后，复合物被转运到细胞表面，呈现给表面表达CD4分子的T细胞。然后，对抗原具有特异性的$CD4^+$ T细胞通过其TCR与APC表面的MHCⅡ类/抗原复合物结合。CD4还与MHCⅡ分子结合，稳定T细胞与APC之间的相互作用。辅助分子，如T细胞上的黏附分子淋巴细胞功能相关抗原1（LFA-1），与APC上的细胞间黏附分子1（ICAM-1）相互作用，是稳定相互作用所必需的。激活黏附复合物，如T细胞上的CD28和APC上的B7-1/2

on the APC, are necessary to stabilize the interaction. Activating adhesion complexes such as CD28 on T cells and B7-1/2 (also known as CD80/86) on APCs are necessary for activation, proliferation, and activation of T cells. Following activation, T cell proliferation is driven by IL-2, which is produced by the activated T cell and stimulates it in an autocrine loop.

Activated CD4$^+$ Th cells (initially called Th0 cells) can be driven by IL-12 and other cytokines to become Th1 cells or by IL-4 and IL-10 to become Th2 cells. Th17 cell differentiation is driven by transforming growth factor-β (TGF-β), IL-6, and IL-23. Th1 cells mediate host defenses against intracellular pathogens such as viruses, bacteria (e.g., *M. tuberculosis*) or parasites (e.g., *Toxoplasma gondii*). They do so by producing γ-interferon, which activates phagocytic cells such as macrophages that then destroy the invading intracellular pathogen, and IL-2, which activates CTLs to lyse infected cells.

Alternatively, activated CD4$^+$ T cells can be driven by IL-4 to become Th2 cells that mediate processes such as antiparasitic immunity. Th2 cells stimulate B cells to produce antibodies against extracellular pathogens through the production of IL-4, and they stimulate proliferation of eosinophils for activity against parasites (e.g., worms) through the production of IL-5.

Th17 cells are stimulated by IL-23 and produce IL-17, which plays an important role in amplifying the inflammatory response by attracting neutrophils to sites of infection caused by extracellular bacteria and possibly fungi. The complexity of these CD4$^+$ T-cell subsets is still being explored.

CD8$^+$ T cells respond to pathogens that initially enter host cells directly, such as viruses. During intracellular replication, viral proteins are degraded in the cytosol by the immunoproteasome, a variant of the proteasome enzyme complex that is typically involved in cellular protein turnover. Resulting peptide chains of 8 to 10 amino acids are transported into the endoplasmic reticulum where they associate with newly synthesized MHC class I molecules and are routed via the Golgi complex to the cell surface. CD8$^+$ CTLs may then bind to the presented MHC class I/antigen complex and lyse the infected cell through release of the pore-forming molecule perforin and apoptosis-inducing enzymes known as granzymes, or through ligation of Fas ligand on the CTL with Fas on the target cell, which also may induce apoptosis. CTLs are generated from naïve CTL precursors through specific association with a dendritic cell (DC) that has been "licensed" through interaction with a CD4$^+$ Th1 cell. Interaction with the DC stimulates the production of IL-2 by the CD4$^+$ Th1 cell and increases B7-1/2 (CD80/86) expression by the DC. The combination of antigen-specific signaling through the TCR, engagement of CD28 on the CD8$^+$ cell by B7-1/2 on the DC, and Th1-derived IL-2 stimulates the CD8$^+$ T cell to proliferate and differentiate into CTLs, which may then lyse infected target cells as described above.

In addition to effector T cells, populations of regulatory T cells modulate the immune response. Most regulatory T cells (Tregs) express CD4, CD25, and the FOXP3 transcription factor and help to temper immune responses, particularly those related to autoimmune diseases but also some infectious diseases.

HOST DEFENSE RESPONSE TO PATHOGENS

Humans are constantly exposed to microbial pathogens. Organisms such as *Streptococcus pneumoniae*, group A streptococci, and respiratory viruses may colonize the respiratory tract. *Staphylococcus aureus*, fungi, and many other organisms live on the skin. Thousands of microbial species have been identified in the gastrointestinal tract; most are benign, many are beneficial, and some are dangerous.

Host defenses need to react continuously and appropriately to breaches in nonimmunologic host defenses. For example, if a person suffers a puncture wound the skin barrier is breached, and pathogens may be inoculated into the subcutaneous tissues. This stimulates inflammatory responses in which cytokines stimulate the expression of adhesion molecules and chemokines on vascular endothelium. Neutrophils in the bloodstream then bind to the endothelium, traverse the vessel walls, and migrate into tissues, where they are attracted by a chemokine gradient to the site of tissue damage and infection.

A second process that breaches nonimmune host defenses results from infection by respiratory viruses. For example, influenza virus may compromise upper and lower respiratory host defenses by damaging the respiratory epithelium, inhibiting ciliary action and mucus production. Bacterial pathogens, most commonly *S. pneumoniae*, that colonize the respiratory tract in normal hosts may then colonize and invade the lower respiratory tract, leading to pneumonia. Organisms such as *M. tuberculosis* may evade upper respiratory and lower respiratory defenses and lodge in alveolar macrophages in the lung, where they can survive and multiply. Interference with alveolar macrophage function (e.g., silica exposure) may increase susceptibility to tuberculosis.

The innate immune system is critical during the early phases of infection. The response is rapid, albeit relatively nonspecific, and eliminates the pathogen or holds it in check until the adaptive immune system has time to respond. Phagocytes such as tissue macrophages patrol the periphery and detect pathogens through pattern receptors such as TLRs. This activates the phagocyte, induces phagocytosis and killing, and stimulates the production of cytokines and chemokines that initiate the inflammatory response and influence the development of the adaptive response.

Complement may be activated innately by pathogens through the alternative and lectin pathways and produce products to attract neutrophils, opsonize pathogens, lyse pathogens, and degranulate mast cells. Vasodilation results from histamine release, and circulating neutrophils are localized to the vascular endothelium nearest the site of invasion by integrins, pass through the vascular wall, and move down a chemokine gradient to the site of infection. Opsonization helps neutrophils, macrophages, and other immune cells ingest and kill the pathogen. These immediate inflammatory and innate immune responses are initiated immediately and increase over hours to days. These responses are highly effective, buying survival time for the host while more specific responses of the adaptive immune system develop.

Immature dendritic cells in peripheral tissues are sentinels for foreign molecules. Through pinocytosis and phagocytosis initiated by TLRs and other receptors, DCs detect pathogens; once they have acquired foreign antigen, DCs migrate to regional lymph nodes. There the DCs mature, process, and present antigen to T cells, initiating the specific adaptive immune response. The type of response depends on the type of pathogen. Intracellular pathogens such as *M. tuberculosis* stimulate a T cell–mediated response, whereas *S. pneumoniae* stimulates primarily a B-cell, antibody-mediated (humoral) response. Most infections produce components of cellular and humoral responses in various degrees that often act in concert. For example, influenza virus induces B-cell and T-cell responses; antibodies neutralize free virus and prevent further infection of respiratory epithelium and CTLs lyse infected epithelial cells.

Humoral Response

Early in infection, preexisting antibodies and complement factors react to pathogens directly and can initiate lysis, opsonization, and neutralization of pathogens. B cells may be activated by T cell–independent antigens or through interaction with CD4$^+$ T cells for T cell–dependent antigens. B-cell populations proliferate and produce IgM antibodies

（也称为 CD80/86）是 T 细胞活化、增殖和激活 T 细胞所必需的。活化后，T 细胞增殖由 IL-2 驱动，IL-2 由活化的 T 细胞产生，并在自分泌环路中刺激 T 细胞。

活化的 $CD4^+$ Th 细胞（最初称为 Th0 细胞）可以在 IL-12 和其他细胞因子的作用下分化为 Th1 细胞，或者在 IL-4 和 IL-10 的作用下分化为 Th2 细胞。Th17 细胞分化由转化生长因子-β（TGF-β）、IL-6 和 IL-23 驱动。Th1 细胞介导宿主对细胞内病原体，如病毒、细菌（例如结核分枝杆菌）的防御或寄生虫（例如刚地弓形虫）。它们通过产生 γ-干扰素和 IL-2 来实现这一目的，γ-干扰素可激活吞噬细胞，如巨噬细胞，进而消灭入侵细胞内的病原体，而 IL-2 则可激活 CTL 来裂解受感染细胞。

此外，活化的 $CD4^+$ T 细胞可以被 IL-4 驱动分化为 Th2 细胞，介导抗寄生虫免疫等。Th2 细胞通过产生 IL-4 刺激 B 细胞产生针对细胞外病原体的抗体，并通过产生 IL-5 刺激嗜酸性粒细胞增殖以对抗寄生虫（如蠕虫）。

Th17 细胞受 IL-23 刺激并产生 IL-17，IL-17 通过将中性粒细胞吸引到由胞外细菌和可能的真菌引起的感染部位，在放大炎症反应中起重要作用。这些 $CD4^+$ T 细胞亚群的复杂性仍在探索中。

$CD8^+$ T 细胞对最初直接进入宿主细胞的病原体（如病毒）产生应答。在细胞内复制过程中，病毒蛋白在胞质中被免疫蛋白酶体降解，免疫蛋白酶体是蛋白酶体复合物的一种变体，通常参与细胞蛋白质的周转。由 8～10 个氨基酸组成的肽链被转运到内质网中，在那里它们与新合成的 MHC Ⅰ类分子结合，并通过高尔基复合体到达细胞表面。然后，$CD8^+$ CTL 可以与呈现的 MHC Ⅰ类/抗原复合物结合，并通过释放成孔分子穿孔素和称为颗粒酶的凋亡诱导酶来裂解感染的细胞，或通过 CTL 上的 Fas 配体与靶细胞上的 Fas 连接也可能诱导细胞凋亡。CTL 是由幼稚的 CTL 前体通过与树突状细胞（DC）的特异性结合产生的，这些树突状细胞（DC）已通过与 $CD4^+$ Th1 细胞的相互作用而获得"许可"。与 DC 的相互作用进而刺激 $CD4^+$ Th1 细胞分泌 IL-2，并增加 DC 对 B7-1/2（CD80/86）的表达，通过 TCR 的抗原特异性信号传导，DC 上的 B7-1/2 与 $CD8^+$ T 细胞上的 CD28 结合以及 Th1 细胞产生的 IL-2 刺激 $CD8^+$ T 细胞增殖并分化成 CTL，然后如上所述裂解受感染的靶细胞。

除效应 T 细胞外，调节性 T 细胞群也能调节免疫应答。大多数调节性 T 细胞（Treg）表达 CD4、CD25 和 FOXP3 转录因子，有助于调节免疫应答，特别是与自身免疫性疾病相关的免疫应答，以及一些感染性疾病。

宿主对病原体的防御反应

人类持续暴露于微生物病原体。肺炎链球菌、A 组链球菌和呼吸道病毒等病原体可在呼吸道定植。金黄色葡萄球菌、真菌和许多其他生物可生活在皮肤上。在胃肠道中已鉴定出数千种微生物；大多数是无害的，许多是有益的，有些是危险的。

宿主防御需要针对非免疫宿主防御的漏洞做出持续和适当的反应。例如，如果一个人被刺伤，皮肤屏障就会被破坏，病原体可能会进入皮下组织中，刺激炎症反应，其中细胞因子刺激血管内皮上黏附分子和趋化因子的表达。然后，血液中的中性粒细胞与内皮结合，穿过血管壁，迁移到组织中，被趋化因子梯度吸引到组织损伤和感染部位。

破坏非免疫宿主防御的第二个过程是由呼吸道病毒感染引起的。例如，流感病毒可能通过破坏呼吸道上皮细胞、抑制纤毛活动和黏液产生来损害上下呼吸道宿主的防御能力。正常宿主的呼吸道定植的细菌病原体，最常见的是肺炎链球菌，可定植并侵入下呼吸道，导致肺炎。结核分枝杆菌等微生物可以逃避上呼吸道和下呼吸道防御，并寄宿在肺部的肺泡巨噬细胞中，在那里它们可以生存和繁殖。干扰肺泡巨噬细胞功能（例如，吸入二氧化硅）可能会增加对结核病的易感性。

先天免疫系统在感染的早期阶段至关重要。此反应是快速的，尽管相对非特异性，但可消除病原体或控制病原体，直到适应性免疫系统做出反应。组织巨噬细胞等吞噬细胞外周巡逻并通过 TLR 等模式受体在检测到病原体，从而激活吞噬细胞，诱导吞噬作用和杀伤作用，并刺激细胞因子和趋化因子的产生，从而启动炎症反应并影响适应性免疫应答的发展。

补体可通过旁路途径和凝集素途径被病原体先天激活，并产生吸引中性粒细胞、调理病原体、裂解病原体和脱颗粒肥大细胞的产物。血管舒张由组胺释放引起，循环中性粒细胞定位于最靠近整合素侵袭部位的血管内皮，穿过血管壁，沿趋化因子梯度移动至感染部位。调理作用有助于中性粒细胞、巨噬细胞和其他免疫细胞摄取并杀死病原体。这些即时炎症和先天免疫应答会立即启动，并在数小时至数天内增加。这些反应非常有效，为宿主争取了生存时间，同时适应性免疫系统产生了更具体的反应。

外周组织中的未成熟树突状细胞是外来分子的哨兵。树突状细胞通过由 TLR 和其他受体引发的胞饮作用和吞噬作用来检测病原体；一旦获得外来抗原，树突状细胞就会迁移到区域淋巴结，在那里，其成熟、加工抗原并将其提呈给 T 细胞，从而启动特异性的适应性免疫应答。应答的类型取决于病原体的类型。细胞内病原体（如结核分枝杆菌）刺激 T 细胞介导的免疫应答，而肺炎链球菌则主要刺激 B 细胞产生抗体介导的（体液）免疫应答。大多数感染产生不同程度的细胞和体液免疫应答，这些免疫应答通常协同发挥作用。例如，流感病毒诱导 B 细胞和 T 细胞应答；抗体可中和游离病毒并防止呼吸道上皮细胞的进一步感染，CTL 可裂解受感染的上皮细胞。

体液免疫应答

在感染早期，预先存在的抗体和补体因子直接与病原体发生反应，并可启动针对病原体的裂解、调理和中和。B 细胞可能被 T 细胞非依赖性抗原激活，也可通过

initially and then with isotype switching produce other types of antibodies, including IgG, IgE, and IgA. Antibodies acting in the extracellular space bind to pathogens or their products, potentially leading to neutralization, agglutination, opsonization, complement fixation, ADCC, and mast cell degranulation.

Cell-Mediated Response

Naïve T cells with specificity for the invading pathogen are activated, proliferate, and produce cytokines. CD4$^+$ T cells produce cytokines that stimulate other T cells such as CTLs, enhance the overall inflammatory response, activate phagocytes for killing, and stimulate antibody production. Previously sensitized memory CD4$^+$ and CD8$^+$ T cells may react rapidly with activation and proliferation on exposure to previously recognized pathogens.

SUGGESTED READINGS

Bennett JE, Dolin R, Blaser M, editors: Mandell, Douglas, and Bennett's principles and practice of infectious diseases, ed 8, Philadelphia, 2015, Saunders.

Medzhitov R, Shevach EM, Trinchieri G, et al: Highlights of 10 years of immunology in nature reviews immunology, Nat Rev Immunol 11:693–702, 2011.

与 CD4$^+$ T 细胞相互作用而被 T 细胞依赖性抗原激活。B 细胞群最初增殖并产生 IgM 抗体，然后通过同种型转换产生其他类型的抗体，包括 IgG，IgE 和 IgA。在细胞外空间起作用的抗体与病原体或其产物结合，可导致中和、凝集、调理作用、补体结合、ADCC 和肥大细胞脱颗粒。

细胞免疫应答

对入侵病原体具有特异性的幼稚 T 细胞被激活、增殖并产生细胞因子。CD4$^+$ T 细胞产生的细胞因子，刺激 CTL 等其他 T 细胞，增强整体炎症反应，激活吞噬细胞进行杀伤，并刺激抗体产生。先前已致敏的记忆 CD4$^+$ 和 CD8$^+$ T 细胞在接触到先前已识别的病原体时会迅速发生活化和增殖反应。

推荐阅读

Bennett JE, Dolin R, Blaser M, editors: Mandell, Douglas, and Bennett's principles and practice of infectious diseases, ed 8, Philadelphia, 2015, Saunders.

Medzhitov R, Shevach EM, Trinchieri G, et al: Highlights of 10 years of immunology in nature reviews immunology, Nat Rev Immunol 11:693–702, 2011.

2

Laboratory Diagnosis of Infectious Diseases

Kimberle Chapin

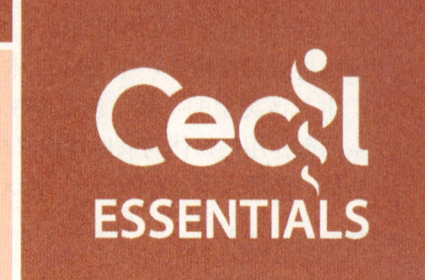

INTRODUCTION

The ability to rapidly and accurately diagnose pathogen-specific infectious diseases and resistance determinants has become the norm in medicine as a result of the continuous introduction of new technologies. In addition, companion diagnostics such as those that assess host-specific biomarker signatures in conjunction with software algorithms to clarify risk (e.g., likelihood of sepsis) or probable pathogen-specific group (e.g., viral vs. bacterial) add a personalized medicine component to infectious disease interpretation.

This chapter highlights significant components of testing for infectious diseases and trends in laboratory medicine and diagnostic technology that affect patient care. The 2018 American Society for Microbiology (ASM) and Infectious Disease Society of America (IDSA) guideline on use of the microbiology laboratory for the diagnosis of infectious diseases is a comprehensive resource summarizing laboratory diagnosis of infectious diseases by basic disease categories (e.g., respiratory, genital) focusing on best-use practice guidelines and containing numerous tables for rapid access of information. The document is well referenced and is updated on a regular basis. Other valued resources exist online for use with uncommonly encountered pathogens, such as the Centers for Disease Control and Prevention (CDC) DPDx (https://www.cdc.gov/dpdx/index.html) for parasitic infections that includes case studies and 360Dx (https://www.360dx.com/) that highlights new infectious diseases technologic advances that are important to track.

DIAGNOSTIC STEWARDSHIP

As infectious disease diagnostic tests and results have become available closer to the time of patient care, the basic concepts of optimal specimen acquisition, test selection, test performance parameters for a given patient population, and result interpretation by providers are admittedly more complex and somewhat overwhelming. Up to 70% of individual patient medical diagnoses are being made with the aid of a laboratory test result. Diagnostic stewardship, a process that promotes a team approach to optimizing microbiology test implementation, provider test choice and interpretation, along with assessment of outcomes to identify value of specific diagnostic tests for patient care have become requisite. For infectious diseases, this includes microbiology diagnostics that have been shown to affect directed patient care, morbidity, mortality, and health care costs. These are now published for a growing list of significant quality measures as shown in Box 2.1.

SPECIMEN COLLECTION AND CANCELLATION OF INAPPROPRIATE SPECIMENS

Collection of the appropriate specimen and its preservation during transportation to a testing site are components of infectious disease diagnosis that are often overlooked. As part of their accreditation and inspection process, laboratories have collection procedures and criteria for rejection of specimens that are deemed inappropriate to process. These evidence-based protocols ensure that results can be used reliably to treat patients and provide reasons for specimen requests not being performed. Examples include cancellation of a nonliquid stool for *Clostridioides difficile* toxin testing because it is inconsistent for a person with *C. difficile* infection (CDI) that produces watery diarrhea; urine specimens for culture received greater than 2 hours after collection and not refrigerated or in preservative, which allows overgrowth of bacteria and uninterpretable mixed organism results; and blood or genital specimens for molecular-based tests submitted in a device that does not preserve the nucleic acid target.

Liquid Media and Self-Collected Specimens

Specimen collection, including surgical tissue specimens, has recently become decentralized. However, the limitations for samples that require culture have been minimized by the use of flocked swabs placed directly into a liquid matrix that preserve both aerobic and anaerobic organisms and nucleic acid targets (e.g., E-swabs [Copan Diagnostics, Inc.]), and dry swabs for molecular analysis. In addition, patient-collected versus provider-collected specimens have been shown to yield equivalent or better test results, increase patient satisfaction, and encourage appropriate use of health care.

Provider Responsibility for Optimizing Results

All personnel (e.g., physicians, physician assistants, nurses, phlebotomists, patients) collecting specimens should be familiar with the appropriate collection devices, recommended collection techniques, testing requirements, including timeliness of transportation to the laboratory or need of fresh tissue (not in formalin) for culture, to ensure optimal identification of the pathogen.

If the practitioner requests a microbiology test not typically performed, such as anaerobic organisms from a cerebral spinal fluid (CSF) specimen, or a test without standardized interpretive criteria (e.g., antimicrobials not FDA-cleared), a call should be made to the laboratory.

RAPID AND/OR DIRECT FROM SPECIMEN DIAGNOSTIC METHODS

Rapid or *STAT* is no longer a term foreign to direct testing for infectious diseases and the microbiology laboratory. All major areas of diagnostic testing, including direct visualization of organisms in specimens, detection of organism-specific antigens, antibodies, proteins, and nucleic acids, as well as cell counts and biomarkers can be performed in 1 to 4 hours. Results are uploaded automatically upon completion into the electronic medical record (EMR) and are often

感染性疾病的实验室诊断

杨帆 译　彭俊平　舒跃龙 审校　刘海鹰 通审

引言

随着高新技术的不断发展融合，快速准确地诊断病原体特异性感染性疾病和耐药性决定因素已经成为医学领域的常态。此外，伴随诊断，例如评估宿主特异性生物标志物特征与软件算法相结合以明确风险（例如感染中毒症的可能性），或可能的病原体特异性组（例如病毒与细菌），为阐述感染性疾病增加了个性化医疗成分。

本章节重点介绍了感染性疾病检测的重要组成部分以及影响患者护理的实验室医学和诊断技术的趋势。2018年美国微生物学会（ASM）和美国传染病学会（IDSA）发布的微生物学实验室在感染性疾病诊断中的应用指南是一个综合性资源，总结了按基本疾病类别（如呼吸系统、生殖系统等）进行的感染性疾病实验室诊断，是聚焦于最佳使用的实践指南，并包含了许多表格以便于快速获取信息。上述文件的参考文献引用规范，并定期更新。其他有价值的在线资源还包括罕见病原体的资源，例如美国疾病控制与预防中心（CDC）的 DPDx（https://www.cdc.gov/dpdx/index.html），其中包括了寄生虫感染的案例研究，以及 360Dx（https://www.360dx.com/），该网站强调了需要追踪的感染性疾病的最新技术进展。

诊断管理

随着感染性疾病诊断检测及其结果越来越接近患者的护理时间，关于最佳样本采集、检测选择、针对特定患者群体的检测性能指标以及检测人员对结果的解释等基本概念显然变得更复杂且令人不知所措。多达70%患者的医学诊断是在实验室检测结果的指导下做出的。诊断管理，即通过团队合作来优化微生物学检测的实施、检测人员的检测选择和结果解读，以及通过评估结果来确定诊断检测对患者护理价值的过程，其已经成为必不可少的环节。对于感染性疾病而言，包括已被证明影响有针对性的患者护理、发病率、死亡率和医疗费用的微生物学诊断。这些现已在越来越多的重要质量衡量指标中公布，如框2.1所示。

样本采集及不规范样本的剔除

将适当样本采集并运输到检测地点的过程中进行保存是感染性疾病诊断中经常被忽视的环节。作为其认证和检查流程的一部分，实验室制定了样本采集程序和对不当样本剔除的标准。这些循证操作流程确保结果可以可靠地用于指导感染性疾病患者的治疗，并提供样本剔除未检的理由。常见案例如下，对用于艰难梭菌毒素检测的非液态粪便样本进行剔除，因为这与艰难梭菌感染（CDI）患者产生水样腹泻的情况不一致；对在采集后超过2 h且未冷藏或未添加防腐剂的尿液样本进行剔除，因为这会导致细菌过度生长和难以解释的混合结果；此外，剔除用于分子检测但储存于不能稳定核酸分子的耗材中的血液或生殖道样本等。

液体介质和自采样本

近年来，包括外科手术组织样本在内的样本采集已逐渐变得去中心化。然而，通过使用直接置于液体基质中的植绒拭子[如 E-swabs（Copan Diagnostics, Inc.）]，可以保存需氧和厌氧生物以及待检核酸靶标，最大限度地减少了需要培养的样本限制，同时也可以使用干拭子进行分子分析。此外，患者自行采集的样本与医务人员采集的样本相比，已被证明能够产生同等或更好的检测结果，提高患者满意度，并鼓励在医疗保健中适当使用。

提供者具有优化检测结果的责任

所有样本采集人员（如医生、医师助理、护士、采血员、患者）都应熟悉符合规定的采集设备、采集技术、检测要求，包括及时将样本送到实验室和对新鲜组织（非福尔马林固定的组织）进行培养，以确保病原体的最佳鉴定结果。如果医生请求进行非常规微生物学检测，例如从脑脊液（CSF）样本中检测厌氧生物，或没有进行标准化的检测（如未获得美国FDA批准的抗微生物药物），则应先与实验室进行协商沟通。

快速和（或）直接从样本中进行诊断的方法

对于直接检测感染性疾病和微生物学实验室，"快速"或"紧急"不再是陌生术语。所有主要的诊断检测领域，包括直接观察样本中的微生物，检测生物特异性的抗原、抗体、蛋白质和核酸，以及细胞计数和生物标志物的识别，都可以在1～4 h完成。结果在完成后会自动上传到电子病历（EMR）中，并且通常在

> **BOX 2.1 Infectious Disease Diagnostics Contributing to Patient Care Quality Measures**
>
> - *Clostridioides difficile* toxin molecular testing and infection control practices
> - Rapid identification and susceptibility for identification and treatment of sepsis to reduce morbidity and mortality
> - Presurgical testing for colonization with methicillin-resistant *Staphylococcus aureus* (MRSA) and *S. aureus* (MSSA), allowing presurgical decontamination and targeted antibiotic therapy in high-risk surgical procedures to reduce surgical site infections
> - Rapid organism identification and resistance determinants to aid in successful anti-infective intervention and stewardship programs
> - PCR technologies for common infections seen in urgent care settings (e.g., GAS and influenza), allowing appropriate therapy, decreasing wait times, and increasing patient satisfaction
> - Multiplex syndromic panels and next-generation sequencing (NGS) allowing rapid identification of public health threats and implementation of risk reduction strategies in outbreak exposures (e.g., GI transmissible pathogens and emerging infections)

available during the time a practitioner is involved with the patient, allowing immediate treatment.

Table 2.1 lists common US Food and Drug Administration (FDA)–cleared or published direct testing methods used in laboratories for primary specimens. Examples include simple stains, such as the Gram stain, to complex nested–polymerase chain reaction (PCR) for syndromic conditions (e.g., infectious disease gastrointestinal panels) and reference tests such as next-generation sequencing (NGS) of cell free DNA.

Direct and *rapid* do not necessarily equate to high predictive values for a true positive or negative test result. Tests commonly used in the past because of ease of use and cost (e.g., viral antigens from throat swabs for influenza and India ink stain in CSF) are not recommended because false-negative and false-positive results, respectively, are common. As well, direct tests that add little value in clarifying the specific diagnosis, such as positive herpes simplex virus 1 and 2 (HSV1/2) antibody in a patient without a vesicle or positive PCR for *C. difficile* toxin in a patient without diarrhea, may in fact be harmful because of misinterpretation about significance.

DIRECT SMEAR INTERPRETATION

A direct smear interpretation can be exceedingly helpful in confirming a suspected infection (e.g., Gram stain of CSF for organisms consistent with pneumococcal meningitis, or fungal elements in tissue) and is performed typically within hours of receipt. Positive sterile specimen smears are reported as critical results. High sensitivity and specificity, however, often depend on specimens being collected appropriately (e.g., obtained before antibiotic administration), providing critical clinical information (e.g., immune status or travel) and experience of the person interpreting the smear.

Special Stains

Specialty staining for a variety of organisms, allowing valuable clinical information, is increasingly being sent off site from clinical care to reference laboratories for either staining or PCR. Most academic medical laboratories still maintain special stain capacity. Fluorescent staining with calcofluor (Fig. 2.1) and auramine have increased sensitivity for direct detection of fungal elements and acid-fast bacilli (AFB), respectively. Direct fluorescent antibody (DFA) staining for *Pneumocystis jirovecii*, more specific and rapid compared with staining of histologic tissue preparations, has some limitations in sensitivity such that

molecular detection is becoming more standard, but when positive, is exceedingly helpful for treatment. Likewise, direct smear interpretation for blood pathogens (e.g., *Babesia* and malaria) is very sensitive for acute disease, but outside of academic medical centers, is typically performed by molecular testing.

CULTURE WITH A BOOST

Despite advances in rapid direct and molecular diagnostics, culture is still a mainstay for infectious disease diagnosis of many specimen types (wounds, urine, blood, tissues), in part because technology to enhance rapid detection and identification of colony growth exist and are cost-effective. Specialized media, such as chromogenic media that are both differential (colony of interest appears a specific color because of added reagents) and selective (incorporated antibiotic allows only desired pathogen to grow), speed detection.

Blood and AFB specimens are incubated in continuously monitoring incubator cabinets that signal when a specimen is positive based on algorithmic growth curves. A positive specimen can be identified at any time of day, pulled and stained immediately after signaling positive, and tested for definitive identification and susceptibility. Many laboratories utilize automated instruments for streaking specimens onto culture plates, allowing consistency better than manual inoculation such that colonies are isolated better and susceptibility can be performed 1 to 2 days earlier. Likewise, incubators that are automated and perform time-lapsed photography on each plate, incorporating comparative differential analysis and artificial intelligence algorithms, can discard "no growth" plates within 24 hours compared to 2 to 5 days. Similarly, rapid identification and antimicrobial susceptibility performed by a combination of fluorescent tagged organisms with specific RNA probes and subsequent time-lapsed photography of organism growth in various antibiotic concentrations allows results 2 days soon than traditional techniques (Accelerate PhenoTest).

Matrix-Assisted Laser Desorption Ionization–Time of Flight Mass Spectrometry

Many laboratories still rely on automated systems that perform identification from organism growth by biochemical and enzymatic phenotypic methods as well as growth methods for determination of antimicrobial susceptibility. However, because these systems require additional growth for reactions to take place, organism identification is delayed another day and susceptibility an additional day. The increased use of matrix-assisted laser desorption ionization–time of flight mass spectrometry (MALDI-TOF MS) is a significant methodologic change that has become standard in many laboratories. This technique relies on the protein spectral analysis of the organism for identification, takes only minutes rather than days, and is very cost-effective. The technique is described in Fig. 2.2. Direct detection from positive blood broth, after a processing step, is also commonly used and allows a more inclusive organism range than molecular panels.

Table 2.2 lists the most common rapid identification methods used from positive broth cultures (e.g., blood) and from colony growth on a culture plate. Use of specific technologies is dependent on expertise in the laboratory, cost, test performance parameters and patient population.

Antibody and Antigen Tests From Blood and Body Fluids

Serology is valuable for confirmation of vaccination and/or response (e.g., rubella), often when a 4-fold rise in antibody titer is an optimal way to clarify if a disease is present, especially if IgM is nonspecific (e.g., *Bartonella*), or the primary technology for diagnosis (e.g., syphilis). Single antibody measurements are rarely helpful in clarifying the disease state (active or past infection) or the mode of transmission and often can be misinterpreted. (e.g., HSV 1/2 antibody).

> **框 2.1　感染性疾病诊断促进患者护理质量的措施**
>
> - 艰难梭菌毒素分子检测和感染控制措施
> - 快速鉴定和药敏试验,有助于减少感染中毒症的发病率和死亡率
> - 手术前检测耐甲氧西林金黄色葡萄球菌(MRSA)和甲氧西林敏感金黄色葡萄球菌(MSSA)的定植,实现在高风险手术过程中进行术前的污染清除和有针对性的抗生素治疗,减少手术部位的感染
> - 快速鉴定微生物和耐药性决定因素有助于成功的抗感染干预和管理程序
> - PCR 技术用于常见感染(如急诊护理中的 A 组链球菌和流感),促进合理医学治疗,减少患者等待时间,提高患者满意度
> - 多重综合征检测试剂盒和二代测序(NGS)可以快速识别公共卫生威胁并在疫情暴发时实施风险降低策略(例如,胃肠道传播病原体和新发感染)

医疗人员对患者做出感染性疾病诊断的时候就已得到检测结果,从而促进了医学治疗的及时性。

表 2.1 列出了美国食品药物监督管理局(FDA)批准和发布的用于实验室常见样本的直接检测方法。包括简单染色,如革兰氏染色,以及用于综合症状诊断(如传染病胃肠道检测试剂盒)的复杂巢式聚合酶链反应(PCR),和参考质控如用于细胞游离 DNA 的二代测序(NGS)等。

直接和快速的检测并不一定意味着对真实阳性或阴性结果具有完美的可信度。在过去,因操作方便和成本低廉而常用的检测方法(如用于流感的咽拭子病毒抗原检测和用于脑脊液的墨汁染色)现不推荐使用,因为会导致常见的假阴性和假阳性结果。同样,直接检测对明确具体诊断几乎没有价值,例如在没有水疱的患者中检测到单纯疱疹病毒 1 型和 2 型(HSV 1/2)抗体阳性或在没有腹泻的患者中检测到艰难梭菌毒素的 PCR 阳性,对上述结果的误判不利于感染性疾病的诊断。

直接涂片

直接涂片对于确认疑似感染非常有帮助(例如,脑脊液革兰氏染色显示与肺炎链球菌脑膜炎相符的病原体,或组织中的真菌成分),并且通常在收到后数小时内进行。阳性无菌样本涂片被报告为关键结果。然而,高敏感性和特异性通常取决于样本是否采集得当(例如,在抗生素给药前采集)、是否提供关键临床信息(例如,免疫状态和旅行史)以及涂片结果分析人员的经验。

特殊染色

针对多种微生物进行特殊染色,从而获得关键的临床诊断信息,越来越多的样本从临床送到标准实验室进行染色或 PCR 检测。大多数学术医学实验室具备特殊染色的能力。使用荧光增白剂(图 2.1)和碱性嫩黄进行荧光染色分别提高了直接检测真菌和抗酸杆菌(AFB)的敏感性。与组织学染色相比,肺孢子虫的直接荧光抗体(DFA)染色更加特异和快速,但由于其敏感性有限,分子检测正逐渐成为标准。然而,当 DFA 检测结果为阳性时,对治疗有极大的帮助。同样,血液中病原体(如巴贝虫和疟原虫)的直接涂片解释对急性疾病非常敏感,但在学术医学中心外,通常通过分子检测进行。

强化培养

尽管快速直接诊断和分子诊断技术具有一些优势,分离培养仍然是许多临床样本类型(如伤口、尿液、血液、组织)感染性疾病诊断的主要方法。部分原因是现有技术可以增强菌落生长的快速检测和鉴定,而且成本效益高。特殊培养基,如显色培养基,既具有区分性(目标菌落因添加的试剂而呈现特定颜色),又具有选择性(加入抗生素只允许所需的病原体生长),加速了基于培养的感染性疾病的诊断。

血液和 AFB 样本被放置在连续监测的培养箱中孵育,通过算法生长曲线在样本为阳性时发出信号。阳性样本可以在一天中的任何时间被识别,发出阳性信号后立即提取并染色,并进行明确的鉴定和药敏试验。许多实验室利用自动化仪器将样本接种到培养板上,比手工接种具有更好的一致性,从而更好地分离菌落并提前 1～2 天进行药敏检测。同样,自动化孵育器对每个培养板进行延时摄影,结合比较差异分析和人工智能算法,可以在 24 h 内丢弃"无生长"的培养皿,而传统方法则需要 2～5 天。同样,通过将荧光标记的微生物与特定的 RNA 探针相结合,并随后对各种抗生素浓度下的微生物生长进行延时摄影,快速鉴定微生物和药敏结果,可以比传统技术(如 Accelerate PhenoTest)早 2 天获得。

基质辅助激光解吸电离飞行时间质谱法

许多实验室仍然依赖自动化系统,通过生化和酶表型的方法以及生长方法来识别微生物,并确定微生物对抗菌药物的敏感性。然而,由于这些系统需要额外的生长时间来进行反应,微生物鉴定会延迟一天,药敏试验又延迟一天。基质辅助激光解吸电离飞行时间质谱(MALDI-TOF MS)的广泛使用,是一项重要的方法学变革,并已逐渐成为标准操作。这种技术依赖于微生物的蛋白质光谱分析进行鉴定,只需几分钟而不是几天且成本效益很高。该技术如图 2.2 所示。经过处理步骤后,从阳性血培养液中直接检测也是一种常用方法,并且比分子组合具有更广泛的生物范围。

表 2.2 列出了从阳性肉汤培养液(如血液)和培养皿上的菌落生长中使用的最常见快速鉴定方法。具体技术的使用取决于实验室的专业知识、成本、检测性能指标和患者人群。

血液和体液中的抗体和抗原检测

血清学诊断在确认疫苗接种和(或)免疫反应(如风疹)方面非常有价值,通常在抗体滴度升高 4 倍时是确认疾病存在的最佳方式,特别是当 IgM 不具有特异性时(如巴尔通体),或者作为诊断的主要技术(如梅毒)。需要注意的是,单次抗体检测很少有助于明确疾病状态(活跃或既往感染)或传播方式,并且常常可能被误诊(如 HSV 1/2 抗体)。

TABLE 2.1 Common Methods of Direct Testing From Specimens

Test Methods[a]	Diagnostic Method	Analyte Detected
Smear stain preparations	Gram stain	Bacteria, fungal elements, including yeast and hyphae
	Fluorescence	DFA: *Pneumocystis jirovecii*, viruses[b]
		Auramine: mycobacteria
		Calcofluor: fungi
	Special: acid-fast (Kinyoun), partial acid-fast (PAF), India ink[c]	Smear use determined by laboratory and based on primary stained specimen[d]
	Wright stain	Leukocyte differentiation and count (e.g., *Plasmodium*, *Babesia*)
	Wright-Giemsa	
Antigen-antibody	Latex agglutination	*Legionella* or *Streptococcus pneumoniae* urinary antigen
		Cryptococcal antigen in serum and CSF
	Lateral flow antibody/antigen	GAS, RSV, influenza A or B, *Plasmodium*
	Serology for IgG, IgM, Western blot	Multiple analytes; detection and/or confirmation of immune status and acute disease
	Biomarkers	Single: Procalcitonin,[e] C-reactive protein
		Combination: multiple biomarkers with algorithmic interpretation (e.g., viral vs. bacterial)
Molecular[f]	Hybridization and signal amplification	Yeast, HPV, bacterial vaginosis or vaginitis
	Amplification of RNA or DNA, single analyte, small or large syndromic panels, direct from specimen or from blood, microbiome based and algorithmic interpreted	Single analytes: Enterovirus, GAS, influenza, RSV; small bundle with ≤5 targets: sexually transmitted pathogens (GC, CT, TV, *Mycoplasma genitalium*)
		Multiplex amplification with ≥5 targets: blood sepsis, respiratory, gastrointestinal, meningitis pathogens, microbiome based: vaginosis/vaginitis
		Chip array: Multiple targets, HPV, HCV genotyping
	Amplification with quantification of nucleic acids	HIV, HCV, HBV
Sequencing	Genotyping	Genetic variants of e.g., HIV, HCV, HPV
Next-generation sequencing (NGS)	16S, 18S, ITS or metagenomic cell free DNA	16S rDNA (prokaryotic); 18S rDNA (eukaryotic), ITS (nontranscribed region of fungal reran) targeted or metagenomics, can differentiate multiple species within one pathogen type/selected organism types or unbiased testing that allows discovery of new pathogens, respectively

CSF, Cerebrospinal fluid; *CT*, *Chlamydia trachomatis*; *DFA*, direct fluorescent antibody; *DNA*, deoxyribonucleic acid; *FDA*, US Food and Drug Administration; *GAS*, group A streptococci; *GC*, *Neisseria gonorrhoeae*; *HBV*, hepatitis B virus; *HCV*, hepatitis C virus; *HIV*, human immunodeficiency virus; *HPV*, human papillomavirus; *Ig*, immunoglobulin; *ITS*, internal transcribed spacer; *RNA*, ribonucleic acid; *RSV*, respiratory syncytial virus; *TV*, *Trichomonas vaginalis*.
[a]One-hour, same-day testing.
[b]Direct fluorescent antibody (DFA) is organism specific (e.g., *P. jirovecii*, varicella zoster, herpes simplex 1 or 2, cytomegalovirus), and better than histologic stains (e.g., silver stain) and Tzanck preparations (e.g., nucleated giant cells), which are not specific and can cause confusion by similar appearances for many infectious causes. Most DFA testing for viruses has been replaced with molecular technologies due to same-day turn-around time and increased sensitivity
[c]Cryptococcal antigen from cerebrospinal fluid (CSF) or serum is the recommended test. India ink often yields false-positive results and is used by the laboratory for confirmation of suspected yeast in a Gram stain of CSF or patients positive by cryptococcal antigen.
[d]For example, partial acid-fast testing is performed if the Gram stain shows branching of gram-positive rods and *Nocardia* is suspected; acid-fast testing may be performed if the auramine-stained sample is positive.
[e]Procalcitonin is a single biomarker used in clarifying bacterial sepsis. Newer combination biomarker tests along with machine learning algorithms suggest greater specificity and sensitivity for sepsis as well as clarifying viral or bacterial disease compared to PCT or traditional C-reactive protein.
[f]Common examples of pathogens are listed for each group, but many more analytes are available.

Cryptococcal antigen from cerebrospinal fluid and blood is the standard of care testing for detection of cryptococcal disease. Likewise, *Legionella* urinary antigen (*L. pneumophila* type 1) and *Histoplasma* urinary antigen are rapid and excellent tests for these conditions.

MOLECULAR DIAGNOSTICS

Use of molecular technology for infectious disease diagnosis is standard of care in microbiology because of ease of use (automation) and the tremendous clinical benefits to patient care (sensitive, specific, and rapid detection). Molecular assays may be performed in either microbiology or core laboratories with overlapping specialty responsibilities (e.g., hematology, chemistry.) The basic categories are shown in Table 2.1.

FDA-cleared direct molecular tests include hybridization and amplification methods. The main difference between these methods is that with hybridization methods, the nucleic acid is not multiplied beyond what is already in the sample. For assays that target DNA, the sensitivity is limited because DNA exists as a single copy. For assays that target proteins or RNA, detection sensitivity is somewhat increased because these components are naturally amplified in the microbe. Familiar hybridization assays include fluorescent in situ hybridization (FISH) for targets in tissue and the protein nucleic acid (PNA) smear. Hybridization assay systems can increase their sensitivity by pairing with signal amplification, such as for human papillomavirus (i.e., Qiagen/Digene HPV test),

表 2.1　样本直接检测的常见方法

检测方法[a]	诊断方法	待检微生物
涂片染色制备	革兰氏染色	细菌、真菌元素，包括酵母和菌丝体
	荧光染色	DFA：肺孢子虫、病毒[b] 碱性嫩黄：分枝杆菌 荧光增白剂：真菌
	特殊染色：抗酸染色（冷染色）、部分抗酸（PAF）、墨汁染色[c]	涂片使用由实验室确定，并基于主要染色样本[d]
	瑞特染色	白细胞分类和计数（例如，疟原虫、巴贝虫）
	瑞氏-吉姆萨染色	
抗原-抗体	乳胶凝集试验	军团菌或肺炎链球菌尿抗原 血清和 CSF 中的隐球菌抗原
	侧流抗体/抗原检测	GAS、RSV、甲型或乙型流感病毒、疟原虫
	血清学检测 IgG、IgM，以及蛋白质印迹法	多重分析物；检测和（或）确认免疫状态和急性疾病
	生物标志物检测	单一生物标志物：如降钙素原[e]、C 反应蛋白 多重生物标志物组合：通过算法解释结果，例如区分病毒感染和细菌感染
分子检测[f]	杂交和信号放大	酵母、HPV、细菌性阴道病或阴道炎
	RNA 或 DNA 扩增：单一分析、小或大综合征检测试剂盒，直接从样本或血液中检测，基于微生物组并通过算法解释	单一分析：肠道病毒、GAS、流感病毒、RSV；小组合（≤5 个）：性传播病原体（GC、CT、TV、生殖支原体） 多重扩增（≥5 个）：血液感染中毒症、呼吸道病原体、胃肠道病原体、脑膜炎病原体、引起阴道病/阴道炎的微生物组 生物芯片技术：多重靶标，HPV、HCV 基因分型
	核酸定量扩增	HIV、HCV、HBV
测序	基因型分型	基因变异，如 HIV、HCV、HPV
二代测序（NGS）	16S、18S、ITS 或宏基因组细胞游离 DNA	16S rDNA（原核生物）；18S rDNA（真核生物）、ITS（真菌的非转录区），目标或宏基因组，可区分一种或多种病原体类型/选择的生物体类型内的多个种类，或无偏检验，可以发现新病原体

CSF，脑脊液；CT，沙眼衣原体；DFA，直接荧光抗体；DNA，脱氧核糖核酸；FDA，美国食品药品监督管理局；GAS，A 组链球菌；GC，淋病奈瑟球菌；HBV，乙型肝炎病毒；HCV，丙型肝炎病毒；HIV，人类免疫缺陷病毒；HPV，人乳头瘤病毒；Ig，免疫球蛋白；ITS，内部转录间隔区；RNA，核糖核酸；RSV，呼吸道合胞病毒；TV，阴道毛滴虫。

[a] 1 h 或当天检测。
[b] 直接荧光抗体（DFA）是特异性的（如肺孢子虫、水痘-带状疱疹病毒、单纯疱疹病毒 1 型或 2 型、巨细胞病毒），比组织学染色（如银染色）和 Tzanck 涂片（如有核巨细胞）更好，这些方法不特异，且因许多感染原因外观相似而引起混淆。大多数病毒的 DFA 检测已被分子技术取代，因其当天可出结果且敏感性提高。
[c] 推荐从脑脊液（CSF）或血清中检测隐球菌抗原。墨汁染色常导致假阳性结果，仅用于实验室确认在脑脊液革兰氏染色或隐球菌抗原阳性的患者中怀疑的酵母菌。
[d] 如果革兰氏染色显示出分枝的革兰氏阳性杆菌且怀疑诺卡菌，则进行部分抗酸染色；如果碱性嫩黄染色样本阳性，则可进行抗酸染色。
[e] 降钙素原（PCT）是用于明确细菌感染中毒症的单一生物标志物。较新的组合生物标志物检测结合机器学习算法比单独使用 PCT 或传统 C 反应蛋白具有更高的特异性和敏感性，可更好地区分病毒性或细菌性疾病。
[f] 每组列出的病原体是常见的例子，但还有许多其他分析物也可用。

脑脊液和血液中的隐球菌抗原检测是检测隐球菌病的标准方法。同样，军团菌尿抗原（嗜肺军团菌 1 型）和组织胞浆菌尿抗原检测是这些疾病快速且优良的检测方法。

分子诊断

由于操作简便（自动化）和对患者照护的巨大临床益处（包括灵敏、特异且快速的检测），分子技术在微生物学中的应用已成为标准方法。分子检测可以在微生物学或交叉专业的核心实验室中进行，后者具有重叠的专业方向（如血液学、化学）。表 2.1 展示了基本的类别。

FDA 批准的直接分子检测包括杂交和扩增。主要区别在于，使用杂交法时，样本中的核酸不会进行扩增。对于以 DNA 为靶标的检测，敏感性有限，因为 DNA 通常以单一拷贝存在。对于以蛋白质或 RNA 为靶标的检测，敏感性有所提高，因为这些成分在微生物中自然放大。常见的杂交检测包括用于组织靶标的荧光原位杂交（FISH）和蛋白质核酸（PNA）涂片。杂交检测系统可以通过与信号放大结合来提高敏感性，例如人乳头瘤病毒（HPV）检测（如 Qiagen/Digene HPV 检

or multiple time point interpretations of probe signal uptake for rapid pathogen identification (i.e., Accelerate PhenoTest).

In contrast, amplification assays increase the original nucleic acid copy number through a variety of processes, including PCR, nested-PCR, transcription-mediated amplification (TMA), and isothermal loop amplification (LAMP). Real-time PCR refers to amplification and detection occurring simultaneously, enabling the analyte to be detected more quickly. Amplification assays can detect a single analyte (e.g., enterovirus from CSF) or a group of pathogens for a disease entity from a single specimen, such as sexually transmitted infections (e.g., *Chlamydia trachomatis*, *Neisseria gonorrhoeae*, and *Trichomonas vaginalis*). They also allow quantification of the viral load for purposes of long-term treatment and assessment of clearance (i.e., human immunodeficiency virus (HIV), hepatitis B virus, and hepatitis C viral loads).

SYNDROMIC ASSAY PANELS

These assays detect a diverse set of pathogens most commonly associated with a specific syndromic condition as well as multiple resistance determinants, (e.g., acute respiratory disease, methicillin susceptibility genes for *S. aureus*). A single specimen aliquoted into a single cartridge is subsequently tested by amplification for multiple targets (multiplexing). FDA-cleared multiplex assays from 3 to 27 targets exist for respiratory syndromes, acute gastroenteritis, sepsis, STIs, bacterial vaginitis/vaginosis, and meningitis. Providers need to be aware of the syndromic panel in use because multiple manufacturers exist and the pathogens reported can vary widely (Fig. 2.3).

16S, 18S AND METAGENOMIC NEXT-GENERATION SEQUENCING FOR PATHOGEN DETECTION

16S and 18S sequencing for prokaryotic and eukaryotic organism identification are in general limited to specific groups of organisms and used in specialty laboratories. Metagenomic cell free DNA analysis is a hypothesis-free diagnostic approach that has the potential to detect nearly any organism from blood. Sequencing is helpful in patients that are immunocompromised, where uncommon pathogens ranging from

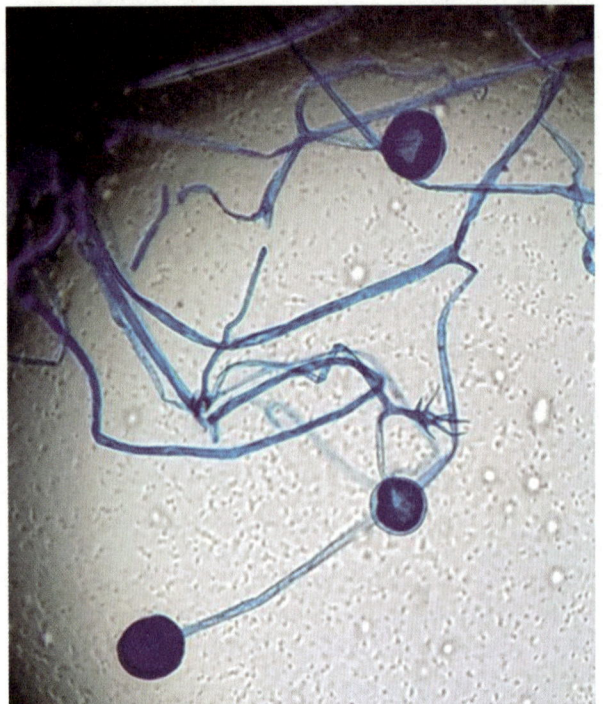

Fig. 2.1 Lactophenol cotton blue depicts fungal hyphae (rhizopus sp.) from a wound specimen.

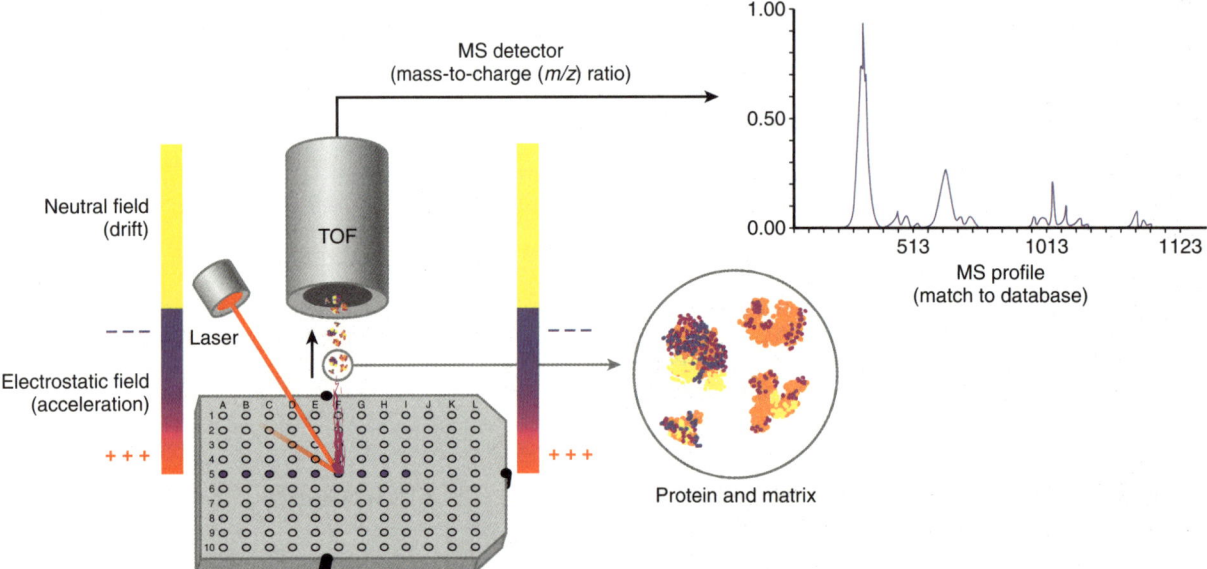

Fig. 2.2 Matrix-assisted laser desorption–time of flight mass spectrometry (MALDI-TOF MS). Bacterial or fungal growth is selected from a culture plate and applied directly onto a MALDI slide. Samples are overlaid with a matrix and dried. Samples are then bombarded by a laser, which results in sublimation and ionization of the sample and the matrix. The ions are separated based on their mass-to-charge ratio in a tube that measures the time it takes the ions to travel. A spectral representation of these ions is generated and analyzed by software that generates a profile that is subsequently compared with a database of reference MS spectra and matched, generating identification. The process takes only minutes. Although the instrumentation is expensive, the technology is US Food and Drug Administration cleared, and it yields rapid, robust, and reliable identification.

测），通过多时间点的探针信号摄取进行快速病原体识别（如 Accelerate PhenoTest）。

相比之下，扩增检测通过多种过程增加原始核酸拷贝数，包括 PCR、巢式 PCR、转录介导扩增（TMA）和等温环扩增（LAMP）。实时 PCR 指的是扩增和检测同时进行，使分析物能够更快被检测到。扩增检测可以检测单一分析物（如脑脊液中的肠道病毒）或单个样本中的一组病原体，如性传播感染（如沙眼衣原体、淋病奈瑟球菌和阴道毛滴虫）。上述方法支持病毒载量的定量，用于长期治疗过程中评估病原体残留量和患者的康复情况（如人类免疫缺陷病毒、乙型肝炎病毒和丙型肝炎病毒载量）。

综合征检测试剂盒

这些试验可以鉴定与特定综合征相关的多种病原体以及多种耐药性决定因素（例如，急性呼吸道疾病，金黄色葡萄球菌的甲氧西林敏感性基因）。一个样本分装到单个试剂盒中，随后通过扩增进行多靶标检测（又名多重检测）。FDA 批准的综合征检测试剂盒涵盖 3 ~ 27 个检测靶标，适用于呼吸系统综合征、急性胃肠炎、感染中毒症、性传播感染、细菌性阴道炎/阴道病和脑膜炎等。检测人员需要了解所使用的综合征检测试剂盒，因为存在多家制造商，靶标病原体可能有很大差异（图 2.3）。

16S、18S 和用于病原体检测的宏基因组二代测序

16S 和 18S 测序方法用于鉴定原核和真核生物，通常限于特定的微生物群体，并在专业微生物学实验室中使用。细胞游离 DNA 宏基因组测序分析是一种无偏检验，具有检测血液中几乎任何微生物的潜力。对于免疫受损的患者，测序技术非常有帮助，因为这类患

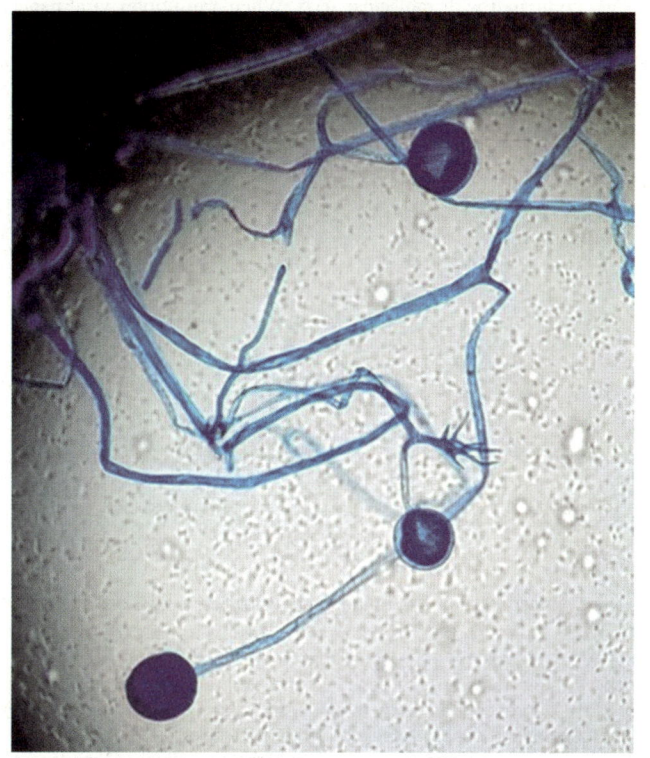

图 2.1　伤口样本乳酚棉蓝染色下的真菌菌丝（根霉属）

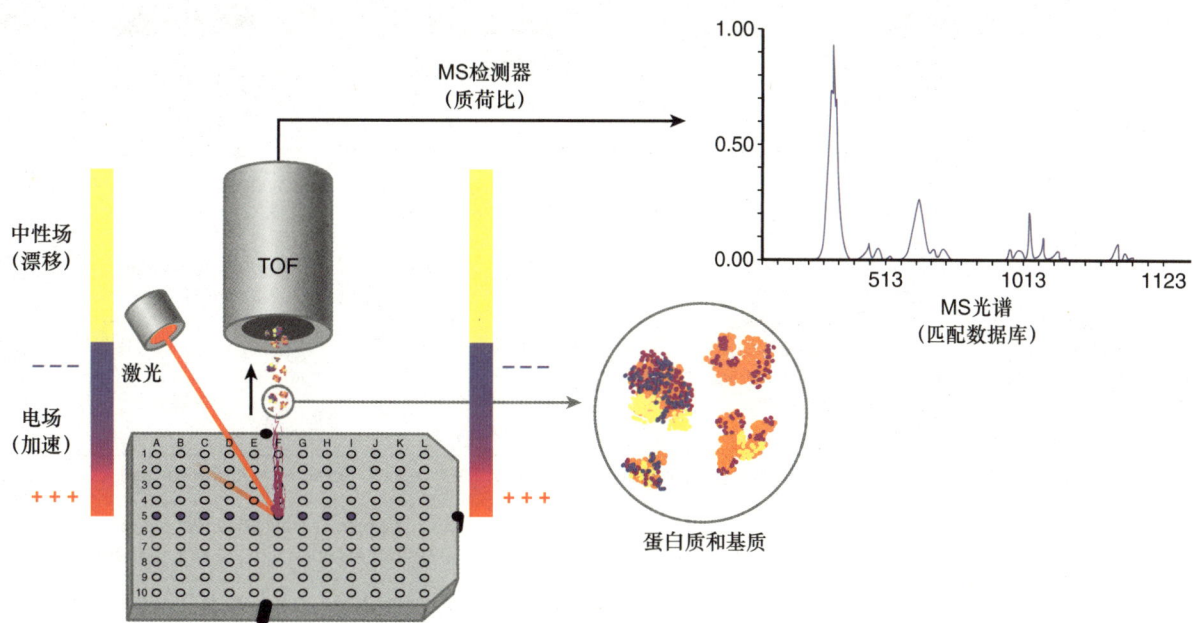

图 2.2　基质辅助激光解吸电离飞行时间质谱法（MALDI-TOF MS）。从培养板中选择细菌或真菌生长物，直接加到 MALDI 载玻片上。样本覆盖上基质并干燥。然后，样本和基质被激光轰击，导致升华和离子化。离子根据它们的质荷比（m/z）在 TOF 管中分离，管内测量离子到达时间。生成这些离子的光谱，并通过软件分析生成一个图谱，然后与参考 MS 光谱数据库进行匹配，从而生成鉴定结果。该过程只需几分钟。尽管仪器昂贵，但该技术已获得美国 FDA 的批准，能够快速、稳健和可靠地进行鉴定

bacteria to viruses, fungi, and parasites may be present and potential infection is not being identified by other methods.

POINT-OF-CARE OR NEAR-PATIENT TESTING

Point-of-care (POC) or near-patient testing offers rapid results, typically while the patient is still in the clinical care setting, allowing directed treatment. This arena will continue to grow as patients shift into urgent care and home use venues. In addition, testing options will begin to replace less sensitive antigen tests with molecular-based tests that are more cost-effective (reducing duplicative testing and decreasing repeat visits) and have short turn-around times (minutes). They will also have an increasing menu outside of the usual urgent care pathogens of group A streptococci (GAS), influenza/RSV, and HIV tests to include other common acute care conditions such as sexually transmitted infections (STIs), bacterial vaginosis (BV), urinary tract pathogens, and biomarkers. The difference in testing diagnostics chosen to be performed in these settings (antigen, PCR, syndromic panel) will depend on the clinical severity of the patient. Urgent care assumes less severe disease and fast directed treatment, optimally with test results within an hour before the patient leaves, whereas emergency department providers may be assessing more critical patients, and testing helps decide admission or discharge to home.

Point-of-Care Testing in Resource-Poor Settings

Importantly, point-of-care testing (POCT) has become feasible for resource poor settings with battery-operated molecular systems or low cost microfluidic systems. Systems exist for diagnosis of tuberculosis and resistance determinants, HIV, human papillomavirus, and resistant STIs.

Point-of-Care Testing Quality Issues

Critically, because of cost, any test used in the POC setting should be reliable enough for the provider to have confidence in the directed treatment. Understanding the predictive values of tests being used, no matter the setting, is critical for interpretation of the result.

POCTs are dependent on the specimen type collected (e.g., nasopharyngeal swab is better than a throat swab for influenza A or B testing), the test analyte (e.g., GAS performance is more reliable than HIV oral testing), and the prevalence of disease at the time of testing as related to the technology of the diagnostic (e.g., influenza antigen-based vs. molecular).

For example, data from the novel H1N1 influenza outbreak demonstrated very poor sensitivity for rapid antigen tests (about 50%) compared with molecular tests. When a multiplex viral panel was used, other viral pathogens were identified as the cause of

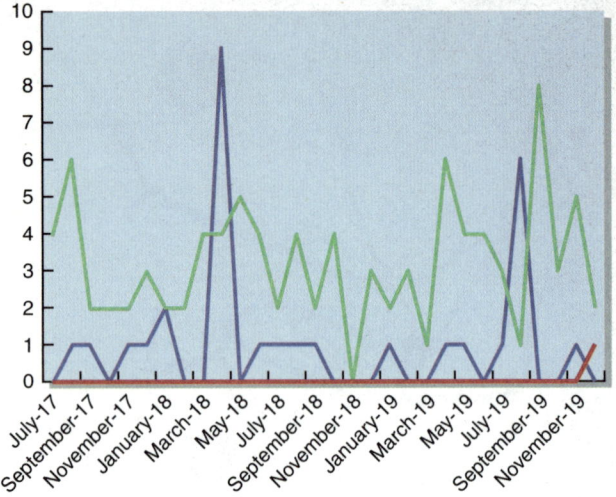

Fig. 2.3 Graph shows results of the parasitic component of a multiplex gastrointestinal PCR panel that identifies pathogens in about 1 hour. Antigen tests are not sensitive and confirmatory parasitic smear or direct fluorescent antibody (DFA) testing takes days to weeks. Two cryptosporidium peaks associated with outbreaks in April 2018 and August 2019 at petting zoos allowed rapid response by the Department of Health, limiting exposures.

TABLE 2.2 Common Rapid Identification Methods From a Positive Culture Broth, Colony, or Tissue[a]

Method	Organisms Detected	Time	Cost	Technical Expertise
PNA fluorescent smear Positive broth	Bacteria, fungi (yeast)	2–4 hr	$$	++
MALDI-TOF MS Colony or positive broth	Bacteria, fungi, mycobacteria	Minutes to 1 hr	$	+
Hybridization probes Colony or positive broth	Bacteria, dimorphic fungi, mycobacteria	4–8 hr	$$$	+++
Amplification[b]	Bacteria, viruses, mycobacteria, parasites	1–4 hr	$$ to $$$$	+ to +++
Next-generation sequencing, whole genome sequencing	Bacteria, fungi, mycobacteria, viruses, environmental	1–3 days	$$$$	+++ to ++++
Combination fluorescent rRNA probe and time-lapsed morphokineteic cellular analysis	Bacterial identification and rapid phenotypic susceptibility	2–8 hr	$$$	++

MALDI-TOF, Matrix-assisted laser desorption ionization-time of flight mass spectrometry; *PNA,* peptide nucleic acid; *$,* relative cost; *+,* relative level of required expertise.
[a]Rapid methods require 2 to 24 hours. Methods presented are US Food and Drug Administration cleared or have had test performance validated in the clinical laboratory. Due to required technical expertise and cost, some of these assays may not be available in the routine laboratory, and providers should inquire about availability
[b]Includes many different technologies, such as polymerase chain reaction (PCR), transcription-mediated amplification (TMA), and isothermal loop amplification (LAMP).

者可能存在和感染了从细菌到病毒、真菌和寄生虫的罕见病原体，而这些病原体可能无法通过其他方法检测。

即时检测或近患者检测

即时检测或近患者检测能够快速地反馈结果，通常在患者仍在临床诊疗环境中时即可获得，从而允许针对性的治疗。随着患者转向急诊护理和家庭使用场所，这一领域将继续增长。此外，检测将开始用分子检测替代敏感性较低的抗原检测，这些分子检测更具成本效益（可减少重复检测和重复就诊）并且耗费较短的周转时间（分钟维度）。检测项目也将不断增加，不仅包括通常的急诊相关病原体如 A 组链球菌（GAS）、流感 / 呼吸道合胞病毒和人类免疫缺陷病毒检测，还将涵盖其他常见的急诊环境，如性传播感染（STI）、细菌性阴道炎（BV）、尿路病原体和生物标志物鉴定等。在这些环境中选择检测诊断方法（抗原、PCR、综合征检测试剂盒）的差异主要取决于患者的临床严重程度。急诊护理通常针对疾病不严重并且需要快速定向治疗的病例，理想情况下在患者离开前 1 h 内获得检测结果，而急诊科医疗人员可能评估更危重的患者，检测有助于决定入院或回家。

医学资源匮乏环境中的即时检测

重要的是，即时检测（POCT）在医学资源匮乏环境中的适用性也在不断提高，例如电池驱动的分子检测系统或低成本的微流控系统。这些系统可以用于诊断结核病及识别其耐药性决定因素、HIV、人乳头瘤病毒和耐药性性传播感染等。

即时检测的质量问题

由于成本问题，保证即时检测环境中使用的任何检测都应足够可靠是至关重要的，以便医务人员对针对性治疗有信心。无论在何种环境中，理解所使用检测手段的可行性及适用性对于感染性疾病的判断至关重要。POCT 的可靠性取决于采集的样本类型（例如，鼻拭子比咽拭子更适合甲型或乙型流感检测）、检测分析物（例如，A 组链球菌口腔检测比 HIV 口腔检测更可靠），以及检测时疾病的流行情况与所使用的诊断技术相关（例如，基于抗原的流感检测与分子检测）。

例如，新型 H1N1 流感暴发期间的数据表明，快速抗原检测的敏感性非常低（约 50%），而分子检测则表现良好。当使用多重病毒检测试剂盒时，超过 50%

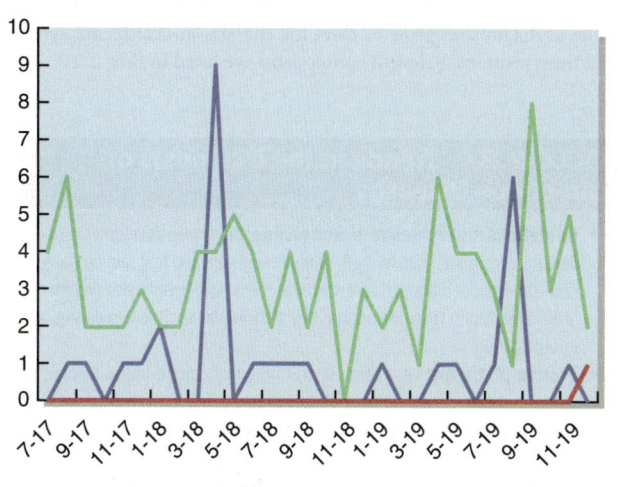

图 2.3 图中展示了一个多重胃肠道 PCR 检测试剂盒检测寄生虫成分的结果，能够在约 1 h 内鉴定病原体。抗原检测不敏感，而确证性寄生虫涂片或直接荧光抗体检测需要数天到数周。2018 年 4 月和 2019 年 8 月在宠物动物园发生的两次隐孢子虫暴发高峰，使卫生部门能够迅速响应，限制了暴露范围

表 2.2 从阳性培养液、菌落或组织中常见的快速鉴定方法[a]				
方法	待检生物	时间	成本	技术专长
PNA 荧光涂片 阳性培养液	细菌、真菌（酵母）	2～4 h	$$	++
MALDI-TOF MS 菌落或阳性培养液	细菌、真菌、分枝杆菌	几分钟到 1 h	$	+
杂交探针 菌落或阳性培养液	细菌、双态性真菌、分枝杆菌	4～8 h	$$$	+++
扩增[b]	细菌、病毒、分枝杆菌、寄生虫	1～4 h	$$～$$$$	+～+++
二代测序，全基因组测序	细菌、真菌、分枝杆菌、病毒、环境	1～3 天	$$$$	+++～++++
组合荧光 rRNA 探针和时间间隔形态动力学细胞分析	细菌鉴定和快速表型药敏	2～8 h	$$$	++

MALDI-TOF，基质辅助激光解吸电离飞行时间质谱；PNA，蛋白质核酸；$，相对成本；+，需要的专业技术的相对水平。
[a] 快速方法需要 2～24 h。所展示的方法已获得美国 FDA 批准或在临床实验室中验证了测试性能。由于需要的技术专长和成本，一些检测可能无法在常规实验室中使用，医务人员应询问可用性。
[b] 包括许多不同的技术，如聚合酶链反应（PCR）、转录介导扩增（TMA）和等温环扩增（LAMP）。

influenza-like illness in more than 50% of patients admitted to hospitals. As a result, amplified testing assays for influenza, RSV, and GAS have been developed by manufacturers as Clinical Laboratory Improvement Amendment (CLIA)–waived tests for use in POC settings. Syndromic panel use in urgent care settings is unusual, but as more systems achieve CLIA-waived status, syndromic panel use will be more common. But urgent care clinics, especially those that serve patients within a specific health care system with more capacity for testing, will likely be able to incorporate greater POC testing, including receipt of self-collected patient specimens. Costs will be balanced by reducing the number of patients getting their care in costly emergency departments.

TRENDS IN THE DIAGNOSIS OF INFECTIOUS DISEASES

The most significant trend in diagnostics is that rapid change will continue as diagnostics grow to meet the changes in health care systems and the consumer. Relevant components are listed in Box 2.2.

BOX 2.2 Trends in the Diagnosis of Infectious Diseases

- **Guidelines and evidence-based testing:** Continued development of evidence-based guidelines for both patient treatment and test reimbursement. Real-time use of diagnostic stewardship teams and health care system test order algorithms to guide appropriate test implementation, ordering, and interpretation.
- **Testing platforms:** Less reliance on traditional culture-based techniques with culture becoming increasingly automated at the front end (processing), aliquoting for MALDI-TOF identification, as well as the back-end components of reading and interpretation (machine algorithms).
- **Molecular technologies:** Wider availability and adoption of syndromic molecular panel assays as well as genetic resistance determinants due to speed and comprehensive menus. Accepted use of cell-free nucleic acid and next-generation sequencing (NGS) detection for low-yield pathogens (e.g., unusual or unexpected) and/or slow growing culture pathogens (e.g., fungi), especially in immunocompromised patients.
- **Antimicrobial resistance and stewardship:** Standardization of rapid phenotypic antimicrobial susceptibility, providing results 48 hours sooner compared to traditional culture susceptibility, aiding in antimicrobial stewardship initiatives.
- **Emerging infections:** Viruses, mycobacteria, mycology, and specialized pathogen culture and susceptibility will continue to move to specialty reference laboratories and public health until more rapid and user-friendly diagnostics are developed. Worldwide increase in fungal diseases will hasten fungal test development. Emergency use authorization (EUA) test systems will be sought by companies for emerging outbreak infections to aid in global strategizing.
- **Point-of-care testing:** Use of rapid and cost-effective molecular tests (microfluidic or similar), battery-operated (or similar), portable platforms developed for POC, including urgent care clinics and resource poor settings.

SUGGESTED READINGS

Barenfanger J, Graham DR, Kolluri L, et al: Decreased mortality associated with prompt Gram staining of blood cultures, Am J Clin Pathol 130(6):870–876, 2008.

Blauwkamp TA, Thair S, Rosen MJ, et al: Analytical and clinical validation of a microbial cell-free DNA sequencing test for infectious disease, Nat Microbiol 4(4):663–674, 2019.

Buss SN, Leber A, Chapin K, et al: Multicenter evaluation of the BioFire FilmArray™ gastrointestinal panel for the etiologic diagnosis of infectious gastroenteritis, J Clin Microbiol 53(3):915–925, 2015.

Clark AE, Kaleta EJ, Arora A, Wolk DM: Matrix-assisted laser desorption ionization-time of flight mass spectrometry: a fundamental shift in the routine practice of clinical microbiology, Clin Microbiol Rev 26(3):547–603, 2013.

Friedman DZP, Schwartz IS: Emerging fungal infections: new patients, new patterns, and new pathogens, J Fungi (Basel) 5(3), 2019.

Gaydos CA: Let's take a "Selfie": self-collected samples for sexually transmitted infections, Sex Transm Dis 45(4):278–279, 2018.

Gu W, Miller S, Chiu CY: Clinical metagenomic next-generation sequencing for pathogen detection, Annu Rev Pathol 14:319–333, 2019.

Herberg J, Kaforou M, Wright VJ, IRIS Consortium, et al: Diagnostic test accuracy of a 2-transcript host RNA signature for discriminating bacterial vs viral infection in febrile children, J Am Med Assoc 316(8):835–845, 2016.

Kamat IS, Ramachandran V, Eswaran H, et al: Procalcitonin to distinguish viral from bacterial pneumonia: a systematic review and meta-analysis, Clin Infect Dis 70(3):538–542, 2020.

Kozel TR, Burnham-Marusich AR: Point-of-Care testing for infectious diseases: past, present, and future, J Clin Microbiol 55(8):2313–2320, 2017.

Mermel LA, Jefferson J, Blanchard K, et al: Reducing clostridium difficile incidence, colectomies, and mortality in the hospital setting: a successful multidisciplinary approach, Jt Comm J Qual Patient Saf 39(7):298–305, 2013.

Messacar K, Parker SK, Todd JK, Dominguez SR: Implementation of rapid molecular infectious disease diagnostics: the role of diagnostic and antimicrobial stewardship, J Clin Microbiol 55(3):715–723, 2017.

Miller JM, Binnicker MJ, Campbell S, et al: A guide to utilization of the microbiology laboratory for diagnosis of infectious diseases: 2018 update by the Infectious Diseases Society of America and the American Society for Microbiology, Clin Infect Dis 67(6):e1–e94, 2018.

Pritt BS, Patel R, Kirn TJ, Thomson Jr RB: Point-counterpoint: a nucleic acid amplification test for Streptococcus pyogenes should replace antigen detection and culture for detection of bacterial Pharyngitis, J Clin Microbiol 54(10):2413–2419, 2016.

Saenger A. Right test, right patient, right time, wrong interpretation? American association for clinical chemistry (AACC) Clinical Laboratory News, 2014.

Saraswat MK, Magruder JT, Crawford TC, et al: Preoperative Staphylococcus aureus screening and targeted decolonization in cardiac surgery, Ann Thorac Surg 104(4):1349–1356, 2017.

Tansarli GS, Chapin KC: Diagnostic accuracy of the Biofire® FilmArray® meningitis/encephalitis panel: a systematic review and meta-analysis, Clin Microbiol Infect(19):30615–30619, S1198-743X, 2019.

van Houten CB, de Groot JAH, Klein A, et al: A host-protein based assay to differentiate between bacterial and viral infections in preschool children (OPPORTUNITY): a double-blind, multicentre, validation study, Lancet Infect Dis 17(4):431–440, 2017.

Weiss ZF, Cunha CB, Chambers AB, et al: Opportunities revealed for antimicrobial stewardship and clinical practice with implementation of a rapid respiratory multiplex assay, J Clin Microbiol 57(10), 2019.

的住院患者的流感样疾病是由其他病毒引起的。因此，制造商开发了适用于即时环境的扩增检测方法，用于流感病毒、呼吸道合胞病毒和A组链球菌检测，这些检测已获得临床实验室改进修正案（CLIA）的豁免资格。在急诊护理环境中，综合征检测试剂盒的使用并不常见，但随着更多系统获得CLIA豁免资格，综合征检测试剂盒的使用将变得更加普遍。急诊诊所，特别是那些为特定医疗系统内的患者提供服务并具有更多检测能力的诊所，可能会更广泛地采用POCT，包括接收患者自行采集的样本。通过减少在昂贵的急诊部门就诊的患者数量来平衡费用。

感染性疾病诊断的趋势

诊断学最显著的趋势是随着诊断技术的不断发展，为适应医疗系统和待检患者的变化和临床现状，感染性疾病诊断的发展与变革也将不断进行。相关内容列在框2.2中。

框2.2 感染性疾病诊断的发展趋势

- **指南和循证检测**：继续开发循证指南，用于指导患者治疗和检测费用报销。实时使用诊断管理团队和卫生保健系统测试算法，指导适当的检测实施、执行和解读。
- **检测平台**：减少对传统培养技术的依赖，培养在前端处理、分装用于MALDI-TOF鉴定，以及后端的读取和解释（如机器算法）变得越来越自动化。
- **分子技术**：由于速度快且覆盖范围全面，综合征检测试剂盒和基因耐药性决定因素的使用更加广泛和普及。细胞游离核酸和二代测序（NGS）检测在低载量病原体（例如不常见或意外病原体）和（或）难培养的病原体（例如真菌）的接受度不断提高，特别是在免疫力低下患者中。
- **抗微生物药物耐药性和管理**：快速表型抗微生物药物敏感性检测的标准化，比传统培养药敏检测提前48 h提供结果，促进抗微生物管理计划的发展。
- **新发感染**：病毒、分枝杆菌、真菌和特殊病原体培养以及药敏检测将继续转移到专业参考实验室和公共卫生领域进行，直到开发出更快速和用户友好的诊断方法。全球真菌疾病的增加将加速真菌检测的发展。企业将寻求新发疫情感染的紧急使用授权（EUA）检测系统，以帮助制定全球战略。
- **即时检测**：在急救诊所和医疗资源匮乏的环境中，使用快速且具有成本效益的分子检测（微流控或类似技术）、电池驱动（或类似技术）便携式平台。

推荐阅读

Barenfanger J, Graham DR, Kolluri L, et al: Decreased mortality associated with prompt Gram staining of blood cultures, Am J Clin Pathol 130(6):870–876, 2008.

Blauwkamp TA, Thair S, Rosen MJ, et al: Analytical and clinical validation of a microbial cell-free DNA sequencing test for infectious disease, Nat Microbiol 4(4):663–674, 2019.

Buss SN, Leber A, Chapin K, et al: Multicenter evaluation of the BioFire FilmArray™ gastrointestinal panel for the etiologic diagnosis of infectious gastroenteritis, J Clin Microbiol 53(3):915–925, 2015.

Clark AE, Kaleta EJ, Arora A, Wolk DM: Matrix-assisted laser desorption ionization-time of flight mass spectrometry: a fundamental shift in the routine practice of clinical microbiology, Clin Microbiol Rev 26(3):547–603, 2013.

Friedman DZP, Schwartz IS: Emerging fungal infections: new patients, new patterns, and new pathogens, J Fungi (Basel) 5(3), 2019.

Gaydos CA: Let's take a "Selfie": self-collected samples for sexually transmitted infections, Sex Transm Dis 45(4):278–279, 2018.

Gu W, Miller S, Chiu CY: Clinical metagenomic next-generation sequencing for pathogen detection, Annu Rev Pathol 14:319–333, 2019.

Herberg J, Kaforou M, Wright VJ, IRIS Consortium, et al: Diagnostic test accuracy of a 2-transcript host RNA signature for discriminating bacterial vs viral infection in febrile children, J Am Med Assoc 316(8):835–845, 2016.

Kamat IS, Ramachandran V, Eswaran H, et al: Procalcitonin to distinguish viral from bacterial pneumonia: a systematic review and meta-analysis, Clin Infect Dis 70(3):538–542, 2020.

Kozel TR, Burnham-Marusich AR: Point-of-Care testing for infectious diseases: past, present, and future, J Clin Microbiol 55(8):2313–2320, 2017.

Mermel LA, Jefferson J, Blanchard K, et al: Reducing clostridium difficile incidence, colectomies, and mortality in the hospital setting: a successful multidisciplinary approach, Jt Comm J Qual Patient Saf 39(7):298–305, 2013.

Messacar K, Parker SK, Todd JK, Dominguez SR: Implementation of rapid molecular infectious disease diagnostics: the role of diagnostic and antimicrobial stewardship, J Clin Microbiol 55(3):715–723, 2017.

Miller JM, Binnicker MJ, Campbell S, et al: A guide to utilization of the microbiology laboratory for diagnosis of infectious diseases: 2018 update by the Infectious Diseases Society of America and the American Society for Microbiology, Clin Infect Dis 67(6):e1–e94, 2018.

Pritt BS, Patel R, Kirn TJ, Thomson Jr RB: Point-counterpoint: a nucleic acid amplification test for Streptococcus pyogenes should replace antigen detection and culture for detection of bacterial Pharyngitis, J Clin Microbiol 54(10):2413–2419, 2016.

Saenger A. Right test, right patient, right time, wrong interpretation? American association for clinical chemistry (AACC) Clinical Laboratory News, 2014.

Saraswat MK, Magruder JT, Crawford TC, et al: Preoperative Staphylococcus aureus screening and targeted decolonization in cardiac surgery, Ann Thorac Surg 104(4):1349–1356, 2017.

Tansarli GS, Chapin KC: Diagnostic accuracy of the Biofire® FilmArray® meningitis/encephalitis panel: a systematic review and meta-analysis, Clin Microbiol Infect(19):30615–30619, S1198-743X, 2019.

van Houten CB, de Groot JAH, Klein A, et al: A host-protein based assay to differentiate between bacterial and viral infections in preschool children (OPPORTUNITY): a double-blind, multicentre, validation study, Lancet Infect Dis 17(4):431–440, 2017.

Weiss ZF, Cunha CB, Chambers AB, et al: Opportunities revealed for antimicrobial stewardship and clinical practice with implementation of a rapid respiratory multiplex assay, J Clin Microbiol 57(10), 2019.

3

Fever and Febrile Syndromes

Maria D. Mileno

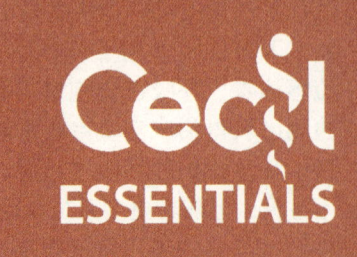

INTRODUCTION

Fever is one of the most common problems requiring medical evaluation. Fever is an elevation in core body temperature greater than normal daily variation, which is 37° C ± 0.4° C (98.6° F ± 0.7° F). Documentation of true fever can be important evidence of infectious processes that warrant investigation. Although fever is characteristic of most infections, it also occurs in noninfectious conditions such as autoimmune and inflammatory diseases, malignancy, and trauma.

This chapter reviews the pathogenesis of the febrile response, the approach to the acutely ill patient with fever, and fever of unknown origin. Fever can be associated with infections, such as those from animal exposures, or with common clinical scenarios in which it may occur as the sole complaint, manifest with rash, or develop with lymphadenopathy. A word of caution about the difference between true and factitious fever is offered at the end of the chapter.

PATHOGENESIS

Thermoregulation of core body temperature is one of the most important mechanisms in mammalian and human physiology. At core temperature the human body's systems work together at their optimum. The hypothalamic heat-regulating set point shifts in response to infection or inflammation mediated primarily by the host's monocytes and macrophages, which are activated as they encounter exogenous bacterial substances, toxins, or the cellular products of trauma.

Monocytes and macrophages produce small proteins called *cytokines*, such as interleukin-1 (IL-1), IL-6, and tumor necrosis factor (TNF). They are collectively known as *endogenous pyrogens* because they actively increase body temperature by increasing the hypothalamic set point, which is the normal temperature for the body that is controlled by the hypothalamus. IL-1 and other endogenous pyrogens are released by macrophages at the site of infection and travel through the bloodstream to the hypothalamus, where they elevate levels of prostaglandin E_2 (PGE_2). Elevated PGE_2 levels increase the set point, and thermoregulatory mechanisms raise the body's core temperature. IL-1 also induces production of PGE_2 in peripheral tissues, which causes the nonspecific myalgias and arthralgias that often accompany fever. Prostaglandin inhibitors such as aspirin or acetaminophen block prostaglandin synthesis and reduce elevated temperatures.

Thermoregulatory control is initiated through sensory neurons in the skin, abdomen, and spinal cord. Central nervous system (CNS) thermoreceptors sense and integrate temperature information. After the hypothalamic set point is raised, the firing rates of neurons in the vasomotor center are altered, causing peripheral vasoconstriction and producing a noticeable cold sensation in the hands and feet. Blood is shunted away from the periphery to the internal organs, and this process is sufficient to raise core body temperature by 1° to 2° C.

Other signaling mechanisms have roles in thermoregulation. The adipocyte-derived hormone leptin actively controls energy homeostasis, and thermogenesis in fat tissue contributes to increasing core temperature. Thermogenesis is important in fighting infection and in responding to cold-induced heat production. Fever has direct antimicrobial effects in some infections such as neurosyphilis and salmonellosis, and elevated temperature augments humoral and cellular immune responses. IL-1 acts independently on two physiologic systems: thermoregulation and iron metabolism. IL-1 can stimulate a wide range of host defenses to conduct a synergistic response to infection.

Fever also can have deleterious effects. It may lead to disorientation and confusion in persons with underlying brain disease and in healthy older individuals. Tachycardia can increase cardiopulmonary work, precipitating congestive heart failure or myocardial infarction in persons with significant cardiopulmonary disease. Fever should be controlled with antipyretics for comfort and to avoid compromising individuals with multiple medical problems. Acetaminophen is preferred for control of fever in children because of the risk of Reye's syndrome with salicylate use.

The terms *fever*, *hyperthermia*, and *hyperpyrexia* are not synonymous. Although most patients with elevated temperature have fever (>38.3° C or 100.9° F), some conditions can increase the body temperature by overriding or bypassing the normal homeostatic mechanism and may even produce body temperatures in excess of 41° C or 105.8° F (i.e., hyperthermia), which can be rapidly fatal and does not respond to antipyretics. Rapid cooling is critical to the patient's survival in hyperthermic conditions such as heat stroke. Even in otherwise healthy individuals, heat stroke can occur after vigorous exercise and prolonged exposure to high environmental temperatures and humidity. Heat stroke is marked by temperatures greater than 40.6° C (105.1° F), altered sensorium or coma, and cessation of sweating. Treatment includes covering the patient with wet compresses followed by intravenous infusion of fluids appropriate to correct fluid and electrolyte losses.

Severe hyperthermia may be a heritable reaction to anesthetics (i.e., malignant hyperthermia) or a response to phenothiazines (i.e., neuroleptic malignant syndrome). Serotonin syndrome, which often includes fever, is classically associated with the simultaneous administration of two serotonergic agents (e.g., selective serotonin reuptake inhibitors plus tramadol). It can also occur after initiation of a single serotonergic drug that increases the serotonin level of individuals who are particularly sensitive to serotonin. Occasionally, persons with CNS disorders such as paraplegia and persons with severe dermatologic conditions are unable to dissipate heat and can experience hyperthermia.

Hyperpyrexia is the term for extraordinarily high fever (>41.5° C or 106.7° F), which can occur in patients with severe infections but is most commonly observed in persons with CNS hemorrhages.

发热和发热性综合征

曹玮 译　李太生　朱华栋 审校　刘海鹰 通审

简述

发热是最常见的需要医学评估的问题之一，是指机体核心体温的升高超过了正常的每日波动范围〔即 37℃ ±0.4℃（98.6℉ ±0.7℉）〕。记录到真实发热可能是感染的重要证据，需要进一步甄别。尽管发热是大部分感染的特征性表现，它也可见于非感染性疾病如自身免疫性疾病及炎性疾病、恶性肿瘤及创伤。

本章综述了发热反应的病理机制、急性发热患者的接诊，以及不明原因发热。发热可为感染的伴随症状，如动物源性暴露所致；或在常见临床情形中作为单一主诉，或与皮疹或淋巴结肿大共同出现。本章最后则提出需警惕真实发热和伪热的鉴别。

发病机制

机体核心体温的调节是哺乳动物和人类最重要的生理机制之一。在核心体温水平，人体系统共同达到最佳运转状态。下丘脑热调节的调定点会因感染或炎症而出现变动，这一变动主要由外源性细菌物质、毒素或损伤的细胞产物激活宿主的单核细胞及巨噬细胞而介导。

单核细胞和巨噬细胞可以产生被称为细胞因子的小蛋白，如白介素-1（IL-1）、IL-6 和肿瘤坏死因子（TNF），统称为内源性致热原，可通过主动提高下丘脑调定点——由下丘脑控制的机体正常体温——而升高体温。IL-1 及其他内源性致热原由巨噬细胞在感染部位释放，经血流抵达下丘脑，并提高前列腺素 E_2（PGE_2）水平。PGE_2 水平升高提升了调定点，而体温调节机制提升了机体的核心体温。IL-1 也可诱导外周组织内产生 PGE_2，导致常伴随发热出现的非特异性肌痛和关节痛。前列腺素抑制剂如阿司匹林或对乙酰氨基酚可阻断前列腺素的合成而降低升高的体温。

体温调节的控制起始于皮肤、腹部和脊髓的感觉神经元。中枢神经系统（CNS）的温度受体感知并整合温度信息。当下丘脑调定点升高后，血管运动中心的神经元激活速率会发生变化，引发外周血管收缩并产生显著的手足畏寒感。血液从外周向内部器官分流，而这一过程足以使核心体温升高 1～2℃。

其他信号机制在体温调节中各司其职。脂肪细胞来源的激素瘦素可主动控制能量平衡，而脂肪组织产热促进核心体温的升高。产热在对抗感染以及应答寒冷诱发的热量产生中至关重要。在某些感染如神经梅毒和沙门菌病中，发热具有直接的抗微生物作用，升高的温度增强了体液和细胞免疫应答。IL-1 可以在热调节和铁代谢两个生理系统中独立发挥作用，能激活较广泛的宿主防御而对发热施加协同应答。

发热也会产生有害作用。在有基础颅脑疾病的人群或健康老年人中，发热可能导致定向力障碍和意识障碍。心动过速可增加心肺负荷，在具有显著心肺疾病的患者中诱发充血性心力衰竭或心肌梗死。应使用退热药物控制发热，以缓解症状并避免诱发多重基础疾病人群进一步恶化。考虑到水杨酸类导致瑞氏综合征的风险，儿童更优选使用对乙酰氨基酚控制体温。

术语"发热""过热"和"超高热"并非同义。尽管大多数体温升高（＞38.3℃或100.9℉）的患者均称为发热，某些情况可因突破正常的平衡机制而导致体温升高甚至造成 41℃或 105.8℉以上的体温（即过热），可迅速致命且对退热药物无应答。在过热情况下，如热射病时，迅速降温是患者存活的关键。即使既往健康的个体，也可在剧烈运动和长时间暴露于高温高湿度环境后出现热射病。其特点包括体温超过 40.6℃（105.1℉）、感觉中枢异常或昏迷，以及停止排汗。治疗包括对患者进行湿敷，继而适当静脉补液以纠正液体和电解质丢失。

严重过热可以是对麻醉药的遗传反应（即恶性高热）或对酚噻嗪类的反应（即神经阻滞剂恶性综合征）。5-羟色胺综合征通常也包括发热，常与同时使用两种 5-羟色胺激动剂（如选择性 5-羟色胺重吸收抑制剂联合曲马多）有关。当对 5-羟色胺特别敏感的人使用一种 5-羟色胺激动剂而提高 5-羟色胺水平时，也可出现 5-羟色胺综合征。偶尔，患 CNS 疾病（如截瘫）的患者以及因严重皮肤病不能散热的患者，也可出现过热。

术语"超高热"是指体温特别高的发热（超过 41.5℃或 106.7℉），可见于严重感染的患者，但最常出现于 CNS 出血的患者。

DIAGNOSTIC APPROACH TO THE ACUTELY ILL PATIENT WITH FEVER

Patterns of fever should be considered when assessing acutely ill, febrile persons. Evaluation includes determining the normal diurnal variation in body temperature, which often persists when patients have fever. Normally, body temperature peaks in the late afternoon or early evening.

Rigors (i.e., bed-shaking chills) often mark the onset of bacterial infection, typically bacteremia, although they may occur in other clinical situations, such as drug-induced fever or transfusion reactions. Wide swings in temperature may indicate an abscess. Malaria should be considered for anyone with fever who has visited or lived in malarious regions or who has relapsing fever accompanied by episodes of shaking chills and high fever separated by 1 to 3 days of normal body temperature and relative well-being. The timing of administration of anti-inflammatory drugs should be assessed because they may alter or blunt the febrile response. Most infectious diseases manifest with fever as an early finding and with subclinical and eventual clinical involvement of specific organ systems.

If fever occurs as the sole complaint or is associated with localized symptoms and signs, the diagnostic approach includes taking a thorough history, including an extensive review of systems, medical and surgical histories, and immunizations, including those from childhood. Antipyretics may be withheld to allow assessment of the fever trajectory. Elderly individuals, persons taking corticosteroids, and patients with chronic liver or renal disease may be less likely to mount a fever. All likely sources of disease, including travel, exposure to *Mycobacterium tuberculosis*, and occupational, hobby, animal, insect, and sexual contacts, should be assessed. Previous itineraries and activities, geographic risks of diseases, and the seasonality and incubation periods of possible disease exposures should be considered in returning travelers.

Viral Infection

Acute febrile illnesses in young healthy adults usually are caused by viral infections, which do not require precise diagnosis because they are self-limited and seldom have therapeutic options. Upper respiratory tract symptoms of rhinorrhea, sore throat, cough, and hoarseness most often result from rhinovirus, coronavirus, parainfluenza virus, and adenoviruses. Adenovirus outbreaks occur among persons living in close quarters such as military barracks or college dormitories. Respiratory syncytial virus, human metapneumovirus, and human bocavirus infections occur in similar conditions and sometimes manifest with pneumonia.

A coronavirus causes the potentially fatal upper respiratory viral infection called *Middle East respiratory syndrome* (MERS). It has caused pneumonia with acute respiratory distress syndrome (ARDS) and death in one half of infected individuals, and it is highly contagious. See Appendix for discussion of COVID-19.

Meningitis symptoms occur predominantly from enterovirus infections during summer months, although the symptom complex warrants urgent treatment of bacterial causes while the diagnostic process occurs. Febrile syndromes without meningitis are more common manifestations of enteroviral infections.

Arthropod-borne viruses such as California encephalitis virus; eastern, western, and Venezuelan equine encephalitis viruses; St. Louis encephalitis virus; and West Nile virus can produce self-limited febrile illnesses and encephalitis. Colorado tick fever is a biphasic illness seen after northwestern and southwestern tick exposures. It is characterized by high fevers and leukopenia. A deer tick virus—Powassan virus—has been associated with numerous cases of fever and encephalitis in New England and the Upper Midwest.

Influenza causes sore throat, cough, myalgias, arthralgias, and headache in addition to fever, and it most often manifests in an epidemic pattern during winter months. It is unusual for fever to persist beyond 5 days in uncomplicated influenza. Prolonged fever in persons with diagnosed influenza warrants investigation and treatment of bacterial superinfection. The epidemics of avian influenza and H1N1 pandemic strains in recent years are sobering reminders that influenza viruses have a remarkable ability to mutate, producing new immune-resistant strains on a regular basis. Preventive yearly influenza vaccination is important.

Mononucleosis syndromes of fever with detectable lymph node enlargement typify infections with Epstein-Barr virus (EBV), cytomegalovirus (CMV), primary human immunodeficiency virus (HIV), and *Toxoplasma gondii* (i.e., toxoplasmosis). Other manifestations of these infections include abnormal liver function test results, respiratory tract symptoms, and neurologic symptoms. Diagnosis of acute HIV infection, which can produce a mononucleosis-like syndrome, is an urgent issue.

Bacterial Infections

Pathogenic bacteria can infect all body parts and can cause a spectrum of localized illness warranting antibiotic therapy. For example, *Staphylococcus aureus* may cause skin abscesses or cellulitis. Highly pathogenic organisms may colonize individuals who have had contact with the health care system. Most concerning is the event of bacteria entering the bloodstream. Obtaining timely blood cultures before administering the antibiotics indicated for presumed bacterial infections in persons with common clinical syndromes can help to identify bloodstream pathogens and define the required course of treatment.

Fever may be the predominant clinical manifestation of *S. aureus* illness. This organism and the methicillin-resistant form (i.e., MRSA) frequently cause sepsis without an obvious primary site of infection. It should be considered in patients undergoing intravenous therapy or hemodialysis and in those who use intravenous drugs or who have severe chronic dermatitis. Bacteremia with staphylococci may cause hematogenous seeding of bones leading to osteomyelitis and heart valves leading to endocarditis in individuals; the bacteremia may also reflect these underlying processes. Other common causes of bacteremia and their sources include *Streptococcus pneumoniae* (i.e., pneumonia), *Escherichia coli* (i.e., urinary tract and gastrointestinal sources), streptococci (i.e., skin), and anaerobes (i.e., gastrointestinal tract).

Listeria monocytogenes bacteremia is seen predominantly in persons with depressed cell-mediated immunity and pregnant women. Although bacteremia is the most common manifestation of listeriosis in these hosts, many with listeriosis may have meningitis and warrant lumbar puncture for cerebrospinal fluid culture. Most cases occur in individuals over age 50.

Typhoid and paratyphoid fever (i.e., enteric fever) are common in many low-income countries. Patients may have fever alone as the primary clinical manifestation. Travelers to six countries account for 80% of US cases: India, Mexico, Philippines, Pakistan, El Salvador, and Haiti. Fever with headache and an insidious onset with an unremarkable physical examination is common, although a faint and transient rash (i.e., rose spots) may appear by the second week of illness. Symptoms may include diarrhea, constipation, vague abdominal discomfort, and sometimes dry cough. Diagnosis depends on the culture of blood or stool.

Fever With Localized Symptoms and Signs

Localized bacterial infection can be apparent, as in cases of abscess, cellulitis, or otitis media, or can be clinically occult. It can develop as

急性发热患者的诊断流程

当评估急性发热患者时，应结合其热型考虑。评估包括确认正常的体温昼夜变化节律，变化节律在发热患者也常常存在。一般情况下，体温在傍晚时分达峰。

寒战（即"打摆子"）往往是发生细菌感染尤其菌血症的标志，不过也可见于其他很多临床情况，如药物热或输血反应。体温大幅波动可能提示脓肿的存在。任何曾前往或居住在疟疾疫区的发热者都应考虑到疟疾的可能，对于周期性发热、间隔1～3天正常体温出现发作性寒战和高热，而一般情况良好的患者也需要考虑疟疾的可能。应评估使用抗炎药物的时间点，这有可能改变或削弱发热反应。大部分感染性疾病早期可表现为发热，随后可出现特定器官系统的亚临床受累直至最终临床受累。

如果发热是唯一主诉或伴随局部症状和体征，诊断流程包括详细询问病史，如广泛全面的系统回顾、既往病史和手术史，以及儿童时期开始的免疫接种史。可以暂缓使用退热药，以评估发热的时间规律。老年人、服用糖皮质激素的人群，以及慢性肝病或肾病患者可能不易出现发热。应评估疾病的所有可能来源，包括旅行、结核分枝杆菌暴露史，以及职业、爱好、动物、昆虫以及性接触。对于旅行者返回后发热，应考虑到患者既往旅行和活动、疾病的地理风险，以及可能疾病暴露的季节性和潜伏期。

病毒感染

既往健康的年轻个体中出现急性发热性疾病，往往是病毒感染所致，这种情况不需要精确诊断，因为疾病具有自限性，几乎没有治疗手段。上呼吸道症状如流涕、咽痛、咳嗽和声嘶，常由鼻病毒、冠状病毒、副流感病毒及腺病毒所致。腺病毒暴发可见于聚集居住的人群如军营或大学宿舍。呼吸道合胞病毒、人偏肺病毒及人博卡病毒感染可在类似场景下出现，有时可表现为肺炎。

一种冠状病毒可引起具有潜在致死性的上呼吸道病毒感染，即中东呼吸综合征（MERS）。它在半数感染者中引发肺炎及急性呼吸窘迫综合征（ARDS）并导致死亡，且具有高度传染性。关于COVID-19的讨论见附录。

夏季时节的脑膜炎症状主要见于肠道病毒感染，但一旦出现该症状群，应在展开诊断流程的同时，及早开始针对细菌性病原的治疗。不伴脑膜炎的发热性综合征是肠道病毒感染更常见的表现。

虫媒病毒，如加利福尼亚脑炎病毒、东方/西方/委内瑞拉马脑炎病毒、圣路易斯脑炎病毒，以及西尼罗河病毒可导致自限性发热疾病及脑炎。科罗拉多蜱传热是在西北及西南地区蜱叮咬后出现的双相性疾病，其特征在于高热和粒细胞减少（缺乏）。鹿蜱携带的病毒——波瓦生病毒，已引起新英格兰和中西部地区北部无数发热及脑炎的病例。

流感除发热外还会引起咽痛、咳嗽、肌痛、关节痛及头痛，常常在冬季呈现出局部流行的特点。在无并发症的流感中，发热很少持续5天以上。流感确诊患者出现热程延长需进一步检查和治疗继发细菌感染。近年来禽流感和H1N1流行株的流行警示我们，流感病毒具有显著的变异能力，产生新的免疫耐受毒株。每年接种预防性流感疫苗至关重要。

出现发热和显性淋巴结肿大的单核细胞增多症是EB病毒（EBV）、巨细胞病毒（CMV）、急性人类免疫缺陷病毒（HIV）以及刚地弓形虫（即弓形虫病的病原体）感染的特征性表现。这些感染的其他表现包括肝功能检测结果异常、呼吸道症状及神经系统症状。急性HIV感染可引起单核细胞增多症综合征，其诊断是紧急的临床情况。

细菌感染

致病性细菌能够感染机体所有部位，引发一系列需要抗生素治疗的局灶性疾病。例如，金黄色葡萄球菌能导致皮肤脓肿或蜂窝织炎。高致病性微生物可以定植在接触医疗系统的个体中。最令人担忧的是细菌进入血流。在有常见临床症状的个体中经验性使用抗生素治疗细菌感染之前及时留血培养，有助于明确血液中的病原菌并确定所需的疗程。

发热可以是金黄色葡萄球菌感染的主要临床表现。金黄色葡萄球菌，包括其对甲氧西林耐药的菌株（即MRSA），常可导致感染中毒症而没有明显的原发感染部位。在使用静脉治疗或血液透析的患者、使用静脉成瘾药物或严重慢性皮炎的患者中应考虑到这一可能。葡萄球菌可经血源性播散至骨导致骨髓炎、至心脏瓣膜导致感染性心内膜炎；菌血症也可能反映了这些潜在过程。菌血症的其他常见病原及其来源包括肺炎链球菌（肺炎）、大肠埃希菌（尿路及胃肠道来源）、链球菌（皮肤）以及厌氧菌（胃肠道）。

单核细胞增生李斯特菌菌血症主要见于细胞免疫力减退者以及孕妇。尽管在这些宿主中菌血症是李斯特菌病最常见的表现，很多李斯特菌病患者可出现脑膜炎，需要进行腰椎穿刺及脑脊液培养。大部分病例为50岁以上的个体。

伤寒和副伤寒（即肠热症）在很多低收入国家很常见。患者的最初临床表现可能仅有发热。80%的美国病例为前往以下6个国家的旅行者：印度、墨西哥、菲律宾、巴基斯坦、萨尔瓦多及海地。发热伴头痛、起病隐匿而体检无明显异常很常见，不过在疾病第二周有可能出现极淡的一过性皮疹（即玫瑰疹）。症状可能还包括腹泻、便秘、轻微腹部不适，偶尔可出现干咳。诊断取决于血或粪便的培养。

发热伴局部症状和体征

局部细菌感染可能表现很直观，如脓肿、蜂窝织炎或中耳炎；也可能临床表现隐匿，仅表现为无差别

TABLE 3.1 Infections Exhibiting Fever as the Sole or Dominant Feature

Infectious Agent or Source	Epidemiologic Exposure and History	Distinctive Clinical and Laboratory Findings
Viruses		
Rhinovirus, adenovirus, parainfluenza	None (adenovirus in epidemics)	Often URI symptoms; throat and rectal cultures; rapid viral antigen testing
Middle East respiratory syndrome (MERS)	Travel to Arabian Peninsula or contact from Middle East	Pneumonia with ARDS; viral antigen testing of sputum; PCR of normally sterile sites (CDC)
Enteroviruses (non-polioviruses: coxsackieviruses, echovirus)	Summer, epidemic	Occasionally aseptic meningitis, rash, pleurodynia, herpangina; serologic or nucleic acid testing (PCR)
Influenza	Winter, epidemic	Headache, myalgias, arthralgias; nasopharyngeal culture, rapid viral antigen testing
EBV, CMV	Close personal contact; blood or tissue exposure; occupational or perinatal exposure	Monospot test, EBV specific antibodies; EBV PCR in immunocompromised; CMV IgM shell vial assay; CMV antigenemia assay; CMV DNA of CSF; culture and histopathology of tissues
Colorado tick fever	Southwest and Northwest regions, tick exposure	Biphasic illness, leukopenia; blood, CSF cultures, serologic or PCR
Powassan virus	New England and Upper Midwest exposure	Altered mentation or encephalitis; serum and CSF IgM (CDC)
Bacteria		
Staphylococcus aureus	IV drug users, IV catheters, hemodialysis, dermatitis	Must exclude endocarditis; blood cultures
Listeria monocytogenes	Depressed cell-mediated immunity	Meningitis may also be present; blood, CSF cultures
Salmonella typhi, Salmonella paratyphi	Food or water contaminated by carrier or patient	Headache, myalgias, diarrhea, or constipation, transient rose spots; blood, marrow, or stool cultures
Streptococci	Valvular heart disease	Low-grade fever, fatigue; blood cultures
Animal Exposure		
Coxiella burnetii (Q fever)	Exposure to infected livestock, parturient animals	Headache, occasionally pneumonitis, hepatitis, culture-negative endocarditis; serologic testing
Leptospira interrogans	Water contaminated by urine from dogs, cats, rodents, small mammals	Headache, myalgias, conjunctival suffusion, biphasic illness, aseptic meningitis; serologic testing

ARDS, Acute respiratory disease syndrome; *CDC*, Centers for Disease Control and Prevention case definition; *CMV*, cytomegalovirus; *CSF*, cerebrospinal fluid; *EBV*, Epstein-Barr virus; *IgM*, immunoglobulin M; *IV*, intravenous; *PCR*, polymerase chain reaction; *URI*, upper respiratory infection.

an undifferentiated febrile syndrome. Careful inspection of mucous membranes and conjunctiva may reveal petechiae, which are clues to meningococcemia or infective endocarditis. Finding heart murmurs in the setting of fever may suggest endocarditis and warrant additional blood cultures. Pulmonary signs in pneumonia include rales and evidence of consolidation, but persons with cryptococcosis, coccidioidomycosis, histoplasmosis, psittacosis, legionellosis, or pneumocystis pneumonia may show few signs. Pyelonephritis and renal abscesses can occur with few localizing signs.

These infections should be suspected based on exposure history and the host's immune status. It is important to assess the size of the liver, spleen, and lymph nodes, particularly in cases of viral infection. A swollen joint may indicate septic arthritis. A complete neurologic examination, including cranial nerves and testing for meningeal signs, may indicate CNS infection.

Malaria, bacterial sepsis, and bacterial infections of the lung, urinary tract, CNS, and intestines with resultant bacteremia warrant urgent initiation of empirical treatment while awaiting final identification and sensitivities. For febrile patients with features suggesting a bacterial infection, evaluation should include complete blood counts with differential and platelet counts, blood smears for those at risk for malaria or babesiosis, urinalysis, throat and blood cultures, and a chest radiograph.

Fevers with rash as a prominent feature warrant exclusion of life-threatening infectious diseases, including meningococcemia, toxic shock syndrome (TSS), and Rocky Mountain spotted fever (RMSF). Characterization of the rash can help. Clues to some of the common infections exhibiting fever as the sole feature and those causing fever with rash are provided in Tables 3.1, 3.2, and 3.3. Tables 3.4 and 3.5 list common syndromes associated with imported fevers when assessing travelers.

FEVER OF UNKNOWN ORIGIN

Most febrile conditions resolve or are readily diagnosed and treated, but some fevers can persist and remain unexplained. Table 3.6 shows the most common causes of unexplained fevers.

The term *fever of unknown origin* (FUO) identifies a pattern of fever with temperatures greater than 38.3° C (101° F) on several occasions over more than 3 weeks after an initial diagnostic work-up for which the diagnosis remains uncertain. Verifying the presence or absence of fever is important; up to 35% of 347 patients admitted to the National Institutes of Health (NIH) for evaluation of prolonged fever were determined not to have significant fever or had fever of factitious origin. Cases of FUO are categorized as classic FUO, health care–associated FUO, neutropenic (immune-deficient) FUO, and HIV-related FUO. Each of these FUO subtypes can have unique causes.

Classic Fever of Unknown Origin

The most common causes of classic FUO are infections, malignancies, and noninfectious inflammatory disorders; miscellaneous causes and undiagnosed cases account for the remaining categories. Historically,

表 3.1 以发热为唯一或主要表现的感染

感染病原体或来源	流行病学暴露及病史	特征性临床及实验室表现
病毒		
鼻病毒、腺病毒、副流感病毒	无（腺病毒流行）	通常为 URI 症状，咽部及直肠培养；快速病毒抗原检测
中东呼吸综合征（MERS）	阿拉伯半岛或中东旅行史	肺炎及 ARDS；痰液病毒抗原检测；常规无菌部位的 PCR（美国 CDC 的病例定义）
肠道病毒（非脊髓灰质炎病毒：柯萨奇病毒、埃可病毒）	夏季，流行性	偶可引起无菌性脑膜炎、皮疹、胸膜性疼痛、疱疹性咽峡炎；血清学或核酸检测（PCR）
流感	冬季，流行性	头痛、肌痛、关节痛；鼻咽分泌物培养，快速病毒抗原检测
EBV、CMV	密切人际接触	单斑试验、EBV 特异性抗体；免疫低下人群行 EBV PCR；CMV IgM 壳病毒测定；CMV 抗原血症测定；CSF 的 CMV DNA；组织培养和组织病理
科罗拉多蜱传热	西南和西北地区，蜱暴露	双相疾病，粒细胞缺乏；血、CSF 培养，血清学或 PCR
波瓦生病毒	新英格兰及中西部北部区域	神志改变或脑炎；血清及 CSF IgM（美国 CDC 的病例定义）
细菌		
金黄色葡萄球菌	静脉药瘾者、静脉导管、血液透析、皮炎	必须除外感染性心内膜炎；血培养
单核细胞增生李斯特菌	细胞免疫低下	有可能存在脑膜炎；血、CSF 培养
伤寒沙门菌、副伤寒沙门菌	携带者或患者污染的食物或水	头痛、肌痛、腹泻或便秘、一过性玫瑰疹；血、骨髓或粪便培养
链球菌	心脏瓣膜病	低热、乏力；血培养
动物暴露		
贝纳柯克斯体（Q 热）	接触感染的家畜、临产的动物	头痛，可有肺炎、肝炎、培养阴性的感染性心内膜炎；血清学检测
问号钩端螺旋体	被狗、猫、啮齿类、小型哺乳动物尿液污染的水	头痛、肌痛、结膜水肿、双相病程、无菌性脑膜炎、血清学检测

ARDS，急性呼吸窘迫综合征；CDC，疾病控制与预防中心；CMV，巨细胞病毒；CSF，脑脊液；EBV，EB 病毒；IgM，免疫球蛋白 M；IV，经静脉；PCR，聚合酶链反应；URI，上呼吸道感染。

的发热性综合征。对黏膜和结膜的细致检查可能会发现瘀点，提示脑膜炎球菌菌血症或感染性心内膜炎。在发热患者中闻及心脏杂音可能提示心内膜炎而需要进行额外的血培养。肺炎的肺部体征包括啰音及实变证据，但罹患隐球菌病、球孢子菌病、组织胞浆菌病、鹦鹉热、军团病或肺孢子虫肺炎的患者可能几乎没有体征。肾盂肾炎及肾脓肿也可能鲜有局部体征。

这些感染的疑诊应基于暴露史和宿主免疫状态。评估肝、脾和淋巴结的大小很重要，尤其是在病毒感染的情况下。关节肿胀可能提示化脓性关节炎。完整的神经系统查体，包括脑神经和脑膜刺激征检查，可能提示 CNS 感染。

疟疾、细菌性感染中毒症，以及肺部、尿路、CNS 和肠道的细菌感染及其继发的菌血症，在等待最终鉴定和药敏结果的同时，应尽快启动经验性抗感染治疗。发热患者如有提示细菌感染的特征，评估应包括全血细胞分类计数和血小板计数、血涂片（有疟疾或巴贝虫病风险者）、尿液分析、咽部及血液培养以及胸部影像学。

发热并以皮疹为突出特征，需要除外危及生命的感染性疾病，包括脑膜炎球菌菌血症、中毒休克综合征（TSS）以及落基山斑点热（RMSF）。皮疹的特征有助于鉴别。某些以发热为唯一表现及导致发热伴皮疹的常见感染，其诊断线索可参考表 3.1、表 3.2 和表 3.3。表 3.4 和表 3.5 列举了评估旅行者输入性发热相关的常见综合征。

不明原因发热

大多数发热疾病可缓解或很快被诊断和治疗，但有些发热可能持续而原因不明。表 3.6 显示了不明原因发热的最常见原因。

术语"不明原因发热（FUO）"是指体温超过 38.3℃（101℉），持续 3 周以上，且经过初步诊断检查后仍不能明确诊断的发热。明确是否存在发热很重要；347 名入住美国国立卫生研究院（NIH）评估为长期发热的患者中，多达 35% 并无显著发热或为伪热。FUO 患者可分为经典型 FUO、医疗机构相关 FUO、中性粒细胞缺乏性（免疫缺陷相关）FUO，以及 HIV 相关 FUO。这些 FUO 的亚型均具有各自特有的病因。

经典型不明原因发热

经典型 FUO 最常见的病因包括感染、恶性肿瘤以及非感染性炎性疾病；此外则为少见原因或无法确诊的

TABLE 3.2 Differential Diagnosis of Infectious Agents Producing Fever and Rash
Maculopapular, Erythematous Lesions
Enterovirus
EBV, CMV, *Toxoplasma gondii*
Acute HIV infection
Colorado tick fever virus
Salmonella typhi
Leptospira interrogans
Measles virus
Rubella virus
Hepatitis B virus
Treponema pallidum
Parvovirus B19
Human herpesvirus 6
Vesicular Lesions
Varicella-zoster virus
Herpes simplex virus
Coxsackievirus A
Vibrio vulnificus
Cutaneous Petechiae
Neisseria gonorrhoeae
Neisseria meningitidis
Rickettsia rickettsii (Rocky Mountain spotted fever)
Rickettsia typhi (murine typhus)
Ehrlichia chaffeensis
Echoviruses
Streptococcus viridans (endocarditis)
Diffuse Erythroderma
Group A streptococci (scarlet fever, toxic shock syndrome)
Staphylococcus aureus (toxic shock syndrome)
Distinctive Rash
Ecthyma gangrenosum: *Pseudomonas aeruginosa*
Erythema migrans: Lyme disease
Mucous Membrane Lesions
Vesicular pharyngitis: coxsackievirus A
Palatal petechiae: rubella, EBV, scarlet fever (group A streptococci)
Erythema: toxic shock syndrome (*Staphylococcus aureus* and group A streptococci)
Oral ulceronodular lesion: *Histoplasma capsulatum*
Koplik spots: measles virus

CMV, Cytomegalovirus; *EBV*, Epstein-Barr virus; *HIV*, human immunodeficiency virus.

infections have made up the largest category, representing 25% to 50% of cases. Abscesses, endocarditis, tuberculosis, complicated urinary tract infections, and biliary tract diseases have consistently been among the most important. Abscesses account for almost one third of infectious causes, and most are intra-abdominal or pelvic in origin. Perforation of a colonic diverticulum or appendicitis can sometimes lead to large, walled-off abdominal abscesses with few localizing signs.

During the past 50 years, the improvement of imaging studies and their greater accessibility have made abdominal or pelvic abscesses and malignancies more easily detected and less likely to be the cause of prolonged, undiagnosed fever. Malignant neoplasms can induce fever directly through the production and release of pyrogenic cytokines and indirectly by undergoing spontaneous or induced necrosis or creating conditions conducive to secondary infections. Endovascular infections are usually detectable by blood cultures, although slow-growing or fastidious organisms may make detection difficult.

Infections, including tuberculosis, typhoid fever, malaria, and amebic liver abscesses, remain the most frequent causes of FUO in developing countries. The incidence of some FUOs varies according to geographic location. Classic FUO may occur as familial Mediterranean fever among Ashkenazi Jews; as Kikuchi disease, which is an unusual form of necrotizing lymphadenitis seen primarily in Japan; and as TNF receptor–associated periodic fever (TRAPS), formerly called familial Hibernian fever, which is an inherited periodic fever syndrome described originally in Ireland.

The proportion of FUOs due to noninfectious inflammatory diseases and undiagnosed conditions has risen. Of the connective tissue diseases, juvenile rheumatoid arthritis (i.e., Still disease), other variants of rheumatoid arthritis, and systemic lupus erythematosus predominate among younger patients. Temporal arteritis and polymyalgia rheumatica syndromes are more common among elderly patients.

Fever may be blunted or absent in up to one third of elderly individuals with serious conditions. Older people may more often have atypical clinical presentations of common infectious and noninfectious diseases. For example, elderly persons may have tuberculosis without cough or fever, infective endocarditis with fatigue and weight loss but without fever, and abdominal abscesses with little abdominal tenderness found on physical examination. Leukocytosis and increased band forms are more likely to be associated with a serious infection. HIV should be considered as a possible cause of FUO in older patients, although it is not usually suspected early in the course of FUO.

Fever in returned travelers is most often caused by common infections, such as malaria and respiratory or urinary tract infections. However, fever caused by dengue, typhoid fever, or amebic liver abscess is increasingly identified, especially among international travelers returning from the tropics. Katayama fever is a febrile syndrome occurring after exposure to fresh water schistosomes in endemic areas. It may resolve spontaneously or may require treatment with antiparasitic agents to prevent sequelae that carry severe morbidity. A travel history should be obtained, and it may redirect the entire work-up.

Health Care–Associated Fever of Unknown Origin

Some FUOs are associated with health care practices, including surgical procedures, urinary and respiratory tract instrumentation, intravascular devices, drug therapy, and immobilization. Quality control measures are set up to minimize and avoid bloodstream infections and decubitus ulcers. Drug-related fever, septic thrombophlebitis, recurrent pulmonary emboli, and *Clostridioides difficile* colitis must be considered in the work-up of hospitalized patients who develop fever greater than 38° C (100.4° F) for more than 3 days if it was not present on admission.

Immune Deficiency–Associated Fever of Unknown Origin

Immunosuppressed individuals have the highest incidence of FUO of any group of patients. Due to impaired immune responses, signs of inflammation other than fever are notoriously absent or diminished, producing atypical clinical manifestations and an absence of radiologic abnormalities for what otherwise would be readily diagnosed infections. In patients with impaired cell-mediated immunity, FUO often results from conditions other than pyogenic bacterial infections (e.g., fungi, CMV).

Neutropenia is a dangerous condition that can be considered a subclass of immunodeficiency. Persons with profound neutropenia are at high risk for bacterial and fungal infections. Episodes of fever

表 3.2　出现发热和皮疹的感染性病原体鉴别诊断

斑丘疹、红斑性皮损
肠道病毒
EBV、CMV、刚地弓形虫
急性 HIV 感染
科罗拉多蜱传热
伤寒沙门菌
问号钩端螺旋体
麻疹病毒
风疹病毒
乙型肝炎病毒
梅毒螺旋体
细小病毒 B19
人疱疹病毒 6 型

水疱性皮损
水痘-带状疱疹病毒
单纯疱疹病毒
柯萨奇病毒 A
创伤弧菌

皮肤瘀点
淋病奈瑟球菌
脑膜炎奈瑟球菌
立氏立克次体（落基山斑点热）
伤寒立克次体（鼠型斑疹伤寒）
查菲埃立克体
埃可病毒
草绿色链球菌（心内膜炎）

弥漫性红皮病
A 组链球菌（猩红热、中毒休克综合征）
金黄色葡萄球菌（中毒休克综合征）

特殊皮疹
坏疽性脓皮病：铜绿假单胞菌
游走性红斑：莱姆病

黏膜病损
疱疹性咽炎：柯萨奇病毒 A
腭瘀点：风疹、EBV、猩红热（A 组链球菌）
红斑：中毒休克综合征（金黄色葡萄球菌和 A 组链球菌）
口腔溃疡结节性病损：荚膜组织胞浆菌
柯氏斑：麻疹病毒

CMV，巨细胞病毒；EBV，EB 病毒；HIV，人类免疫缺陷病毒。

病例。长期以来，感染病因占比最大，占 25%～50%。脓肿、心内膜炎、结核病、复杂性尿路感染以及胆道疾病一直是最重要的病因。脓肿约占感染性病因的 1/3，腹腔或盆腔来源的脓肿最常见。结肠憩室穿孔或阑尾炎有时可导致大的包裹性腹腔脓肿而局部体征不明显。

近 50 年来，影像学技术的进步和可及性改善，使腹腔或盆腔脓肿及肿瘤更容易被发现，其导致长期不明原因发热的可能性下降。恶性肿瘤可通过产生和释放炎性细胞因子而直接导致发热，也可因不断的自发性或诱导性坏死，或产生易继发感染的情况而间接导致发热。血管内感染通常可由血培养发现，但慢生长或苛养性微生物的检测可能较困难。

感染，包括结核病、伤寒、疟疾以及阿米巴肝脓肿，仍是发展中国家最常见的 FUO 病因。FUO 的某些类型发病率因地理位置而有所差异。经典型 FUO 的病因在德系犹太人中可能是家族性地中海热，在日本可能是菊池病——主要见于日本的一种坏死性淋巴结炎的少见类型；TNF 受体相关周期性发热（TRAPS），以前又称为家族性寒冷性发热，则是一种最早报道于爱尔兰的遗传性周期性发热综合征。

由非感染性炎性疾病及未诊断疾病所致 FUO 的比例有所上升。在结缔组织病中，幼年型类风湿关节炎（即斯蒂尔病）、类风湿关节炎的其他变种以及系统性红斑狼疮是年轻患者中最主要的病因。颞动脉炎和风湿性多肌痛综合征在老年患者中更为常见。

在多达 1/3 患严重疾病的老年人中，发热可能很不明显或甚至不出现。老年人患常见感染性或非感染性疾病时，更易出现不典型的临床表现。例如，老年人患结核病可能不咳嗽或发热，患感染性心内膜炎可能出现疲劳和体重下降但不发热，患腹腔脓肿时查体几乎没有腹部压痛。白细胞增多及杆状核增多更有可能与严重感染相关。老年人 FUO 的可能原因应当考虑到 HIV，尽管它在 FUO 过程中不是早期的鉴别诊断。

归来的旅行者出现发热最常由常见感染所致，如疟疾和呼吸道或尿路感染。然而，登革热、伤寒或阿米巴肝脓肿引起的发热在增加，尤其在从热带地区返回的国际旅行者中。片山热是在流行区接触淡水血吸虫后出现的一种发热性综合征，有可能自发缓解也有可能需要抗寄生虫药物治疗以避免后遗的严重并发症。应询问患者旅行史，其信息有可能改变整个临床评估的方向。

医疗机构相关不明原因发热

部分 FUO 与医疗处置相关，包括手术操作、尿路和呼吸道植入器械、血管内装置、药物治疗和制动等。设立质控措施以减少和避免血流感染和压疮。住院患者如果入院时不发热，在院内发热超过 38℃（100.4℉）达 3 天以上，在其鉴别诊断中应考虑到药物热、感染中毒性血栓性静脉炎、复发性肺栓塞以及艰难梭菌性结肠炎。

免疫缺陷相关不明原因发热

在所有患者中，免疫低下患者 FUO 发生率最高。由于免疫应答受损，除发热之外的炎症表现广泛缺失或减弱，导致在一般情况下很容易诊断的感染临床表现不典型、影像学异常缺失。在细胞免疫受损的患者中，FUO 常由化脓性细菌感染之外的原因所致（如真菌或 CMV）。

中性粒细胞减少是可被归为一种免疫缺陷亚型的高危情形。有显著中性粒细胞减少的患者细菌和真菌感染的风险较高。中性粒细胞减少患者出现发热非常

TABLE 3.3 Fever and Rash in Viral Infection

Virus	Disease Features	Incubation and Early Symptoms
Coxsackie, ECHO virus	Maculopapular rubelliform, 1–3 mm, faint pink, begins on face, spreading to chest and extremities Herpetiform vesicular stomatitis with peripheral exanthema (papules and clear vesicles on an erythematous base), including palms and soles (hand, foot, and mouth disease)	Summertime No itching or lymphadenopathy Multiple cases in household or community-wide epidemic Mostly diseases of children
Measles	Erythematous, maculopapular rash begins on upper face and spreads down to involve extremities, including palms and soles. Koplik spots are blue-gray specks on a red base found on buccal mucosa near second molars. Atypical measles occurs in individuals who received killed vaccine and then are exposed to measles. The rash begins peripherally and is urticarial, vascular, or hemorrhagic.	Incubation period 10–14 days First, severe upper respiratory symptoms, coryza, cough, and conjunctivitis; then Koplik spots, then rash
Rubella	Maculopapular rash beginning on face and moving down; petechiae on soft palate	Incubation 12–23 days Adenopathy; posterior auricular, posterior cervical, and suboccipital
Varicella	Generalized vesicular eruption; pruritic lesions in different stages from erythematous macules to vesicles to crusted; spread from trunk centrifugally; zoster lesions are painful and often dermatomal	Incubation 14–15 days; late winter, early spring Herpes zoster is a reactivation, occurs any season
Herpes simplex virus	Oral primary: small vesicles on pharynx, oral mucosa that ulcerates; painful and tender Recurrent: vermilion border, one or few lesions, genital; may be asymptomatic or appear similar to oral lesions on genital mucosa	Incubation 2–12 days
Hepatitis B and C virus	Prodrome in one fifth; erythematous, maculopapular rash, urticaria Leukocytoclastic vasculitis occurs in hepatitis C	Arthralgias, arthritis; abnormal liver function test results; hepatitis B antigenemia
Epstein-Barr virus	Erythematous, maculopapular rash on trunk and proximal extremities Occasionally urticarial or hemorrhagic	Transiently occurs in 5–10% of patients during first week of illness
Human immunodeficiency virus	Maculopapular truncal rash may occur as early manifestation of infection	Associated fever, sore throat, and lymph node enlargement may persist for 2 or more weeks

TABLE 3.4 Common Syndromes and Diseases Associated With Fever in Returned Travelers

Sore Throat	Cough	Abdominal Pain	Arthralgia or Myalgia	Diarrhea
Bacterial pharyngitis	Amebiasis (hepatic)	Amebiasis (intestinal)	Arboviruses	Amebiasis (intestinal)
Diphtheria	Anthrax	Anthrax	Dengue	Anthrax
Infectious mononucleosis	Bacterial pneumonia	*Campylobacter enteritis*	Yellow fever	*Campylobacter enteritis*
HIV seroconversion	Filarial fever	Legionnaires disease	Babesiosis	HIV seroconversion
Lyme disease	TPE	Malaria	Bartonellosis	Legionnaires disease
Poliomyelitis	Histoplasmosis	Measles	Brucellosis	Malaria melioidosis
Psittacosis	Legionnaires disease	Melioidosis	Erythema nodosum leprosum	Plague
Tularemia	Leishmaniasis (visceral)	Plague	Hepatitis (viral)	Relapsing fever
Viral hemorrhagic fever (Lassa)	Loeffler syndrome	Relapsing fevers	Histoplasmosis	Salmonellosis
Nonspecific viral URTI	Malaria	Salmonellosis	HIV seroconversion	Schistosomiasis (acute)
	Measles	Schistosomiasis (acute)	Legionnaires disease	Shigellosis
	Melioidosis	Shigellosis	Leptospirosis	Typhoid in children
	Plague	Typhoid fever	Lyme disease	Viral hemorrhagic fevers
	Q fever	Viral hemorrhagic fevers	Malaria	Yersiniosis
	Relapsing fever	Yersiniosis	Plague	
	Schistosomiasis (acute)		Poliomyelitis	
	Toxocariasis		Q fever	
	Trichinosis		Relapsing fevers	
	Tuberculosis		Secondary syphilis	
	Tularemia		Toxoplasmosis	
	Typhoid and paratyphoid		Trichinosis	
	Typhus		Trypanosomiasis (African)	
	Viral hemorrhagic fevers		Tularemia	
	Nonspecific viral URTIs		Typhoid and paratyphoid	
			Typhus	
			Viral hemorrhagic fevers	

HIV, Human immunodeficiency virus; *TPE,* tropical pulmonary eosinophilia; *URTI,* upper respiratory tract infection.
From Beeching N, Fletcher T, Wijaya L: Returned travelers. In Zuckerman JN, editor: Principles and practice of travel medicine, ed 2, Boston, 2013, Wiley-Blackwell, p 271.

表 3.3 病毒感染的发热和皮疹

病毒	疾病特征	潜伏期和早期症状
柯萨奇病毒、埃可病毒	斑丘红疹状，1～3 mm，淡红色，头面部向胸部及四肢蔓延 疱疹样水疱性口炎伴外周皮疹（丘疹和红斑基底上的透明水疱），包括手心和足心（手足口病）	夏季时节 无瘙痒或淋巴结肿大 家中多个病例或社区内小流行 绝大多数为儿童患病
麻疹	红斑性、斑丘疹，自上面部向下蔓延至肢体，包括手心和足心。柯氏斑为颊黏膜近第二磨牙处红色基底上的蓝灰色斑点 不典型麻疹可见于接受灭活疫苗的个体暴露于麻疹时。皮疹从四肢起病，为荨麻疹、水疱或出血性皮疹	潜伏期 10～14 天 先出现严重的上呼吸道症状、鼻塞、咳嗽和结膜炎；随后出现柯氏斑，然后出现皮疹
风疹	斑丘疹，自面部开始向下蔓延；软腭上可见瘀点	潜伏期 12～23 天 耳后、颈后和枕下淋巴结肿大
水痘	广泛性水疱疹；从红斑疹到水疱到结痂等不同阶段的瘙痒性皮损；从躯干向外离心性分布；带状疱疹皮损通常疼痛且按皮节分布	潜伏期 14～15 天；深冬及初春 带状疱疹是再激活病变，发生于任何季节
单纯疱疹病毒	口腔原发感染：咽部及口腔黏膜小水疱，可形成溃疡；疼痛且有压痛 复发：红色边界，一个或多个病损，生殖器区域；可无症状或在生殖器黏膜上出现与口腔病损类似的皮损	潜伏期 2～12 天
乙型肝炎病毒和丙型肝炎病毒	1/5 患者有前驱症状；红色斑丘疹，荨麻疹；白血病碎裂性血管炎可见于丙型肝炎	关节痛、关节炎；肝功能结果异常；乙肝抗原血症
EB 病毒	躯干和近端肢体的红色斑丘疹，偶有荨麻疹或出血疹	在 5%～10% 患者的疾病第 1 周一过性出现
人类免疫缺陷病毒	躯干斑丘疹，可作为感染的早期表现出现	伴有发热、咽痛及淋巴结肿大，可持续 2 周以上

表 3.4 旅行者发热的常见症状和疾病

咽痛	咳嗽	腹痛	关节痛或肌痛	腹泻
细菌性咽炎	阿米巴病（肝）	阿米巴病（肠道）	虫媒病毒	阿米巴病（肠道）
白喉	炭疽	炭疽	登革热	炭疽
传染性单核细胞增多症	细菌性肺炎	弯曲杆菌肠炎	黄热病	弯曲杆菌肠炎
HIV 血清转换	丝虫热	军团病	巴贝虫病	HIV 血清转换
莱姆病	TPE	疟疾	巴尔通体病	军团病
脊髓灰质炎	组织胞浆菌病	麻疹	布鲁氏菌病	疟疾
鹦鹉热	军团病	类鼻疽	麻风结节性红斑	类鼻疽
土拉菌病	黑热病（内脏利什曼病）	鼠疫	肝炎（病毒性）	鼠疫
病毒性出血热（拉沙热）	吕弗勒（Loeffler）综合征	回归热	组织胞浆菌病	回归热
非特异性病毒性 URTI	疟疾	沙门菌感染	HIV 血清转换	沙门菌感染
	麻疹	血吸虫病（急性）	军团病	血吸虫病（急性）
	类鼻疽	志贺菌感染	钩端螺旋体病	志贺菌感染
	鼠疫	伤寒	莱姆病	儿童伤寒
	Q 热	病毒性出血热	疟疾	病毒性出血热
	回归热	耶尔森菌感染	鼠疫	耶尔森菌感染
	血吸虫病（急性）		脊髓灰质炎	
	弓蛔虫病		Q 热	
	旋毛虫病		回归热	
	结核病		二期梅毒	
	土拉菌病		弓形虫病	
	伤寒和副伤寒		旋毛虫病	
	斑疹伤寒		锥虫病（美国）	
	病毒性出血热		土拉菌病	
	非特异性病毒性 URTI		伤寒和副伤寒	
			斑疹伤寒	
			病毒性出血热	

HIV，人类免疫缺陷病毒；TPE，热带性肺嗜酸细胞浸润症；URTI，上呼吸道感染。

引自 Beeching N, Fletcher T, Wijaya L: Returned travelers. In Zuckerman JN, editor: Principles and practice of travel medicine, ed 2, Boston, 2013，Wiley-Blackwell, p 271.

TABLE 3.5 Common Clinical Findings and Associated Infections After Tropical Travel

Clinical Findings	Infections
Fever and rash	Dengue, chikungunya, rickettsial infections, enteric fever (skin lesions may be sparse or absent), acute HIV infection, measles, acute schistosomiasis
Fever and abdominal pain	Enteric fever, amebic liver abscess
Undifferentiated fever and normal or low white blood cell count	Dengue, malaria, rickettsial infection, enteric fever, chikungunya
Fever and hemorrhage	Viral hemorrhagic fevers (dengue and others), meningococcemia, leptospirosis, rickettsial infections
Fever and eosinophilia	Acute schistosomiasis; drug hypersensitivity reaction; fascioliasis and other parasitic infections (rare)
Fever and pulmonary infiltrates	Common bacterial and viral pathogens; legionellosis, acute schistosomiasis, Q fever, melioidosis
Fever and altered mental status	Cerebral malaria, viral or bacterial meningoencephalitis, African trypanosomiasis
Mononucleosis syndrome	Epstein-Barr virus, cytomegalovirus, toxoplasmosis, acute HIV infection
Fever persisting >2 weeks	Malaria, enteric fever, Epstein-Barr virus, cytomegalovirus, toxoplasmosis, acute HIV, acute schistosomiasis, brucellosis, tuberculosis, Q fever, visceral leishmaniasis (rare)
Fever with onset >6 weeks after travel	Vivax malaria, acute hepatitis (B, C, or E), tuberculosis, amebic liver abscess

HIV, Human immunodeficiency virus.
Modified from Centers for Disease Control and Prevention: CDC health information for international travel 2012, New York, 2012, Oxford University Press.

are common in patients with neutropenia. Many episodes are short lived because they respond quickly to treatment or are manifestations of rapidly fatal infections.

Bacteremia and sepsis can cause rapid deterioration in neutropenic patients, and empirical, broad-spectrum antibiotics should be administered promptly without waiting for the results of cultures. However, only about 35% of prolonged episodes of febrile neutropenia respond to broad-spectrum antibiotic therapy. If fevers persist after 3 days of treatment with broad-spectrum antibiotics, diagnostic tests to explore fungal causes should be considered along with empirical antifungal treatment.

Human Immunodeficiency Virus–Related Fever of Unknown Origin

The advent of highly active antiretroviral therapy (ART) with the achievable suppression of the HIV viral load has greatly reduced the frequency of FUO in HIV-infected patients. High vigilance is warranted to test for new HIV in a matter-of-fact manner in the primary care setting. The primary phase of HIV infection can be asymptomatic or sometimes be characterized by a mononucleosis-like illness in which fever is a prominent feature (see Chapter 16). After symptoms of the primary phase of HIV infection resolve, patients enter a long period of subclinical infection during which they are usually afebrile. In the later phases of untreated HIV infection, episodes of fever become common, often signifying a superimposed illness. Many of these are potentially devastating opportunistic infections, which tend to manifest in atypical fashion because of the severe immunodeficiency. Patients with untreated acquired immunodeficiency syndrome (AIDS) can have multiple infections simultaneously, which highlights the importance of treating and documenting adherence with ART. After initiating effective ART the HIV viral load is effectively suppressed and the frequency of FUO in HIV-infected patients falls markedly.

Approach to the Patient With Fever of Unknown Origin

Evaluation of a patient with FUO typically includes verification that the patient has fever, consideration of the fever pattern, a comprehensive history, repeated physical examinations, appropriate laboratory investigations, key imaging studies, and invasive diagnostic procedures. The physical examination should scrutinize the patient more closely than usual because key physical abnormalities in patients with FUO are subtle and require repeated examinations to be appreciated.

Work-up of a patient with an FUO should focus on the history, physical examination, and initial laboratory data. In place of rational diagnostic thinking, there is a temptation to order multiple comprehensive laboratory and imaging studies. Rather than leading to a diagnosis, this shotgun approach may result in enormous expense, false-positive results, and unnecessary additional investigations that may obfuscate the true diagnosis.

A fundamental principle in the management of classic FUO is that therapy should be withheld, whenever possible, until the cause of the fever has been determined, so that treatment can be tailored to a specific diagnosis. The exception is in the setting of the immunocompromised host because rapid empirical treatment is most often needed.

If fevers persist after an exhaustive work-up there may be a role for fluorodeoxyglucose positron emission tomography (18 FDG-PET/CT) imaging, if available. This allows enhancement of acute and chronic inflammatory processes by uptake of FDG in all activated leukocytes and provides the necessary spatial resolution that may substantially contribute to finding the cause of FUO. The radiation exposure and cost and the degree of incremental improvement in detection over other methods must be carefully considered.

Cardiac ECHO can be helpful if culture-negative endocarditis or atrial myxoma is suspected in patients with cardiac murmurs. The most invasive tests such as lymph node biopsies, bone marrow biopsies, and temporal artery biopsies should be undertaken only with strong clinical suspicion and based on physical findings or those found on imaging. Persons who reside in the southeastern part of the United States and immigrants from world regions endemic for *Strongyloides stercoralis* should have a *S. stercoralis* titre—whether or not they have a fever—to identify and eradicate risk for overwhelming strongyloidiasis.

SPECIFIC CONDITIONS AND EXPOSURES CAUSING FEVER

Fever After Animal Exposures
Q Fever

Q fever is a widespread zoonotic infection caused by the pathogen *Coxiella burnetii* that has acute and chronic manifestations. The primary source of infection is infected cattle, sheep, and goats. The organism can exist for months in soil and can become airborne. The onset of disease is typically abrupt, and high-grade fever (40° C or 104° F),

表 3.5　热带旅行后常见的临床表现及其相关感染

临床表现	感染
发热伴皮疹	登革热、奇昆古尼亚热、立克次体感染、肠热症（皮肤病损可能较少或不出现）、急性 HIV 感染、麻疹、急性血吸虫病
发热伴腹痛	肠热症、阿米巴肝脓肿
非特异性发热，白细胞正常或偏低	登革热、疟疾、立克次体感染、肠热症、奇昆古尼亚热
发热伴出血	病毒性出血热（登革热及其他）、脑膜炎球菌血症、钩端螺旋体病、立克次体感染
发热伴嗜酸性粒细胞增多	急性血吸虫病；药物过敏反应；片形吸虫病及其他寄生虫感染（罕见）
发热伴肺部浸润影	常见细菌及病毒病原体；军团菌；急性血吸虫病；Q 热、类鼻疽
发热伴神志改变	脑型疟、病毒或细菌性脑膜脑炎、非洲锥虫病
单核细胞增多症	EB 病毒、巨细胞病毒、弓形虫病、急性 HIV 感染
发热持续 > 2 周	疟疾、肠热症、EB 病毒、巨细胞病毒、弓形虫病、急性 HIV、急性血吸虫病、布鲁氏菌病、结核病、Q 热、内脏利什曼病（罕见）
旅行后 6 周以上出现发热	间日疟、急性病毒性肝炎（甲型、乙型或戊型）、结核病、阿米巴肝脓肿

HIV，人类免疫缺陷病毒
改编自 Centers for Disease Control and Prevention：CDC health information for international travel 2012，New York，2012，Oxford University Press.

普遍。很多发热持续时间不长，因为它们或是对治疗迅速产生应答，或是快速致命性感染的表现。

菌血症和感染中毒症能导致粒细胞缺乏患者的迅速恶化，无需等待培养结果回报，就应及时予以经验性广谱抗生素治疗。然而，仅有约 35% 持续时间较长的发热性中性粒细胞减少会对广谱抗生素治疗产生应答。如使用广谱抗生素治疗 3 天以上发热仍不缓解，需考虑开展真菌病因的诊断检查并启动经验性抗真菌治疗。

HIV 相关不明原因发热

高效抗逆转录病毒治疗（ART）的进步能够抑制 HIV 病毒载量，极大地降低了 HIV 感染者出现 FUO 的可能性。初级医疗机构应具有高度警惕性，按需检测筛查新的 HIV 感染。HIV 感染的急性期阶段可无临床症状，或有时表现为单核细胞增多症样疾病，并以发热为突出特征（见第 16 章）。在 HIV 感染急性期症状缓解后，患者进入一个相对较长的亚临床感染阶段，此时通常不发热。在未经治疗的 HIV 感染晚期阶段，发热变得常见，通常提示继发的疾病。其中很多是具有潜在致命性的机会性感染，但由于严重免疫缺陷而易表现不典型。未经治疗的获得性免疫缺陷综合征（AIDS）患者可同时合并多种感染，凸显了 ART 治疗和依从性记录的重要性。在启动有效 ART 后，HIV 病毒载量能够得到有效抑制，HIV 感染者 FUO 的发生率显著下降。

不明原因发热患者的接诊

对 FUO 患者的评估通常包括确认发热的存在、对热型的考虑、详细的病史采集、反复的体格检查、恰当的实验室检测、关键的影像学检查，以及侵入性诊断操作。体格检查对患者的观察应比通常情况下更细致，因为在 FUO 患者中关键的体格检查异常非常微小，需要反复检查才能发现。

FUO 患者的诊断评估应聚焦病史、体格检查和初始实验室结果。与理性诊断思路不同，一种观点倾向于进行多种全面的实验室和影像学检查。但这种大撒网式的检查方式并不一定能获得诊断，却可能造成大额花费、假阳性结果和不必要的额外检查而忽略了真实诊断。

经典型 FUO 临床处理的基本原则，是在可能的情况下在明确发热病因前不进行治疗，这样能够根据特定诊断进行相应治疗。例外是免疫低下宿主的 FUO，因为此时迅速的经验性治疗通常十分必要。

如果在进行广泛的检查后发热仍未缓解，条件允许时行氟脱氧葡萄糖正电子发射计算机断层成像（18FDG-PET/CT）可能会有帮助。这一检查基于所有活化白细胞摄取 FDG 而强化显示急性和慢性炎症过程，从而提供必要的空间分辨，对寻找 FUO 的病因可能会有极大帮助。这一检查的辐射暴露、花费以及在其他检查基础上检测再提升的程度，是需要慎重考虑的问题。

有心脏杂音的患者怀疑培养阴性的心内膜炎或心房黏液瘤，超声心动图有助于其诊断。最具侵袭性的检查如淋巴结活检、骨髓活检和颞动脉活检仅应在临床高度怀疑时进行，并需基于体格检查结果或影像学结果。居住在美国东南部的人群以及从全球其他粪类圆线虫流行区域迁入的移民，不论发热与否，都应检测粪类圆线虫滴度，以明确或除外全身粪类圆线虫病的可能。

导致发热的特定情况和暴露

动物暴露后的发热

Q 热

Q 热是由贝纳柯克斯体引起的广泛传播的人畜共患感染，可表现为急性或慢性感染。原发感染来源为感染的牛、绵羊和山羊。微生物可以在土壤中存活数月，也可通过空气传播。该病通常为急性起病，高热（40℃或 104℉）、疲乏、头痛及肌痛是最常见的症状。

TABLE 3.6 Common Causes of Fever of Unknown Origin

Infections
Abscesses
Brucellosis
Catheter infections
Cytomegalovirus
Coccidioidomycosis
Histoplasmosis
Human immunodeficiency virus (HIV) infection
Infective endocarditis
Intra-abdominal, subdiaphragmatic, and pelvic disease
Liver and biliary tract disease
Lyme disease
Mycobacterium tuberculosis
Osteomyelitis
Sinusitis
Toxoplasmosis
Urinary tract infection

Autoimmune Conditions
Adult Still disease
Familial Mediterranean
Sarcoidosis
Rheumatoid arthritis
Systemic lupus erythematosus
Temporal arteritis

Malignancy
Hepatocellular carcinoma
Leukemia
Metastatic cancers
Pancreatic cancer
Renal cell carcinoma

Miscellaneous Causes
Deep vein thrombosis, pulmonary embolism
Hyperthyroidism
Kikuchi disease
Periodic fever (tumor necrosis factor receptor associated)

---

fatigue, headache, and myalgias are the most common symptoms. Acute Q fever is usually a mild disease that resolves spontaneously within 2 weeks. Q fever endocarditis usually occurs in patients with previous valvular damage or immunocompromise, and it is often the predominant manifestation of chronic infection.

An immunofluorescence assay is the reference method for the serodiagnosis of Q fever. Consideration of doxycycline therapy is warranted only for patients who are symptomatic.

Leptospirosis

Leptospirosis is a zoonotic infection with protean manifestations caused by the spirochete *Leptospira interrogans*. It is distributed worldwide, but most clinical cases occur in the tropics. The organism infects rodents, cattle, swine, dogs, horses, sheep, and goats, and it is shed in the urine. Humans most often become infected after exposure to environmental sources, such as contaminated water.

Leptospirosis may manifest as a subclinical illness followed by seroconversion, a self-limited systemic infection, or a severe, potentially fatal illness accompanied by multiorgan failure. Acute illness manifests with the abrupt onset of fever, rigors, myalgias, and headache in 75% to 100% of patients. Conjunctival suffusion in a patient with a nonspecific febrile illness accompanied by lymphadenopathy, hepatomegaly, and splenomegaly points to a diagnosis of leptospirosis.

During the second phase of illness, fever is less pronounced, but headache and myalgias can be severe, and aseptic meningitis is an important manifestation. In some patients with leptospirosis, the clinical course may be complicated by jaundice (although liver failure is rare), renal failure, uveitis, hemorrhage, ARDS, myocarditis, and rhabdomyolysis (i.e., Weil syndrome).

Because the clinical features and routine laboratory findings of leptospirosis are not specific, a high index of suspicion must be maintained. The diagnosis is usually made by serologic testing for *L. interrogans*. Symptomatic individuals warrant treatment with doxycycline.

Brucellosis

Brucellosis is a zoonotic infection caused by *Brucella melitensis*. It is transmitted to humans by contact with fluids from infected animals (e.g., sheep, cattle, goats, pigs) or derived food products such as unpasteurized milk and cheese.

Clinical manifestations of brucellosis include fever, night sweats, malaise, anorexia, arthralgias, fatigue, weight loss, and depression. Patients may have fever and a multitude of complaints but no other objective findings. The onset of symptoms may be abrupt or insidious, developing over several days to weeks. The musculoskeletal and genitourinary systems are the most common sites of involvement. Neurobrucellosis, endocarditis, and hepatic abscesses occur in 1% to 2% of cases.

The diagnosis of brucellosis should be considered for an individual with otherwise unexplained fever and nonspecific complaints who has had a possible exposure. Ideally, the diagnosis is made by culture of the organism from blood or other sites, such as bone marrow. Serologic tests include tube agglutination and enzyme-linked immunosorbent assay (ELISA). For adults with nonfocal disease, treatment with doxycycline and rifampin is suggested.

Fever and Rash

The most concerning diseases associated with fever and rash are meningococcemia, staphylococcal TSS, and RMSF.

Bacterial Meningitis

Neisseria meningitidis is the leading cause of bacterial meningitis in children and young adults in the United States. Recent experience in New York City identified HIV patients as being at increased risk for meningococcal disease.

Manifestations of meningococcal disease can range from transient fever and bacteremia to fulminant disease, with death ensuing within hours of the onset of clinical symptoms. Acute systemic meningococcal disease may manifest as one of three syndromes: meningitis alone, meningitis with accompanying meningococcemia, and meningococcemia without clinical evidence of meningitis.

The typical initial symptoms of meningitis due to *N. meningitidis* consists of the sudden onset of fever, nausea, vomiting, headache, decreased ability to concentrate, and myalgias in an otherwise healthy patient. A petechial rash appears as discrete lesions 1 to 2 mm in diameter, most frequently occurring on the trunk and lower portions of the body. More than 50% of patients have petechiae at clinical presentation. Petechiae can coalesce into larger purpuric and ecchymotic lesions.

Staphylococcal Toxic Shock Syndrome

S. aureus strains produce exotoxins that cause three syndromes: food poisoning, caused by ingestion of *S. aureus* enterotoxin; scalded skin syndrome, caused by exfoliative toxin; and TSS, caused by toxic shock syndrome toxin 1 (TSST-1) and other enterotoxins. About one half

表 3.6　不明原因发热的常见原因
感染
脓肿
布鲁氏菌病
导管感染
巨细胞病毒感染
球孢子菌病
组织胞浆菌病
人类免疫缺陷病毒（HIV）感染
感染性心内膜炎
腹腔内、膈下及盆腔脓肿
肝及胆道疾病
莱姆病
结核分枝杆菌感染
骨髓炎
鼻窦炎
弓形虫病
尿路感染
自身免疫病
成人斯蒂尔病
家族性地中海热
结节病
类风湿关节炎
系统性红斑狼疮
颞动脉炎
恶性肿瘤
肝细胞癌
白血病
转移癌
胰腺癌
肾细胞癌
其他病因
深静脉血栓、肺栓塞
甲状腺功能亢进
菊池病
周期热（肿瘤坏死因子受体相关）

急性 Q 热通常临床较轻，可在 2 周内自发缓解。Q 热心内膜炎通常见于有既往瓣膜损害或免疫抑制的患者，常是慢性感染最主要的表现。

免疫荧光检测是 Q 热血清学诊断的参考方法。仅对有症状的患者考虑尽快使用多西环素治疗。

钩端螺旋体病

钩端螺旋体病是由问号钩端螺旋体引起的人畜共患感染，临床表现千变万化。该病在全球范围内均有分布，但绝大多数临床病例发生于热带地区。这种微生物可以感染啮齿类、牛、猪、狗、马、绵羊及山羊，可通过尿液排出。人类常在接触环境源如污染的水源后发生感染。

钩端螺旋体病的表现包括亚临床疾病继之血清转换、自限性的全身感染，或严重的伴多脏器衰竭的致命性疾病。75%～100% 的急性感染患者表现为骤起发热、寒战、肌痛和头痛。非特异性发热伴淋巴结肿大、肝脾大的患者如出现结膜充血，提示钩端螺旋体病的可能。

在疾病的第二阶段，发热有所缓解，但头痛和肌痛可能很严重，无菌性脑膜炎是该阶段的重要表现。在某些钩端螺旋体病的患者中，临床病程中可并发黄疸（尽管肝衰竭少见）、肾功能不全、葡萄膜炎、出血、ARDS、心肌炎及横纹肌溶解（即 Weil 综合征）。

由于钩端螺旋体病的临床特征和常规实验室检查都不特异，应对本病保持高度警惕。通常通过问号钩端螺旋体的血清学检测做出诊断。有症状的患者应接受多西环素治疗。

布鲁氏菌病

布鲁氏菌病是由马耳他布鲁氏菌引起的人畜共患感染。通过接触感染动物（如绵羊、牛、山羊、猪）的体液，或其相关食物制品如未经巴氏消毒的牛奶和奶酪，而传染给人类。

布鲁氏菌病的临床表现包括发热、盗汗、不适、厌食、关节痛、疲乏、体重下降和抑郁。患者可能存在发热和一系列主诉，但没有其他客观发现。症状可急骤或隐匿起病，发展数日或数周。肌肉骨骼和泌尿生殖系统是最常见的受累系统。1%～2% 患者可能出现神经布鲁氏菌病、心内膜炎及肝脓肿。

在发热伴非特异性症状的患者中，如除外其他病因又有可能的暴露史，应考虑布鲁氏菌病诊断的可能。血或其他部位如骨髓培养阳性是理想的诊断依据。血清学检测包括试管凝集试验和酶联免疫吸附试验（ELISA）。对于无局部病灶的成人患者，推荐使用多西环素和利福平治疗。

发热和皮疹

发热和皮疹相关的最紧要的疾病为脑膜炎球菌血症、葡萄球菌 TSS 和 RMSF。

细菌性脑膜炎

脑膜炎奈瑟球菌是美国儿童和青年细菌性脑膜炎的首要病因。纽约市近期的经验表明 HIV 患者患脑膜炎球菌病的风险升高。

脑膜炎球菌病可出现从一过性发热和菌血症，到暴发型疾病等不同表现，后者在临床症状出现后数小时内即死亡。急性全身性脑膜炎球菌病可表现为以下三种综合征之一：单纯脑膜炎、脑膜炎伴脑膜炎球菌血症，以及无脑膜炎临床证据的脑膜炎球菌血症。

脑膜炎奈瑟球菌脑膜炎在既往健康者中的典型初期症状包括骤起发热、恶心、呕吐、头痛、注意力不集中以及肌痛。可出现分散性瘀点皮疹，直径 1～2 mm，最常见于躯干和躯体下部。50% 以上患者临床会出现瘀点。瘀点也可相互融合形成更大的紫癜或瘀斑型皮损。

葡萄球菌中毒性休克综合征

金黄色葡萄球菌菌株产生的外毒素可导致三种综合征：食物中毒——进食金黄色葡萄球菌外毒素所致；烫伤样皮肤综合征——由剥脱毒素引起；以及 TSS——由中毒休克综合征毒素 1（TSST-1）及其他外毒素引起。

of reported TSS cases are menstrual, associated with bacterial growth on highly absorbent tampons. Non-menstrual TSS has been associated with surgical and postpartum wound infections, mastitis, septorhinoplasty, sinusitis, osteomyelitis, arthritis, burns, cutaneous and subcutaneous lesions (especially of the extremities, perianal area, and axillae), and respiratory infections after influenza. Some MRSA strains can produce TSST-1, and patients infected with these strains may develop TSS.

The Centers for Disease Control and Prevention (CDC) case definition for a confirmed case includes several criteria. Patients must have fever greater than 38.9° C, hypotension, diffuse erythroderma, desquamation (unless the patient dies before desquamation can occur), and involvement of at least three organ systems. Although 80% to 90% of TSS patients have *S. aureus* isolated from mucosal or wound sites, the isolation of *S. aureus* is not required for the diagnosis of staphylococcal TSS.

Rickettsial Infections

RMSF is a potentially lethal but usually curable tick-borne disease. Most cases of RMSF occur in the spring and early summer in endemic areas, particularly in the south central and southeastern states, when outdoor activity is most common. The etiologic agent, *Rickettsia rickettsii*, is a gram-negative, obligate intracellular bacterium that is usually transmitted through a tick bite. Up to one third of patients with proven RMSF do not recall a recent tick bite or recent tick contact.

In the early phases of illness, most patients have nonspecific signs and symptoms such as fever, headache, malaise, myalgias, arthralgias, and nausea with or without vomiting. Most patients with RMSF develop a rash between the third and fifth days of illness. The rash typically begins with pink, blanching macules that evolve to a deep red color and then become hemorrhagic. The lesions begin at the wrists, forearms, and ankles and then spread to the arms, thighs, trunk, and face.

The diagnosis of RMSF is based on a constellation of symptoms and signs in an appropriate epidemiologic setting (e.g., endemic area in the spring or early summer). In later illness, the diagnosis can be made by skin biopsy and confirmed serologically.

Murine typhus is a worldwide illness caused by *Rickettsia typhi* organisms that are transmitted by fleas. It produces a moderately severe illness characterized by fever, rash, and headache. Disease in the United States has been reported in Texas and Southern California.

Rickettsia africae, the cause of African tick-bite fever, occurs in travelers returning from East Africa. It produces a large eschar with a febrile syndrome similar to RMSF. Rickettsial infections respond to treatment with doxycycline and warrant rapid initiation of treatment.

Lyme Disease

Lyme disease is a tick-borne illness caused by pathogenic species of the spirochete *Borrelia burgdorferi* in the United States. Other species in Europe and Asia can cause more aggressive presentations. Localized disease includes erythema migrans in 80% of patients and nonspecific findings that resemble a viral syndrome. Erythema migrans is an expanding macule that forms an annular lesion with a clearing middle.

Early disseminated Lyme disease with acute neurologic or cardiac involvement usually occurs weeks to several months after the tick bite and may be the first manifestation of the disease. Nonspecific symptoms (e.g., headache, fatigue, arthralgias) may persist for months after treatment of Lyme disease. There is no evidence that these persistent subjective complaints represent ongoing active infection. Co-infection with *Babesia* and *Ehrlichia* is common, and these infections should be considered in persons diagnosed with Lyme disease.

Human Ehrlichiosis

The principal vector of *Ehrlichia chaffeensis*, the agent that causes human monocytic ehrlichiosis (HME), is the Lone Star tick (*Amblyomma americanum*). Patients typically have an acute illness that has an incubation period of 1 to 2 weeks. Most patients are febrile and have nonspecific symptoms such as malaise, myalgia, headache, and chills.

One feature that may distinguish HME from human granulocytic anaplasmosis (HGA), another tick-borne illness caused by *Anaplasma phagocytophilum*, is a rash (macular, maculopapular, or petechial). This rash occurs in about 30% of patients with HME but is rare in patients with HGA.

The preferred and most widely available diagnostic method for ehrlichiosis is the indirect fluorescent antibody test. The diagnosis should be considered in all patients with Lyme disease or babesiosis. Treatment with doxycycline should be initiated for all patients suspected of having ehrlichiosis or anaplasmosis.

Viral Infections Associated With Rash

The typical manifestations of viral infections associated with rash may unequivocally establish the cause of a febrile syndrome. For example, varicella-zoster virus infection manifests with distinctive lesions of chickenpox or herpes zoster (i.e., shingles). The resurgence of measles mandates the ability to recognize its rash.

Acute onset of high fever characterizes viral hemorrhagic fevers, along with bleeding complications and high mortality rates in some cases. Arthropods often transmit viral infections, including dengue, which is one of the most common causes of fever in returned travelers.

Fever With Lymphadenopathy

Generalized and localized lymphadenopathy can be major manifestations of some infectious diseases, such as in mononucleosis syndromes, tuberculosis, HIV infection, and pyogenic infections.

Infectious mononucleosis is characterized by a triad of fever, tonsillar pharyngitis, and lymphadenopathy. EBV is a widely disseminated herpesvirus that is spread by intimate contact between susceptible persons and EBV shedders. Lymph node involvement in infectious mononucleosis is typically symmetrical and more commonly involves the posterior cervical than the anterior chains. The posterior cervical nodes are deep beneath the sternocleidomastoid muscles and must be carefully palpated. The nodes may be large and moderately tender. Lymphadenopathy may also become more generalized including enlargement of the spleen, which distinguishes infectious mononucleosis from other causes of pharyngitis.

Lymphadenopathy peaks in the first week and then gradually subsides over 2 to 3 weeks. Splenomegaly is seen in 50% of patients with infectious mononucleosis and usually begins to recede by the third week of the illness.

Patients with a clinical picture of infectious mononucleosis should have a white blood cell count with differential and a heterophile (Monospot) test. If the heterophile test result is positive, no further testing is necessary when the clinical scenario is compatible with typical infectious mononucleosis. If the heterophile test result is negative but there is still a strong clinical suspicion of EBV infection, the Monospot test can be repeated because results can be negative early in clinical illness.

If the clinical syndrome is prolonged or the patient does not have a classic EBV syndrome, immunoglobulin M (IgM) and immunoglobulin G (IgG) viral capsule antigen (VCA) and Epstein-Barr nuclear antigen (EBNA) antibodies should be measured. IgG EBNA detected within 4 weeks of symptom onset excludes acute primary EBV infection as an explanation and should prompt consideration of EBV-negative causes of mononucleosis.

Cytomegalovirus

The spectrum of human illness caused by CMV is diverse and mostly depends on the host. CMV infection in the immunocompetent host

约半数报道的 TSS 病例发生于经期，与高吸力卫生棉条的细菌繁殖有关。非经期相关的 TSS 多与手术及产后伤口感染、乳腺炎、鼻中隔成形术、鼻窦炎、骨髓炎、关节炎、烧伤、表皮和皮下病灶（尤其是肢端、肛周及腋窝区域）以及流感后呼吸道感染等相关。某些 MRSA 菌株可产生 TSST-1，而感染这些菌株的患者可发生 TSS。

美国 CDC 对确诊病例的定义包括若干条标准。患者需具备发热超过 38.9℃、低血压、弥漫性红皮病、皮肤脱屑（除非患者在进入皮肤脱屑阶段前死亡），并累及至少三个器官系统。尽管 80%～90% TSS 患者可从黏膜或伤口部位分离到金黄色葡萄球菌，分离阳性并非葡萄球菌性 TSS 诊断的必要条件。

立克次体感染

落基山斑点热（RMSF）是潜在致命但可治疗的蜱传疾病。大多数 RMSF 病例发生于春季和初夏等户外活动频繁时节的流行区，尤其是美国中南部和东南部州。其病原体立氏立克次体，是一种革兰氏阴性的专性胞内菌，常通过蜱叮咬传播。多达 1/3 确诊 RMSF 的患者并未回忆出近期的蜱叮咬或蜱接触史。

在疾病的早期阶段，大部分患者表现为非特异性症状和体征，如发热、头痛、不适、肌痛、关节痛及恶心伴或不伴呕吐。多数 RMSF 患者在病程的第 3～5 天会出现皮疹。典型的皮疹初为粉色、是压之褪色的斑疹，逐渐变为深红色、出血性皮疹。皮损起始于腕部、前臂、踝部，随后扩展至上臂、大腿、躯干和面部。

RMSF 的诊断是基于合理流行场景下（如流行区的春季或初夏季节）临床症状体征的集合。在病程晚期，诊断可以通过皮肤活检及血清学检测确诊。

鼠型斑疹伤寒是由斑疹伤寒立克次体引发的全球分布性疾病，经虱传播。会引起中度严重的疾病，以发热、皮疹和头痛为主要特征。美国在田纳西州和加利福尼亚州南部有病例报道。

非洲立克次体是非洲蜱咬热的病原体，在东非返回的旅行者中可有出现。该病会产生较大焦痂，并出现与 RMSF 类似的发热性综合征。立克次体感染对多西环素治疗的反应良好，需快速启动治疗。

莱姆病

莱姆病是美国由伯氏疏螺旋体中致病种类导致的蜱传疾病。欧洲和亚洲的其他品种可能导致更具侵袭性的临床表现。局灶性疾病中约 80% 患者可出现游走性红斑，也可出现与病毒感染综合征相似的非特异性改变。游走性红斑是扩大性斑疹，形成其中央苍白圈的环形病损。

早期播散性莱姆病伴急性神经系统或心脏受累，通常发生于蜱叮咬后的数周至数月，脏器受累可以作为该病的首发表现。非特异性症状（如头痛、疲劳、关节痛）在莱姆病治疗后仍可持续数月。尚无证据表明这些持续的主观症状提示持续的活动性感染。与巴贝虫病和埃立克体的合并感染很常见，在已诊断为莱姆病的患者中也应考虑到这些感染。

人埃立克体病

查菲埃立克体是导致人单核细胞埃立克体病（HME）的主要病原，其传播的主要媒介为孤星蜱（美国钝眼蜱）。患者通常为急性病程，潜伏期 1～2 周。多数患者出现发热及非特异性症状如不适、肌痛、头痛和寒战。

区别 HME 与人嗜粒细胞无形体病（HGA，由嗜吞噬细胞无形体导致的另一种蜱传疾病）的特征之一是皮疹（斑疹、斑丘疹或瘀点）。皮疹在约 30% 的 HME 患者中出现，但在 HGA 患者中罕见。

优选及最广泛开展的埃立克体病诊断方法是间接荧光抗体检测。在所有莱姆病或巴贝虫病的患者中均应考虑这一诊断的可能。对所有怀疑埃立克体病或无形体病的患者均应启动多西环素治疗。

出疹性病毒感染

出疹性病毒感染的典型表现可以明确诊断发热性综合征的病因。例如，水痘-带状疱疹病毒感染表现为水痘或带状疱疹（俗称"缠腰龙"）的特征性皮疹。麻疹的再度流行则对其皮疹识别能力提出了要求。

急性起病的高热是病毒性出血热的特征表现，可合并出血并发症，某些病例的病死率较高。节肢动物常传播病毒感染，包括登革热，这也是旅行者返回后发热最常见的原因之一。

发热伴淋巴结肿大

全身及局部淋巴结肿大可成为某些感染性疾病的主要临床表现，如单核细胞增多症、结核病、HIV 感染及化脓性感染。

传染性单核细胞增多症以发热、扁桃体咽炎及淋巴结肿大三联征为特征。EBV 是广泛存在的疱疹病毒，主要通过易感者与 EBV 排毒者密切接触而传播。传染性单核细胞增多症中淋巴结的受累通常是对称的，颈后部淋巴结的受累较颈前部更为常见。颈后淋巴结位于胸锁乳突肌的深部，需要仔细触诊。淋巴结可出现增大和轻度压痛。淋巴结肿大可更为广泛，包括出现脾大，这也是传染性单核细胞增多症与其他原因咽炎的鉴别点。

淋巴结肿大在第 1 周时达到高峰，随后 2～3 周逐渐消退。脾大可见于 50% 的传染性单核细胞增多症患者，通常在病程第 3 周开始逐渐缓解。

具有传染性单核细胞增多症临床表现的患者应当进行白细胞分类计数以及嗜异性抗体检测。如嗜异性抗体检测为阳性，且临床症状符合典型的传染性单核细胞增多症，则不需要再进行其他检查。如嗜异性抗体检测为阴性但临床仍高度怀疑 EBV 感染，可以再重复嗜异性抗体检测，因疾病早期其结果可能为阴性。

如临床症状迁延或患者不具备典型 EBV 综合征表现，应检测病毒衣壳蛋白（VCA）及 EB 核抗原（EBNA）的免疫球蛋白 M（IgM）和免疫球蛋白 G（IgG）抗体。起

usually is asymptomatic or may manifest as a mononucleosis-like syndrome. Transmission occurs through multiple routes.

The mononucleosis syndrome associated with CMV infection has been described as typhoidal because systemic symptoms and fever predominate, and signs of enlarged cervical nodes and splenomegaly are not as commonly seen as they are in EBV infection. Diarrhea, fever, fatigue, abdominal pain, and mildly abnormal liver enzymes are common findings. Immunocompromised patients, such as those who have received transplants, may have serious, life-threatening infections such as pneumonitis, hepatitis, colitis, and retinitis. Serology provides indirect evidence of recent CMV infection based on changes in antibody titers at different time points during the clinical illness. Serologies are also helpful in determining past exposure to CMV. This information is particularly relevant for monitoring immunosuppressed hosts at risk for CMV reactivation syndromes.

Primary Human Immunodeficiency Virus Infection

Most cases of new HIV infection are passed asymptomatically, and routine testing of sexually active persons should be performed as part of good primary care. All patients with mononucleosis syndromes should undergo HIV testing. Published series consistently report that the most common findings of acute HIV are fever, generalized lymphadenopathy, sore throat, rash, myalgia or arthralgia, and headache when symptomatic.

Toxoplasmosis

Toxoplasmosis, an infection with a worldwide distribution, is caused by the intracellular protozoan parasite *T. gondii*. Humans can acquire *Toxoplasma* organisms through ingestion of contaminated meat, vertical transmission, blood transfusion, exposure to oocysts from cat feces, or organ transplantation.

Immunocompetent persons with primary infection are usually asymptomatic, but latent infection can persist for the life of the host. When symptomatic infection does occur, the most common manifestation is bilateral, symmetrical, nontender cervical adenopathy. Patients may have headache, fever, and fatigue. Symptoms usually resolve within several weeks. In AIDS patients or other immunocompromised hosts who have been previously infected, *T. gondii* infection may reactivate in the brain, causing abscesses and encephalitis.

Infections Causing Regional Lymphadenopathy

Scrofula (i.e., tuberculous cervical adenitis) develops in a subacute to chronic pattern. Low-grade fever is usually associated with a large mass of matted cervical lymph nodes. In children, *M. tuberculosis* is the etiologic agent, but in adults, *Mycobacterium avium* complex and *Mycobacterium scrofulaceum* are more commonly found. Surgical excision is the treatment of choice.

Cat-Scratch Disease

Cat-scratch disease, a condition caused by *Bartonella henselae*, is characterized by self-limited regional lymphadenopathy after a cat scratch or transmission from another vector. Other manifestations can include visceral organ, neurologic, and ocular involvement. In 85% to 90% of children, cat-scratch disease manifests as a localized cutaneous and lymph node disorder near the site of organism inoculation. In some individuals, the organisms disseminate and infect the liver, spleen, eye, bone, or CNS. Patients with localized disease usually have a self-limited illness, whereas those with disseminated disease can have life-threatening complications. *B. henselae* infection should be considered in the initial evaluation of FUO in children.

The diagnosis of cat-scratch disease is based on typical clinical findings (i.e., lymphadenopathy) associated with probable exposure to cats or fleas. Laboratory testing that supports the diagnosis includes a positive *B. henselae* antibody titer or biopsy of a lymph node with a positive Warthin-Starry stain or polymerase chain reaction (PCR) analysis of tissue.

Pyogenic Infection

S. aureus and group A streptococcal (GAS) infections can produce acute, suppurative lymphadenitis. Enlarged and tender lymph nodes usually are found in the submandibular, cervical, axillary, or inguinal areas. Patients have fever and leukocytosis. Pyoderma, pharyngitis, and periodontal infections are usually the primary sites of infection. Management includes drainage and antibiotics.

Plague

Bubonic plague is a bacterial syndrome caused by *Yersinia pestis* that usually consists of fever, headache, and a large mat of inguinal, axillary, or cervical lymph nodes. Lymph nodes suppurate and drain spontaneously. The diagnosis should be considered for acutely ill patients in the southwestern United States with possible exposure to fleas and rodents. Gram-negative coccobacilli can be seen in lymph node aspirates. The characteristic safety-pin appearance of *Y. pestis* with dark blue staining of polar bodies is seen with Wayson stain.

Sexually Transmitted Diseases

Inguinal lymphadenopathy associated with sexually transmitted diseases can be unilateral or bilateral. In primary syphilis, enlarged nodes are discrete, firm, and nontender. Tender lymphadenopathies with matting are seen in lymphogranuloma venereum. The lymphadenopathy of chancroid is most often unilateral and manifests with pain and fused lymph nodes. Primary genital herpes infection also causes tender inguinal lymphadenopathy.

FACTITIOUS FEVER AND SELF-INDUCED ILLNESS

In most case series, factitious fever or self-induced illness is a relatively uncommon cause of FUO, but it may occur more often than generally appreciated. Patients with these conditions are often young women, and 50% have had training in some aspect of health care. They are often well educated, cooperative, articulate, and manipulative of family and caregivers. Patients can no longer manipulate thermometers because electronic or infrared thermometry is used, and causing factitious fever is difficult. Clues to the factitious fever diagnosis include absence of a toxic appearance despite high temperature readings, lack of tachycardia, and absent diurnal variation. Patients may appear well between episodes of fever.

Genuine fever can be induced if an individual injects or ingests pyrogenic substances such as bacterial suspensions, urine, or feces. Although intermittent polymicrobial bacteremia may suggest a diagnosis of intra-abdominal abscess, it represents self-induced infection. The discovery of needles and substances for injection in the patient's belongings may help in the diagnosis.

In most cases, a psychogenic basis for the behavior is assumed. However, one study with detailed psychological patient analyses found no evidence of major psychiatric diagnoses among individuals with self-induced or simulated illnesses. Munchausen syndrome and Munchausen by proxy are the most extreme forms of factitious fever. Patients often agree stoically to numerous highly invasive procedures to diagnose and treat themselves or their children (i.e., proxy). All of these individuals require objective but complete, tactful, and compassionate assessments and considerable psychiatric care.

病4周内检测到 IgG EBNA 可排除急性原发 EBV 感染的可能，而需考虑 EBV 以外的单核细胞增多症病因。

巨细胞病毒感染

CMV 可引起的人类疾病谱多样，主要取决于宿主本身。免疫正常宿主的 CMV 感染通常无症状，也可表现为单核细胞增多症样综合征。传播有多种途径。

CMV 感染相关的单核细胞增多症也被描述为"伤寒样的"，因为其主要表现为全身症状和发热，而淋巴结肿大和脾大的体征不如 EBV 感染常见。腹泻、发热、疲乏、腹痛及轻度肝酶异常较为常见。免疫功能低下宿主，如移植后人群，可出现严重而危及生命的感染如肺炎、肝炎、结肠炎和视网膜炎。基于病程不同时间点的抗体滴度变化，血清学检测可提供近期 CMV 感染的间接证据。血清学检测也有助于确定既往 CMV 暴露。这一信息特别适用于监测免疫抑制宿主发生 CMV 再活化综合征的风险。

急性 HIV 感染

绝大多数新发 HIV 感染病例是无症状的，对性活跃人群的常规检测应当成为良好初级保健的一部分。所有出现单核细胞增多症表现的患者均应进行 HIV 检测。发表的病例系列一致报道急性 HIV 感染最常见的症状为发热、全身淋巴结肿大、咽痛、皮疹、肌痛或关节痛，以及头痛。

弓形虫病

弓形虫病是一种由胞内寄生原虫刚地弓形虫导致的感染，呈全球性分布。人类可因摄入污染的肉类、垂直传播、输血、接触猫粪中卵囊，或器官移植而感染弓形虫。

免疫正常个体的原发感染往往无症状，但潜伏感染可持续宿主终身。发生症状性感染时，最常见的症状为双侧、对称性、无痛性的颈部淋巴结肿大。患者可出现头痛、发热和疲乏。症状通常在数周后可自行缓解。在 AIDS 患者或其他免疫低下人群中，刚地弓形虫感染可能在脑中再活化，导致脓肿和脑炎。

导致局部淋巴结肿大的感染

瘰疬（即结核性颈部淋巴结炎）为亚急性或慢性病程，常出现低热伴大块成堆的颈部淋巴结。儿童中病原体为结核分枝杆菌，但成人中更常见鸟分枝杆菌复合群和瘰疬分枝杆菌。手术切除是治疗之选。

猫抓病

猫抓病由汉赛巴尔通体引起，以猫抓伤或其他媒介传染后出现自限性的区域淋巴结肿大为特征。其他表现可包括内脏器官、神经及眼受累。85%～90%的儿童中，猫抓病表现为微生物接种部位附近局限性的皮肤及淋巴结肿大。在某些个体中，病原体播散而感染肝、脾、眼、骨或 CNS。局灶性疾病的患者通常为自限性疾病，而播散性病变的患者可能出现危及生命的并发症。在儿童 FUO 的初始评价中应考虑到汉赛巴尔通体感染。

猫抓病的诊断取决于典型的临床症状（如淋巴结肿大）伴可能的猫或蚤类接触史。支持诊断的实验室检测包括汉赛尔巴通体抗体滴度阳性，或淋巴结活检沃森-斯塔里银染色或组织聚合酶链反应（PCR）为阳性。

化脓性感染

金黄色葡萄球菌和 A 组链球菌（GAS）感染可出现急性化脓性淋巴结炎。常可在颌下、颈部、腋窝或腹股沟区域见增大伴压痛的淋巴结。患者可出现发热和白细胞增高。皮肤脓肿、咽炎及牙周感染通常为原发感染部位。治疗包括引流和抗生素治疗。

鼠疫

腺鼠疫是一种由鼠疫耶尔森菌引起的细菌性综合征，常出现发热、头痛及增大融合的腹股沟、腋窝或颈部淋巴结。淋巴结可出现自发的化脓和破溃。美国西南部地区急性起病的患者，如可能有蚤和啮齿类接触史，需要考虑疑诊。淋巴结抽吸液中能发现革兰氏阴性的球杆菌。使用魏森染色能观察到特征性的带深蓝色极体的别针样菌体。

性传播疾病

性传播疾病相关的腹股沟淋巴结肿大可为单侧或双侧。在一期梅毒中，肿大淋巴结分散、坚硬且无痛。成堆的痛性淋巴结肿大可见于性病性淋巴肉芽肿。软下疳的淋巴结肿大最常见为单侧，伴疼痛和淋巴结融合。原发生殖器疱疹感染也常引起痛性腹股沟淋巴结肿大。

伪热和自身诱发的疾病

在多数病例系列中，伪热或自身诱发的疾病是 FUO 相对少见的病因，但实际可能比想象中更常见。出现此类情况的患者往往是年轻女性，其中 50% 曾接受过健康照护某些方面的训练，通常教育良好、具有合作性、表达清晰且可操纵家庭成员及护理员。由于电子或红外测温计的使用，患者现在无法操纵体温计，使得造出伪热更加困难。伪热的诊断线索包括体温读数较高时无中毒症状、无心动过速、缺失昼夜变化等。患者发热后往往状态良好。

注射或服用化脓性介质如细菌混悬液、尿或粪便，可诱发出真性发热。尽管间断的复数菌菌血症可能提示腹腔内脓肿，这也是人为感染的表现。在个人物品中发现针头以及注射针剂可能有助于诊断。

多数情况下，认为该行为存在精神性根源。然而，一项研究进行了详细的患者心理分析，并未发现在自身诱发的疾病的患者中存在显著的精神性疾病诊断。孟乔森综合征以及代理型孟乔森综合征是伪热的最极端形式。患者往往同意忍受无数高度有创的操作以诊断和治疗自己或自己的孩子（即代理型）。这些个体均需要客观但完整、有灵活度和有同情心的评估，也需要很多精神心理照护。

SUGGESTED READINGS

Aduan RP, Fauci AS, Dale DC, et al: Factitious fever and self-induced infection: a report of 32 cases and review of the literature, Ann Intern Med 90:230–242, 1979.

Aduan RP, Fauci AS, Dale DC, et al: Prolonged fever of unknown origin (FUO): a prospective study of 347 patients, Clin Res 26:558A, 1978.

Brown I, Finnigan NA: Fever of unknown origin (FUO). In StatPearls [Internet], Treasure Island (FL), 2019, StatPearls Publishing. [Updated 2018 Nov 18]. Available from: https://www.ncbi.nlm.nih.gov/books/NBK532265.

Cannon J: Perspective on fever: the basic science and conventional medicine, Complement Ther Med 21(Suppl 1):S54–S60, 2013.

Osilla EV, Sharma S: Physiology, temperature regulation. In StatPearls [Internet], Treasure Island (FL), 2019, StatPearls Publishing. [Updated 2019 Mar 16]. Available from: https://www.ncbi.nlm.nih.gov/books/NBK507838.

Weber D, Cohen M, Rutala W: The acutely ill patient with fever and rash. In Bennett JE, Dolin R, Blaser M, editors: MandellDouglas and Bennett's principles and practice of infectious diseases, ed 8, Elsevier, 2015, pp 732–747.

推荐阅读

Aduan RP, Fauci AS, Dale DC, et al: Factitious fever and self-induced infection: a report of 32 cases and review of the literature, Ann Intern Med 90:230–242, 1979.

Aduan RP, Fauci AS, Dale DC, et al: Prolonged fever of unknown origin (FUO): a prospective study of 347 patients, Clin Res 26:558A, 1978.

Brown I, Finnigan NA: Fever of unknown origin (FUO). In StatPearls [Internet], Treasure Island (FL), 2019, StatPearls Publishing. [Updated 2018 Nov 18]. Available from: https://www.ncbi.nlm.nih.gov/books/NBK532265.

Cannon J: Perspective on fever: the basic science and conventional medicine, Complement Ther Med 21(Suppl 1):S54–S60, 2013.

Osilla EV, Sharma S: Physiology, temperature regulation. In StatPearls [Internet], Treasure Island (FL), 2019, StatPearls Publishing. [Updated 2019 Mar 16]. Available from: https://www.ncbi.nlm.nih.gov/books/NBK507838.

Weber D, Cohen M, Rutala W: The acutely ill patient with fever and rash. In Bennett JE, Dolin R, Blaser M, editors: MandellDouglas and Bennett's principles and practice of infectious diseases, ed 8, Elsevier, 2015, pp 732–747.

4

Bacteremia and Sepsis

Russell J. McCulloh, Steven M. Opal

DEFINITION

Sepsis is a leading cause of morbidity and death among hospitalized patients. The disease process results from a complex interplay of host immune responses and infectious microorganisms. In 2016 an international panel of experts released an updated definition of sepsis, specifying it as life-threatening organ dysfunction caused by a dysregulated host response to infection. Manifestations can include fever, altered mental status, and abnormalities in inflammation and coagulation. Severe cases can progress to multiple organ system dysfunction followed by organ failure and death.

Diagnostic criteria for sepsis are provided in Table 4.1. The term "severe sepsis," once recognized as a separate entity defined by more severe organ dysfunction, is now synonymous with the current definition of sepsis and should no longer be used. Septic shock is a combination of sepsis and persistent hypotension and tissue hypoperfusion despite adequate fluid resuscitation or the need to use vasopressors to maintain a mean arterial pressure (MAP) at 65 mm Hg or greater and in addition an elevated serum lactate greater than 2 mmol/L. The continuum of disease manifestations from localized infection to multiorgan failure and refractory septic shock is depicted in Fig. 4.1.

Sepsis is a situation in which the infection-induced systemic inflammatory and coagulopathic responses have become injurious to the host. Sepsis is an infectious process characterized by tissue injury from hypoperfusion and immune dysregulation. *Severe infection* should be used to describe an infection that is accompanied by systemic inflammation but without evidence of organ dysfunction remote from the site of infection (i.e., the former definition of sepsis). Whether these revised definitions can resolve the current confusion in terminology remains to be seen.

Understanding the pathophysiology of sepsis syndrome has proved helpful in differentiating and treating severe inflammatory processes that manifest with symptoms similar to sepsis, including pancreatitis, severe trauma, thermal burns, and certain toxin or environmental exposures. These processes can produce a systemic inflammatory response syndrome (SIRS), but they lack the component of infection needed to establish a diagnosis of sepsis. The remarkable clinical similarity between these severe "sterile" inflammations and septic shock reflects their molecular profiles. Identical signaling pathways for the immune response are activated by highly conserved pathogen-associated molecular patterns (PAMPs), which are molecular motifs recognized by cells of the host's innate immune system. Damage-associated molecular patterns (DAMPs) are molecules released by injured host cells that act as endogenous danger signals to promote the inflammatory response (see "Pathophysiology of Septic Shock" later in this chapter).

EPIDEMIOLOGY

The worldwide incidence of sepsis is difficult to assess due to limited data from developing countries. In industrialized countries, reported rates of sepsis range from 22 to 300 cases per 100,000 people. Sepsis may account for up to 6% of adult deaths. In the United States, more than 750,000 cases of sepsis and 200,000 sepsis-related deaths occur annually. The risk of mortality depends on the severity of illness and multiple host factors (discussed later). Overall, estimates of death from sepsis range from 20% of mild to moderate cases to more than 60% of patients with septic shock.

The financial impact of sepsis cases is immense. Each episode of sepsis costs approximately $50,000 in health care expenditures, for a total of more than $24 billion dollars in 2016 in the United States alone.

Bacterial infections are the most common cause of sepsis. Bloodstream infections due to bacteria account for the largest proportion of hospitalizations. The rates are highest for premature infants, the advanced elderly (especially those older than 85 years of age), and patients with intravenous catheters, implanted devices, or severe medical morbidities such as severe burns or hematologic malignancies.

Pathogens most commonly identified in bloodstream infections include staphylococci (e.g., *Staphylococcus aureus*), group A streptococci, *Escherichia coli*, *Klebsiella* species, *Enterobacter* species, and *Pseudomonas aeruginosa*. Immunocompromised patients and patients with long-term intravascular catheters are at increased risk for fungal bloodstream infections from *Candida* species, and some species may be resistant to commonly used antifungal medications. Given the broad variety of potential pathogens, clinicians face the dual challenges of an accurate and timely diagnosis and choice of appropriate empirical therapy.

Several epidemiologic factors can guide the clinician in cases of sepsis when a source has not been identified. Table 4.2 lists microorganisms that are associated with certain host factors that predispose a patient to infection and sepsis. Host factors associated with worse outcomes include extremes of age, use of immunomodulating medications, and concomitant chronic medical conditions.

Several diagnostic and treatment factors are associated with severity of illness and clinical outcome. Delay in effective antimicrobial therapy correlates with worse outcomes. Infection with multidrug-resistant organisms may cause a delay in effective therapy, and for some organisms, particularly gram-negative enteric rods, the delay may be independently related to worse outcomes. Certain organisms (e.g., *P. aeruginosa, Staphylococcus aureus*) are more virulent. The primary infection site also is important; respiratory sites are the most common, and the central nervous system often is the most lethal site of infection. The number of organ systems involved plays a role, with mortality increasing as the number of dysfunctional organ systems increases.

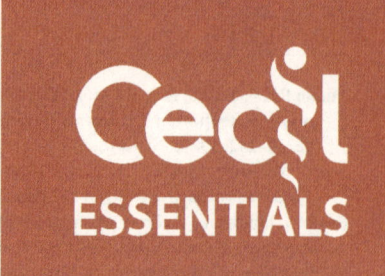

菌血症和感染中毒症

韩宁 译 肖江 张福杰 王芳 审校 张福杰 通审

定义

感染中毒症是住院患者发病和死亡的主要原因。该疾病过程源于宿主免疫反应和传染性微生物的复杂相互作用,2016年,一个国际专家小组发布了感染中毒症的最新定义,将其明确为由宿主感染反应失调引起的危及生命的器官功能障碍。临床表现可能包括发热、精神状态改变以及炎症和凝血方面的异常。严重的病例可能会发展为多器官系统功能障碍,并导致器官衰竭和死亡。

表4.1提供了感染中毒症的诊断标准。曾经的"严重感染中毒症"一词,被认定为由更严重器官功能障碍定义的单独的疾病,现在与当前感染中毒症的定义相同,不应再被使用。感染中毒性休克包含感染中毒症和持续性低血压和组织灌注不足,即使进行充分的液体复苏或需要使用血管升压素来保持65 mmHg或更高的平均动脉压(MAP),此外血清乳酸升高大于2 mmol/L。图4.1显示了从局部感染到多器官衰竭和难治性感染中毒性休克的连续性的疾病表现。

感染中毒症是指感染引发的系统性炎症和凝血反应,从而对宿主造成伤害。感染中毒症是一种感染性过程,其特征是灌注不足和免疫失调而造成的组织损伤。应使用严重感染来描述伴随全身炎症的感染,但没有证据表明远离感染部位的器官功能障碍(即以前感染中毒症的定义)。这些新修改的定义是否能够解决目前术语学上疑惑还有待进一步观察。

理解感染中毒症综合征的病理生理学已被证实有助于鉴别和治疗表现为类似于感染中毒症症状的严重炎症过程,包括胰腺炎、严重创伤、热烧伤以及某些毒素或环境暴露。这些过程可以造成全身炎症反应综合征(SIRS),但它们缺乏确定感染中毒症诊断所需的感染性的成分。这些严重的"无菌性"炎症和感染中毒性休克之间的显著临床相似性反映了它们的分子学特征。免疫反应的相同信号通路由高度保守的病原体相关分子模式(PAMP)激活,这些模式是宿主先天免疫系统细胞识别的分子基序。损伤相关分子模式(DAMP)是受伤的宿主细胞释放的分子,作为内源性危险信号,以促进炎症反应的发生(见本章后文的"感染中毒性休克的病理生理学"部分)。

流行病学

由于发展中国家的数据有限,全球感染中毒症发病率难以评估。在工业化国家,报告的感染中毒症发病率为每10万人22~300例不等。感染中毒症可能占成人死亡人数的6%。在美国,每年发生超过75万例感染中毒症病例和20万例感染中毒症相关死亡。死亡风险取决于疾病的严重程度和多种宿主因素(稍后讨论)。总体而言,感染中毒症死亡估计从轻度到中度病例的20%到感染中毒性休克患者的60%以上不等。

感染中毒症病例的财务影响是巨大的。每次感染中毒症发作的医疗保健支出约为5万美元,仅在美国,2016年的相关支出总计超过240亿美元。

细菌感染是感染中毒症最常见的原因。细菌引起的血流感染在住院人数中所占比例最大。早产儿、高龄老人(特别是85岁以上的人)以及带有静脉导管、植入性装置或严重医疗疾病(如重度烧伤或血液恶性肿瘤)的患者,发病率最高。

血流感染中最常见的病原体包括葡萄球菌(如金黄色葡萄球菌)、A组链球菌、大肠埃希菌、克雷伯菌、肠杆菌和铜绿假单胞菌。免疫功能低下的患者和长期携带血管内导管的患者患上念珠菌真菌血流感染的风险增加,一些病原体可能对常用的抗真菌药物有耐药性。鉴于潜在的病原体种类繁多,临床医生面临着准确和及时的诊断以及选择适当的经验疗法的双重挑战。

在尚未确定来源的情况下,几个流行病学因素可以指导临床医生治疗感染中毒症。表4.2列出了与某些宿主因素相关的微生物,这些宿主因素使患者容易发生感染和感染中毒症。与更差的结果相关的宿主因素包括高龄、免疫调节药物的使用以及伴随的慢性疾病。

几个诊断和治疗因素与疾病的严重程度和临床结果有关。有效抗菌治疗的延迟使用与更差的结果相关。多药耐药菌种的感染可能会导致有效治疗的延迟,对于一些病原体,特别是革兰氏阴性肠杆菌,延迟可能与更差的结果独立相关。某些病原体(如铜绿假单胞菌、金黄色葡萄球菌)更具有毒性。原发感染部位也很重要,呼吸道感染是最常见的,中枢神经系统通常是最致命的感染部位。所涉及的器官系统数量也有影响,死亡率随着功能失调的器官系统数量的增加而增加。

TABLE 4.1 Diagnostic Criteria for Sepsis[a]

General Criteria
Life-threatening organ dysfunction caused by a dysregulated response to infection

Organ Dysfunction Criteria
Change in Sequential (Sepsis-related) Organ Failure Assessment (SOFA)[b] score of ≥2 points. It can be used to measure the severity of organ dysfunction.

SOFA Scoring (Range 0–4 Per Category, 0–24 Total Score Range)

Criterion	0	1	2	3	4
Respiration; Pao_2/Fio_2 (torr)	>400	≤400	≤300	≤200 with respiratory support	≤100 with respiratory support
Platelets (×10³/mm³)	>150	≤150	≤100	≤50	≤20
Bilirubin (mg/dL)	<1.2	1.2–1.9	2.0–5.9	6.0–11.9	>12.0
Glasgow Coma Scale	15	13–14	10–12	6–9	<6
Hypotension[c]	None	MAP <70 mm Hg	Dopamine ≤5 or dobutamine (or any dose of vasopressin)	Dopamine >5 or epi ≤0.1 or norepi ≤0.1 (or phenylephrine 100–300 mcg bolus	Dopamine >15 or epi >0.1 or norepi >0.1 (or phenylephrine>300 mcg bolus
Creatinine (mg/dL) or urine output (mL/day)	<1.2	1.2–1.9	2.0–3.4	3.5–4.9 <500 mL/day	>5.0 <200 mL/day

Septic Shock Criteria
Vasopressor requirement to maintain a mean arterial pressure of 65 mm Hg or greater, AND
Hyperlactatemia (serum lactate >2 mmol/L [>18 mg/dL])

From Singer M, Deutschman CS, Seymour CW, et al: The Third International Consensus Definitions for Sepsis and Septic Shock (Sepsis-3), JAMA 315(8):801-10, 2016.
Fio_2, Fraction of inspired oxygen; INR, international normalized ratio; MAP, mean arterial pressure; Pao_2, partial pressure of oxygen.
[a]The criteria include documented or suspected infection and some of the variables listed.
[b]Assuming baseline SOFA of 0 in most cases.
[c]Adrenergic agents must be administered for at least 1 hour to count; doses are in mcg/kg/min.

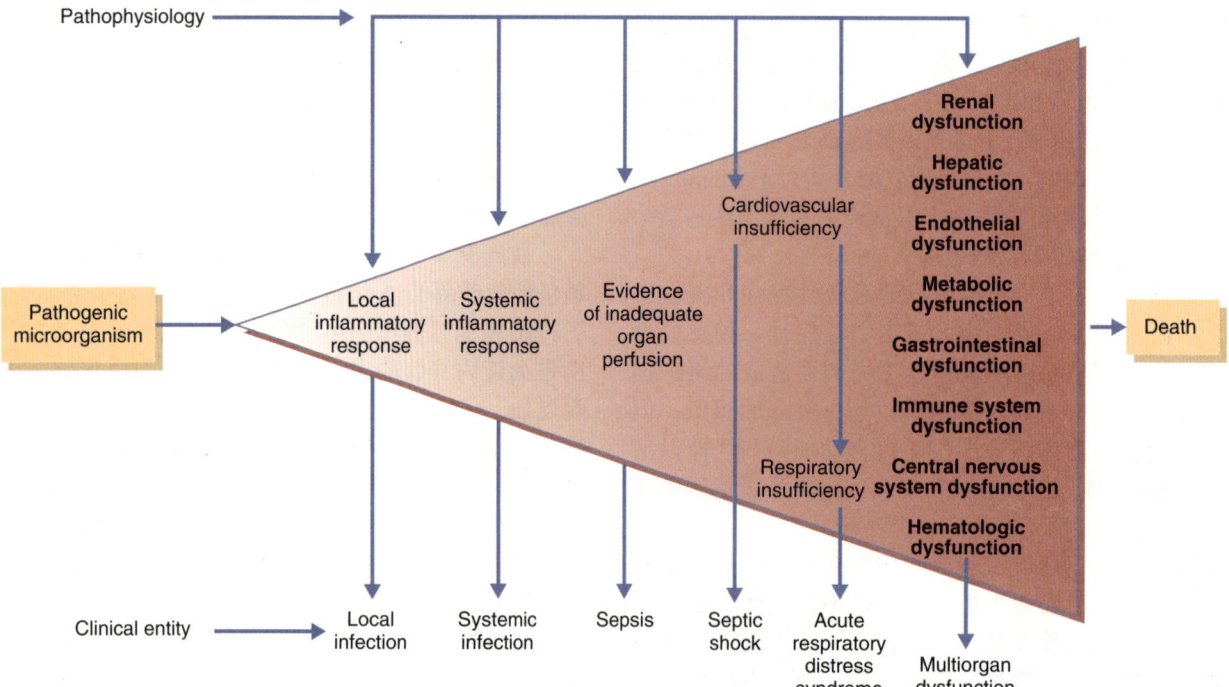

Fig. 4.1 The spectrum of illness and nomenclature for sepsis pathophysiology.

PATHOLOGY AND IMMUNOPATHOGENESIS

The pathologic findings of fatal septic shock are often rather bland on gross examination and even histologic examination of tissue samples. The most common finding is increased tissue edema in the interstitial spaces and excess lung fluid and pleural fluid. Signs of hyaline membrane formation and fibrin deposition in the alveoli are common and

表 4.1 感染中毒症的诊断标准 [a]

总体标准
对感染的异常调节造成的危及生命的器官功能障碍

器官功能障碍的标准
感染中毒症相关性器官功能衰竭评价（SOFA）[b]的改变大于等于 2 分。它可以用于器官功能障碍严重程度的评价

SOFA 评分（每级 0～4 分，总分 0～24 分）

标准	0	1	2	3	4
呼吸系统 PaO_2/FiO_2	>400	<400	<300	呼吸支持时<200	呼吸支持时<100
血小板（$\times 10^3/mm^3$）	>150	≤150	≤100	≤50	≤20
胆红素（mg/dl）	<1.2	1.2～1.9	2.0～5.9	6.0～11.9	>12.0
格拉斯哥昏迷指数	15	13～14	10～12	6～9	<6
低血压[c]	无	MAP<70 mmHg	多巴胺≤5 或多巴酚丁胺（或任何剂量的血管升压素）	多巴胺>5 或肾上腺素≤0.1 或去甲肾上腺素≤0.1（或去氧肾上腺素 100～300 μg 冲击剂量）	多巴胺>15 或肾上腺素>0.1 或去甲肾上腺素>0.1（或去氧肾上腺素>300 μg 冲击剂量）
肌酐（mg/dl）或尿量（ml/d）	<1.2	1.2～1.9	2.0～3.4	3.5～4.9	>5.0

感染中毒性休克的标准
需要升压药维持平均动脉压 65 mmHg 或更高，且
高乳酸血症［血清乳酸>2 mmol/L（>18 mg/dl）］

引自 Singer M, Deutschman CS, Seymour CW, et al：The Third International Consensus Definitions for Sepsis and Septic Shock (Sepsis-3), JAMA 315（8）：801-10，2016.
FiO_2，吸入氧浓度；INR，国际标准化比值；MAP，平均动脉压；PaO_2，氧分压。
[a] 标准包括确定的或疑似的感染以及某些所列的情况。
[b] 假定大多数情况下基线 SOFA 0 分。
[c] 肾上腺素类药物必须至少应用 1 h，剂量的单位为 μg/(kg·min)。

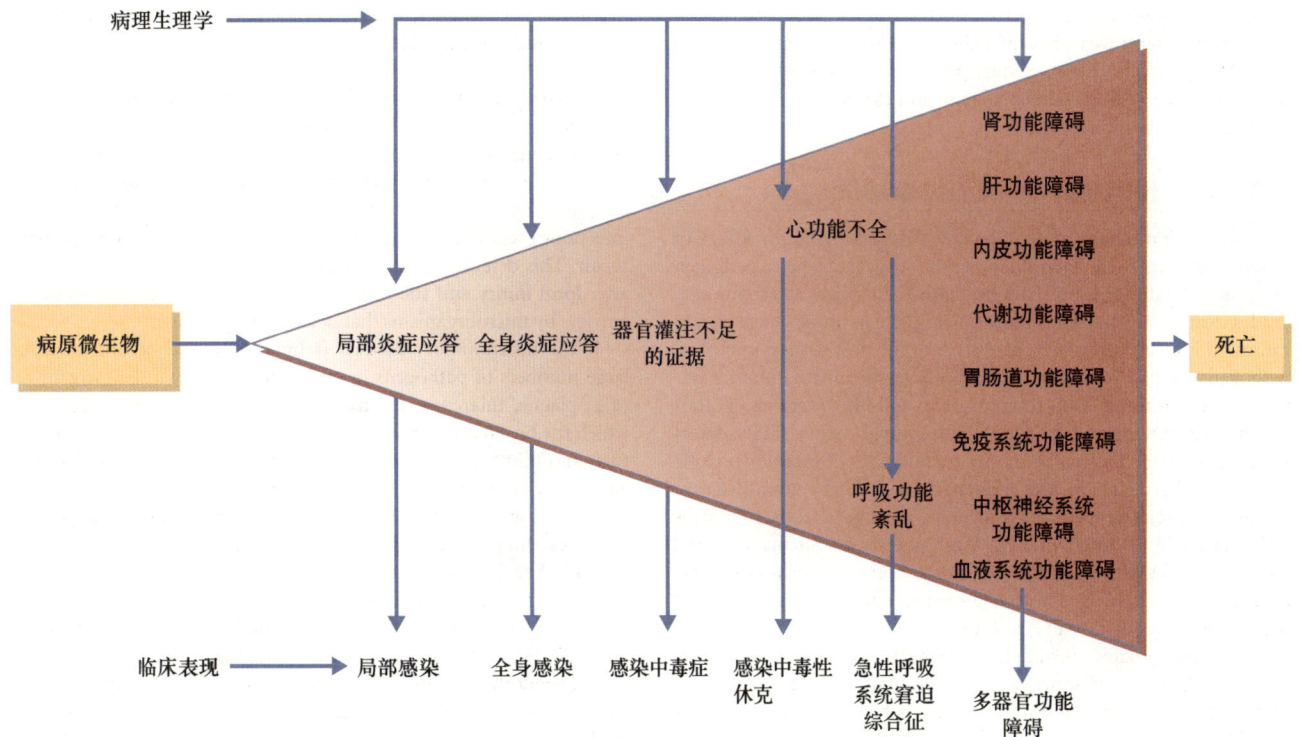

图 4.1 感染中毒症病理生理学相关疾病及命名谱

病理学和免疫发病机制

致命性的感染中毒性休克的病理学表现在大体检查和组织样本检查中都表现不明显。最常见的发现是间质间隙中组织水肿增加，肺部液体和胸膜液体过量。在肺泡中形成透明膜和纤维蛋白沉积的迹象很常见，

TABLE 4.2	Microorganisms Commonly Identified in Septic Patients Based on Host Factors
Host Factor	Organisms to Consider
Asplenia	Encapsulated organisms, particularly *Streptococcus pneumoniae, Haemophilus influenzae, Neisseria meningitidis, Capnocytophaga canimorsus*
Cirrhosis	*Vibrio, Salmonella,* and *Yersinia* species; encapsulated organisms, other gram-negative rods
Alcohol abuse	*Klebsiella* species, *S. pneumoniae*
Diabetes	Mucormycosis, *Pseudomonas* species, *Escherichia coli,* group B streptococci
Neutropenia	Enteric gram-negative rods, *Pseudomonas, Aspergillus, Candida, Mucor* species, *Staphylococcus aureus,* streptococcal species
T-cell dysfunction	*Listeria, Salmonella,* and *Mycobacterium* species, herpesviruses (including herpes simplex, cytomegalovirus, varicella-zoster virus)
Acquired immunodeficiency syndrome	*Salmonella* species, *S. aureus, Mycobacterium avium* complex, *S. pneumoniae,* group B streptococci

indicate the fibroproliferative stage of acute respiratory distress syndrome (ARDS). Occasionally, punctate or macroscopic evidence can be detected in the adrenal tissues. Diffuse petechiae in tissues and mucosal surfaces may indicate disseminated intravascular coagulation (DIC).

The kidneys usually appear normal, and necrosis of kidney tissues is distinctly uncommon. The term *acute tubular necrosis* is a misnomer, and the term *acute kidney injury* (AKI) is more appropriate for describing the functional and usually reversible loss of kidney function found in septic shock without accompanying evidence of glomerular or tubular necrosis.

An important finding at autopsy is identification of the infectious focus that caused septic shock. The focal infection that precipitated sepsis is readily identifiable in most deceased patients despite days to weeks of seemingly appropriate antimicrobial therapy directed against the pathogens. If careful histochemical studies are performed shortly after a patient succumbs to sepsis, excessive apoptosis (but not necrosis) of immune effector cells is identifiable in lung, spleen, lymph nodes, and hepatic tissues. Electron microscopy of tissues after death from sepsis often reveals loss of tight junctions along epithelial and endothelial surfaces. Electron microscopy also demonstrates diffuse mitochondrial swelling and degradation and clearance of intracellular organelles (i.e., autophagy).

PATHOPHYSIOLOGY OF SEPTIC SHOCK

The molecular mechanisms that underlie the basic pathophysiology of septic shock have been determined. Sepsis is triggered when a pathogen or cluster of pathogens breaches the epithelial barriers at a tissue site, evades clearance by humoral and cellular innate immune defenses, and causes an invasive infection. On entry into the host tissues, microbial pathogens are first sensed by myeloid cells of the innate immune system by pattern recognition receptors (e.g., toll-like receptors [TLRs]) on the cell surface and in endosomal compartments. TLRs detect highly conserved molecular motifs of microbes. Examples include lipopolysaccharide (LPS), the endotoxin produced by gram-negative bacteria; bacterial lipopeptides from gram-positive bacteria; β-glucans of the cell wall of fungi; viral RNA genomes and proteins; bacterial flagella; and DAMPs released from injured host cells, including intracellular structures such as histone proteins, mitochondrial DNA, and high-mobility group box 1 (Fig. 4.2).

TLRs and related intracellular pattern recognition receptors, including the inflammasome elements, retinoic acid–inducible gene 1 *(RIG1)*–like helicases, and cytoplasmic microbial TLR4, alert the host to infection. TLR4 is the long-sought-after LPS receptor of the human innate immune system. LPS is released from the cell membrane of gram-negative bacteria on their destruction. LPS is first bound to a carrier protein, LPS-binding protein, and the LPS monomer is then delivered to a membrane-associated, multiligand, pattern recognition receptor, CD14. LPS monomers are then passed to a soluble protein (i.e., myeloid differentiation factor 2 [MD2]) and bind to the ectodomain of TLR4. After this LPS/MD2/TLR4 complex is completed and dimerized, intracellular signaling alerts the host to the invasive infectious challenge. The pathway induces a series of phosphorylation events of adaptor proteins and signaling molecules that terminate in the activation and translocation of transcriptional activating factors such as nuclear factor-κB (NF-κB) into the nucleus. The transcription factors bind to promoter sites of the acute phase protein network, resulting in an acute outpouring of inflammatory, host defense, and coagulation components.

Other TLRs, such as TLR5 (i.e., bacterial flagella) and the TLR2/TLR1 and TLR2/TLR6 heterodimers (i.e., bacterial lipopeptides, lipoteichoic acid, and other elements of bacteria and fungi), are expressed on the cell surface of immune effector cells that recognize different molecular patterns. Nucleic acid recognition–specific TLRs reside in endosomal vacuoles, where they detect microbial DNA (TLR9), single-stranded RNA (TLR7 and TLR8), and double-stranded RNA (TLR3).

An array of complement elements, cytokines, chemokines, prostaglandins, vasoactive peptides, platelet-activating factor, and proteases are generated, resulting in activation of neutrophils, neutrophil extracellular traps (NETs), monocytes, macrophages, dendritic cells, lymphocytes, and endothelial cells in a combined effort to wall off the infectious process, clear the pathogens, and begin the process of tissue repair. This defense system efficiently clears pathogens from the host after local injury and the inevitable minor breaches of the epithelial barriers by microorganisms that occur over a lifetime.

If the inflammatory process is unchecked and accompanied by large numbers of pathogens or even a few highly virulent organisms (e.g., plague, tularemia, anthrax, and hemorrhagic fever viruses) to which the host has no preexisting immunity, a generalized, inflammatory, and injurious process known as *sepsis* evolves over a short time, and it can be deleterious or lethal to the host. The same inflammatory response that can be life-saving in localized infection can become life-threatening if it becomes sustained and generalized.

Endothelial membranes throughout the body are activated and become pro-adherent and pro-coagulant surfaces that promote neutrophil and platelet adherence. Neutrophils release proteases, cytokines, NETs, reactive oxygen radicals, and vasoactive prostanoids that damage endothelial cells and their function. Cytokine-inducible nitric oxide synthase is upregulated, resulting in massive generation of nitric oxide (NO). NO is a potent vasodilator, and in combination with other vasoactive peptides and phospholipid mediators, it promotes diffuse opening of capillary beds and increased permeability, with loss of

第4章 菌血症和感染中毒症

表4.2 根据宿主因素在感染中毒症患者中常见的微生物	
宿主因素	需要考虑的病原体
无脾	包膜菌，特别是肺炎链球菌、流感嗜血杆菌、脑膜炎奈瑟球菌、犬咬二氧化碳嗜纤维菌
肝硬化	弧菌、沙门菌和耶尔森菌；包膜菌、其他革兰氏阴性杆菌
酗酒	克雷伯菌、肺炎链球菌
糖尿病	毛霉菌、假单胞菌、大肠埃希菌、B组链球菌
中性粒细胞缺乏	肠道革兰氏阴性杆菌、假单胞菌、曲霉菌、念珠菌、毛霉菌病、金黄色葡萄球菌、链球菌
T细胞功能不全	李斯特菌、沙门菌和分枝杆菌、疱疹病毒（包括单纯疱疹病毒、巨细胞病毒、水痘-带状疱疹病毒）
获得性免疫缺陷综合征	沙门菌、金黄色葡萄球菌、鸟分枝杆菌复合群、肺炎链球菌、B组链球菌

这表明急性呼吸窘迫综合征（ARDS）的纤维增生阶段。偶尔，肾上腺组织中可以检测到点状或宏观证据。组织和黏膜表面的弥漫性瘀点可能表明弥散性血管内凝血（DIC）。

肾通常显示正常，肾组织坏死非常罕见。"急性肾小管坏死"这个术语是不合适的，而"急性肾损伤（AKI）"一词更适合描述在感染中毒性休克中发现的功能性的且通常可逆性的肾功能丧失，而不伴有肾小球或肾小管坏死的证据。

通过尸检，从而获得的一个重要发现是确定导致感染中毒性休克的感染性病灶。尽管针对病原体进行了数天至数周的看似适当的抗菌治疗，但诱发的感染中毒症的局灶性感染在大多数死亡患者中很容易识别。如果在患者死于感染中毒症后不久进行仔细的组织化学研究，则在肺、脾、淋巴结和肝组织中可以识别出免疫效应细胞的过度凋亡（而非坏死）。感染中毒症死亡后组织的电子显微镜检查通常显示上皮和内皮表面的紧密连接的丧失。电子显微镜还展示了弥漫性线粒体肿胀和降解以及细胞内细胞器的清除（即自噬）。

感染中毒性休克的病理生理学

感染中毒性休克基本病理生理学的分子机制已经确定。当病原体或一簇病原体突破组织部位的上皮屏障，逃避体液和细胞先天免疫防御的清除，并导致侵入性感染时，就会引发感染中毒症。进入宿主组织后，微生物病原体首先通过细胞表面和内部部分的模式识别受体［如Toll样受体（TLR）］由先天免疫系统的髓样细胞感知。TLR检测微生物的高度保守的分子基序。包括革兰氏阴性菌产生的内毒素脂多糖（LPS）、革兰氏阳性菌的细菌脂肽、真菌细胞壁的β-葡聚糖、病毒RNA基因组和蛋白质、细菌鞭毛，以及从受损宿主细胞释放的DAMP，包括细胞内结构，如组蛋白、线粒体DNA和高迁移率组蛋白质1（图4.2）。

TLR和相关的细胞内模式识别受体，包括炎症性元素、视黄酸诱导基因1（RIG1）样螺旋酶和细胞质微生物TLR4，提醒宿主感染。TLR4是人类先天免疫系统长期寻求的LPS受体。LPS在革兰氏阴性菌的细胞膜中释放出来，首先与载体蛋白——LPS结合蛋白结合，然后LPS单体被传递到一个与膜相关的多配体模式识别受体CD14。接着，LPS单体被传递到可溶性蛋白质，即骨髓分化因子2（MD2），并结合到TLR4的外域。在这个LPS/MD2/TLR4复合物完成并且二聚化后，细胞内信号传导会提醒宿主注意存在侵入性感染性挑战。该途径诱发一系列适配蛋白和信号分子的磷酸化事件，这些事件终止于核因子-κB（NF-κB）等转录激活因子进入核的易位。转录因子与急性期蛋白网络的启动子位点结合，导致炎症、宿主防御和凝血成分的急性大量释放。

其他TLR，如TLR5（即细菌鞭毛）和TLR2/TLR1和TLR2/TLR6异二聚体（即细菌脂肽、脂质酸和其他细菌和真菌元素）在识别不同分子模式的免疫效应细胞的细胞表面表达。核酸识别特异性TLR驻留在内体囊泡中，在那里它们探测到微生物DNA（TLR9）、单链RNA（TLR7和TLR8）和双链RNA（TLR3）。

一系列补体成分、细胞因子、趋化因子、前列腺素、血管活性肽、血小板激活因子和蛋白酶，从而激活中性粒细胞、中性粒细胞胞外诱捕网（NET）、单核细胞、巨噬细胞、树突细胞、淋巴细胞和内皮细胞，共同作用隔离传染性的过程，清除病原体，并开始组织修复过程。在微生物造成局部损伤和必然的轻微破坏上皮屏障后，这种防御系统可以有效地清除宿主体内的病原体。

如果炎症过程未被监测到且不受控制，并伴有大量病原体甚至一些高毒力病原微生物（如鼠疫、土拉菌病、炭疽和出血热病毒），而如果宿主没有预先存在的免疫力，那么被称为感染中毒症的泛化、炎症性的有害过程会在短时间内发生和进展，它可能对宿主有害或者致命。在局部感染中可以挽救生命的同样的炎症反应，如果持续和逐步泛化加重，可能会危及生命。

全身的内皮细胞膜被激活，并成为促黏附和促凝集的表面，促进中性粒细胞和血小板黏附。中性粒细胞释放蛋白酶、细胞因子、NET、活性氧自由基和血管活性前列腺素，破坏内皮细胞及其功能。细胞因子诱导的一氧化氮合酶被上调，导致大量产生一氧化氮（NO）。NO是一种有效的血管扩张剂，与其他血管活性肽和磷脂介质相结合，它促进毛细血管床的弥漫性打开和增加通透性，并造成血管内液体无法进入间

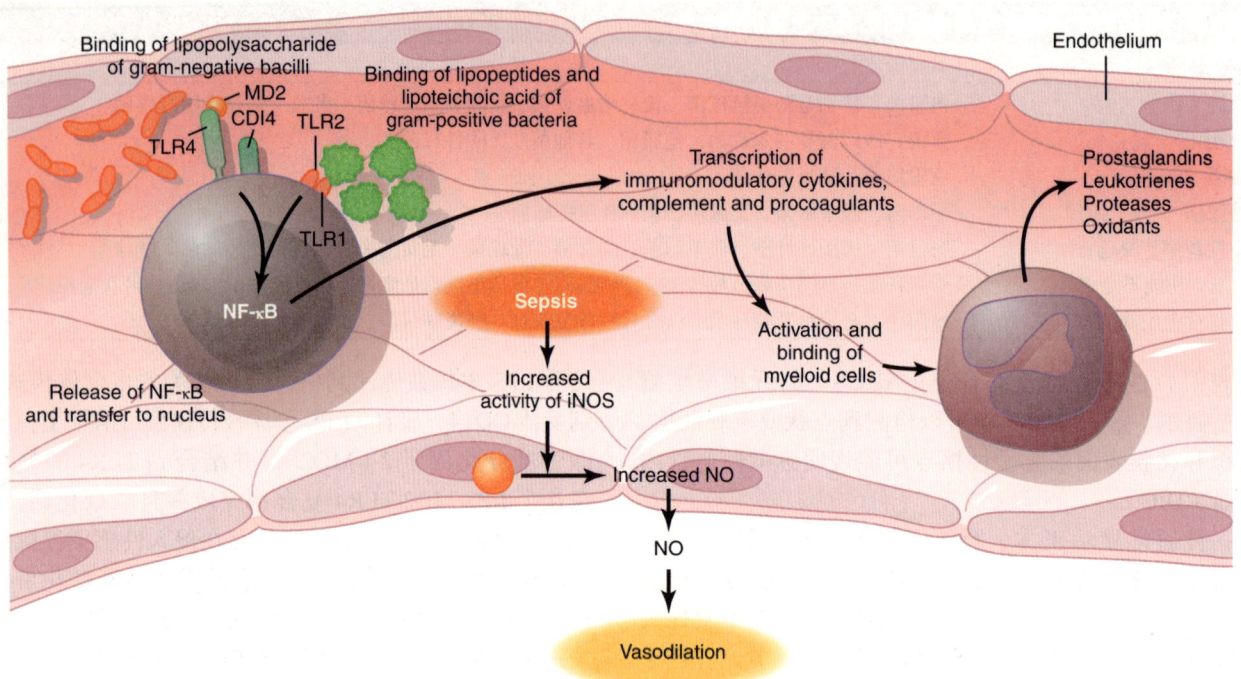

Fig. 4.2 Immunopathogenesis of sepsis. Early recognition of bloodstream infection begins with sensing by pattern recognition receptors: toll-like receptor 4 (TLR4); cluster determinant 14 (CD14); myeloid differentiation factor 2 (MD2) for gram-negative bacterial lipopolysaccharide and TLR2 for lipoteichoic acid and other elements from gram-positive bacteria. Engagement of the TLRs by their ligands signals transcription of the acute phase response genes by nuclear factor-κB (NF-κB). Septic shock is initiated by systemic release of an array of vasoactive mediators, including nitric oxide (NO) produced by cytokine-inducible NO synthase (iNOS).

intravascular fluids into the interstitial spaces. Reactive oxygen species combine with NO to generate highly injurious reactive nitrogen intermediates (e.g., peroxynitrite) that damage mitochondrial function and induce apoptosis. Systemic hypotension rapidly develops, and septic shock ensues. Immediate action by the clinician is mandatory to correct the hemodynamic status and resolve the underlying infection.

CLINICAL PRESENTATION

Despite the vast improvements in understanding the pathophysiologic basis of sepsis, clinical diagnosis remains limited to the medical history, symptomatic assessment, and nonspecific laboratory and hemodynamic criteria. Compounding the problem is the need for prompt institution of appropriate antimicrobial therapy, making early recognition of sepsis critically important. Patients with clinical findings as outlined in Table 4.1 should undergo thorough and prompt evaluation for a possible infectious cause, including bacterial cultures of blood and (when indicated) other body fluids. Localizing signs and symptoms should prompt a thorough physical examination and directed imaging to identify a nidus of infection. Defects of natural defensive barriers, such as transcutaneous devices or intravascular catheters, should be assessed for infection and removed if suspected to be the origin of the septic process. To minimize the potential delay in prompt recognition and management of sepsis resulting from obtaining laboratory data, the Sepsis-3 recommendations included a bedside quick SOFA (qSOFA) scoring system. The qSOFA allows for repeated bedside evaluations of patients at risk for developing sepsis and relies on three clinical criteria, each worth 1 point: (a) Respiratory rate 22/min or greater; (b) altered mentation; and (c) systolic blood pressure less than 100 mm Hg. A qSOFA score of 2 or greater should prompt further investigation into infectious causes and organ dysfunction as well as initiation or escalation of therapy, as appropriate. Despite its clinical logic and its simplicity, the experience thus far with its predictive value has been mixed. General clinical presentation of sepsis varies widely. Many patients have fever or chills, but older patients and those on immunomodulating medications may not mount a fever. Hypothermia portends a worse prognosis or more severe illness. Tachypnea may be an indicator of respiratory compensation for underlying metabolic acidosis or the early signs and symptoms of ARDS.

Mental status changes can result from metabolic derangements caused by sepsis, hypoglycemia, the underlying infectious process, or concomitant hypotension. This symptom can be difficult to identify in the elderly patient with dementia, and caution should be exercised in the evaluation and treatment of the otherwise stable elderly patient with possible mental status changes.

Skin findings (e.g., cellulitis, abscess) can provide clues to the cause of sepsis and may indicate the state of peripheral systemic perfusion. Several microorganisms can cause specific skin manifestations in systemic infection. *S. aureus* and streptococci can cause diffuse erythroderma, bullous lesions, or generalized desquamation. Bacteremia caused by several gram-negative organisms, including *P. aeruginosa* and enteric organisms, can result in ecthyma gangrenosum, particularly in immunocompromised patients. These lesions are round and 1 to 15 cm in diameter, and they have a central area of necrosis and peripheral erythema. Infection with *Neisseria meningitidis* can result initially in lower extremity petechiae progressing to diffuse purpura, which likely portends septic shock and a high risk of death. A similar clinical presentation can be observed in other unusual infectious diseases, such as

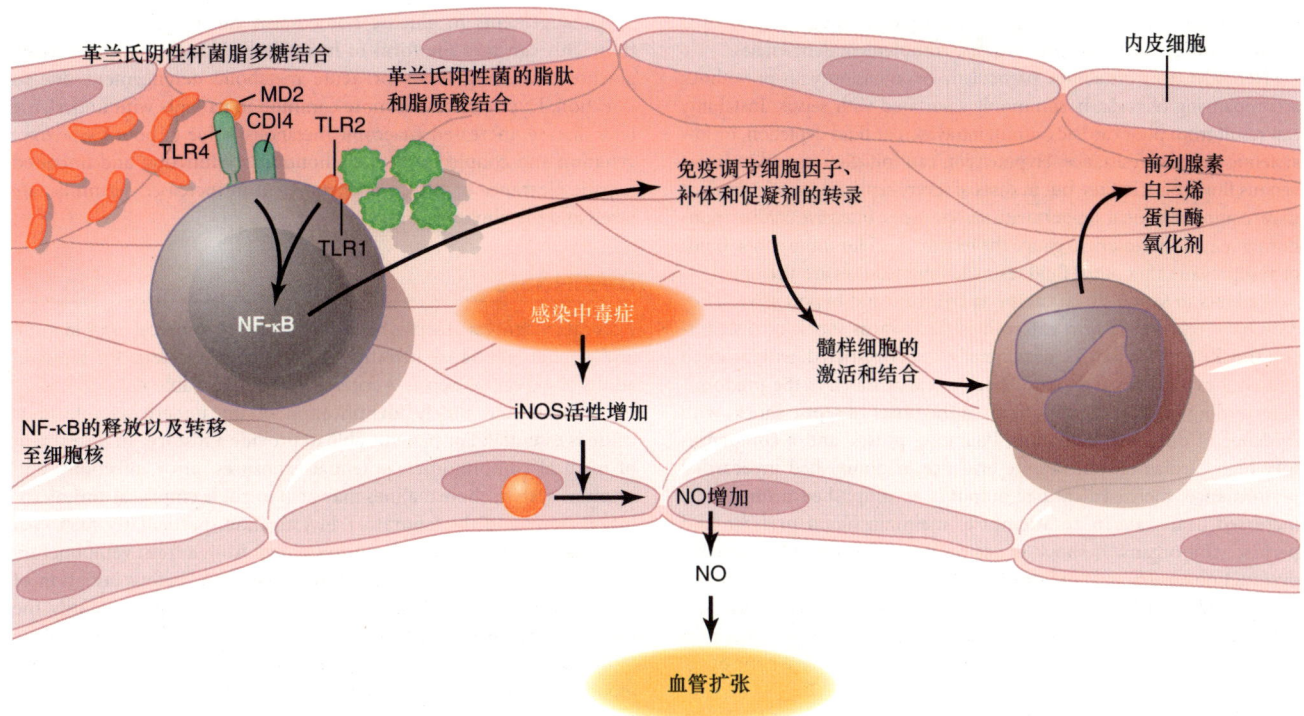

图 4.2 感染中毒症的免疫学致病机制。通过识别受体的感知早期识别血流感染：Toll 样受体 4（TLR4）、簇点 14（CD14）、髓样细胞分化因子 2（MD2）用于识别革兰氏阴性菌的脂多糖，以及 TLR2 用于识别革兰氏阳性菌的脂壁酸和其他成分。TLR 与其配体的结合通过核因子-κB（NF-κB）信号传导，触发急性期反应基因的转录。感染中毒性休克是由一系列血管活性介质的系统释放引发的，包括由细胞因子诱导的一氧化氮合酶（iNOS）

质部位。活性氧与 NO 结合，产生高破坏性活性氮中间体（例如过氧亚硝酸盐），破坏线粒体功能并诱导凋亡。全身低血压迅速发展，感染中毒性休克随之而来。临床医生必须立即采取行动，以纠正血流动力学状态并解决潜在的感染问题。

临床表现

尽管在了解感染中毒症的病理生理学基础方面取得了巨大进步，但临床诊断仍然仅限于病史、症状评估以及非特异性实验室和血流动力学标准。需要及时进行适当的抗菌治疗，因此及早识别感染中毒症至关重要。具有表 4.1 中概述的临床结果的患者应对可能的感染原因进行彻底和及时的评估，包括血液的细菌培养和（如有指征）其他体液。定位体征和症状应促使进行全面的体检以直接确定感染的原因。天然防御屏障的缺陷，如经皮装置或血管内导管，应评估是否感染，如果怀疑是感染中毒症的起源，则应将其去除。为了尽量减少因获取实验室数据而导致的迅速识别和处理感染中毒症的潜在延迟，感染中毒症-3 建议包括床旁快速 SOFA（qSOFA）评分系统。qSOFA 允许对有感染中毒症风险的患者进行反复的床边评估，并依赖于三个临床标准，每个标准都值 1 分：(a) 呼吸频率 22 次 / 分或更高；(b) 心率改变；(c) 收缩压小于 100 mmHg。qSOFA 评分为 2 分或更高应进一步调查感染原因和器

官功能障碍，并酌情启动或升级治疗。尽管其具有临床逻辑和简单性，但迄今为止的经验及其预测价值参差不齐。感染中毒症的一般临床表现差异很大。许多患者发热或寒战，但老年患者和服用免疫调节药物的患者可能不会发热。体温过低预示着预后更差或更严重的疾病。呼吸暂停可能是潜在代谢性酸中毒或 ARDS 早期体征和症状的呼吸补偿指标。

精神状态变化可能由感染中毒症、低血糖、潜在的传染过程或伴随的低血压引起的代谢紊乱引起。患有痴呆的老年患者中可能很难识别这种症状，因此在评估和治疗可能存在意识状态改变的原本稳定的老年患者时应谨慎行事。

皮肤表现（例如蜂窝织炎、脓肿）可以提供感染中毒症原因的线索，并可能表明周围全身灌注的状态。几种微生物可以在全身感染中引起特定的皮肤表现。有些病原微生物可以造成特异性的皮肤表现。金黄色葡萄球菌和链球菌可以引起弥漫性红皮病、大疱性病变或全身脱屑。由几种革兰氏阴性菌（包括铜绿假单胞菌和肠道细菌）引起的菌血症可能导致坏疽性深脓疱，特别是在免疫功能低下的患者中。这些病变呈圆形，直径为 1～15 cm，它们有中心区域的坏死和周围性红斑。感染脑膜炎奈瑟球菌最初会导致下肢瘀点发展为弥漫性紫癜，这可能预示着感染中毒性休克和高死亡风险。在其他不寻常的感染性疾病中可以观察到类似的临床表现，例如脾切除患者严重肺炎球菌感染

overwhelming pneumococcal sepsis in the asplenic host or disseminated neisserial infections in patients with late complement deficiencies.

Hemodynamic instability, particularly hypotension with or without accompanying oliguria, is commonly associated with sepsis. Instability can result from poor cardiac output, intravascular fluid depletion, or low systemic vascular resistance. Hypotension can initially respond to intravenous fluid resuscitation, but in cases of severe sepsis and septic shock, it may require additional support with vasopressors. Intensive cardiac monitoring may be necessary to gauge the relative need for intravenous fluids or vasopressors after initial fluid resuscitation measures are attempted.

Patients in septic shock can be tachycardic and hypotensive. They may have relatively warm extremities (i.e., warm shock or distributive shock), or they may be peripherally vasoconstricted, with mottled and cool extremities (i.e., cold shock). Warm shock is the predominant finding in most adult patients at the onset of septic shock, with evidence of diffuse vasodilation, bounding pulses, and a compensatory high cardiac output despite evidence of diminished myocardial performance. Increased cardiac output is accomplished primarily by increased heart rate in an attempt to maintain blood pressure and perfuse vital organs. If shock is not promptly corrected, myocardial dysfunction ensues and cold shock evolves over the next several hours. Older patients with limited cardiac reserves tolerate shock poorly and are more likely to develop cold shock. Evidence of septic shock at presentation that is refractory to early resuscitation portends a poor prognosis, with mortality rates exceeding 70%.

Besides hypotension, oliguria can represent developing AKI. It can arise from a combination of the disease process, infecting organism, and medications. Inflammatory cytokines, microbial toxins, systemic hypotension, and iatrogenic renal injury from medications can result in AKI. Other causes of renal injury include interstitial injury from infection or medications and immune complex–mediated injury, as seen in cases of endocarditis.

Besides tachypnea, pulmonary symptoms seen in septic patients include marked hypoxia due to interstitial edema, inflammation, or hemodynamic instability. ARDS is defined as an arterial partial pressure of oxygen less than 50 mm Hg despite fractional inspired oxygen of greater than 50%, together with diffuse alveolar infiltrates and a pulmonary capillary wedge pressure of less than 18 mm Hg. ARDS occurs in up to 40% of septic patients. The diffuse pulmonary inflammation in ARDS results in increased pulmonary vascular permeability, which complicates fluid resuscitation efforts because excessive fluid can exacerbate pulmonary edema and hypoxia. Altered mental status and sepsis-related myopathy also result in airway compromise and weak respiratory effort, necessitating invasive ventilatory support.

Patients with sepsis can have marked hematologic changes. They may have neutrophilic leukocytosis, which is often accompanied by increased immature cell counts, or they can be markedly leukopenic (particularly lymphopenic), often in cases of severe septic shock. Transient neutropenia is often seen in the early phase of septic shock and results from activation and adherence of neutrophils along endothelial surfaces in the microcirculation. This is rapidly followed by prolonged neutrophilia as sepsis-induced inflammatory cytokines stimulate bone marrow synthesis of new white blood cells.

Thrombocytopenia and coagulopathy can occur, and patients have petechiae or purpura at presentation. Severe derangements in coagulation can produce DIC, which can lead to thrombin deposition throughout the microcirculation. Excessive activation and degradation of clotting factors can deplete coagulation factors, resulting in diffuse hemorrhage. Excessive mucosal bleeding around airway tubes and prolonged bleeding from venipuncture sites presage internal bleeding events. Massive gastrointestinal hemorrhage can occur, which can cause or exacerbate hypotension and shock.

Derangements in glucose homeostasis can be seen at presentation. This can take the form of hyperglycemia in diabetics receiving glucose-containing fluids or acute metabolic derangement due to infection. Hypoglycemia is more common in patients with underlying liver disease. Increased anaerobic metabolism due to poor tissue oxygenation and coupled with mitochondrial dysfunction and impaired hepatic clearance of lactic acid may result in increased serum lactate levels and metabolic acidosis.

DIAGNOSIS

Accurate diagnosis of sepsis relies on the history, physical examination, and general laboratory investigation. Diagnostic criteria for sepsis in adults based on the Sepsis-3 criteria are listed in Table 4.1.

Accurate and timely identification of the underlying infectious cause is essential. For patients able to provide a history, an assessment of medical comorbidities, potential exposures, prior infections, and immune system abnormalities may help to guide empirical antimicrobial therapy and the laboratory investigation, particularly microbial cultures. Two sets of blood cultures drawn from a fresh venipuncture and from existing indwelling intravascular lines (before initiation of empirical antimicrobial therapy when possible) help to identify the causative organism in many cases. A recent study in over 3000 patients reinforces the value of obtaining diagnostic, pre-antibiotic treatment, blood cultures. The diagnostic yield was nearly 50% higher for blood cultures obtained in the pre-antibiotic treatment group compared to the post-antibiotic treatment blood cultures (sampled up to 120 minutes after the start of antibiotic therapy). Symptomatic assessment and physical examination should suggest a location of focal infection that can help to guide radiologic studies and interventions to drain pus.

Beyond microbial cultures, several other laboratory studies can help to define the severity of illness and provide baseline data for monitoring the response to therapy. Basic laboratory testing, including a complete blood count with differential, chemistries, and creatinine and aminotransferase levels, can help to identify significant organ dysfunction. Oxygen saturation by pulse oximetry should be measured promptly to identify gas exchange capacity and the need for ventilatory support. Coagulation studies should be obtained, particularly for patients with evidence of DIC and those who are thrombocytopenic. For patients with altered mental status or marked respiratory difficulty, arterial blood gas sampling can help define the underlying derangement and physiologic compensation and can indirectly gauge the severity of illness.

Levels of inflammatory markers, including C-reactive protein and procalcitonin, usually are elevated. An elevated procalcitonin level can help to differentiate septic shock from other causes of shock and provide some prognostic data and a measure of response to therapy. In cases of sepsis due to pneumonia, serial measurement of procalcitonin can help to guide the duration of antibiotic therapy.

Other testing should be directed toward identifying the potential cause. Patients with severe diarrhea should undergo testing for antibiotic-associated *Clostridioides difficile* infection. Imaging studies should focus on identifying infectious sources and facilitate drainage of fluid collections or abscesses. Computed tomography may be of use in such circumstances, although for the critically ill patient who is not stable for transport, bedside radiographic studies, especially ultrasound, should be considered.

Multiple tests of physiologic function and advanced microbiologic diagnostic tests are increasingly used in clinical practice. They include polymerase chain reaction (PCR)–based assays for identifying bacteria and viruses and various assays of inflammatory cytokines and other biomarkers alone and in combination as potential diagnostic and prognostic aids.

中毒症或晚期补体缺陷患者的播散性奈瑟球菌感染。

血流动力学不稳定，特别是低血压伴随着或不伴随着少尿，通常与感染中毒症有关。血流动力学不稳定是由于心输出量下降、血管内液体容量减少或全身血管阻力低。低血压最初会对静脉液体复苏有反应，但在严重感染中毒症和感染中毒性休克的情况下，可能需要血管升压素的额外支持作用。在尝试初步液体复苏措施后，可能需要进一步加强心脏监测，以评价是否需要进一步静脉输液或使用血管升压素。

感染中毒性休克患者可以发生心动过速和低血压。他们的四肢相对温暖（即暖休克或分布性休克），或者他们可能发生外周血管收缩，四肢皮肤发花及肢体湿冷（即冷休克）。暖休克是大多数成年患者在感染中毒性休克开始时的主要表现，尽管有证据表明患者的心肌性能下降，但亦有广泛的血管扩张、洪脉和代偿性高心输出量。增加心输出量主要是通过提高心率来实现的，以维持血压和重要器官的灌注。如果休克没有及时纠正，心肌功能障碍会随之而来，会在接下来的几个小时内发展为冷休克。心脏储备有限的老年患者对休克的耐受性很差，更容易发生冷休克。早期复苏难治性感染中毒性休克的证据预示着预后不佳，病死率超过70%。

除了低血压，少尿代表发生了急性肾损伤（AKI）。它是综合疾病过程，病原微生物以及治疗等因素而形成的。炎症性细胞因子、微生物毒素、全身性低血压和药物引起的医源性肾损伤可能导致AKI。肾损伤的其他原因包括感染或药物引起的间质损伤和免疫复合体介导的损伤，如在心内膜炎病例所见到的。

除了呼吸暂停外，在感染中毒症患者中出现的肺部症状包括由于间质性水肿、炎症或血流动力学不稳定而导致的明显的低氧血症。ARDS被定义为尽管FiO$_2$大于50%，但动脉氧分压仍低于50 mmHg，并且伴有弥漫性肺泡浸润和肺毛细血管楔压小于18 mmHg。高达40%的感染中毒症患者会发生ARDS。ARDS中的弥漫性肺泡炎症导致肺血管渗透性增加，这使液体复苏工作复杂化，因为过多的液体会加剧肺水肿和缺氧。精神状态的改变和与感染中毒症相关的肌病也会导致气道受损和呼吸力减弱，需要有创性的通气支持。

感染中毒症患者可能会有明显的血液学变化。他们可以发生中性白细胞增多，通常伴随着未成熟细胞计数的增加，或者他们可能发生明显的白细胞减少（特别是淋巴细胞减少），这通常见于严重感染中毒性休克的情况下。短暂性中性粒细胞减少经常出现在感染中毒性休克的早期阶段，这是微循环中中性粒细胞沿内皮表面激活和黏附的结果。随之而来的是长期的中性粒细胞升高，因为感染中毒症诱导的炎症细胞因子刺激骨髓合成新的白细胞。

血小板减少症和凝血功能障碍也会发生，患者可以出现瘀点瘀斑。凝血的严重紊乱可以造成DIC，这可能导致整个微循环中的凝血酶沉积。凝血因子的过度激活和降解会耗尽凝血因子，导致弥漫性出血。气道周围黏膜出血过多以及静脉穿刺部位长时间出血预示着内出血事件的发生。可能会发生胃肠道大出血，这会导致或加剧低血压和休克。

在感染中毒症患者初次就诊时，葡萄糖稳态的紊乱是常见的。可能表现为接受含葡萄糖液体的糖尿病患者的高血糖，或感染引起的急性代谢紊乱。低血糖在有基础肝病的患者中更为常见。由于组织氧合不良导致的增加的无氧代谢，再加上线粒体功能障碍和肝清除乳酸能力的损害，可能导致血清乳酸水平升高和代谢性酸中毒。

诊断

感染中毒症的准确诊断取决于病史、体格检查和一般实验室检查。基于感染中毒症-3标准的成人感染中毒症诊断标准列于表4.1。

准确及时地识别潜在的感染原因至关重要。对于能够提供病史的患者，评估医学共病、潜在暴露、既往感染和免疫系统异常可能有助于指导经验性抗菌治疗和实验室检查，特别是微生物培养。从静脉穿刺和现有的静脉置管（在开始经验性抗菌治疗之前）中提取的两套血培养有助于在许多病例里的病原体的识别。最近对3000多名患者进行的一项研究证实了在为了明确诊断、使用抗生素治疗前的血培养的价值。与抗生素治疗后血培养相比，抗生素治疗前组获得的血培养的诊断结果比抗生素治疗后（在抗生素治疗开始后120 min内取样）的诊断结果高出近50%。通过症状评估和体格检查可以提示感染的病灶，这有助于指导影像学的检查和采取措施来进行脓液的引流。

除了微生物培养外，其他几项实验室检查可以帮助确定疾病的严重程度，并为监测治疗反应提供基线数据。基本的实验室检测，包括全血细胞分类计数、生化、肌酐和转氨酶水平检查，可以帮助识别严重的器官功能障碍。应及时测量脉搏血氧饱和度，以确定气体交换能力和对通气支持的需求。应进行凝血方面的检查，特别是对有DIC证据的患者和血小板减少症患者。对于精神状态改变或呼吸明显困难的患者，动脉血气检查可以帮助确定潜在异常和生理性的代偿，并可以间接评价疾病的严重程度。

炎症标志物的水平，包括C反应蛋白和，通常会升高。降钙素原水平升高有助于区分感染中毒性休克和其他休克，并提供一些预后数据以及对治疗反应进行评价。在肺炎引起的感染中毒症的病例中，对降钙素原的连续测量可以帮助指导抗生素治疗的持续时间。

其他的检测应当针对识别可能的原因。严重腹泻患者应接受抗生素相关艰难梭菌感染的检测。影像学检查应侧重于确定感染来源，并帮助进行液体收集或脓肿的引流。尽管对于不稳定、不宜搬运的危重患者，应该考虑床旁放射学研究，特别是超声检查，CT检查可能在这种情况下亦是必要的。

多种生理功能测试和先进的微生物诊断检测越来越多地用于临床实践。它们包括基于聚合酶链反应（PCR）的检测，用于识别细菌和病毒，还包括单独或结合作为潜在诊断和预后辅助工具的炎症细胞因子和其他生物标志物的各种检测。

TABLE 4.3 Recommended Initial Management of Sepsis in Adults

- Start resuscitation immediately in patients with hypotension or serum lactate level >2 mmol/L.
- Obtain appropriate cultures before starting antibiotics if doing so does not significantly delay therapy.
- Evaluate for a focus of infection amenable to source control (e.g., abscess drainage).
- Remove intravascular catheters if potentially infected.
- Begin broad-spectrum antibiotics within the first hour of severe sepsis and septic shock. Initial antibiotic regimen is based on likely source of sepsis, likely pathogens, and local antibiotic susceptibility patterns of common pathogens.
- Begin fluid resuscitation using crystalloids as the first choice. If colloids are used, avoid starches and consider albumin in selected patients who have hypoalbuminemia or require large-volume fluid resuscitation.
- Give fluid challenge of up to 30 mL/kg of crystalloids over 15–30 min in septic patients with suspected volume depletion; larger volumes of fluids may be needed in some patients. The goals for resuscitation should be a central venous pressure of 8–12 mm Hg, a mean arterial pressure (MAP) ≥65 mm Hg, and a superior vena cava oxygen saturation ≥70% or mixed venous oxygen saturation ≥65%.
- Maintain targeted MAP of ≥65 mm Hg; if fluids are not effective in reestablishing adequate blood pressure, begin vasopressors. After hemodynamic parameters are stabilized, limit fluid therapy to prevent pulmonary fluid accumulation and exacerbation of hypoxemia.
- Use norepinephrine, centrally administered, as the vasopressor of choice. Epinephrine is the second choice, followed by vasopressin as salvage therapy. Dobutamine may be useful if an inotrope is needed. Avoid dopamine except for special situations (i.e., low risk of tachyarrhythmia and persistent bradycardia).
- Give red blood cells when the hemoglobin concentration decreases to <7 g/dL; target hemoglobin level is 7–9 g/dL.
- Target a tidal volume of 6 mL/kg in patients with acute respiratory distress syndrome.
- Give low-molecular-weight heparin or unfractionated heparin for deep vein thrombosis prophylaxis; use graduated pressure stockings or intermittent compression devices if heparin therapy is contraindicated.
- Provide stress ulcer prophylaxis using histamine H_2-blockers or a proton pump inhibitor.
- Provide expert supportive care; provide low-dose nutrition for the first week; consider stress-dose steroids if refractory septic shock occurs; maintain blood glucose in the 110-180 mg/dL range.

Data from Dellinger RP, Levy MM, et al: Surviving Sepsis Campaign: international guidelines for the management of severe sepsis and septic shock, 2012, Crit Care Med 41:580-637, 2013.

TABLE 4.4 Initial Antibiotic Recommendations for Adult Patients With Sepsis

Indication	Recommended Dosages[a]
Empirical coverage (source unknown)	Vancomycin 15 mg/kg q12h plus piperacillin-tazobactam[b] 3.375 g IV q6h or imipenem 0.5 g IV q6h or meropenem 1.0 g IV q8h with or without an aminoglycoside (e.g., tobramycin 5 mg/kg IV q24)[c]
Community-acquired pneumonia (CAP)	Ceftriaxone 1 g IV q24h plus azithromycin 500 mg IV q24h or a fluoroquinolone (e.g., moxifloxacin 400 mg IV q24h or levofloxacin 750 mg IV q24h)[d]
Community-acquired urosepsis	Piperacillin-tazobactam 3.375 g IV q6h or ciprofloxacin 400 mg IV q12h
Meningitis	Vancomycin 15 mg/kg IV q6h plus ceftriaxone 2 g IV q12h plus dexamethasone 0.15 mg/kg IV q6h × 2–4 days, preferably before antibiotics; add ampicillin 2 g IV q4h if listeria is suspected.
Nosocomial pneumonia	Vancomycin 15 mg/kg q12h plus piperacillin-tazobactam 4.5 g IV q6h or imipenem 0.5 g IV q6h or meropenem 1 g IV q8h or cefepime 2 g IV q8h plus an aminoglycoside (e.g., amikacin 15 mg/kg IV q24h or tobramycin 5–7 mg/kg IV q24h) or levofloxacin 750 mg IV q24h. Some authorities substitute linezolid 600 mg IV q12h for vancomycin if MRSA is a significant concern or known to be the cause.
Neutropenia	Cefepime 2 g IV q8h; add vancomycin 15 mg/kg IV q12h if a central line is present and infection is a concern. Add antifungal coverage with caspofungin 70 mg IV × 1, then 50 mg IV q24h if fever persists ≥5 days. For suspected or proven invasive aspergillosis, voriconazole 6 mg/kg IV q12h × 2, then 4 mg/kg IV q12h should be used.
Cellulitis and skin infections	Vancomycin 15 mg/kg IV q12h. Add piperacillin-tazobactam 3.375 g IV q6h in diabetics and immunocompromised patients. If necrotizing fasciitis is suspected, add clindamycin 900 mg. IV; surgical debridement is crucial.

IV, Intravenous; *MRSA*, methicillin-resistant *Staphylococcus aureus*.
[a]Assumes normal renal function; dose adjustments are required with impaired creatinine clearance.
[b]Substitute aztreonam 2 g IV q8h if patient is allergic to penicillin.
[c]Monitor drug levels of aminoglycosides (i.e., peak and trough).
[d]Substitute cefepime or a carbapenem and azithromycin ± an aminoglycoside if the patient has severe CAP or health care–associated pneumonia.

TREATMENT

Septic shock is a medical emergency. Immediate attempts to reestablish physiologic hemodynamics, vital organ support, and oxygen delivery to tissues should accompany early diagnosis and treatment of infection. Patients should be transferred to the intensive care unit as soon as possible to receive optimal monitoring, hemodynamic support, and expert supportive care.

Early recognition, prompt resuscitation, and early institution of appropriate antimicrobial agents are the most important determinants of a successful outcome. If appropriate, draining infectious foci (i.e., source control) should be done as soon as possible. Key elements of the 2016 Surviving Sepsis Campaign guidelines are summarized in Table 4.3.

An essential element in the treatment of sepsis is early administration of antibiotics active against the causative pathogen. Treatment is best given within 1 hour of the onset of septic shock, and an empirical, broad-spectrum antimicrobial regimen is usually employed until the results of cultures of blood and the site of infection become available. A suggested initial treatment regimen is provided in Table 4.4. Failing

表4.3　成人感染中毒症的推荐初步管理措施

- 低血压或血清乳酸水平＞2 mmol/L 的住院患者立即开始复苏。
- 如果不会显著延迟治疗，在开始使用抗生素之前获得适当的培养结果。
- 评估感染灶以进行源头控制（例如，脓肿引流）。
- 如果有感染的可能，拔除血管内导管。
- 在严重感染中毒症和感染中毒性休克的第1 h 内开始使用广谱抗生素。最初的抗生素方案是基于可能的感染中毒症原因、可能的病原体以及当地常见病原体对抗生素的敏感性等。
- 以晶体液为首选，开始液体复苏。如果使用胶体，请避免使用含淀粉的液体，并考虑在患有低白蛋白血症或需要大量液体复苏的相应患者中使用白蛋白。
- 对于怀疑有液体不足的感染中毒症患者，在15～30 min，给予高达30 ml/kg 的晶体液。某些患者可能需要更大剂量的液体。复苏的目标应该是中心静脉压为8～12 mmHg，平均动脉压（MAP）≥65 mmHg，上腔静脉氧饱和度≥70%或混合静脉氧饱和度≥65%。
- 保持目标 MAP≥65 mmHg；如果足够的液体不能有效地恢复足够的血压，就开始使用升压药物。在血流动力学指标稳定之后，限制液体治疗的入量，防止发生肺水肿及低氧血症的加重。
- 作为首选的升压药，通过中心静脉使用去甲肾上腺素。在血管升压素作为抢救疗法后，肾上腺素是第二种选择。如果需要使用正性肌力药物，多巴酚丁胺可能有效。除特殊情况外，避免使用多巴胺（存在心动过速和持续性心动过缓的低风险）。
- 当血红蛋白浓度降至＜7 g/dl 时，输注红细胞；目标血红蛋白水平为7～9 g/dl。
- 针对急性呼吸窘迫综合征住院患者的潮气量为6 ml/kg。
- 给予低分子量肝素或普通肝素，用于深静脉血栓形成的预防；如果肝素治疗禁忌，请使用压力弹力袜或间歇性加压装置。
- 使用组胺 H_2 阻滞剂或质子泵抑制剂进行应激性溃疡预防。
- 提供专业的对症支持治疗；在第一周提供低剂量营养治疗；如果发生难治性感染中毒性休克，应考虑使用应激剂量类固醇；将血糖保持在110～180 mg/dl 范围内。

数据引自 Dellinger RP, Levy MM, et al: Surviving Sepsis Campaign: international guidelines for the management of severe sepsis and septic shock, 2012, Crit Care Med 41: 580-637, 2013.

表4.4　成年感染中毒症患者的初始抗生素推荐

适应证	治疗推荐[a]
经验性覆盖（来源不详）	万古霉素 15 mg/kg q12 h 加哌拉西林-他唑巴坦[b] 3.375 g IV q6 h 或亚胺培南 0.5 g IV q6 h 或美罗培南 1.0 g IV q8 h 联用或不联用氨基糖苷类药物（如妥布霉 5 mg/kg q24 h）[c]
社区获得性肺炎（CAP）	头孢曲松 1 g IV q24 h 加阿奇霉素 500 mg IV q24 h 或氟喹诺酮（如莫西沙星 400 mg IV q24 h 或左氧氟沙星 750 mg IV q24 h）[d]
社区获得性尿血液感染中毒症	哌拉西林-他唑巴坦 3.375 g IV q6 h 或环丙沙星 400 mg IV q12 h
脑膜炎	万古霉素 15 mg/kg IV q6 h 加头孢曲松 2 g IV q12 h 加地塞米松 0.15 mg/kg IV q6 h×2～4 天，在应用抗生素之前；如果怀疑李斯特菌感染，加用氨苄西林 2 g IV q4 h
医院内肺炎	万古霉素 15 mg/kg q12 h 加哌拉西林-他唑巴坦 4.5 g q6 h 或亚胺培南 0.5 g IV q6 h 或美罗培南 1 g IV q8 h 或头孢吡肟 2 g IV q8 h 加氨基糖苷（如阿米卡星 15 mg/kg IV 24 h 或妥布霉素 5～7 mg/kg IV q24 h）或左氧氟沙星 750 mg IV q24 h。如果考虑为 MRSA 感染，一些机构建议应用利奈唑胺 600 mg IV q12 h 替代万古霉素
中性粒细胞减少	头孢吡肟 2 g IV q8 h；如果存在中心静脉导管并且担心感染，加用万古霉素 15 mg/kg IV q12 h。如果发热超过5天，加用卡泊芬净 70 mg IV 1 次，之后 50 mg IV q24 h 覆盖真菌感染。对于怀疑和确认侵袭性曲霉菌的感染，应用伏立康唑 6 mg/kg IV q12 h 2 次，之后 4 mg/kg IV q12 h
蜂窝织炎和皮肤感染	万古霉素 15 mg/kg q12 h，在糖尿病患者和免疫缺陷的患者，加哌拉西林-他唑巴坦 3.375 g IV q6 h。如果怀疑坏死性筋膜炎，应用克林霉素 900 mg IV. 外科手术是非常重要的

IV，静脉注射；MRSA，耐甲氧西林金黄色葡萄球菌。
[a] 假定肾功能正常；肾功能不全时根据受损的肌酐清除率进行剂量的调整。
[b] 如果患者对青霉素过敏，换用氨曲南 2 g IV q8 h。
[c] 监测氨基糖苷类药物的浓度（包括峰、谷浓度）。
[d] 如果患者有严重的 CAP 或医疗相关肺炎，换用头孢吡肟或者碳青霉烯类药物和阿奇霉素±一种氨基糖苷类药物。

治疗

感染中毒性休克是医学急症。需要早期的诊断及抗感染的治疗。需要即刻采取措施恢复患者生理性的血流动力学、重要器官的支持以及组织的氧气供应。患者应当尽快转至ICU接受更好的监测，血流动力学的支持以及专业支持治疗。

早期识别、及时复苏和早期使用适当的抗菌药物是成功治疗结果的最重要决定因素。如果必要的话，尽早的进行感染性病灶（及源头控制）的引流。2016年版《挽救感染中毒症运动指南》中关键内容总结在表4.3。

感染中毒症的治疗核心内容是早期使用对病原微生物有效的抗生素。最好在出现感染中毒性休克1 h 内进行治疗。通常在血培养结果出来之前以及感染部位明确治疗，经验性地使用广谱的抗生素治疗。表4.4提供了初

to treat the causative pathogen until its identity and susceptibility profile become available days later is associated with adverse outcomes. After the pathogen is identified, de-escalation to the simplest monotherapy to which it is susceptible is important.

PROGNOSIS

Despite advances in clinical practice and treatment, sepsis mortality rates remain high, ranging from 20% to 30% among relatively healthy adults to more than 80% among the elderly, immunocompromised, and those with significant chronic medical comorbidities. Patients may experience significant weakness, wasting, and debilitation due to severe catabolism, poor nutrition, and prolonged hospitalization. Prolonged rehabilitation in a skilled facility after the initial hospitalization and additional home-based therapy may be required. Patients may have permanent disabilities, including impaired renal function or persistent debilitation from procedures required to treat the underlying infection.

SUGGESTED READINGS

Anand V, Zhang Z, Kadri SS, et al: Epidemiology of quick sequential organ failure assessment criteria in undifferentiated patients and association with suspected infection and sepsis, Chest 156(2):289–297, 2019.

Angus D, van der Poll T: Severe sepsis and septic shock, N Engl J Med 369:840–851, 2013.

Cheng MP, Stenstrom R, Paqette K, et al: Blood culture results before and after antimicrobial administration in patients with severe manifestations of sepsis: a diagnostic study, Ann Intern Med, 2019. https://doi.org/10.7326/M19-1696.

Hotchkiss RS, Coopersmith CM, McDunn JE, et al: The sepsis seesaw: tilting toward immunosuppression, Nat Med 15:496–497, 2009.

Howell MD, Davis AM: Management of sepsis and septic shock, J Am Med Assoc 317(8):317, 2017.

Melamed A, Sorvillo FJ: The burden of sepsis-associated mortality in the United States from 1999 to 2005: an analysis of multiple-cause-of-death data, Crit Care 13:R28, 2009.

Rhee C, Dantes R, Epstein L, et al: Incidence and trends of sepsis in US hospitals using clinical vs claims data, 2009-2014, J Am Med Assoc 318(13):1241–1249, 2017.

Singer M, Deutschman CS, Seymour CW, et al: The third international consensus definitions for sepsis and septic shock (sepsis-3), J Am Med Assoc 315(8):801–810, 2016.

Vincent JL, Opal SM, Marshall JC, et al: Sepsis definitions: time for a change, Lancet 381:774–775, 2013.

始治疗方案的建议。在病原确定和药物敏感性确定后才开始治疗会使得治疗延误，效果不佳。在病原体明确后，可以根据耐药的结果进行抗生素的降级使用单药治疗。

预后

虽然临床实践和治疗已经取得了进步，感染中毒症的病死率仍然很高。相对健康的成年人群中的病死率是20%～30%，在老年人、免疫缺陷人群以及有严重慢性合并症的人群中超过80%。由于严重的分解代谢、营养不良以及住院时间的延长，患者会出现严重的虚弱状态、消耗状态，以及衰弱状态。患者出院后仍需要居家的进一步的治疗和康复。患者可能面临着永久性的失能，包括由于治疗感染所致的肾功能损伤或持久的衰弱状态，

推荐阅读

Anand V, Zhang Z, Kadri SS, et al: Epidemiology of quick sequential organ failure assessment criteria in undifferentiated patients and association with suspected infection and sepsis, Chest 156(2):289–297, 2019.

Angus D, van der Poll T: Severe sepsis and septic shock, N Engl J Med 369:840–851, 2013.

Cheng MP, Stenstrom R, Paqette K, et al: Blood culture results before and after antimicrobial administration in patients with severe manifestations of sepsis: a diagnostic study, Ann Intern Med, 2019. https://doi.org/10.7326/M19-1696.

Hotchkiss RS, Coopersmith CM, McDunn JE, et al: The sepsis seesaw: tilting toward immunosuppression, Nat Med 15:496–497, 2009.

Howell MD, Davis AM: Management of sepsis and septic shock, J Am Med Assoc 317(8):317, 2017.

Melamed A, Sorvillo FJ: The burden of sepsis-associated mortality in the United States from 1999 to 2005: an analysis of multiple-cause-of-death data, Crit Care 13:R28, 2009.

Rhee C, Dantes R, Epstein L, et al: Incidence and trends of sepsis in US hospitals using clinical vs claims data, 2009-2014, J Am Med Assoc 318(13):1241–1249, 2017.

Singer M, Deutschman CS, Seymour CW, et al: The third international consensus definitions for sepsis and septic shock (sepsis-3), J Am Med Assoc 315(8):801–810, 2016.

Vincent JL, Opal SM, Marshall JC, et al: Sepsis definitions: time for a change, Lancet 381:774–775, 2013.

5

Infections of the Central Nervous System

Su N. Aung, Allan R. Tunkel

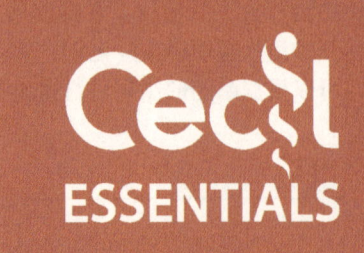

INTRODUCTION

Infections of the central nervous system (CNS) can be caused by a number of pathogens, including viruses, bacteria, fungi, and parasites (i.e., protozoa and helminths). These infectious agents can penetrate the CNS by direct seeding or hematogenous spread and cause a constellation of symptoms. The clinical presentation of a CNS infection varies depending on the virulence of the offending pathogen, the location of the infection, and underlying host factors. CNS infections can impact structures contained in the cranium or spinal cord and may be associated with significant morbidity and mortality. This chapter focuses on meningitis, encephalitis, and focal intracranial and paraspinal infections, as well as prion diseases.

MENINGITIS

Definition

Meningitis, defined as inflammation of the leptomeninges that cover the brain and spinal cord, is identified by an abnormal increase in the number of white blood cells in cerebrospinal fluid (CSF). Inflammation can be caused by many infectious agents (i.e., bacteria, viruses, fungi, and parasites) and also can occur as a result of noninfectious conditions, including tumors or cysts, medications (e.g., nonsteroidal anti-inflammatory drugs, antimicrobial agents), systemic illnesses (e.g., systemic lupus erythematosus, Behçet disease, sarcoidosis), or neurologic procedures (e.g., neurosurgery, spinal anesthesia, intrathecal injections, retained devices).

The clinical presentation may be acute, subacute, or chronic based on the virulence of the infecting agent and patient characteristics. Acute meningitis is a syndrome characterized by the onset of symptoms within hours to several days, whereas chronic meningitis is usually characterized by abnormal clinical and CSF findings that persist for at least 4 weeks. Acute meningitis is most often caused by bacteria and viruses, whereas chronic meningitis is most often caused by spirochetes, mycobacteria, and fungi. The clinical presentation may also vary depending on the age of the patient, underlying health conditions, predisposing factors (e.g., head trauma, recent neurosurgery, presence of a CSF shunt or other retained devices), and immunosuppression.

Epidemiology and Etiology
Bacterial Meningitis

Bacterial meningitis is associated with high morbidity and mortality and requires prompt clinical recognition and treatment. Over 1.2 million cases of bacterial meningitis are diagnosed each year worldwide with incidence and mortality rates varying by region, pathogen, and age. CSF findings commonly include pleocytosis (CSF white blood cell count in the hundreds to thousands range) usually associated with neutrophilic predominance, low glucose, and elevated protein.

Based on a prior surveillance study in the United States from 2003 to 2007, the most common pathogens causing bacterial meningitis were *Streptococcus pneumoniae* (58% of cases), *Streptococcus agalactiae* (18% of cases), *Neisseria meningitidis* (14% of cases), *H. influenzae* (7% of cases), and *Listeria monocytogenes* (3% of cases). Specific etiologic agents may be identified based on the patient's age and various risk factors (Table 5.1).

In the United States, *S. pneumoniae* is the most common etiologic agent of bacterial meningitis. The incidence has declined since the introduction of pneumococcal conjugate vaccines PCV7 and later PCV13, but mortality remains high, ranging from 18% to 26%. Among survivors, high rates of neurologic sequelae and systemic complications occur, especially in those over 60 years of age. Conditions associated with severe pneumococcal meningitis include asplenia or splenic dysfunction, multiple myeloma, hypogammaglobulinemia, alcoholism, malnutrition, chronic liver or kidney disease, and diabetes mellitus. Patients often have contiguous or distant foci of infection such as pneumonia, otitis media, mastoiditis, sinusitis, and endocarditis. Head trauma, with a CSF leak, is an important risk factor for recurrent pneumococcal meningitis.

The group B streptococcus (i.e., *S. agalactiae*) is a common etiologic agent of meningitis in neonates, with 52% of cases occurring during the first year of life. Mortality in the United States ranges from 7% to 27% with substantial long-term morbidity seen among survivors. Group B streptococcal meningitis can also occur in adults. Risk factors in adults include age older than 60 years, pregnancy or the postpartum state, diabetes mellitus, and other chronic diseases and immunosuppressed states but may also occur in adults without underlying conditions.

Neisseria meningitidis usually causes meningitis in children and young adults. Most cases in the United States are caused by serogroups B, C, and Y; serogroups A and W seldom occur in the United States. Patients with deficiencies in the terminal complement components (C5 to C8, and perhaps C9) and properdin are at increased risk for meningococcal infections, including meningitis with significantly higher rates of neurologic sequelae. Outbreaks of meningitis due to *N. meningitidis* may occur in persons living in close quarters, such as among household members, in daycare centers, college dormitories, and among the incarcerated. One outbreak of serogroup C disease was reported in New York City among men who have sex with men, and outbreaks caused by serogroup B have been reported at college campuses,

中枢神经系统感染

王芳 译 田地 韩宁 审校 张福杰 通审

引言

诸多病原体可导致中枢神经系统（CNS）感染，包括病毒、细菌、真菌及寄生虫（例如原生动物和蠕虫）。这些病原体可以直接侵犯或通过血流进入CNS并引起一系列症状。CNS感染的临床表现取决于致病病原体的毒力、感染的位置和潜在的宿主因素。CNS感染可影响颅内或脊髓中的组织结构，造成严重的后果。本章重点介绍脑膜炎、脑炎、局灶性颅内和颅旁感染以及朊病毒疾病。

脑膜炎

定义

脑膜炎是指覆盖大脑和脊髓的软脑膜的炎症，可通过脑脊液（CSF）中白细胞数量的增加来识别。可引起脑膜炎的病原体很多，如细菌、病毒、真菌及寄生虫，也可能由非感染性疾病引起，包括肿瘤或囊肿、药物（如非甾体抗炎药、抗菌药物）、全身性疾病（如系统性红斑狼疮、白塞综合征、结节病）或神经系统手术（如神经外科手术、脊髓麻醉、鞘内注射、置入物）。

根据感染病原体的毒力和患者的特征，临床上可表现为急性、亚急性或慢性。急性脑膜炎是一种以数小时至数天内出现症状为特征的综合征，而慢性脑膜炎通常以持续至少4周的异常临床和脑脊液检查结果为特征。急性脑膜炎多由细菌和病毒引起，而慢性脑膜炎多由螺旋体、分枝杆菌和真菌引起。临床表现也会因患者的年龄、基本健康状况、易感因素（如头部外伤、近期神经外科手术、存在脑脊液分流管或其他留置装置）和免疫抑制情况而有所不同。

流行病学和病因

细菌性脑膜炎

细菌性脑膜炎的发病率和死亡率较高，需要及时诊断和治疗。全世界每年诊断的细菌性脑膜炎病例超过120万例，发病率和死亡率因地区、病原体和年龄而异。脑脊液表现通常为细胞数增多（脑脊液白细胞计数在数百到数千），以中性粒细胞为主，脑脊液糖降低，蛋白升高。

2003—2007年美国一项监测研究显示，引起细菌性脑膜炎的最常见病原体为肺炎链球菌（58%）、无乳链球菌（18%）、脑膜炎奈瑟球菌（14%）、流感嗜血杆菌（7%）和单核细胞增生李斯特菌（3%）。一些特定的病原可根据患者的年龄和各种危险因素来确定（表5.1）。

在美国，肺炎链球菌是细菌性脑膜炎最常见的病原体。自引入肺炎链球菌结合疫苗PCV7及其后的PCV13以来，细菌性脑膜炎发病率有所下降，但死亡率仍高达18%～26%。幸存者常有神经系统后遗症及全身并发症，60岁以上老年患者后遗症发生率更高。重症肺炎链球菌性脑膜炎的危险因素包括无脾或脾功能障碍、多发性骨髓瘤、低丙种球蛋白血症、酒精中毒、营养不良、慢性肝肾疾病和糖尿病。患者常有肺炎、中耳炎、乳突炎、鼻窦炎、心内膜炎等相邻或远处感染灶。头颅创伤伴有脑脊液漏是复发性肺炎链球菌性脑膜炎的重要危险因素。

B组链球菌（即无乳链球菌）是新生儿脑膜炎的常见病原体，其中52%发生在出生后第一年。美国报道的死亡率为7%～27%，幸存者中有相当大比例出现长期残疾。B组链球菌性脑膜炎也可发生于成人。成人患者的危险因素包括60岁以上、孕产妇、糖尿病和其他慢性疾病和免疫功能低下，但也可能发生在没有基础疾病的成年人中。

脑膜炎奈瑟球菌通常引起儿童和年轻成年人的脑膜炎。美国报道，大多数病例是由血清型B群、C群和Y群引起的；血清型A群和W群在美国少见。末端补体成分（C5～C8，可能还有C9）和备解素缺乏的患者发生脑膜炎奈瑟球菌感染的风险增加，出现脑膜炎并多伴神经系统后遗症。脑膜炎奈瑟球菌引起的脑膜炎暴发可出现在群居于狭窄空间的人群中，例如家庭成员之间、日托中心、大学宿舍和被监禁者中。纽约男男同性性行为者中曾出现C群脑膜炎奈瑟球菌感染暴发，大学校园中也有B群脑膜炎奈瑟球菌的暴发，

TABLE 5.1 Common Bacterial Pathogens and Factors Predisposing to Meningitis

Predisposing Factor	Bacterial Pathogens
Age	
<1 mo	*Streptococcus agalactiae, Escherichia coli, Listeria monocytogenes*
1–23 mo	*S. agalactiae, E. coli, Haemophilus influenzae, Streptococcus pneumoniae, Neisseria meningitidis*
2–50 yr	*S. pneumoniae, N. meningitidis*
>50 yr	*S. pneumoniae, N. meningitidis, L. monocytogenes*, aerobic gram-negative bacilli
Immunocompromised state	*S. pneumoniae, N. meningitidis, L. monocytogenes*, aerobic gram-negative bacilli (including *Pseudomonas aeruginosa*)
Basilar skull fracture	*S. pneumoniae, H. influenzae*, group A β-hemolytic streptococci
Head trauma; post neurosurgery	*Staphylococcus aureus*, coagulase-negative staphylococci (especially *Staphylococcus epidermidis*), aerobic gram-negative bacilli (including *P. aeruginosa*)

From Hasbun R, van de Beek D, Brouwer MC, Tunkel AR: Acute meningitis. In Bennett JE, Dolin R, Blaser M, editors: Mandell, Douglas, and Bennett's principles and practice of infectious diseases, ed 9, Philadelphia, 2020, Saunders.

most recently at the Rutgers University, Columbia University, and University of California San Diego (Centers for Disease Control and Infection [CDC], May 2019). Risk is also increased in patients who are taking eculizumab (inhibits complement).

Prophylaxis is indicated for people in the same household, roommates, young adults exposed in dormitories, travelers who had direct contact with respiratory secretions from an index patient or was seated next to an index patient during a prolonged flight, and individuals who were exposed to oral secretions (e.g., intimate kissing, or health care workers who performed mouth-to-mouth resuscitation or endotracheal intubation on the index patient). Chemoprophylaxis should be administered as soon as possible if indications are met, ideally within 24 hours after identification of the index case, and is usually not beneficial beyond 14 days. Recommended antimicrobials for prophylaxis include rifampin, ciprofloxacin, and ceftriaxone. Currently, there are vaccines that cover serogroups A, C, W, Y (MenACWY) and serogroup B (MenB). Vaccination with the quadrivalent meningococcal vaccine against serogroups A, C, W, and Y is recommended for children ages 11 to 18 years of age and individuals 2 months or older with risk factors including anatomic or functional asplenia, persistent complement deficiency, HIV infection, individuals taking eculizumab, travelling to certain countries where vaccine is recommended (e.g., Saudi Arabia, Mecca, or Hajj), at-risk exposure during outbreaks, and microbiologists who work with the meningococcus bacteria. Two meningococcal B vaccines were approved in 2015 for persons aged 10 to 25 years; the recommendation from the Advisory Committee on Immunization Practices is that adolescents and young adults, ages 16 to 23 years, may be vaccinated for short-term protection against most strains of *N. meningitidis* serogroup B, but that the risk of infection in the United States is currently low.

Among typable strains, *Haemophilus influenzae* serotype b (Hib) was a common cause of meningitis and epiglottis among children prior to the widespread use of the conjugate vaccine against *H. influenzae* type b. The incidence of meningitis due to *H. influenzae* has declined more than 90% since the introduction of vaccination. Isolation of this microorganism in older children and adults suggests certain underlying conditions, such as sinusitis, otitis media, epiglottitis, pneumonia, structural lung disease, diabetes mellitus, alcoholism, splenectomy or asplenic states, head trauma with CSF leak, immune deficiency, hematopoietic stem cell transplantation, and chemotherapy or radiation therapy. In the post-Hib vaccination era, nontypable *H. influenzae* has emerged as a cause of invasive infections, including meningitis, particularly among the elderly and young children.

Meningitis caused by *Listeria monocytogenes* is most common in neonates, adults older than 50 years, alcoholics, immunosuppressed adults, pregnancy, conditions associated with iron overload, and in patients with chronic conditions such as diabetes mellitus, collagen vascular disease, liver disease, and renal disease. Given the likely gastrointestinal portal of entry for this microorganism, outbreaks of *Listeria* infection have been associated with ingestion of contaminated coleslaw, raw vegetables, milk, and cheese. Sporadic cases have been linked to contaminated turkey franks, alfalfa tablets, cantaloupe, diced celery, hog's head cheese, and processed meats. *Listeria* CNS infection has been associated with rhombencephalitis, which refers to inflammation of the hindbrain (brainstem and cerebellum) with concomitant findings on brain imaging and is more commonly seen in immunocompetent persons.

Meningitis caused by aerobic gram-negative pathogens (e.g., *Klebsiella* sp, *Escherichia coli*, *Serratia marcescens*, *Pseudomonas aeruginosa*, *Acinetobacter* sp) are becoming more important as etiologies, particularly in patients with a history of head trauma or neurosurgical procedures. At-risk individuals include neonates, older adults, immunosuppressed patients, those with gram-negative sepsis, and rarely in disseminated strongyloidiasis associated with the hyperinfection syndrome.

Staphylococcus aureus meningitis is usually found in the early period after neurosurgery or recent head trauma, in those with CSF shunts, or in patients with underlying conditions such as diabetes mellitus, alcoholism, chronic kidney disease requiring hemodialysis, injection-drug use, and malignancies. *S. aureus*, particularly methicillin-resistant strains, is most commonly seen in health care–associated ventriculitis and meningitis. Community-acquired *S. aureus* meningitis is found in patients with sinusitis, osteomyelitis, and pneumonia.

Viral Meningitis

Viral meningitis is the most common type of meningitis. The CSF profile of viral meningitis usually includes pleocytosis with elevated WBCs in the tens to hundreds range, lymphocytic predominance, normal glucose, and elevated protein. Overall, meningitis due to a viral etiology is often less severe than bacterial meningitis, and symptoms usually self-resolve. Risk factors for severe infection include young age (less than 5 years) and immunosuppression.

Enteroviruses are the leading identifiable cause of the *aseptic meningitis syndrome*, a term used to define any meningitis (particularly with lymphocytic pleocytosis) for which a cause is not apparent after initial evaluation, routine CSF stains, and cultures. The CDC estimate that 10 to 15 million symptomatic enteroviral infections occur annually in the United States; of these, 30,000 to 75,000 are meningitis cases, although this is likely an underestimation.

Many other viruses can cause the aseptic meningitis syndrome, including mumps virus (in unimmunized populations), human immunodeficiency virus (HIV), several arboviruses (e.g., St. Louis encephalitis virus, the California encephalitis group of viruses, Colorado tick fever virus, West Nile virus), and herpesviruses (including Epstein-Barr virus, the herpes simplex viruses, and varicella-zoster virus). The

第5章 中枢神经系统感染

表 5.1　脑膜炎常见细菌病原体及易感因素

易感因素	细菌病原体
年龄	
＜1个月	无乳链球菌、大肠埃希菌、单核细胞增生李斯特菌
1~23个月	无乳链球菌、大肠埃希菌、流感嗜血杆菌、肺炎链球菌、脑膜炎奈瑟球菌
2~50岁	肺炎链球菌、脑膜炎奈瑟球菌
＞50岁	肺炎链球菌、脑膜炎奈瑟球菌、单核细胞增生李斯特菌、需氧革兰氏阴性杆菌
免疫缺陷状态	肺炎链球菌、脑膜炎奈瑟球菌、单核细胞增生李斯特菌、需氧革兰氏阴性杆菌（包括铜绿假单胞菌）
颅底骨折	肺炎链球菌、流感嗜血杆菌、A组链球菌
头部创伤；神经外科术后	金黄色葡萄球菌、凝固酶阴性葡萄球菌（尤其是表皮葡萄球菌）、需氧革兰氏阴性杆菌（包括铜绿假单胞菌）

引自 Hasbun R, van de Beek D, Brouwer MC, Tunkel AR: Acute meningitis. In Bennett JE, Dolin R, Blaser M, editors: Mandell, Douglas, and Bennett's principles and practice of infectious diseases, ed 9, Philadelphia, 2020, Saunders.

罗格斯大学、哥伦比亚大学和加州大学圣地亚哥分校近期均有病例报道（美国CDC，2019年5月）。使用依库珠单抗（补体抑制剂）的住院患者患病风险也会增加。

脑膜炎奈瑟球菌感染患者的共同居住者、室友、同宿舍的年轻人、直接接触患者呼吸道分泌物或与患者相邻而坐的长途飞行旅客，以及暴露于患者口腔分泌物的人（例如亲密接吻，或对患者进行口对口复苏或气管插管的医护人员）需要进行脑膜炎奈瑟球菌药物预防。有以上指征的人群，应尽快进行化学预防，最好在确定接触患者后2 h内进行，超过14天后通常无益。推荐的预防性抗菌药物包括利福平、环丙沙星和头孢曲松。现有疫苗可预防血清型A群、C群、W群、Y群（MenACWY）和血清型B群（MenB）脑膜炎奈瑟球菌。建议11~18岁的儿童和2个月或2个月以上存在解剖或功能性无脾、持续补体缺乏、HIV感染、服用依库珠单抗、前往某些推荐接种疫苗的国家/地区（例如，沙特阿拉伯、麦加或朝觐）、暴发期间有风险暴露，以及接触脑膜炎奈瑟球菌的研究人员接种针对血清型A群、C群、W群、Y群四价脑膜炎奈瑟球菌疫苗。2015年，两种B群脑膜炎奈瑟球菌疫苗获批用于10~25岁的人群；免疫接种咨询委员会建议16~23岁的青少年和年轻人可以接种疫苗，以短期预防大多数脑膜炎奈瑟球菌B群菌株，但目前美国的感染风险很低。

在广泛应用针对b型流感嗜血杆菌的结合疫苗之前，b型流感嗜血杆菌（Hib）是儿童脑膜炎和会厌炎的常见病因。自引入疫苗接种以来，流感嗜血杆菌引起的脑膜炎发病率下降超过90%。在年龄较大的儿童和成人中分离出这种微生物提示某些潜在疾病，例如鼻窦炎、中耳炎、会厌炎、肺炎、肺结构病变、糖尿病、酗酒、脾切除术或无脾状态、头外伤造成的脑脊液漏、免疫缺陷、造血干细胞移植以及化疗或放疗。在开展Hib疫苗接种后，未分型的流感嗜血杆菌已成为侵袭性感染（包括脑膜炎）的病因，特别是在老年人和幼儿中。

单核细胞增生李斯特菌引起的脑膜炎最常见于新生儿、50岁以上的成年人、酗酒者、免疫抑制的成人、妊娠期、与铁超负荷相关的疾病以及糖尿病、胶原血管疾病、肝病和肾病等慢性疾病患者。鉴于这种微生物可能进入胃肠道入侵，李斯特菌感染的暴发与摄入受污染的凉拌卷心菜、生蔬菜、牛奶和奶酪有关。散发病例与受污染的火鸡肉、苜蓿、哈密瓜、芹菜丁、猪头奶酪和加工肉类有关。李斯特菌中枢神经系统感染可引起脑干脑炎，指后脑（脑干和小脑）炎症，伴有相应影像改变，多见于免疫功能正常的人。

由需氧革兰氏阴性菌（如克雷伯菌属、大肠埃希菌、黏质沙雷菌、铜绿假单胞菌、不动杆菌）引起的脑膜炎作为病因变得越来越重要，尤其是有头部外伤或神经外科手术史的住院患者。高危人群包括新生儿、老年人、免疫抑制患者、革兰氏阴性感染中毒症患者、类圆线虫高度感染综合征的患者。

金黄色葡萄球菌性脑膜炎通常见于神经外科术后早期或近期头部外伤、脑脊液分流的患者，或者有基础疾病如糖尿病、酗酒、需要血液透析的慢性肾病、注射药物使用和恶性肿瘤的患者。金黄色葡萄球菌，尤其是MRSA，是最常见的院内感染的脑室炎和脑膜炎病原体。社区获得性金黄色葡萄球菌脑膜炎见于鼻窦炎、骨髓炎和肺炎患者。

病毒性脑膜炎

病毒性脑膜炎是最常见的脑膜炎类型。病毒性脑膜炎的脑脊液检查通常可见白细胞升高达到数十至数百个，以淋巴细胞为主，糖正常，蛋白质升高。总体而言，病毒性脑膜炎通常不如细菌性脑膜炎严重，并且症状通常可自行缓解。严重感染的危险因素包括低龄（小于5岁）和免疫抑制。

肠道病毒是无菌性脑膜炎的最主要的病因，无菌性脑膜炎定义为初步诊断（通过脑脊液常规染色及培养）病因不明的脑膜炎（尤其是伴有脑脊液淋巴细胞增多的脑膜炎）。美国疾病预防控制中心估计，美国每年有1000万~1500万例有症状的肠道病毒感染；其中，保守估计脑膜炎患者有30 000~75 000例。

许多其他病毒可引起无菌性脑膜炎综合征，包括流行性腮腺炎病毒（在未免疫人群中）、人类免疫缺陷病毒（HIV）、虫媒病毒（如圣路易斯脑炎病毒、加利福尼亚病毒、科罗拉多蜱传热病毒、西尼罗病毒）和

syndrome of herpes simplex virus (HSV) meningitis is most commonly associated with primary genital infection. The DNA of HSV has been detected in the CSF of patients with the syndrome of recurrent benign lymphocytic meningitis (previously known as Mollaret meningitis), with almost all cases caused by herpes simplex virus type 2 (HSV-2).

Spirochetal Meningitis

The most common spirochetes associated with meningitis are *Treponema pallidum* (the etiologic agent of syphilis) and *Borrelia burgdorferi* (the etiologic agent of Lyme disease). The incidence of syphilitic meningitis is greatest in the first 2 years after initial infection, occurring in 0.3% to 2.4% of untreated cases. The overall incidence of neurosyphilis has increased, with the majority of cases reported in patients with HIV infection. Based on the CDC surveillance data from 2008 to 2015, approximately 12.5% of cases of Lyme disease had neurologic manifestations, including facial palsy (8.4%), radiculoneuropathy (3.8%), lymphocytic meningitis (1.3%), and encephalitis (<1%).

Tuberculous Meningitis

Mycobacterium tuberculosis can lead to pulmonary and extrapulmonary disease, including involvement of the CNS. Tuberculous meningitis accounts for approximately 15% of cases of extrapulmonary tuberculosis in the United States. CNS disease is much more common in less developed areas of the world. Factors associated with reactivation of latent foci and progression to the syndrome of late generalized tuberculosis include advanced age, immunosuppressive drug therapy, HIV/AIDS, transplantation, malignancy, gastrectomy, pregnancy, chronic medical conditions, and close contacts to individuals with active infection. The epidemiology of tuberculosis has been influenced by the advent of HIV infection, in which extrapulmonary disease (including CNS infection) occurs in more than 70% of cases with co-infection.

Fungal Meningitis

The incidence of fungal meningitis has risen dramatically in recent years due to the increasing numbers of immunosuppressed patients and broad usage of immunosuppressive drugs. *Cryptococcus neoformans* is the most common etiologic agent of clinically recognized fungal meningitis, most commonly diagnosed in persons who are immunosuppressed or have chronic medical conditions; HIV-infected patients are in the highest-risk group. Cases have also been documented in immunocompetent healthy individuals.

Coccidioides immitis is a thermal dimorphic fungus that is endemic in the semiarid regions of the Americas and desert areas of the southwestern United States (e.g., California, Arizona, New Mexico, Texas), where about one third of the population is infected. Less than 1% of patients develop disseminated infection, and one third to one half of those with disease have meningeal involvement.

Other fungi less commonly cause CNS infection. *Histoplasma capsulatum* is endemic to fertile river valleys, principally the Mississippi and Ohio River basins. *Blastomyces dermatitidis* is also distributed in the Mississippi and Ohio River basins, as well as regions around the Great Lakes and along the Saint Lawrence River. *Candida* meningitis is uncommon and occurs as a manifestation of disseminated candidiasis, usually in premature neonates, individuals with ventricular drainage devices, and as isolated chronic meningitis.

Clinical Presentation
Acute Meningitis

Adult patients with acute meningitis typically seek medical attention within hours to days of illness. Patients with acute bacterial meningitis classically exhibit fever, headache, meningismus, and signs of cerebral dysfunction (i.e., confusion, delirium, or a declining level of consciousness ranging from lethargy to coma). The presentation may vary based on age, underlying disease status, and specific pathogen involved. The etiology can be very challenging to distinguish early in the onset of illness. In bacterial meningitis, the meningismus may be subtle, marked, or accompanied by Kernig sign or Brudzinski sign, although the sensitivity of these signs is only 5% in adults. Cranial nerve palsies (especially involving cranial nerves III, IV, VI, and VII) and focal cerebral signs are seen in 10% to 20% of cases. Seizures occur in about 30% of patients. Older adult patients with bacterial meningitis, especially those with underlying conditions (e.g., diabetes mellitus, cardiopulmonary disease), may have disease that manifests insidiously with lethargy or obtundation, no fever, and various signs of meningeal inflammation. Older adult patients may have an antecedent or concurrent bronchitis, pneumonia, or paranasal sinusitis.

Viral meningitis is typically a self-limited illness, but symptoms can be difficult to distinguish from bacterial meningitis, particularly early in the disease course. The clinical manifestations of enteroviral meningitis, the most common etiology of viral meningitis, depend on host age and immune status. In adolescents and adults, more than one half of the patients have nuchal rigidity. Adults usually present with headache, which is often severe and frontal. Photophobia is also common in older patients. Nonspecific symptoms and signs include vomiting, anorexia, rash, diarrhea, cough, upper respiratory findings (especially pharyngitis), and myalgias. Other clues to the diagnosis of enteroviral disease are the time of year (more prevalent in summer and autumn months) and known epidemic disease in the community. The duration of illness of enteroviral meningitis is usually less than 1 week, and many patients report improvement after lumbar puncture, presumably from the reduction in intracranial pressure.

Meningitis associated with HSV-2 infections is usually characterized by stiff neck, headache, and fever. Patients with recurrent benign lymphocytic meningitis characteristically develop a few to 10 episodes of meningitis lasting 2 to 5 days, followed by spontaneous recovery. These patients have acute onset of headache, fever, photophobia, and meningism; about 50% of patients have transient neurologic manifestations, including seizures, hallucinations, diplopia, cranial nerve palsies, or altered consciousness. Unlike HSV encephalitis, HSV meningitis is usually benign and resolves without treatment. The second most common herpesvirus causing aseptic meningitis is varicella-zoster virus (VZV) and can occur in the absence of the typical vesicular rash. Epstein-Barr virus (EBV) meningitis can be seen in the presence of concomitant mononucleosis-like picture with rash, pharyngitis, lymphadenopathy, and splenomegaly.

West Nile virus (WNV) causes neuroinvasive disease in approximately 1% of patients with WNV infections, which is most often seen during summer months in the United States. WNV meningitis symptoms typically include fever, headache, nausea, vomiting, stiff neck, photophobia, and occasionally a maculopapular rash. Patients may experience persistent symptoms and exhibit abnormal neurologic findings for years following the acute infection.

In patients infected with mumps virus, CNS infection causes fever, vomiting, and headache. Fevers are usually high and last for 72 to 96 hours. These symptoms usually occur about 5 days after the onset of parotitis, which can be present in about 50% of cases. In uncomplicated cases, defervescence typically leads to clinical recovery; the total duration of illness is usually 7 to 10 days.

Subacute or Chronic Meningitis

Meningitis caused by spirochetes, mycobacteria, or fungi in the adult patient can linger for weeks to years after clinical presentation. The patient may initially have no overt symptoms, suffer from low-grade headaches and fever, or experience gradual mental status and other neurologic changes.

Syphilitic meningitis (neurosyphilis) caused by *Treponema pallidum* usually manifests in a manner similar to that of other forms of aseptic

疱疹病毒（包括 EB 病毒、单纯疱疹病毒和水痘-带状疱疹病毒）。单纯疱疹病毒（HSV）脑膜炎主要由原发生殖器感染引起。在复发性良性淋巴细胞脑膜炎综合征（以前称莫拉雷脑膜炎）患者的脑脊液中检测到 HSV 的 DNA，几乎均由单纯疱疹病毒 2 型（HSV-2）引起。

螺旋体脑膜炎

最常见引起脑膜炎的螺旋体是苍白密螺旋体（梅毒的病原体）和伯氏疏螺旋体（莱姆病的病原体）。梅毒性脑膜炎的发病率在初次感染后的前 2 年最高，在未经治疗的病例中发生率为 0.3%～2.4%。HIV 感染住院患者中神经梅毒总体发病率有所增加。根据美国 CDC 2008—2015 年的监测数据，大约 12.5% 的莱姆病患者有神经系统表现，包括面瘫（8.4%）、神经根病（3.8%）、淋巴细胞性脑膜炎（1.3%）和脑炎（＜1%）。

结核性脑膜炎

结核分枝杆菌可导致肺部和肺外疾病，包括中枢神经系统受累。在美国，结核性脑膜炎约占肺外结核病例的 15%。中枢神经系统疾病多见于全世界的欠发达地区。潜伏病灶再激活和进展为晚期全身性结核病综合征的危险因素包括高龄、免疫抑制药物治疗、HIV/AIDS、移植、恶性肿瘤、胃切除术、妊娠、慢性疾病以及与活动性结核患者密切接触。结核病的流行病学受到 HIV 感染的影响，HIV 合并结核感染者中超过 70% 为肺外疾病（包括中枢神经系统感染）。

真菌性脑膜炎

近年来，由于免疫缺陷患者逐渐增多和免疫抑制药物的广泛使用，真菌性脑膜炎的发病率显著上升。新型隐球菌是临床最常见的真菌性脑膜炎的病原体，多见于免疫抑制或慢性疾病患者；其中 HIV 感染者风险最高。但免疫功能正常的健康人也有发病的报道。

粗球孢子菌是一种热二态性真菌，在美洲的半干旱地区和美国西南部的沙漠地区（例如，加利福尼亚州、亚利桑那州、新墨西哥州、得克萨斯州）流行，那里约有 1/3 的人口受到感染。其中有不到 1% 患者为播散性感染，1/3～1/2 的患者出现脑膜炎。

其他真菌较少引起中枢神经系统感染。荚膜组织胞浆菌流行于肥沃河谷地区，主要流行于密西西比河和俄亥俄河流域。皮炎芽生菌也分布在密西西比河和俄亥俄河流域，以及五大湖周围和圣劳伦斯河沿岸地区。念珠菌性脑膜炎少见，是播散性念珠菌病的一种表现，通常见于早产儿、心室引流装置患者，也可表现为单纯性慢性脑膜炎。

临床表现
急性脑膜炎

成人急性脑膜炎患者通常在发病后数小时至数天内就医。急性细菌性脑膜炎患者通常表现为发热、头痛、脑膜刺激征和脑功能障碍的体征（即意识模糊、谵妄或意识水平下降，从嗜睡到昏迷轻重不等）。临床表现可能因年龄、基础疾病和感染病原体不同而异。在发病早期明确感染病原可能非常困难。细菌性脑膜炎的脑膜刺激征可能很微妙或很明显，成人患者有 5% 伴有克尼格征或巴宾斯基征。10%～20% 的患者出现脑神经麻痹（尤其是累及第Ⅲ、Ⅳ、Ⅵ和Ⅶ脑神经）和局灶性脑体征。大约 30% 患者出现癫痫发作。老年细菌性脑膜炎患者，尤其是有基础疾病（例如糖尿病、心肺疾病）的患者可隐袭起病，表现为嗜睡、反应迟钝，无发热和其他脑膜炎体征。老年患者的细菌性脑膜炎可能继发于支气管炎、肺炎或鼻旁窦炎。

病毒性脑膜炎通常是一种自限性疾病，但其症状可能难以与细菌性脑膜炎区分开来，尤其是在病程早期。肠道病毒是病毒性脑膜炎最常见的病因，其临床表现取决于宿主的年龄和免疫状态。在青少年和成人中，超过一半的患者有颈强直。成人通常表现为严重的额部头痛。老年患者常有畏光。非特异性症状和体征包括呕吐、厌食、皮疹、腹泻、咳嗽、上呼吸道表现（尤其是咽炎）和肌痛。诊断肠道病毒性疾病的依据还有发病季节（夏秋季更多发）和在流行地区起病。肠道病毒引起的脑膜炎的病程通常少于 1 周，许多患者在腰椎穿刺后病情有所改善，可能是由于腰穿后颅内压降低。

HSV-2 感染引起的脑膜炎通常有颈强直、头痛和发热。复发性良性淋巴细胞脑膜炎患者的特征性表现是脑膜炎反复发作数次至 10 次，每次持续 2～5 天，随后自行恢复。这些患者有急性发作的头痛、发热、畏光和脑膜刺激征；约 50% 的患者有短暂的神经系统表现，包括癫痫发作、幻觉、复视、脑神经麻痹或意识改变。与单纯疱疹病毒脑炎不同，单纯疱疹病毒脑膜炎通常是良性的，无须治疗，可以自愈。引起无菌性脑膜炎的第二大常见疱疹病毒是水痘-带状疱疹病毒（VZV），可不伴典型水疱疹。EB 病毒（EBV）脑膜炎可伴有皮疹、咽炎、淋巴结肿大和脾大的单核细胞增多症样表现。

约有 1% 的西尼罗病毒（WNV）感染者会出现神经侵袭性疾病，美国夏季常见。西尼罗病毒脑膜炎的症状通常包括发热、头痛、恶心、呕吐、颈强直、畏光，偶尔还会出现斑丘疹。患者可能在急性感染后数年内持续有症状及异常的神经系统表现。

流行性腮腺炎病毒感染中枢神经系统会引起发热、呕吐和头痛。通常为高热，持续 72～96 h。通常发生在腮腺炎起病后约 5 天，约 50% 腮腺炎患者会出现。没有并发症的患者，热退后病情缓解；总病程 7～10 天。

亚急性或慢性脑膜炎

成人螺旋体、分枝杆菌或真菌性脑膜炎的症状可持续数周至数年。患者病初可能没有明显症状，可表现为轻微头痛和发热，或逐渐出现精神状态和其他神经系统变化。

梅毒性脑膜炎（神经梅毒）由苍白密螺旋体引起，临床表现与其他原因引起的无菌性脑膜炎相似，患者主诉头痛、恶心和呕吐。其他发现包括颈强直、发热、

meningitis. Patients complain of headache, nausea, and vomiting. Other findings include stiff neck, fever, seizures, cranial nerve palsies, and less commonly, other focal neurologic abnormalities (e.g., hemiplegia, aphasia, and mental status changes). Meningovascular syphilis occurs as a result of focal syphilitic arteritis. Most patients experience symptoms including headache, vertigo, personality changes, behavioral changes, insomnia, seizures, or focal neurologic deficits that can last for weeks to months. In rare cases, if untreated, the focal deficits can progress to stroke with irreversible neurologic deficits.

Meningitis is the most important neurologic abnormality of acute disseminated Lyme disease and usually occurs 2 to 10 weeks following erythema migrans. Headache is the most common symptom of Lyme meningitis. Other symptoms include photophobia, nausea, vomiting, and stiff neck. About 50% of patients with Lyme meningitis have mild cerebral symptoms consisting most commonly of somnolence, emotional lability, depression, impaired memory and concentration, and behavioral symptoms. Approximately 50% of patients may exhibit cranial neuropathies, with facial nerve palsy occurring in 80% to 90% of cases.

Patients with tuberculous meningitis experience an insidious prodrome characterized by malaise, lassitude, low-grade fever, intermittent headache, and personality changes. Within 2 to 3 weeks, the meningitic phase manifests as protracted headache, photophobia, stiff neck, vomiting, and confusion. In some adults, the initial prodromal stage may take the form of a slowly progressive dementia, whereas others may have a rapidly progressive meningitis syndrome indistinguishable from pyogenic bacterial meningitis. Fever is an inconstant finding on physical examination (50% to 98% of cases). Meningismus and signs of meningeal irritation are not uniform findings and can be absent in 25% to 80% of patients. Focal neurologic signs frequently consist of unilateral or, less commonly, bilateral cranial nerve palsies; cranial nerve VI is most commonly affected.

The time course of fungal meningitis depends on the clinical setting. Cases may manifest acutely, subacutely, or chronically; some of the fungal meningitides may cause symptoms that persist for years in the absence of antifungal treatment. In contrast, the same organisms can produce severe symptoms and signs within a few days and without clinical signs of meningeal irritation, particularly in the immunocompromised patient. In patients without acquired immunodeficiency syndrome (AIDS), cryptococcal meningitis typically manifests as a subacute process after days to weeks of symptoms. Headache is the most frequent complaint. Fever, stiff neck, photophobia, and personality changes may also occur; confusion, irritability, and other personality changes reflecting meningoencephalitis occur in about 50% of patients. Ocular abnormalities occur in about 40% of patients and include papilledema and cranial nerve palsies.

In AIDS patients, manifestation of cryptococcal meningitis can be subtle, with minimal or no symptoms. AIDS patients may report only headache and lethargy. Although fever is common, meningeal signs occur in a minority of these patients.

Patients with meningeal coccidioidomycosis usually complain of headache, low-grade fever, weight loss, and mental status changes. About one half of patients develop disorientation, lethargy, confusion, or memory loss. Meningeal signs are uncommon. The presenting symptoms of *Histoplasma* meningitis are nonspecific. Symptoms usually include headache and fever. Only about one half of patients have focal neurologic mental status symptoms. Candidal meningitis also manifests with nonspecific findings and is seen as an extension of disseminated disease in at-risk individuals.

Diagnosis

Clinically suspected meningitis is diagnosed by analysis of CSF obtained by lumbar puncture (Table 5.2). Table 5.3 illustrates general CSF findings for patients with meningitis based on cause, and the following sections detail specific methods for establishing an etiologic diagnosis.

Bacterial Meningitis

Gram stain examination of CSF permits rapid, accurate identification of the causative microorganism in 60% to 90% of patients with bacterial meningitis, and it has a specificity of nearly 100%. CSF culture is the gold standard in diagnosis and is positive in 80% to 90% of patients with community-acquired bacterial meningitis if CSF is obtained before the start of antimicrobial therapy. The probability of identifying the organism decreases for patients who received prior antimicrobial therapy. CSF sterilization may occur more rapidly after initiation of parenteral antimicrobial therapy than previously suggested, with complete sterilization of CSF containing meningococcus within 2 hours and the beginning of sterilization of pneumococcus by 4 hours following initiation of antimicrobial therapy.

TABLE 5.2 Cerebrospinal Fluid Tests for Patients With Suspected Central Nervous System Infection

Routine Tests
WBC count with differential
RBC count[a]
Glucose concentration[b]
Protein concentration
Gram stain
Bacterial culture

Selected Tests Based on Clinical Suspicion
Viral culture[c]
Smears and culture for acid-fast bacilli
Venereal Disease Research Laboratory (VDRL) test
India ink preparation
Cryptococcal polysaccharide antigen
Fungal culture
Antibody tests (IgM or IgG, or both)[e]
Nucleic acid amplification tests (e.g., PCR)[f]
Cytology[g]
Flow cytometry

From Hasbun R, Tunkel AR: Approach to the patient with central nervous system infection. In Bennett JE, Dolin R, Blaser M, editors: Mandell, Douglas, and Bennett's principles and practice of infectious diseases, ed 9, Philadelphia, 2020, Saunders.
CSF, Cerebrospinal fluid; IgG, immunoglobulin G; IgM, immunoglobulin M; PCR, polymerase chain reaction; RBCs, red blood cells; WBCs, white blood cells.

[a]Check in the first and last tubes; in patients with a traumatic tap, there should be a decrease in the number of RBCs with continued flow of CSF. The following formula can be used for determining whether the numbers of CSF red blood cells and white blood cells are consistent with a traumatic tap (all units are number of cells/cubic mm):

$$\text{Adjusted WBCs in CSF} = \text{Actual WBCs in CSF} - \frac{\text{WBCs in blood} \times \text{RBCs in CSF}}{\text{RBCs in blood}}$$

[b]Compare with serum glucose concentration measured just before lumbar puncture.
[c]Yield of viral culture may be low.
[e]May be useful for specific causes of meningitis and encephalitis.
[f]Most useful for specific viral causes of encephalitis and causes of chronic meningitis.
[g]In patients with suspected malignancy.

癫痫发作、脑神经麻痹，较少见局灶性神经系统异常（如偏瘫、失语和精神状态改变）。局灶性梅毒性动脉炎导致脑血管梅毒。大多数患者出现头痛、眩晕、性格改变、行为异常、失眠、癫痫发作或局灶性神经功能缺损等症状，可持续数周至数月。在极少数情况下，如果不及时治疗，局灶性神经功能受损可发展为卒中，造成不可逆转的神经功能缺损。

脑膜炎是急性播散性莱姆病最重要的神经系统异常表现，通常在发生游走性红斑后的 2～10 周。头痛是莱姆病脑膜炎最常见的症状。其他症状还有畏光、恶心、呕吐和颈强直。约 50% 的莱姆病脑膜炎患者有轻微的脑部症状，最常见的是嗜睡、易激动、抑郁、记忆力和注意力减退以及行为异常。约 50% 患者会出现脑神经病变，80%～90% 的病例会出现面神经麻痹。

结核性脑膜炎起病隐袭，前驱症状表现为乏力、倦怠、低热、间歇性头痛和性格改变。2～3 周进入脑膜炎期，表现为持续头痛、畏光、颈强直、呕吐和意识障碍。一些成年人，前驱期可能表现为缓慢进展的痴呆，而另一些人则可能出现迅速进展的脑膜炎综合征，与化脓性细菌性脑膜炎难以区分。体格检查中，50%～98% 病例有发热。25%～80% 的患者可能没有脑膜刺激征。局灶性神经系统体征通常是单侧脑神经麻痹，少部分患者有双侧脑神经麻痹表现；第 Ⅵ 对脑神经受累最常见。

真菌性脑膜炎的病程临床差异较大，患者可表现为急性、亚急性或慢性；在没有抗真菌治疗的情况下，一些真菌性脑膜炎患者的症状可持续数年之久。还有患者感染相同真菌可在几天内出现严重的症状和体征，而没有脑膜刺激表现，尤其是在免疫力低下的患者中。在没有获得性免疫缺陷综合征（AIDS）的患者中，隐球菌性脑膜炎通常在出现症状几天到几周后表现为亚急性过程。最常见表现为头痛，还可伴有发热、颈强直、畏光和性格改变；约 50% 的患者会出现意识障碍、易激惹和性格改变等脑膜脑炎表现。约 40% 的患者会出现视觉异常，包括视乳头水肿和脑神经麻痹。

AIDS 患者隐球菌性脑膜炎的表现可能不明显，症状极轻或没有症状。AIDS 患者可能仅表现为头痛和嗜睡。发热常见，但只有少数患者会出现脑膜刺激征。

脑膜球孢子菌病患者通常主诉头痛、低热、体重减轻和精神状态改变。约一半的患者会出现定向力下降、嗜睡、意识障碍或记忆丧失。脑膜刺激征不常见。组织胞浆菌脑膜炎症状为非特异性的，通常包括头痛和发热。只有约一半患者有局灶性神经精神症状。念珠菌性脑膜炎也表现为非特异性症状，为高危人群感染后播散至中枢神经系统所致。

诊断

临床疑似脑膜炎需要经过腰椎穿刺检查 CSF 进行诊断（表 5.2）。表 5.3 说明了不同病因所致脑膜炎的

表 5.2　疑似中枢神经系统感染患者的 CSF 检测

常规检查
WBC 分类计数
RBC 计数[a]
脑脊液糖水平[b]
脑脊液蛋白水平
革兰氏染色
细菌培养

根据临床情况选择
病毒培养[c]
抗酸杆菌涂片和培养
性病研究实验室（VDRL）试验
墨汁染色
隐球菌多糖抗原
真菌培养
抗体检测［IgM 和（或）IgG］[e]
核酸扩增检测（如 PCR）[f]
细胞学检查[g]
流式细胞学检测

引自 Hasbun R, Tunkel AR: Approach to the patient with central nervous system infection. In Bennett JE, Dolin R, Blaser M, editors: Mandell, Douglas, and Bennett's principles and practice of infectious diseases, ed 9, Philadelphia, 2020, Saunders.

CSF，脑脊液；IgG，免疫球蛋白 G；IgM，免疫球蛋白 M；PCR，聚合酶链反应；RBC，红细胞；WBC，白细胞。

[a] 对比第一管和最后一管；对于腰椎穿刺损伤的患者，随着 CSF 持续流出，红细胞数量应有所减少。以下公式可用于判断 CSF 红细胞和白细胞的数量是否与穿刺损伤有关（所有单位均为细胞数 / 立方毫米）：

$$\text{调整后 CSF 中的 WBC} = \text{CSF 中的实际 WBC} - \frac{\text{外周血中的 WBC} \times \text{CSF 中 RBC}}{\text{外周血中 RBC}}$$

[b] 与腰椎穿刺前测量的血清葡萄糖浓度进行比较。
[c] 病毒培养阳性率很低。
[e] 可用于特定病因的脑膜炎和脑炎。
[f] 对特定病毒引起的脑炎和慢性脑膜炎最有用。
[g] 疑似恶性肿瘤患者。

CSF 的一般特点。下文将详细介绍不同病原引起的脑膜炎诊断的具体方法。

细菌性脑膜炎

对脑脊液进行革兰氏染色检查可快速、准确地鉴定出 60%～90% 的细菌性脑膜炎患者的致病微生物，特异性接近 100%。脑脊液培养是诊断的金标准，如果在开始抗菌治疗前进行脑脊液培养，社区获得性细菌性脑膜炎的阳性率可达 80%～90%。对于之前接受过抗菌治疗的患者，检出病原体的阳性率降低。静脉应用抗菌治疗后，CSF 中细菌转阴的速度可能比以前认为的更快，CSF 中脑膜炎奈瑟球菌可在抗感染治疗 2 h 内完全消失，而肺炎链球菌则可在开始抗菌治疗后 4 h 内消失。

TABLE 5.3	Cerebrospinal Fluid Findings for Patients With Infectious Causes of Meningitis			
Cause of Meningitis	White Blood Cell Count (cells/mm³)	Primary Cell Type	Glucose (mg/dL)	Protein (mg/dL)
Viral	50–1000	Mononuclear[a]	>45	<200
Bacterial	1000–5000[b]	Neutrophilic[c]	<40[d]	100–500
Tuberculous	50–300	Mononuclear[e]	<45	50–300
Cryptococcal	20–500[f]	Mononuclear	<40	>45

From Hasbun R, Tunkel AR: Approach to the patient with central nervous system infection. In Bennett JE, Dolin R, Blaser M, editors: Mandell, Douglas, and Bennett's principles and practice of infectious diseases, ed 9, Philadelphia, 2020, Saunders.
[a]May be neutrophilic early in presentation.
[b]May range from <100 to >10,000 neutrophils/mm³.
[c]About 10% of patients have a cerebrospinal fluid (CSF) lymphocyte predominance.
[d]Should always be compared with a simultaneous serum glucose level; ratio of CSF to serum glucose is ≤0.4 in most cases.
[e]A therapeutic paradox may exist in which a mononuclear predominance becomes neutrophilic during antituberculosis therapy.
[f]More than 75% of patients with acquired immunodeficiency syndrome have <20 cells/mm³.

Several rapid diagnostic tests have been developed to aid in the etiologic diagnosis of bacterial meningitis. Latex agglutination techniques detect the antigens of *H. influenzae* type b, *S. pneumoniae*, *N. meningitidis*, *E. coli* K1, and the group B streptococci. However, because bacterial antigen testing does not appear to modify the decision to administer antimicrobial therapy and false-positive results have been reported, routine use of this modality for rapid determination of the bacterial cause of meningitis is not recommended. It can, however, be considered for patients who have been pretreated with antimicrobial therapy and when CSF Gram stain and culture results are negative.

Nucleic acid amplification tests, such as polymerase chain reaction (PCR), have been used to amplify DNA from patients with meningitis caused by up to 14 meningeal pathogens including bacterial, viral, and fungal agents in one test known as the Meningitis/Encephalitis Panel or BioFire, which has very high sensitivity and specificity. Despite the more comprehensive and rapid identification potential, use of this testing should be reserved for patients with high likelihood of meningitis or encephalitis without an identified pathogen on initial testing. Prior to considering this test, patients should still have CSF sent for routine Gram stain, culture, and testing for other common pathogens (i.e., PCR for herpes simplex viruses and enteroviruses) based on epidemiology, patient risk factors, and season. Therefore, this comprehensive test is commonly reserved for patients with negative initial tests despite clinical correlation or due to prior antimicrobial therapy.

Differentiation of Bacterial From Viral Meningitis

In patients without a positive CSF Gram stain or culture, the diagnosis of acute bacterial meningitis is often difficult to establish or reject. A combination of clinical features, with or without test results, has been assessed to develop models in an attempt to accurately predict the likelihood of bacterial meningitis compared with other potential causes (most often viruses). In a published meta-analysis of bacterial meningitis score validation studies in which 5312 patients were identified from eight studies, 4896 (92%) had sufficient clinical data to calculate the bacterial meningitis score, which identified children with CSF pleocytosis who were at very low risk for bacterial meningitis. Low-risk features were a negative CSF Gram stain, a CSF absolute neutrophil count less than 1000 cells/mm³, a CSF protein level less than 80 mg/dL, and a peripheral absolute neutrophil count less than 10,000 cells/mm³. Despite the potential utility of this meta-analysis and other similar studies, decisions related to empiric therapy should be based on clinical judgment.

Several proteins have been examined for their usefulness in the diagnosis of acute bacterial meningitis. C-reactive protein (CRP) detected in serum or CSF and serum procalcitonin concentrations have been elevated in patients with acute bacterial meningitis and may be useful in discriminating between bacterial and viral meningitis. In patients with meningitis in whom the CSF Gram stain result is negative and analysis of other parameters is inconclusive, serum concentrations of CRP or procalcitonin that are normal or below the limit of detection have a high negative predictive value in the diagnosis of bacterial meningitis.

PCR is the most promising alternative to viral culture for the diagnosis of enteroviral meningitis. Enteroviral reverse transcription PCR (RT-PCR) has been tested in clinical settings and found to be more sensitive than culture for the detection of enterovirus; the sensitivity has ranged from 86% to 100% and specificity from 92% to 100% for the diagnosis of enteroviral meningitis. For patients with HSV-2 meningitis, PCR is the recommended test for diagnosis. In patients with recurrent benign lymphocytic meningitis, detection of HSV-2 has been strongly associated with typical cases in patients without symptoms or signs of genital infection.

Spirochetal Meningitis

For the diagnosis of neurosyphilis, no single routine laboratory test is definitive. The specificity of the CSF Venereal Disease Research Laboratory (VDRL) test for the diagnosis of neurosyphilis is high, but the sensitivity is low (30% to 70%). A reactive CSF VDRL test result in the absence of blood contamination is sufficient to diagnose neurosyphilis; a nonreactive result does not exclude the diagnosis. The diagnosis of neurosyphilis is based on elevated CSF concentrations of white blood cells or protein, or both, in the appropriate clinical and serologic setting.

The best currently available laboratory test for the diagnosis of Lyme disease is demonstration of specific serum antibody to *B. burgdorferi*, and this positive test result for a patient with a compatible neurologic abnormality is strong evidence for the diagnosis. However, these tests are not standardized, and marked variations are seen between laboratories.

Tuberculous Meningitis

The identification of tuberculous organisms in CSF by specific stains is difficult due to the small population of organisms. In many series, less than 25% of specimens were smear positive and less than 50% were culture positive. The technique of PCR for detecting fragments of mycobacterial DNA in CSF specimens appears to be a promising tool. The Gen-Probe technique is based on amplification of ribosomal RNA derived from *Mycobacterium tuberculosis* using a labeled DNA probe. A 5-year retrospective study of the performance of this test found a sensitivity and specificity of 94% and 99%, respectively, for patients with positive CSF cultures.

Fungal Meningitis

Conclusive proof of a fungal etiology for meningitis requires identification of the fungus in CSF, although CSF cultures are not always

表 5.3　感染性脑膜炎患者的脑脊液检查结果

脑膜炎病因	白细胞计数（/mm³）	主要细胞类型	糖（mg/dl）	蛋白（mg/dl）
病毒性	50～1000	单核细胞[a]	>45	<200
细菌性	1000～5000[b]	中性粒细胞[c]	<40[d]	100～500
结核性	50～300	单核细胞[e]	<45	50～300
隐球菌性	20～500[f]	单核细胞	<40	>45

引自 Hasbun R, Tunkel AR: Approach to the patient with central nervous system infection. In Bennett JE, Dolin R, Blaser M, editors: Mandell, Douglas, and Bennett's principles and practice of infectious diseases, ed 9, Philadelphia, 2020, Saunders.

[a] 早期可以中性粒细胞为主。
[b] 中性粒细胞在＜100～＞10000/mm³。
[c] 约10%的患者CSF中以淋巴细胞为主。
[d] 应始终与同时检测的血清葡萄糖水平进行比较；在大多数情况下，脑脊液与血清葡萄糖的比值≤0.4。
[e] 在抗结核治疗过程中，以单核为主会变成以中性粒细胞为主。
[f] 75%以上的获得性免疫缺陷综合征患者的细胞数小于20/mm³。

目前已开发出几种快速诊断检测方法进行细菌性脑膜炎的病因诊断。乳胶凝集技术可检测b型流感嗜血杆菌、肺炎链球菌、脑膜炎奈瑟球菌、大肠埃希菌K1和B组链球菌的抗原。但细菌抗原检测似乎并不影响抗菌治疗的决策，并且也存在假阳性结果的报道，因此不建议常规使用这种方法来快速检测脑膜炎细菌。然而对于已接受抗菌治疗的患者，以及脑脊液革兰氏染色和培养结果呈阴性的患者，可以考虑使用这种方法。

核酸扩增检测，如聚合酶链反应（PCR），已被用于扩增脑膜炎患者的DNA，包括细菌、病毒和真菌等多达14种病原体（即脑膜炎/脑炎检测板或BioFire，其敏感性及特异性均很高）。尽管该检测具有更全面、更快速的鉴定能力，但应仅限于在初次检测中未发现病原体的脑膜炎或脑炎疑诊患者。在进行该检测方法之前，患者仍应进行CSF常规革兰氏染色、培养，并根据流行病学、患者高危因素和季节进行其他常见病原体的检测（如PCR检测单纯疱疹病毒和肠道病毒）。因此，这种全面检测通常只适用于有临床症状但初步检测结果为阴性的患者，或曾接受过抗菌治疗的患者。

细菌性脑膜炎与病毒性脑膜炎鉴别

脑脊液革兰氏染色或培养阴性的患者，往往难以确定急性细菌性脑膜炎的诊断。为了准确预测细菌性脑膜炎与其他潜在病因（最常见的是病毒）相比的可能性，我们对临床特征（无论是否有检测结果）进行了综合评估，并建立了模型。在一项已发表的细菌性脑膜炎评分验证研究的荟萃分析中，8项研究中5312名患者，其中4896名（92%）患者有足够的临床数据来计算细菌性脑膜炎评分，该评分可确定脑脊液细胞增多患儿患细菌性脑膜炎的风险极低。低风险特征包括CSF革兰氏染色阴性、CSF中性粒细胞绝对值小于1000/mm³、CSF蛋白水平小于80 mg/dl、外周中性粒细胞绝对数小于10 000/mm³。尽管这项荟萃分析和其他类似研究具有潜在的实用性，但仍应根据临床具体情况决定是否进行经验性治疗。

检测某些蛋白有助于急性细菌性脑膜炎的诊断。急性细菌性脑膜炎患者血清或脑脊液中的C反应蛋白（CRP）和血清降钙素原浓度升高，可能有助于鉴别细菌性脑膜炎和病毒性脑膜炎。在脑脊液革兰氏染色结果为阴性且其他参数分析不确定的脑膜炎患者中，正常或低于检测限的CRP或降钙素原血清浓度在细菌性脑膜炎诊断中具有很高的阴性预测值。

对于诊断肠道病毒脑膜炎的患者，PCR检测比病毒培养更可行。肠道病毒逆转录PCR（RT-PCR）在临床中的应用，证实它比病毒培养对肠道病毒的检测更敏感；其敏感性达86%～100%，特异性92%～100%。对于HSV-2脑膜炎患者，推荐使用PCR进行诊断。在复发性良性淋巴细胞性脑膜炎患者中，不伴生殖器感染症状或体征的典型脑膜炎病例常常可检出HSV-2。

螺旋体脑膜炎

不能通过单一常规实验室检测诊断神经梅毒。脑脊液性病研究实验室（VDRL）检测对神经梅毒诊断的特异性较高，但敏感性较低（30%～70%）。在没有血液污染的情况下，脑脊液VDRL检测阳性结果足以诊断神经梅毒；阴性结果不能排除诊断。有临床表现和血清学检查提示时，脑脊液中白细胞或蛋白质浓度升高，或两者同时升高可以诊断神经梅毒。

目前诊断莱姆病的最佳实验室检测方法是检测血清中的伯氏疏螺旋体特异性抗体，对于具有相符的神经系统异常的患者，阳性检测结果为诊断提供了有力证据。然而，这些检测并没有标准化，不同实验室之间存在显著差异。

结核性脑膜炎

由于脑脊液结核分枝杆菌数量较少，因此很难通过特异性染色鉴定。在许多系列研究中，只有不到25%的涂片呈阳性，不到50%的培养呈阳性。在CSF标本中检测分枝杆菌DNA片段的PCR技术可能是一种很可行的方法。Gen-Probe技术的基础是使用标记的DNA探针扩增结核分枝杆菌的核糖体RNA。一项为期5年的回顾性研究发现，对于CSF培养阳性的患者，该检测方法的敏感性和特异性分别为94%和99%。

真菌性脑膜炎

确诊真菌性脑膜炎需要在CSF中鉴定出真菌，但真菌性脑膜炎病例中脑脊液培养常呈阴性。无论患者

positive in cases of fungal meningitis. The yield of CSF culture in cryptococcal meningitis is excellent for non-AIDS and AIDS patients. CSF India ink examination remains a rapid, effective test that is positive in 50% to 75% of cases; the yield increases up to 88% among patients with AIDS. In contrast, only 25% to 50% of patients with other causes of fungal meningitis have positive CSF cultures.

Because cultures may be negative or require long periods before yielding positive results for patients with fungal meningitis, adjunctive studies (particularly serologic tests) may be helpful for the diagnosis. The latex agglutination test for cryptococcal polysaccharide antigen is sensitive and specific for the diagnosis of cryptococcal meningitis. Cryptococcal polysaccharide antigen also can be found in the serum and CSF, usually in severely immunosuppressed patients such as those with AIDS. Serologic antibody tests (i.e., coccidioidal and histoplasmal antigens) and antigen urine tests (i.e., histoplasmal antigen) may be useful in other cases of fungal meningitis. Because fungal meningitis is often an indication of disseminated disease, other serologic assays that help in identification of fungal infection, such as galactomannan (component of the cell wall of the mold *Aspergillus* that is released during growth) and 1,3-β-D-glucan (cell wall component of various medically important fungi), may also aid in diagnosis.

Treatment

Initial Treatment of the Patient With Acute Meningitis

Acute bacterial meningitis is a life-threatening illness, and early detection, work-up, and antimicrobial therapy are imperative to reduce morbidity and mortality. The initial management of a patient with presumed bacterial meningitis includes performance of a lumbar puncture to determine whether CSF findings are consistent with the diagnosis (Fig. 5.1). If meningitis is suspected, institution of antimicrobial therapy should be based on the results of Gram staining that suggest an etiologic pathogen (Table 5.4). However, if no etiologic agent can be identified by this means or performance of the lumbar puncture is delayed, institution of empirical antimicrobial therapy after obtaining blood cultures should be based on the patient's age and underlying disease status (Table 5.5).

It is reasonable to proceed with the lumbar puncture without computed tomography (CT) of the head if the patient does not meet any of the following criteria: new-onset seizures, an immunocompromised state, signs that are suspicious for space-occupying lesions (i.e., papilledema or focal neurologic signs, not including cranial nerve palsy), or moderate to severe impairment of consciousness. Patients at risk should undergo CT of the head before lumbar puncture to evaluate for increased intracranial pressure (i.e., result of an intracranial mass lesion or generalized brain edema) due to the potential risk of herniation if a lumbar puncture is performed. In this setting, emergent empirical antimicrobial therapy and adjunctive dexamethasone therapy (if indicated), after obtaining blood cultures, should be initiated before obtaining neuroimaging.

Specific Antimicrobial Therapy for Meningitis

After the infecting meningeal pathogen is isolated and susceptibility testing results are known, antimicrobial therapy can be modified for optimal treatment of patients with bacterial meningitis (Table 5.6). Recommended dosages of antimicrobial agents for adults with infections of the CNS are shown in Table 5.7.

One pathogen requires special discussion. Specific therapy for pneumococcal meningitis depends on the in vitro susceptibility of the organism to penicillin and the third-generation cephalosporins. Based on the reduced susceptibility of meningitis strains of pneumococcus to penicillin (approximately one third of isolates in the United States), penicillin is not recommended as empirical therapy in patients with

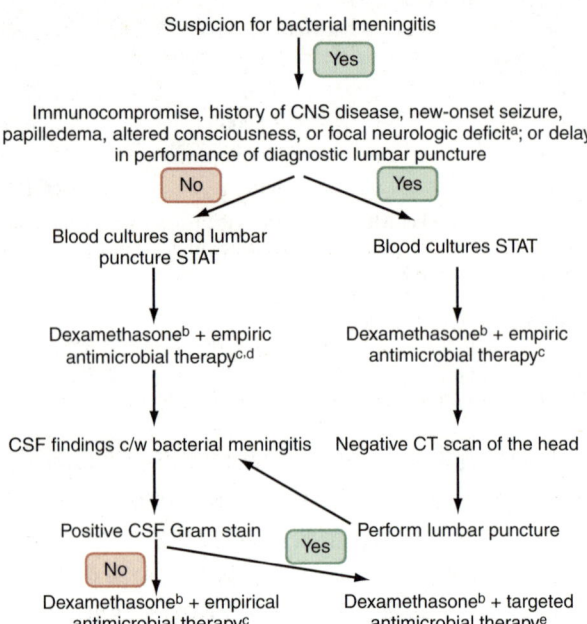

Fig. 5.1 Management algorithm for adults with suspected bacterial meningitis. [a]Palsy of cranial nerve VI or VII is not an indication to delay lumbar puncture. [b]See text for recommendations for use of adjunctive dexamethasone in patients with bacterial meningitis. [c]See Table 5.5. [d]Dexamethasone and antimicrobial therapy should be administered immediately after CSF is obtained. [e]See Table 5.4. *CNS*, Central nervous system; *CT*, computed tomography; *c/w*, consistent with; *STAT*, intervention should be done emergently. (From Tunkel AR, Hartman BJ, Kaplan, SL, et al: Practice guidelines for the management of bacterial meningitis, Clin Infect Dis 39:1267-1284, 2004.)

suspected pneumococcal meningitis. The combination of vancomycin plus a third-generation cephalosporin (i.e., cefotaxime or ceftriaxone) is recommended as an empirical regimen. After susceptibility studies of the isolated pneumococcus are performed, antimicrobial therapy can be modified for optimal treatment (see Table 5.7).

Viral meningitis is usually a benign self-limited illness. Recovery of patients with HSV-2 meningitis is usually complete without neurologic sequelae, and it is not clear whether antiviral treatment alters the course of mild meningitis.

The preferred antimicrobial regimen for the treatment of CNS syphilis is intravenous aqueous crystalline penicillin G at a dosage of 18 to 24 million units daily in divided doses every 4 hours or by continuous infusion for 10 to 14 days. Alternatively, procaine penicillin (2.4 million units intramuscularly daily) plus probenecid (500 mg orally four times daily), both for 10 to 14 days, can be used.

Parenteral antimicrobial therapy is usually needed to treat the neurologic manifestations of Lyme disease, including meningitis. The current recommendation is to treat most patients with Lyme meningitis with intravenous ceftriaxone at a dosage of 2 g daily for 14 days (range, 10 to 28 days); no evidence supports treatment durations longer than 4 weeks.

In patients with tuberculous meningitis, the most important principle of therapy is early initiation on the basis of strong clinical suspicion; it should not be delayed until proof of infection has been obtained. Identification can take weeks due to indolent culture growth. The American Thoracic Society, in conjunction with the CDC and the Infectious Diseases Society of America, recommend 2 months of isoniazid, rifampin, ethambutol, and pyrazinamide, followed by 7 to 10 months of isoniazid and rifampin for patients with drug-sensitive

是否合并 AIDS，隐球菌性脑膜炎 CSF 培养的阳性率都非常高。CSF 墨汁染色仍然是一种快速、有效的检测方法，50%～75% 的病例呈阳性；在 AIDS 患者中，阳性率最高可达 88%。相比之下，只有 25%～50% 的其他真菌性脑膜炎患者的 CSF 培养呈阳性。

真菌性脑膜炎患者的培养可能呈阴性或需要很长时间才能得到阳性结果，需要辅助检查（尤其是血清学检测）协助诊断。隐球菌多糖抗原乳胶凝集试验对诊断隐球菌性脑膜炎具有较高的敏感性和特异性。血清和脑脊液中隐球菌多糖抗原可呈阳性，患者通常伴有严重免疫抑制，如 AIDS。其他真菌性脑膜炎患者中，进行血清抗体检测（即球孢子菌抗原抗体和组织胞浆菌抗原抗体）和尿中抗原检测（即组织胞浆菌抗原）可有助于明确病因。由于真菌性脑膜炎通常是播散性真菌病的表现，其他血清学检测有助于鉴别诊断，如半乳糖甘露聚糖（曲霉菌细胞壁的成分，在生长过程中释放）和 1,3-β-D-葡聚糖（很多重要致病真菌的细胞壁成分）。

治疗

急性脑膜炎患者的初始治疗

急性细菌性脑膜炎常可危及生命，早期发现、早期检查和抗菌治疗是降低发病率和死亡率的当务之急。对可疑细菌性脑膜炎的患者的初步治疗包括进行腰椎穿刺，检测 CSF 协作诊断（图 5.1）。如果怀疑是脑膜炎，应根据革兰氏染色结果显示的病原体（表 5.4）进行抗菌治疗。但是，如果通过这种方法无法确定病原体，或无法及时进行腰椎穿刺术，则应根据患者的年龄和基础疾病状况（表 5.5），在获得血液培养后进行经验性抗菌治疗。

如果患者不符合以下任何条件：新发癫痫发作、免疫功能低下、有可疑占位性病变的体征（即乳头状脑水肿或局灶性神经系统体征，不包括脑神经麻痹）或中度至重度意识障碍，可以不进行头部计算机断层成像（CT）而进行腰椎穿刺。高危患者在腰椎穿刺前应进行头部 CT 检查，以评估颅内压是否增高（即颅内肿块病变或全身因素所致脑水肿引起的颅内压增高），因为如果进行腰椎穿刺，有可能导致脑疝形成。在这种情况下，应在进行神经影像学检查前，在获得血液培养结果后开始紧急经验性抗菌治疗和地塞米松辅助治疗（如有指征）。

脑膜炎针对性抗感染治疗

在分离出导致脑膜炎的病原体并得知药敏试验结果后，可对抗菌治疗进行调整，以优化细菌性脑膜炎患者的治疗（表 5.6）。表 5.7 列出了中枢神经系统感染成人的抗菌药物推荐剂量。

需要特别注意的是，肺炎链球菌脑膜炎的具体治疗方法取决于病菌对青霉素和第三代头孢菌素的体外敏感性。由于肺炎链球菌脑膜炎菌株对青霉素的敏感性降低（美国约有 1/3 的分离菌株对青霉素敏感），对于疑似肺炎链球菌性脑膜炎患者不建议将青霉素作为

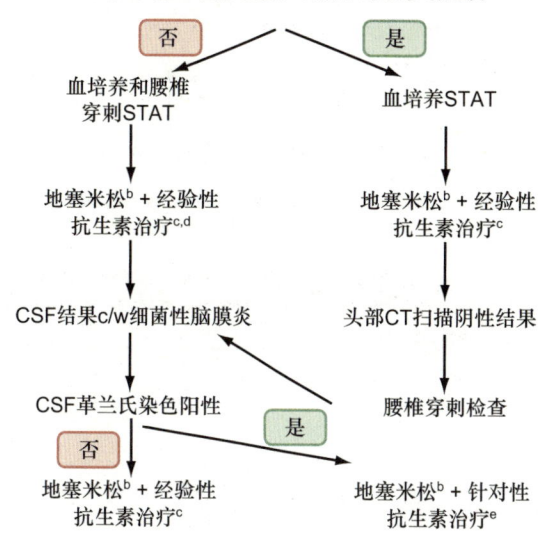

图 5.1 成人疑似细菌性脑膜炎患者的处理流程。[a] 第Ⅵ或第Ⅶ脑神经麻痹不是推迟腰椎穿刺的指征。[b] 有关细菌性脑膜炎患者辅助使用地塞米松的建议，参见正文。[c] 见表 5.5。[d] 留取 CSF 后，应立即使用地塞米松和抗菌药物。[e] 见表 5.4。CNS，中枢神经系统；CT，计算机断层成像；c/w，符合；STAT，应紧急进行干预（引自 Tunkel AR, Hartman BJ, Kaplan, SL, et al: Practice guidelines for the management of bacterial meningitis, Clin Infect Dis 39: 1267-1284, 2004.）

经验性疗法。推荐将万古霉素加第三代头孢菌素（如头孢噻肟或头孢曲松）作为经验性治疗方案。在对分离出的肺炎链球菌进行药敏试验后，可调整抗菌疗法，以达到最佳治疗效果（表 5.7）。

病毒性脑膜炎通常是一种良性自限性疾病。HSV-2 脑膜炎患者通常可以完全康复，不会留下神经系统后遗症，目前尚不清楚抗病毒治疗是否会改变轻度脑膜炎的病程。

治疗中枢神经系统梅毒的首选抗菌方案是静脉注射水溶性青霉素 G，剂量为每日 1800 万～2400 万单位，每 4 h 一次，连续输注 10～14 天。或者，也可以使用普鲁卡因青霉素（每天 240 万单位，肌内注射）加丙磺舒（每天 500 mg，分 4 次口服），疗程均为 10～14 天。

莱姆病神经系统病变包括脑膜炎的治疗通常需要肠外抗菌治疗。目前推荐头孢曲松静脉注射治疗，剂量为每天 2 g，持续 14 天（范围 10～28 天）；没有证据支持治疗时间超过 4 周。

如临床高度怀疑结核性脑膜炎，最重要的治疗原则是及早开始治疗；在获得病原学证据之前，不应拖延治疗，因为结核分枝杆菌生长缓慢，培养需要数周时间。美国胸科学会与美国疾病控制与预防中心（CDC）和美国传染病学会推荐对药物敏感的结核性脑膜炎患者应用异烟肼、利福平、乙胺丁醇和吡嗪酰胺，疗程 2 个月，然后再使用 7～10 个月的异烟肼和利福平。结

TABLE 5.4 Recommended Antimicrobial Therapy for Acute Bacterial Meningitis

Microorganism[a]	Antimicrobial Therapy
Haemophilus influenzae type b	Third-generation cephalosporin[b]
Neisseria meningitidis	Third-generation cephalosporin[b]
Streptococcus pneumoniae	Vancomycin plus a third-generation cephalosporin[b,c]
Listeria monocytogenes	Ampicillin or penicillin G[d]

Modified from Tunkel AR, Hartman BJ, Kaplan, SL, et al: Practice guidelines for the management of bacterial meningitis, Clin Infect Dis 39:1267-1284, 2004.
[a]Pathogen presumptively identified by positive Gram stain.
[b]Cefotaxime or ceftriaxone.
[c]Some experts would add rifampin if dexamethasone is also given.
[d]Addition of an aminoglycoside should be considered.

TABLE 5.5 Empirical Therapy for Purulent Meningitis

Predisposing Factor	Antimicrobial Therapy
Age	
<1 mo	Ampicillin plus cefotaxime or cefepime; or ampicillin plus an aminoglycoside
1–23 mo	Vancomycin plus a third-generation cephalosporin[a,b]
2–50 yr	Vancomycin plus a third-generation cephalosporin[a,b,c]
>50 yr	Vancomycin plus ampicillin plus a third-generation cephalosporin[a]
Immunocompromised state	Vancomycin plus ampicillin plus cefepime or meropenem
Basilar skull fracture	Vancomycin plus a third-generation cephalosporin[a]
Head trauma; after neurosurgery	Vancomycin plus ceftazidime, cefepime, or meropenem

Modified from Tunkel AR, Hartman BJ, Kaplan, SL, et al: Practice guidelines for the management of bacterial meningitis, Clin Infect Dis 39:1267-1284, 2004.
[a]Cefotaxime or ceftriaxone.
[b]Some experts add rifampin if dexamethasone is also given.
[c]Add ampicillin if meningitis caused by Listeria monocytogenes is suspected.

tuberculous meningitis. Therapy for tuberculous meningitis may need to be individualized, with longer durations of therapy used for patients with more severe illness or HIV.

Therapy for cryptococcal meningitis in patients with AIDS is usually an amphotericin B preparation (i.e., amphotericin B deoxycholate, liposomal amphotericin B, or amphotericin B lipid complex) plus flucytosine for 2 weeks, followed by consolidation therapy with fluconazole for 8 weeks. For non-AIDS patients with cryptococcal meningitis, the optimal use of fluconazole is less clear.

In a retrospective review of HIV-negative patients with CNS cryptococcosis, the patients were more likely to receive an induction regimen containing amphotericin B and subsequent therapy with fluconazole. Most experts recommend high-dose fluconazole (800 to 1200 mg daily) as first-line therapy for coccidioidal meningitis.

The current recommended treatment for Histoplasma meningitis is liposomal amphotericin B for 4 to 6 weeks, followed by itraconazole for at least 1 year. Amphotericin B, alone or in combination with flucytosine, also is the treatment of choice for Candida meningitis.

Adjunctive Therapy

For adult patients with bacterial meningitis, adjunctive dexamethasone should be administered to those with suspected or proven pneumococcal meningitis. This recommendation is based on a prospective, randomized, double-blind trial enrolling 301 adults with bacterial meningitis. Adjunctive dexamethasone was associated with a reduction in the proportion of patients who had unfavorable outcomes (15% vs. 25%, $P = .03$) and in the proportion of patients who died (7% vs. 15%, $P = .04$). The benefits were most striking for the subgroup of patients with pneumococcal meningitis and those with moderate to severe disease as assessed by the admission Glasgow Coma Scale.

Dexamethasone is administered at a dosage of 10 mg intravenously every 6 hours for 4 days in adults. The first dose should be given concomitantly with or just before the first dose of an antimicrobial agent for maximal attenuation of the subarachnoid space inflammatory response. Adjunctive dexamethasone should not be used in patients who have already received antimicrobial therapy or the meningitis is found not to be caused by S. pneumoniae. Despite the positive benefits of adjunctive dexamethasone for adults with bacterial meningitis described previously, the routine use of adjunctive dexamethasone for patients with bacterial meningitis in the developing world has been controversial.

Tuberculous meningitis is associated with significant morbidity and mortality despite the availability of effective antituberculous chemotherapy. Use of adjunctive corticosteroids has abrogated the signs and symptoms of disease, and early treatment with adjunctive dexamethasone should be used in all patients with tuberculous meningitis.

Patients with cryptococcal meningitis may have increased intracranial pressure or hydrocephalus, or both. For patients with neurologic deficits and evidence of increased intracranial pressure (usually an opening pressure >25 cm H_2O), daily lumbar puncture is recommended. Rarely, in cases of persistent opening pressure despite frequent lumbar punctures with removal of CSF, surgical CSF shunting may be required.

ENCEPHALITIS

Definition

Encephalitis is inflammation of the brain parenchyma that is associated with neurologic dysfunction. In the absence of pathologic evidence of brain inflammation, an inflammatory response in the CSF

表 5.4 急性细菌性脑膜炎的推荐抗菌疗法

微生物[a]	抗菌疗法
b 型流感嗜血杆菌	第三代头孢菌素[b]
脑膜炎奈瑟球菌	第三代头孢菌素[b]
肺炎链球菌	万古霉素联合第三代头孢菌素[b,c]
单核细胞增生李斯特菌	氨苄西林或青霉素 G[d]

改编自 Tunkel AR, Hartman BJ, Kaplan, SL, et al: Practice guidelines for the management of bacterial meningitis, Clin Infect Dis 39: 1267-1284, 2004.
[a] 通过革兰氏染色阳性初步确定的病原体。
[b] 头孢噻肟或头孢曲松。
[c] 一些专家认为,如果同时使用地塞米松,可加用利福平。
[d] 应考虑添加氨基糖苷类药物。

表 5.5 化脓性脑膜炎的经验疗法

易感因素	抗菌治疗
年龄	
< 1 个月	氨苄西林加头孢噻肟或头孢吡肟;或氨苄西林加氨基糖苷类药物
1～23 个月	万古霉素加第三代头孢菌素[a,b]
2～50 岁	万古霉素加第三代头孢菌素[a,b,c]
> 50 岁	万古霉素加氨苄西林加第三代头孢菌素[a]
免疫抑制状态	万古霉素加氨苄西林加头孢吡肟或美罗培南
颅底骨折	万古霉素加第三代头孢菌素[a]
头部创伤;神经外科术后	万古霉素加头孢噻肟、头孢吡肟或美罗培南

改编自 Tunkel AR, Hartman BJ, Kaplan, SL, et al: Practice guidelines for the management of bacterial meningitis, Clin Infect Dis 39: 1267-1284, 2004.
[a] 头孢噻肟或头孢曲松。
[b] 一些专家认为,如果同时使用地塞米松,可加用利福平。
[c] 如果怀疑是由单核细胞增生李斯特菌引起的脑膜炎,可加用氨苄西林。

核性脑膜炎的治疗可能需要因人而异,病情较重或感染 AIDS 的患者需要更长的治疗时间。

AIDS 患者隐球菌性脑膜炎的治疗通常采用两性霉素 B 制剂(即两性霉素 B 脱氧胆酸盐、两性霉素 B 脂质体或两性霉素 B 脂质复合物)加氟胞嘧啶治疗 2 周,然后再用氟康唑巩固治疗 8 周。对于非 AIDS 隐球菌性脑膜炎患者,氟康唑的最佳使用方法不明确。

针对 HIV 阴性的中枢神经系统隐球菌病患者进行的回顾性研究中,患者更有可能接受含有两性霉素 B 的诱导疗法,随后再接受氟康唑治疗。大多数专家推荐应用大剂量氟康唑(每天 800～1200 mg)作为球孢子菌性脑膜炎的一线疗法。

目前推荐的组织胞浆菌脑膜炎治疗方法是使用两性霉素 B 脂质体,疗程为 4～6 周,然后使用伊曲康唑,疗程至少 1 年。两性霉素 B 单独使用或与氟胞嘧啶联合使用也是治疗念珠菌性脑膜炎的首选方法。

辅助治疗

对于细菌性脑膜炎的成人患者,疑似或确诊为肺炎链球菌脑膜炎的患者应使用地塞米松辅助治疗。一项前瞻性、随机、双盲试验,共招募了 301 名细菌性脑膜炎成人患者。研究显示,辅助使用地塞米松可降低患者的不良预后比例(15% vs. 25%,$P = 0.03$)和死亡比例(7% vs. 15%,$P = 0.04$)。肺炎链球菌脑膜炎患者亚群和根据入院格拉斯哥昏迷量表评估为中度至重度患者亚群的获益最为显著。

成人每 6 h 静脉注射地塞米松 10 mg,连续 4 天。第一剂应在给予抗菌药物的同时或稍早给予,以最大限度地减轻蛛网膜下腔炎症反应。对于已经接受过抗菌治疗或明确脑膜炎并非由肺炎链球菌引起的患者,不宜辅助使用地塞米松。尽管地塞米松对成人细菌性脑膜炎患者的辅助治疗效果显著,但在发展中国家,对细菌性脑膜炎患者常规使用地塞米松仍存在争议。

即使应用有效的抗结核药物,结核性脑膜炎的发病率和死亡率仍很高。使用皮质类固醇辅助治疗可减轻疾病的症状和体征,所有结核性脑膜炎患者都应尽早使用地塞米松辅助治疗。

隐球菌性脑膜炎患者可能会出现颅内压增高或脑积水,或两者兼而有之。对于有神经功能障碍和颅内压增高证据的患者(开放压通常 > 25 cmH$_2$O),建议每天进行腰椎穿刺。在极少数情况下,尽管频繁进行腰椎穿刺放脑脊液,但脑脊液开放压仍持续高,则可能需要进行 CSF 分流手术。

脑炎

定义

脑炎是脑实质炎症并有神经功能障碍。在没有脑组织炎症病理证据的情况下,脑脊液中的炎症反应或

TABLE 5.6 Antimicrobial Therapy for Patients With Meningitis

Microorganism	Therapy of Choice
Bacteria	
Haemophilus influenzae	
β-Lactamase negative	Ampicillin
β-Lactamase positive	Ceftriaxone or cefotaxime
Neisseria meningitidis	
Penicillin MIC <0.1 µg/mL	Penicillin G or ampicillin
Penicillin MIC 0.1–1.0 µg/mL	Ceftriaxone or cefotaxime
Streptococcus pneumoniae	
Penicillin MIC ≤0.06 µg/mL	Penicillin G or ampicillin
Penicillin MIC ≥0.12 µg/mL	
Ceftriaxone or cefotaxime MIC <1.0 µg/mL	Ceftriaxone or cefotaxime
Ceftriaxone or cefotaxime MIC ≥1.0 µg/mL	Vancomycin[a] plus ceftriaxone or cefotaxime
Enterobacteriaceae[b]	Ceftriaxone or cefotaxime
Pseudomonas aeruginosa	Ceftazidime or cefepime
Acinetobacter baumannii[b]	Meropenem
Listeria monocytogenes	Ampicillin or penicillin G[c]
Streptococcus agalactiae	Ampicillin or penicillin G[c]
Staphylococcus aureus	
Methicillin-sensitive	Nafcillin or oxacillin
Methicillin-resistant	Vancomycin[a]
Staphylococcus epidermidis	Vancomycin[a]
Spirochetes	
Treponema pallidum	Penicillin G
Borrelia burgdorferi	Ceftriaxone or cefotaxime
Mycobacteria	
Mycobacterium tuberculosis	Isoniazid + rifampin + pyrazinamide + ethambutol
Fungi	
Cryptococcus neoformans	Amphotericin B preparation[d] + flucytosine
Coccidioides immitis	Fluconazole
Mucormycosis	Liposomal amphotericin B
Histoplasma capsulatum	Liposomal amphotericin B
Candida species	Amphotericin B preparation[d] ± flucytosine

MIC, Minimum inhibitory concentration.
[a]Addition of rifampin may be considered; see text for indications.
[b]The choice of a specific antimicrobial agent must be guided by in vitro susceptibility testing.
[c]Addition of an aminoglycoside should be considered.
[d]Amphotericin B deoxycholate, liposomal amphotericin B, or amphotericin B lipid complex.

or parenchymal abnormalities on neuroimaging are often used as surrogate markers of brain inflammation; however, encephalitis can occur without significant CSF pleocytosis or demonstrable neuroimaging abnormalities. Encephalitis and meningitis share many features. Both syndromes can manifest with fever, headache, and altered mental status, although the encephalitis patient may suffer from more severe alterations in mental status.

There is also clinical overlap between encephalitis and encephalopathy. Patients with encephalopathy, however, exhibit confusion early in the course of their illness that can quickly progress to obtundation. Causes of encephalopathy include metabolic disturbances, hypoxia, ischemia, intoxications, organ dysfunction, paraneoplastic syndromes, and systemic infections.

Epidemiology and Etiology

Encephalitis is characterized by inflammation of the brain in conjunction with symptoms and signs of neurologic dysfunction. Encephalitis results in substantial morbidity and mortality, and it confers considerable burden on the health care system. The hospital admission rate in one study was 7.3 per 100,000 people. The case-fatality rate among patients with encephalitis varies from 3.8% to 7.4% and is significantly higher among patients also infected with HIV. There is high morbidity among survivors of encephalitis, with resultant loss of productivity, function, and the need for prolonged rehabilitation or skilled nursing care.

Infectious causes of encephalitis are diverse and include viruses (most common), bacteria, fungi, and parasites. Clues in the patient's history that aid identification include seasonal variation, geographic location, prevalence of disease in the local community, travel history, recreational activities, occupational exposures, insect contact, animal contact, vaccination history, and immune status of the patient.

The most commonly identified viral causes of encephalitis in the United States are herpes simplex virus type 1 (HSV-1), West Nile virus, and the enteroviruses, followed by other herpesviruses (e.g., varicella-zoster virus). Other agents may be highly endemic regionally (e.g., La Crosse virus in the Midwest) or internationally (e.g., rabies virus, Japanese encephalitis virus). Bacterial agents, including *Ehrlichia*

表 5.6　脑膜炎患者的抗菌治疗

微生物	治疗选择
细菌	
流感嗜血杆菌	
β-内酰胺酶阴性	氨苄西林
β-内酰胺酶阳性	头孢曲松或头孢噻肟
脑膜炎奈瑟球菌	
青霉素 MIC ＜ 0.1 μg/ml	青霉素 G 或氨苄西林
青霉素 MIC 0.1 ～ 1.0 μg/ml	头孢曲松或头孢噻肟
肺炎链球菌	
青霉素 MIC ≤ 0.06 μg/ml	青霉素 G 或氨苄西林
青霉素 MIC ≥ 0.12 μg/ml	
头孢曲松或头孢噻肟 MIC ＜ 1.0 μg/ml	头孢曲松或头孢噻肟
头孢曲松或头孢噻肟 MIC ≥ 1.0 μg/ml	万古霉素[a]加头孢曲松或头孢噻肟
肠杆菌科[b]	头孢曲松或头孢噻肟
铜绿假单胞菌	头孢噻肟或头孢吡肟
鲍曼不动杆菌[b]	美罗培南
单核细胞增生李斯特菌	氨苄西林或青霉素 G[c]
无乳链球菌	氨苄西林或青霉素 G[c]
金黄色葡萄球菌	
甲氧西林敏感	萘夫西林或奥沙西林
耐甲氧西林	万古霉素[a]
表皮葡萄球菌	万古霉素[a]
螺旋体	
苍白螺旋体	青霉素 G
伯氏疏螺旋体	头孢曲松或头孢噻肟
分枝杆菌	
结核分枝杆菌	异烟肼＋利福平＋吡嗪酰胺＋乙胺丁醇
真菌	
新型隐球菌	两性霉素 B 制剂[d]＋氟胞嘧啶
球孢子菌	氟康唑
毛霉菌	两性霉素 B 脂质体
组织胞浆菌	两性霉素 B 脂质体
假丝酵母菌属	两性霉素 B 制剂[d]±氟胞嘧啶

MIC，最低抑菌浓度。
[a] 可考虑加用利福平；适应证见正文。
[b] 具体抗菌剂的选择必须以体外药敏试验为指导。
[c] 应考虑添加氨基糖苷类药物。
[d] 两性霉素 B 脱氧胆酸盐、脂质体两性霉素 B 或两性霉素 B 脂质复合物。

神经影像学脑实质异常通常提示脑组织炎症；但脑炎时可能没有脑脊液细胞增多或明显的神经影像学异常。脑炎和脑膜炎有许多共同特征。均可出现发热、头痛和精神状态改变，但脑炎患者的精神状态改变可能更为严重。

临床上脑炎和脑病通常也需要鉴别。脑病患者在病程早期会表现出意识障碍，很快进展为反应迟钝。脑病的病因包括代谢紊乱、缺氧、缺血、中毒、器官功能障碍、副肿瘤综合征和全身感染。

流行病学和病因学

脑炎是脑组织炎症并伴有神经功能障碍的症状和体征。脑炎死亡率很高，并给医疗系统造成巨大负担。一项研究显示，每 10 万人中入院 7.3 人。脑炎患者的病死率为 3.8% ～ 7.4%，AIDS 患者脑炎的病死率更高。脑炎幸存者后遗症发生率高，导致劳动力及功能丧失，需要长期康复或专业护理。

感染性脑炎的病因多种多样，包括病毒（最常见）、细菌、真菌和寄生虫。患者病史包括季节、地域及当地疾病流行情况、旅行史、娱乐活动、职业暴露、昆虫及动物接触史、疫苗接种史及免疫功能状态有助于明确病因。

在美国，导致病毒性脑炎最常见的病因是 1 型单纯疱疹病毒（HSV-1）、西尼罗病毒和肠道病毒，其次是其他疱疹病毒（如水痘-带状疱疹病毒）。拉克罗斯病毒有明显的地方性，在美国中西部地区流行，国际上广泛流行的则包括狂犬病病毒、流行性乙型脑炎病毒。细

TABLE 5.7 Recommended Dosages of Antimicrobial Agents for Meningitis in Adults With Normal Renal and Hepatic Function

Antimicrobial Agent	Total Daily Dose[a]	Dosing Interval (hr)
Amikacin[b]	15 mg/kg	8
Amphotericin B deoxycholate	0.6–1.0 mg/kg	24
Amphotericin B lipid complex	5 mg/kg	24
Ampicillin	12 g	4
Cefepime	6 g	8
Cefotaxime	8–12 g	4–6
Ceftazidime	6 g	8
Ceftriaxone	4 g	12–24
Ethambutol[d]	15 mg/kg	24
Fluconazole	400–800 mg[c]	24
Flucytosine[d,e]	100 mg/kg	6
Gentamicin[b]	5 mg/kg	8
Isoniazid[d,f]	300 mg	24
Liposomal amphotericin B	5–7.5 mg/kg	24
Meropenem	6 g	8
Nafcillin	12 g	4
Oxacillin	12 g	4
Penicillin G	24 million units	4
Pyrazinamide[d]	15–30 mg/kg	24
Rifampin[d]	600 mg	24
Tobramycin[b]	5 mg/kg	8
Sulfamethoxazole-trimethoprim	10–20 mg/kg[g]	6–12
Vancomycin[h]	30–45 mg/kg	8–12
Voriconazole[i]	8 mg/kg	12

[a]Unless indicated, therapy is administered intravenously.
[b]Need to monitor peak and trough serum concentrations.
[c]Dose of 800–1200 mg is recommended for patients with coccidioidal meningitis.
[d]Oral administration.
[e]Maintain serum concentrations of 50–100 µg/mL.
[f]Initiate therapy at a dose of 10 mg/kg.
[g]Dosage based on trimethoprim component; many experts would use a dose of 5 mg/kg every 8 hours.
[h]Maintain serum trough concentrations of 15–20 µg/mL.
[i]IV loading dose of 6 mg/kg every 12 hours for two doses; maintain serum trough concentrations of 2–5 µg/mL.

species and *Rickettsia rickettsii*, are potentially treatable causes of encephalitis, and prompt administration of appropriate antimicrobial therapy may be life-saving.

Perhaps the most challenging aspect of encephalitis is that no pathogen is identified in 50% to 70% of cases. Another difficulty is the relevance of an identification of an infectious agent outside of the CNS in a patient with encephalitis; these agents may cause a systemic illness that also involves neurologic symptoms but does not necessarily invade the CNS directly. Additionally, it may be challenging to distinguish infectious encephalitis from postinfectious or postimmunization encephalitis or encephalomyelitis; the latter process is usually mediated by an immunologic response to a preceding infection or immunization. Up to 10% of patients have a noninfectious cause; examples include paraneoplastic syndromes, vasculitis, or collagen vascular disorders.

Antibody-mediated encephalitis refers to a group of inflammatory brain diseases associated with antibodies against neuronal cell-surface proteins, ion channels, or receptors resulting in neuropsychiatric symptoms. This group of diseases is distinct from traditional autoimmune disorders such as systemic lupus erythematosus. Autoimmune encephalitis may be the third most common cause of encephalitis, and the most common form of autoimmune encephalitis is the type with antibodies against the N-methyl-D-aspartate receptor (NMDAR). In contrast to paraneoplastic syndromes, which are associated with antibodies against intracellular neural antigens, the antibodies bind to extracellular epitopes of cell-surface proteins in autoimmune encephalitis. Common receptors include NMDAR, α-amino-3-hydroxy-5-methyl-4-isoxazolepropionic acid receptor (AMPAR), γ-aminobutyric acid (GABA) receptor, and glioma-inactivated 1 (LG1) receptor. Two potential triggers of autoimmune encephalitis are tumors and viral encephalitis. However, most cases occur with no apparent immunologic triggers, which may suggest a genetic predisposition to these disorders.

Clinical Presentation

Because encephalitis is infrequently confirmed by pathologic means, the signs and symptoms of neurologic dysfunction are used as surrogate markers, and they are often nonspecific. The clinical signs and symptoms of encephalitis are determined by the specific area of the brain involved and by the severity of the infection. Some organisms show neurotropism for particular anatomic sites. HSV-1 infection almost universally involves the temporal lobe, and the clinical presentation typically includes temporal lobe seizures. Associated signs include personality changes, decreasing consciousness, focal neurologic findings (including dysphagia), paresthesias and weakness, and focal seizures. Sudden onset of fever and headache can also accompany these mental status changes.

Diffuse brain involvement is frequently seen with arboviral infections, and it is associated with global impairment in neurologic

表 5.7 肝肾功能正常成人脑膜炎抗菌药物的推荐剂量

抗菌药物	每日总剂量[a]	治疗间隔（h）
阿米卡星[b]	15 mg/kg	8
两性霉素 B 脱氧胆酸盐	0.6～1.0 mg/kg	24
两性霉素 B 脂质复合物	5 mg/kg	24
氨苄西林	12 g	4
头孢吡肟	6 g	8
头孢噻肟	8～12 g	4～6
头孢他啶	6 g	8
头孢曲松	4 g	12～24
乙胺丁醇[d]	15 mg/kg	24
氟康唑	400～800 mg[c]	24
氟胞嘧啶[d, e]	100 mg/kg	6
庆大霉素[b]	5 mg/kg	8
异烟肼[d, f]	300 mg	24
两性霉素 B 脂质体	5～7.5 mg/kg	24
美罗培南	6 g	8
纳夫西林	12 g	4
奥沙西林	12 g	4
青霉素 G	24 万单位	4
吡嗪酰胺[d]	15～30 mg/kg	24
利福平[d]	600 mg	24
妥布霉素[b]	5 mg/kg	8
甲氧苄啶-磺胺甲噁唑	10～20 mg/kg[g]	6～12
万古霉素[h]	30～45 mg/kg	8～12
伏立康唑[i]	8 mg/kg	12

[a] 除非有说明，否则均采用静脉注射疗法。
[b] 需要监测血清浓度的峰值和谷值。
[c] 建议球孢子菌性脑膜炎患者服用 800～1200 mg。
[d] 口服给药。
[e] 保持血清中药物浓度 50～100 μg/ml。
[f] 起始剂量 10 mg/kg。
[g] 根据甲氧苄啶的成分确定剂量；许多专家使用的剂量为 5 mg/kg 每 8 h 一次。
[h] 保持血清谷浓度在 15～20 μg/ml。
[i] 负荷剂量 6 mg/kg 每 12 h 一次，共两次；保持血清谷浓度 2～5 μg/ml。

菌病原体，包括埃立克体和立克次体是可以治疗，及时采取适当的抗菌治疗可能会挽救生命。

50%～70% 的脑炎病例无法明确病原体。此外脑炎患者中发现中枢神经系统以外的感染源也十分困难；这些感染源可能会引起全身性疾病，也会出现神经系统症状，但不一定会直接侵入中枢神经系统。此外，将感染性脑炎与感染后或免疫后脑炎或脑脊髓炎鉴别也很困难；后者通常是由对之前感染或免疫的免疫反应介导的。多达 10% 的脑炎患者是非感染性的，如副肿瘤综合征、血管炎或胶原血管疾病。

抗体介导的脑炎是指一组炎症性脑病，由神经元细胞表面蛋白、离子通道或受体抗体导致神经精神症状。这类疾病有别于系统性红斑狼疮等传统的自身免疫性疾病。自身免疫性脑炎可能是导致脑炎的第三大常见病因，而最常见的自身免疫性脑炎是具有 N-甲基-D-天冬氨酸受体（NMDAR）抗体的类型。与针对细胞内神经抗原的抗体相关的副肿瘤综合征不同，这种抗体会与细胞内的神经抗原结合，从而导致脑炎。在自身免疫性脑炎中，这些受体与细胞表面蛋白的胞外表位有关。常见的受体包括 NMDAR、α-氨基-3-羟基-5-甲基-4-异噁唑丙酸受体（AMPAR）、γ-氨基丁酸（GABA）受体和胶质瘤失活 1（LG1）受体。肿瘤和病毒性脑炎可能是自身免疫性脑炎的诱因。然而，大多数病例的发生并无明显的免疫学诱因，这可能表明这些疾病有遗传倾向。

临床表现

脑炎很少能通过病理手段确诊，而是由神经功能障碍的体征和症状作为诊断依据，但它们往往是非特异性的。脑炎的临床症状和体征取决于大脑病变的特定区域和感染的严重程度。有些病原体有好发的病变部位。HSV-1 感染几乎普遍累及颞叶，典型临床上为颞叶癫痫发作。相关症状包括性格改变、意识模糊、局灶性神经功能异常（包括吞咽困难）、麻痹和虚弱以及局灶性癫痫发作。突然发热和头痛也可伴随这些精神状态变化。

虫媒病毒感染经常会导致脑部弥漫性受累，并伴有神经系统的全面损伤和昏迷。发热和头痛常常发生

function and coma. Fever and headache frequently precede the onset of altered mental status, which can range from mild confusion to obtundation. Other neurologic manifestations may include behavioral changes (e.g., psychosis), focal paresis or paralysis, cranial nerve palsies, and movement disorders (e.g., chorea). About 80% of patients infected with West Nile virus are asymptomatic, and about 20% have only fever. Symptomatic patients may have fever, headache, myalgia, and flaccid paralysis. A maculopapular rash is seen in 50% of patients.

VZV is an important cause of acute encephalitis in adults, often associated with viral reactivation and leading to a CNS vasculopathy. Importantly, CNS reactivation may occur in the absence of skin lesions. Children, on the contrary, exhibit CNS symptoms concurrently with varicella or in a postinfectious form.

Evidence of inflammation or infection at sites distant from the CNS may be useful in making a microbiologic diagnosis for patients with encephalitis. For instance, rickettsial diseases, varicella-zoster virus, and West Nile virus often have associated skin manifestations. Stomatitis and ulcerative lesions in the mouth or an exanthem in a peripheral distribution can suggest enterovirus infection. Patients with tuberculous and fungal meningoencephalitis may have suggestive pulmonary findings.

A syndrome frequently misclassified as encephalomyelitis, based on the similar clinical presentation, is post-inflammatory encephalomyelitis. The most widely cited example is acute disseminated encephalomyelitis (ADEM), which is seen primarily in children and adolescents. ADEM is characterized by poorly defined white matter lesions on magnetic resonance imaging (MRI) that enhance after gadolinium administration. Post-inflammatory encephalomyelitis is likely mediated by an immunologic response to an antecedent antigenic stimulus such as infection or immunization. Viral infections associated with ADEM include measles, mumps, rubella, varicella-zoster, Epstein-Barr, cytomegalovirus, herpes simplex, hepatitis A, and coxsackieviruses. Immunizations temporally associated with ADEM include vaccines for Japanese encephalitis, yellow fever, measles, influenza, smallpox, anthrax, and rabies, but a direct causal association with these vaccines is difficult to establish. ADEM usually begins between 2 days and 4 weeks after the antigenic stimulus, and patients develop rapid onset of encephalopathy, with or without meningeal signs. The neurologic features depend on the location of the lesions.

In patients with anti-NMDAR encephalitis, prodromal symptoms, including low-grade fever, headache, and malaise, may occur in approximately 60% of patients. Common clinical features include behavioral changes, psychosis, seizures, memory and cognitive deficits, dysautonomia, abnormal movements, and altered consciousness. Females diagnosed with anti-NMDAR encephalitis will have an ovarian teratoma 50% of the time. Symptoms are more often neurologic in children and psychiatric in adults, but in most cases, symptoms progress to a similar syndrome. In contrast, patients with limbic encephalitis are generally older than 45 years and have symptoms including confusion, seizures, behavioral changes, and distinct memory deficits in which they have trouble forming new memories but old ones are preserved.

Diagnosis

The initial laboratory testing of an individual should include a complete blood count, tests of renal and hepatic function, coagulation studies, and serum and urine toxicology studies. A low white blood cell count, low platelet count, and elevated liver transaminase levels may suggest *Ehrlichia* or *Anaplasma* infection. A baseline chest radiograph should be obtained because a focal infiltrate can suggest particular pathogens (e.g., fungal or mycobacterial infections).

Neuroimaging studies are important to perform for all patients with encephalitis; MRI is more sensitive at detecting abnormalities than CT, and it is the preferred study. Diffusion-weighted MRI is superior to conventional MRI for the detection of early signal abnormalities in viral encephalitis caused by HSV, enterovirus 71, and West Nile virus. In patients with HSV encephalitis, there may be significant edema and hemorrhage in the temporal lobes. Patients with flavivirus (e.g., West Nile virus, Japanese encephalitis virus) encephalitis may display characteristic patterns of mixed-intensity or hypodense lesions on T1-weighted images of the thalamus, basal ganglia, and midbrain. MRI findings with linear T2-weighted regions of high signal involving the internal and external capsules (also termed the "parentheses" sign) has been associated with Eastern equine encephalitis (an arbovirus infection) compared to other viral encephalitides, although the frequency of this finding is unclear given the rarity of this infection. In patients with ADEM, MRI usually reveals multiple focal or confluent areas of signal abnormality in the subcortical white matter and, sometimes, in subcortical gray matter on T2-weighted and fluid attenuation inversion recovery (FLAIR) sequences; the lesions are usually enhancing and display similar stages of evolution. MRI of the head is abnormal in 30% of patients with antibody-mediated encephalitis. Positive findings include increased FLAIR signal involving the cortical, subcortical, or cerebellar regions.

Electroencephalography is rarely specific for a given pathogen in patients with encephalitis, but results can be helpful in identifying the degree of cerebral dysfunction by detecting subclinical seizure activity, and it may provide information about the specific area of the brain involved. In more than 80% of patients with HSV encephalitis, there is a temporal lobe focus with periodic lateralizing epileptiform discharges (PLEDs).

Lumbar puncture with CSF analysis (i.e., cell count and differential, glucose and protein levels) and a measurement of the opening pressure should be performed in all patients with encephalitis unless there is a specific contraindication. Most patients with viral encephalitis have a mononuclear cell pleocytosis with cell counts ranging from 10 to 1000/mm^3. Early in the disease process, CSF pleocytosis may be absent, or there may be an elevation in neutrophils. While lymphocytic predominance is seen with progression of the viral infection, persistent neutrophilic pleocytosis has been observed in patients with West Nile virus encephalitis. The CSF protein concentration is typically elevated, but usually less than 100 to 200 mg/dL, whereas the CSF glucose concentration is typically normal. Patients may have high RBCs in the CSF due to hemorrhagic encephalitis. CSF viral cultures are usually not recommended. Up to 10% of patients with viral encephalitis will have completely normal CSF findings. The presence of eosinophils in the CSF may suggest certain etiologies, specifically encephalitis caused by helminths. A decreased CSF glucose concentration is indicative of bacterial, fungi, or protozoal etiology. CSF profiles of patients with ADEM are similar to patients with viral encephalitis with lymphocytic pleocytosis (though less marked compared to infectious encephalitis), high protein concentration, and normal glucose concentration. Additionally, oligoclonal bands and elevated IgG index and synthesis may be present.

Brain biopsy has largely been replaced by CSF molecular tests. For certain types of infections, however, brain biopsy may be diagnostic. In rabies infections, for example, Negri bodies are a distinctive histopathologic feature. Intranuclear eosinophilic amorphous bodies surrounded by a halo may be seen in diseases such as HSV encephalitis. Biopsy of skin lesions should be performed in encephalitis patients with concomitant rash including maculopapular or petechial lesions, which can be high yield in identifying the responsible agent (e.g., *R. rickettsii*).

在精神状态改变之前,精神状态改变的范围从轻度意识障碍到昏迷不等。其他神经系统表现可能包括行为异常(如精神症状)、局灶性麻痹或瘫痪、脑神经麻痹和运动障碍(如舞蹈症)。约 80% 的西尼罗病毒感染者无症状,约 20% 仅有发热。脑炎的患者可能会发热、头痛、肌痛和弛缓性麻痹。50% 的患者会出现斑丘疹。

VZV 是成人急性脑炎的重要病因,通常与病毒再激活有关,并导致中枢神经系统血管病变。病毒在中枢神经系统再激活可没有皮疹表现。儿童在感染水痘的同时或感染后会出现中枢神经系统症状。

中枢神经系统以外部位的炎症或感染可有助于对脑炎患者明确病因。例如,立克次体病、水痘-带状疱疹病毒和西尼罗病毒常常伴有皮肤表现。口腔炎和口腔溃疡或外周皮疹可提示肠道病毒感染。结核性脑膜脑炎和真菌性脑膜脑炎患者可能有相应的肺部表现。

炎症后脑脊髓炎是一种经常被误诊为脑脊髓炎的综合征,其临床表现与炎症后脑脊髓炎相似。最常见的例子是急性播散性脑脊髓炎(ADEM),主要见于儿童和青少年。急性播散性脑脊髓炎的特点是磁共振成像(MRI)上的白质病变界线不清,钆造影后增强。炎症后脑脊髓炎很可能是对前驱感染或免疫接种等抗原刺激的免疫反应介导的。与 ADEM 相关的病毒感染包括麻疹病毒、腮腺炎病毒、风疹病毒、水痘-带状疱疹病毒、EB 病毒、巨细胞病毒、单纯疱疹病毒、甲型肝炎病毒和柯萨奇病毒。与 ADEM 在时间上相关的免疫接种包括流行性乙型脑炎疫苗、黄热病疫苗、麻疹疫苗、流感疫苗、天花疫苗、炭疽疫苗和狂犬病疫苗,但与这些疫苗的直接因果关系难以确定。ADEM 通常在抗原刺激后 2 天至 4 周开始发病,患者会迅速出现脑病,伴或不伴有脑膜刺激症状。神经系统表现取决于病变的部位。

大约 60% 的抗 NMDAR 脑炎患者会出现前驱症状,包括低热、头痛和乏力。常见的临床表现包括行为异常、精神症状、癫痫发作、记忆和认知障碍、自主神经功能障碍、运动异常和意识改变。50% 抗 NMDAR 脑炎的女性患者会出现卵巢畸胎瘤。儿童的症状多为神经系统症状,成人则多为精神症状,但在大多数情况下,症状最终进展相似。相比之下,边缘型脑炎患者的年龄一般在 45 岁以上,症状包括意识模糊、癫痫发作、行为异常和明显的记忆障碍,即难以形成新的记忆,但既往记忆保留。

诊断

初步实验室检测应包括全血细胞计数、肝肾功能检测、凝血功能检测以及血清和尿液毒理学检测。白细胞计数低、血小板减少和肝转氨酶水平升高提示感染埃立克体或无形体的可能性大。胸部 X 线检查显示局灶性浸润可能提示特定的病原体(如真菌或分枝杆菌感染)。

神经影像学检查对所有脑炎患者都很重要;首选 MRI,其比 CT 敏感,更能发现病变。对于 HSV、肠道病毒 71 和西尼罗病毒引起的病毒性脑炎的早期病变,弥散加权 MRI 优于传统 MRI。HSV 脑炎患者颞叶可出现明显的水肿和出血。黄病毒(如西尼罗病毒、流行性乙型脑炎病毒)脑炎患者可能会在丘脑、基底节和中脑的 T1 加权图像上显示出特征性的混合强度或低密度病变。与其他病毒性脑炎相比,东部马脑炎(一种虫媒病毒感染)MRI 更容易出现内囊和外囊区线性 T2 加权高信号(也称为"括号"征),这种感染很少见,因此这种发现的敏感性和特异性尚不清楚。在 ADEM 患者中,MRI T2 加权和液体抑制反转恢复(FLAIR)序列上显示皮层下白质中的多个局灶性或融合性信号异常区域,有时也会显示皮层下灰质中的信号异常区域;病变通常会增强,并呈现相似的变化过程。30% 的抗体介导的脑炎患者头部 MRI 异常,包括皮质、皮质下或小脑区域的 FLAIR 信号增高。

脑电图对感染性脑炎患者的诊断不具有特异性,但可通过检测亚临床癫痫发作活动来帮助确定脑功能障碍的程度,并可帮助进行定位诊断。80% 以上的 HSV 脑炎患者,颞叶病灶伴有周期性一侧癫痫样放电(PLED)。

除非有明确的禁忌证,否则所有脑炎患者都应进行腰椎穿刺,并对 CSF 进行分析(即细胞分类计数、葡萄糖和蛋白质水平)和测量脑脊液开放压力。大多数病毒性脑炎患者会出现单核细胞增多,细胞计数为 10 ~ 1000/mm^3。在病程早期,CSF 可能没有细胞增多的表现,或者中性粒细胞增多。随着病毒感染的进展,淋巴细胞增多占据优势,但在西尼罗病毒性脑炎患者中也可观察到持续的中性粒细胞增多。脑脊液蛋白质浓度通常升高,但通常不超过 100 ~ 200 mg/dl,而脑脊液葡萄糖通常正常。出血性脑炎患者脑脊液中的红细胞可能较高。通常不推荐脑脊液病毒培养。多达 10% 的病毒性脑炎患者的脑脊液检查结果完全正常。脑脊液中出现嗜酸性粒细胞可能提示某些病因,特别是由蠕虫引起的脑炎。CSF 葡萄糖降低则提示细菌、真菌或原虫感染。ADEM 患者的 CSF 与病毒性脑炎患者相似,都有淋巴细胞增多(但增多没有感染性脑炎明显)、蛋白升高和正常葡萄糖浓度。此外,还可能出现寡克隆区带、IgG 指数和合成升高。

脑活检在很大程度上已被脑脊液分子检测取代。但是某些感染,例如,狂犬病感染中,内氏小体是一个特征性的组织病理学表现。在 HSV 脑炎等疾病中,核内嗜酸性粒细胞不规则体伴周围晕环。对于同时伴有皮疹(包括斑丘疹或瘀斑)的脑炎患者,应进行皮肤病变活检,对确定病原体(如立克次体)有利。

Testing for specific agents includes laboratory methods such as antigen detection, culture, serology, and molecular diagnostics. HSV encephalitis is a treatable and relatively common cause of encephalitis, and an HSV PCR should be performed on the CSF of all patients with a clinical diagnosis of encephalitis. False-negative PCR test results can occur within the first 72 hours after onset, and if HSV encephalitis is strongly suspected (e.g., in a patient with temporal lobe involvement), a repeat HSV PCR on a second sample of CSF within 3 to 7 days is recommended. For enterovirus and varicella encephalitis, CSF PCR testing is recommended; however, detection of antibodies to varicella-zoster virus in the CSF appears to have greater sensitivity than detection of viral DNA. Concomitant serum viral studies are sometimes helpful in diagnosing viral encephalitis. In one report of an enterovirus 71 outbreak, only 31% of cases had a positive CSF result with higher yields from throat and stool PCR specimens; viral shedding from the gastrointestinal tract may occur for weeks following infection. Similarly, for Epstein-Barr virus encephalitis, serum serology including antiviral capsid antigens (VCA), immunoglobulin M/ immunoglobulin G (IgM/IgG), and anti-Epstein-Barr nuclear antigen (EBNA) are recommended in addition to CSF PCR due to false positive and false negative results associated with the PCR test.

Testing for other agents should be individualized with consideration of the patient's exposures, travel, season of the year, and clinical and laboratory characteristics. Many infections require acute and convalescent (i.e., paired) serum samples to determine a diagnosis. A serum specimen collected during the acute phase of the illness should be stored and tested in parallel when the convalescent serum sample is drawn. Immunoglobulin M (IgM) and immunoglobulin G (IgG) capture enzyme-linked immunosorbent assays (ELISAs) have become useful and widely available for the diagnosis of arboviral encephalitis. Detection of intrathecal IgM antibody is a specific and sensitive method for the diagnosis of West Nile virus infection. There is substantial cross-reactivity among the flaviviruses (e.g., West Nile virus, St. Louis encephalitis virus, Japanese encephalitis virus); plaque-reduction neutralization assays may be helpful in distinguishing which flavivirus is involved in the event of elevated titers.

Serologic testing for *Rickettsia*, *Ehrlichia*, and *Anaplasma* species should be performed for all encephalitis patients during the appropriate season and with travel to or residence in endemic areas, especially because these are treatable causes. In addition to serologies, concurrent serum PCR testing for *Anaplasma* is recommended, because a positive result may be more indicative of an acute infection. Empiric therapy should not be withheld from patients with a compatible clinical presentation because antibodies are not always detectable early in the course of illness.

Identification of NMDAR antibodies confirms the diagnosis of anti-NMDAR encephalitis. Obtaining both serum and CSF antibodies is also recommended. Diagnosis should lead to the search for a tumor in female patients; the tumor is almost always an ovarian teratoma.

Treatment

One of the most important first steps in managing encephalitis is to consider treatable causes. Specific antiviral therapy is usually limited to infections caused by herpesviruses (especially HSV-1 and varicella-zoster virus) and HIV. Therefore, acyclovir (10 mg/kg intravenously every 8 hours in adults with normal renal function) should be administered to patients with encephalitis. Empirical therapy for acute bacterial meningitis should be initiated when clinical and laboratory testing is compatible with bacterial infection. If rickettsial or ehrlichial infections are suspected, empirical doxycycline should be administered. The management of West Nile virus infection is supportive care.

In patients with suspected postinfectious encephalomyelitis (i.e., ADEM), high-dose intravenous corticosteroids (1 g of methylprednisolone intravenously daily for at least 3 to 5 days) are usually recommended, followed by an oral taper for 3 to 6 weeks. In patients with autoimmune encephalitis, the current approach includes immunotherapy and removal of the immunologic trigger. Most patients are treated with glucocorticoids, intravenous immune globulin, or plasma exchange. If there is no clinical response to these treatments, then rituximab or cyclophosphamide may be used. Rituximab may be helpful in reducing the risk of clinical relapse. Additionally, early identification and removal of this trigger is important for achieving a good outcome (i.e., removal of an ovarian teratoma in patients with anti-NMDAR encephalitis). Time to recovery, degree of residual deficit, and risk of relapse vary depending on the type of autoimmune encephalitis. Spontaneous clinical improvement is rare. Prompt institution of immunotherapy is associated with favorable outcomes.

BRAIN ABSCESS

Definition

A *brain abscess* is a focal intracerebral infection that begins as a localized area of cerebritis followed by the formation of a pus collection.

Pathology and Pathophysiology

Brain abscesses produce symptoms and findings similar to those of other space-occupying lesions (e.g., brain tumors), but they often progress more rapidly and affect meningeal structures more frequently than tumors. Brain abscesses may arise from several mechanisms, the most common of which is spread from a contiguous focus of infection; examples include infections of the middle ear, mastoid cells, paranasal sinuses, as well as dental infections. A second mechanism is hematogenous dissemination from a distant focus of infection. Brain abscesses resulting from hematogenous spread are usually multiple and mutliloculated, and they are associated with higher mortality. Original foci of infection include chronic pyogenic lung disease (e.g., lung abscesses, bronchiectasis, empyema, and cystic fibrosis), skin and soft tissue infections, osteomyelitis, intraabdominal infections, infectious endocarditis, cyanotic heart disease, and pulmonary arteriovenous malformations often linked with hereditary hemorrhagic telangiectasia. Traumas, particularly those involving dural breach, and invasive neurosurgical procedures, are also a pathogenic mechanism of brain abscess development. In 10% to 35% of patients, brain abscess is cryptogenic.

The infection is often polymicrobial, and the pathogen(s) involved depend on the mechanism of spread as well as the host characteristics. Commonly isolated pathogens are aerobic and microaerobic streptococci and gram-negative anaerobes such as *Bacteroides* and *Prevotella*. Less common are gram-negative aerobes and *Staphylococcus*. *Actinomyces*, *Nocardia*, and *Candida* are even less prevalent. In immunosuppressed individuals, *Aspergillus* and *Toxoplasma* are important causes of abscesses. Surgical specimens are culture positive in 70% of antibiotic-treated patients and 95% of patients undergoing surgery before antibiotic administration.

Clinical Presentation

The clinical course of brain abscess ranges from indolent to fulminant. The classic clinical picture is composed of signs of systemic infection (e.g., fever), those related to focal brain involvement, and those due to an increased intracranial pressure and mass effect. Elements of one or two categories are often absent in a given case, particularly early in the disease course. For example, almost one half of patients may not have a fever or leukocytosis. The classic triad of fever, headache, and focal neurologic deficit is found only in about 20% of patients on admission. Recent

特异性病原体的检测包括抗原检测、培养、血清学和分子诊断等实验室方法。HSV脑炎是一种可治疗且相对常见的脑炎病因，所有临床诊断为脑炎的患者的脑脊液都应进行HSV PCR检测。如果强烈怀疑是HSV脑炎（如颞叶受累的患者），建议在3～7天内对第二份CSF样本重复进行HSV PCR检测，因为起病72 h内的脑脊液HSV PCR可能为假阴性。对于肠道病毒和水痘脑炎，建议进行CSF PCR检测；但检测CSF中的水痘-带状疱疹病毒抗体似乎比检测病毒DNA更灵敏。同时进行的血清病毒检查有时有助于诊断病毒性脑炎。在一份关于暴发性肠道病毒71感染脑炎的报告中，只有31%的病例CSF检测阳性，而咽喉和粪便PCR标本的阳性率更高；胃肠道的病毒脱落可能会在感染后数周内出现。同样，对于EB病毒脑炎，由于PCR检测存在假阳性和假阴性结果，因此除CSF PCR外，还建议检测血清，包括抗病毒衣壳抗原（VCA）、IgM/IgG和抗EB病毒核抗原（ENA）。

根据患者的接触史、旅行史、季节性以及临床和实验室特征，对其他病原体的检测应因人而异。许多感染需要急性期和恢复期（即配对）的血清样本才能确定诊断。在疾病急性期采集的血清样本应储存起来，并在抽取恢复期血清样本时同时进行检测。IgM和IgG捕获酶联免疫吸附试验（ELISA）已成为诊断虫媒病毒性脑炎的有用方法，并得到广泛应用。检测鞘内IgM抗体是诊断西尼罗病毒感染的一种特异而灵敏的方法。黄病毒（如西尼罗病毒、圣路易斯脑炎病毒、流行性乙型脑炎病毒）之间存在很多交叉反应；如果滴度升高，斑块还原中和试验可能有助于区分哪种黄病毒感染。

在相应的季节，或在流行地区居住或有旅行史时，应对所有脑炎患者进行立克次体、埃立克体和无形体属血清学检测，因为这些都是可以治疗的疾病。除血清学检查外，推荐同时进行无形体血清PCR检测，阳性结果支持急性感染。临床表现符合要求的患者不应延误治疗，因为在病程早期并不总能检测到抗体。

NMDAR抗体阳性可确诊抗NMDAR脑炎。建议同时检测血清和脑脊液抗体。女性患者确诊后应排查肿瘤；肿瘤几乎都是卵巢畸胎瘤。

治疗

脑炎最重要的第一步就是治疗病因。特异性抗病毒治疗通常仅限于由疱疹病毒（尤其是HSV-1和水痘-带状疱疹病毒）和HIV引起的感染。因此，脑炎患者应使用阿昔洛韦（10 mg/kg，肾功能正常的成人每8 h静脉注射一次）。当临床和实验室检测结果支持细菌感染时，应开始对急性细菌性脑膜炎进行经验性治疗。如果怀疑是立克次体或埃立克体感染，则应根据经验使用多西环素。西尼罗病毒感染的治疗方法是对症治疗。

对于疑似感染后脑脊髓炎（即ADEM）患者，通常建议静脉注射大剂量皮质类固醇（每天静脉注射1 g甲泼尼龙，至少3～5天），然后改口服减量应用3～6周。对于自身免疫性脑炎患者，目前的治疗方法包括免疫治疗和去除免疫诱因。大多数患者接受糖皮质激素、静脉注射免疫球蛋白或血浆置换治疗。如果这些治疗无效，则可能使用利妥昔单抗或环磷酰胺。利妥昔单抗可能减少临床复发。此外，及早发现并去除诱因对预后也很重要（例如，切除抗NMDAR脑炎患者的卵巢畸胎瘤）。根据自身免疫性脑炎类型的不同，康复时间、后遗症程度和复发风险也各不相同。自发临床好转的情况很少见。及时进行免疫治疗可获得良好的疗效。

脑脓肿

定义

脑脓肿是一种局灶性脑内感染，起初是局部区域性脑膜炎，随后形成脓液聚集。

病理学和病理生理学

脑脓肿产生的症状和检查结果与其他占位性病变（如脑肿瘤）相似，但脑脓肿通常进展更快，更容易影响脑膜结构。脑脓肿可能由几种机制引起，其中最常见的是由毗连的感染灶扩散，例如中耳、乳突小房、鼻旁窦以及牙源性感染。第二种机制是来自远处感染灶的血源性传播。血源性传播导致的脑脓肿通常是多发性的，而且是多部位的，死亡率较高。原发感染灶包括慢性化脓性肺病（如肺脓肿、支气管扩张、肺水肿和囊性纤维化）、皮肤和软组织感染、骨髓炎、腹腔内感染、感染性心内膜炎、发绀型心脏病以及通常与遗传性出血性毛细血管扩张症有关的肺动静脉畸形。外伤，尤其是涉及硬脑膜破损的外伤和侵入性神经外科手术，也是脑脓肿发病的一个致病机制。10%～35%的脑脓肿患者病因不明。

感染通常是多微生物的，病原体取决于传播机制和宿主情况。常见培养出的病原体是需氧和微需氧链球菌以及革兰氏阴性厌氧菌，如乳酸杆菌和普雷沃菌。较少见的是革兰氏阴性需氧菌和葡萄球菌。放线菌、诺卡菌和念珠菌则更少见。在免疫抑制人群中，曲霉菌和弓形虫是导致脓肿的重要原因。在接受抗生素治疗的患者中，70%的手术标本培养呈阳性；在使用抗生素前接受手术的患者中，95%的标本培养呈阳性。

临床表现

脑脓肿的临床表现轻重不等，可隐袭起病，也可暴发起病，典型的临床表现包括全身感染症状（如发热）、与受累部位有关的症状以及颅内压增高和占位效应引起的症状。某些病例，尤其是在病程早期，往往缺乏其中一两种表现。例如，近一半的患者可能没有发热或白细胞增多。只有约20%的患者在入院时才会

TABLE 5.8	Location and Clinical Presentation of Brain Abscesses
Location	Clinical Presentation
Frontal lobe	Headache, drowsiness, inattention, deterioration of mental status, hemiparesis with unilateral motor signs, and motor speech disorder
Temporal lobe	Ipsilateral headache and aphasia (dominant side); visual defect
Cerebellum	Ataxia, nystagmus, vomiting, and dysmetria
Brainstem	Fever, headache, facial weakness, hemiparesis, dysphagia, and vomiting

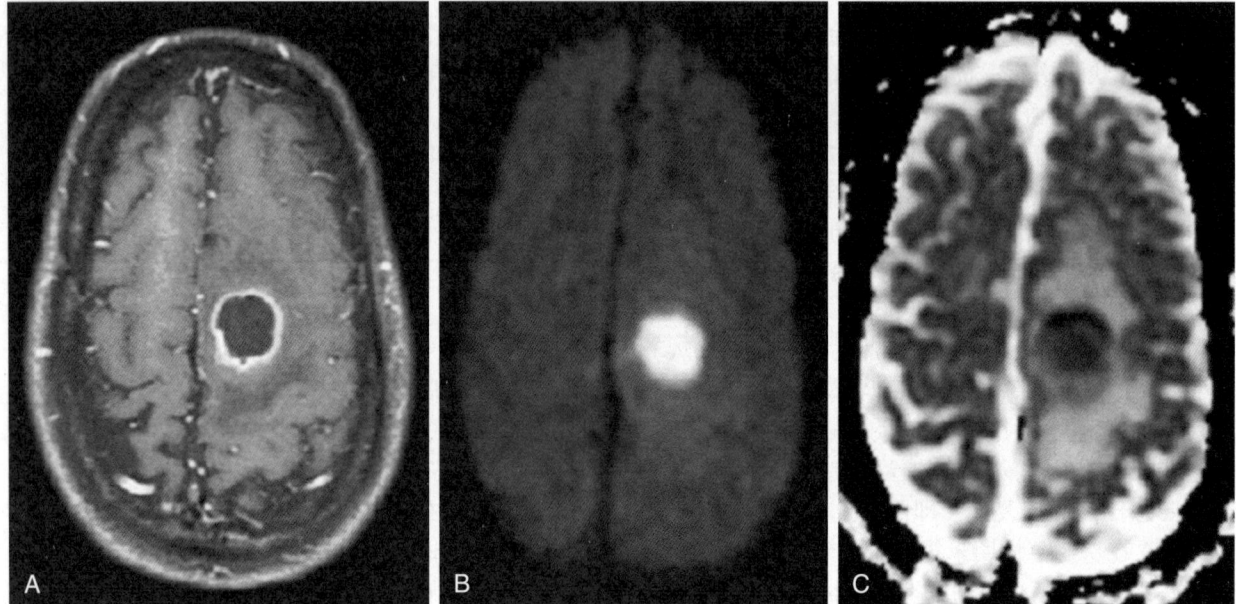

Fig. 5.2 Magnetic resonance imaging features of a brain abscess. (A) Contrast-enhanced scan shows a ring-enhancing lesion in the left frontal lobe. (B) The diffusion-weighted image shows restricted diffusion in the cavity due to viscous pus and cellular material. (C) Corresponding apparent diffusion coefficient map shows dark, viscous material in the cavity and surrounding edema.

onset of a headache is the most common symptom, which may increase in severity associated with focal signs related to the location of the abscess (e.g., hemiparesis, aphasia), followed by obtundation and coma. However, headache may be moderate to severe and hemicranial or generalized but often lacks distinguishing features. Seizures precede the diagnosis in 30% of cases. *Toxoplasma* abscesses are often associated with movement disorders due to their propensity for the basal ganglia. The period of evolution may be as brief as hours or as long as days to weeks with more indolent organisms. The location of the brain abscess can correlate with clinical presentation (Table 5.8). A worrisome complication of brain abscess is rupture. Sudden worsening of a headache with new onset of meningismus may signify rupture of the abscess into the ventricular space. This is associated with a high mortality, up to 85% in some series.

Diagnosis

CSF examination should be avoided; it is seldom diagnostic, and results can be normal. Lumbar puncture in the setting of a mass lesion carries the risk of transtentorial herniation. Because the brain abscess is seeded from a peripheral site of infection, a search for other sites of infection can help to identify the causative organisms and determine appropriate treatment.

MRI with intravenous gadolinium provides better soft tissue visualization than CT and is the imaging of choice in diagnosing brain abscesses. MRI is particularly useful for detecting multiple abscesses and posterior fossa abscesses. It can demonstrate cerebritis, the extent of a mass effect, and associated venous thrombosis. Repeat or serial imaging can be used to determine response to therapy. In the early cerebritis stage, CT results may be normal, but the MRI FLAIR sequence is very sensitive for visualization of brain edema. On T1-weighted images, the area of cerebritis is seen initially as a low-signal-intensity, ill-defined area. T1-weighted images in the later stages of infection may show the formation of a rim of slightly higher signal intensity and central necrosis. Contrast administration typically shows ring enhancement with central necrosis. This area of central necrosis appears bright on diffusion-weighted images and dark on apparent diffusion coefficient (ADC) images (Fig. 5.2). MRI of tumors shows the opposite features. Differentiating a brain abscess from tumor is important for the stereotactic approach to ring-enhancing lesions before biopsy or surgical excision. An abscess should be drained centrally, whereas a tumor should be biopsied along its rim.

Patient risk factors, location of the brain abscess, and characteristic findings on CT or MRI imaging can help implicate the responsible pathogen. *Nocardia* brain abscesses are often mutilobulated. *Listeria* brain abscesses are often located in the brain stem. Findings of cerebral infarcts that develop into single or multiple brain abscesses usually in the frontal or temporal lobes in a patient with risk factors for invasive aspergillosis should suggest that diagnosis. CT or MRI findings of sinus opacification, erosion of bone, and obliteration of deep fascial planes may indicate rhinocerebral mucormycosis. Rounded isodense or hypodense lesions with ring enhancement seen on contrast imaging are consistent with CNS toxoplasmosis in the appropriate patient.

表 5.8 脑脓肿的部位和临床表现	
部位	临床表现
额叶	头痛、嗜睡、注意力不集中、精神状态恶化、偏瘫伴单侧运动症状和运动性语言障碍
颞叶	同侧头痛和失语（优势侧）；视力缺陷
小脑	共济失调、眼球震颤、呕吐和构音障碍
脑干	发热、头痛、面部无力、偏瘫、吞咽困难和呕吐

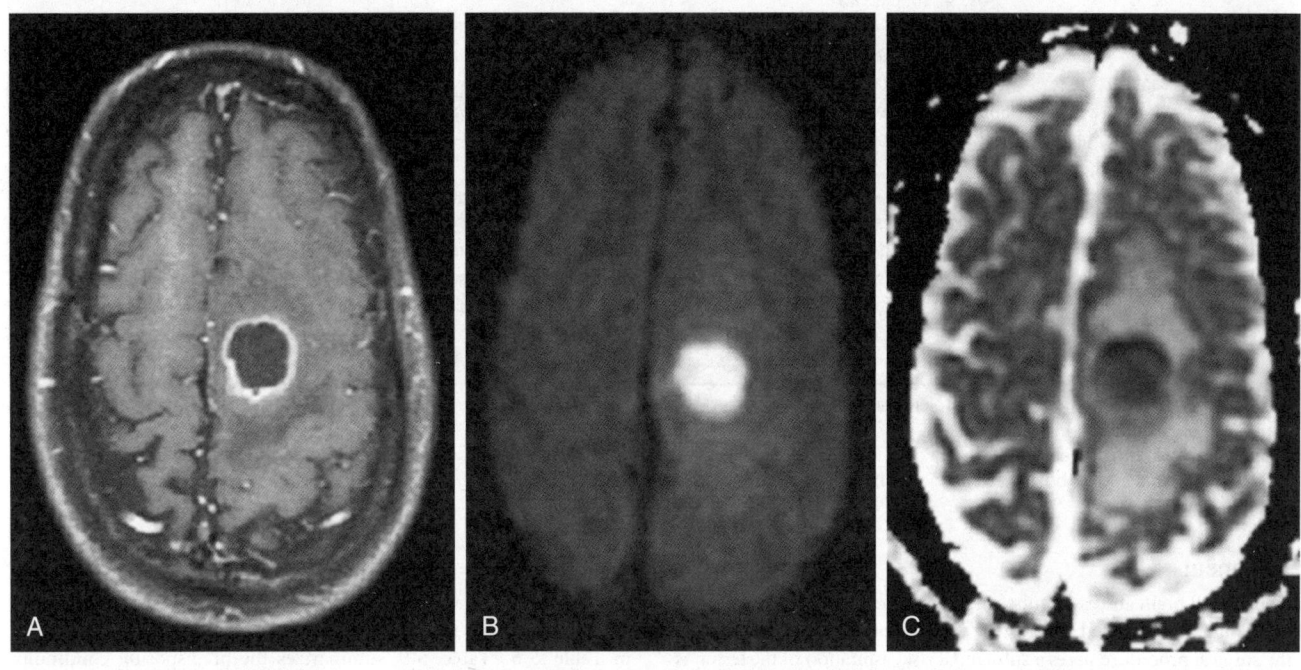

图 5.2 脑脓肿的磁共振成像特征。（A）对比增强扫描显示左侧额叶有环形强化病灶。（B）弥散加权图像显示，由于黏稠的脓液和细胞物质，腔内的弥散受限。（C）相应的表观弥散系数图显示，脓腔内有深色黏稠物质，周围水肿

出现发热、头痛和局灶性神经功能缺损的典型三联征。头痛是最常见的症状，并逐渐加重，伴有与脓肿位置有关的局灶性体征（如偏瘫、失语），随后出现反应迟钝和昏迷。头痛为中度到重度、偏头痛或全脑痛，但往往缺乏明显特征。30% 的病例在确诊前会出现癫痫发作。由于弓形虫脓肿易侵犯基底神经节，因此常伴有运动障碍。病情进展可能短至数小时，也可能长至数天至数周。脑脓肿的位置可能与临床表现相关（表 5.8）。脑脓肿的严重并发症是脓肿破裂，表现为头痛突然加重并伴有新发脑膜炎可能意味着脓肿破裂进入脑室。有报道脓肿破裂患者死亡率高达 85%。

诊断

应避免 CSF 检测：脑脓肿时脑脊液检测结果可能是正常的，对诊断通常无帮助，存在脑内占位病变腰椎穿刺可能造成脑疝。由于脑脓肿是从外周感染部位播散而来，因此寻找其他感染部位有助于确定致病菌并确定适当的治疗方法。

与 CT 相比，钆增强 MRI 软组织显像更清晰，是诊断脑脓肿的首选成像技术。MRI 更适合检测多发性脓肿和后窝脓肿。也适合于诊断脑炎，评估占位效应的程度，以及继发静脉血栓。重复或连续成像可评估治疗的反应。在脑炎早期，CT 结果可能正常，但 MRI FLAIR 序列对脑水肿的显示非常敏感。在 T1 加权图像中，脑炎区域最初表现为低信号强度、边界不清晰的病变。感染后期的 T1 加权图像可显示病灶边缘信号强度稍高和中心坏死。造影剂增强后通常会显示病灶中心坏事伴环状强化。DWI 显示中心坏死区亮信号而表观扩散系数（ADC）上病灶显示为暗信号（图 5.2）。肿瘤的 MRI 则显示出相反的特征。区分脑脓肿和肿瘤对于环形强化病灶在立体定向活检或手术切除非常重要。脓肿应从病灶中心引流，而肿瘤则应沿其边缘进行活检。

患者的危险因素、脑脓肿的位置、CT 或 MRI 成像的特征性发现有助于确定病原体。诺卡菌脑脓肿形态不规则，呈分叶状，李斯特菌脑脓肿通常位于脑干。在有侵袭性曲霉菌病危险因素的患者中，如果发现位于额叶或颞叶的脑梗死进展为单个或多个脑脓肿，通常提示诊断侵袭性曲霉菌。CT 或 MRI 发现窦腔浑浊、骨侵蚀和深筋膜平面阻塞，可能提示鼻脑毛霉病。增强扫描发现圆形等密度或低密度病变并伴有环状强化，在特定患者中提示中枢神经系统弓形虫病。

TABLE 5.9 Predisposing Conditions, Microbiology, and Empiric Treatment[a] of Brain Abscesses

Predisposing Condition	Usual Organism	Antimicrobial Regimen
Otitis media or mastoiditis	Streptococci (anaerobic and aerobic), *Bacteroides* and *Prevotella* sp, Enterobacteraceae	Metronidazole + a third-generation cephalosporin[b]
Sinusitis	Streptococci, *Bacteriodes* sp, Enterobacteriaceae, *Staphylococcus aureus*, *Haemophilus* sp	Vancomycin + a third-generation cephalosporin[b] + metronidazole
Dental infection	Mixed *Fusobacterium*, *Prevotella*, *Actinomyces*, and *Bacteriodes* sp, streptococci	Metronidazole + a third-generation cephalosporin[b]
Lung abscess, empyema, bronchiectasis	*Fusobacterium*, *Actinomyces*, *Bacteriodes*, and *Prevotella* sp, streptococci, *Nocardia* sp	Third-generation cephalosporin[b] + metronidazole + trimethoprim-sulfamethoxazole
Bacterial endocarditis	*S. aureus*, streptococci	Vancomycin[c]
Congenital heart disease	Streptococci, *Haemophilus* sp	Third-generation cephalosporin[b]
Penetrating trauma or invasive neurosurgical procedure	*S. aureus*, streptococci, Enterobacteriaceae, *Clostridioides* sp	Vancomycin + a third- or fourth-generation cephalosporin
Neutropenia	Aerobic gram-negative bacilli, *Aspergillus* sp, Mucorales, *Candida* sp, *Scedosporium* sp	Vancomycin + cefepime; consider antifungals
HIV infection	*Toxoplasma gondii*, *Nocardia* sp, *Mycobacterium* sp, *Listeria monocytogenes*, *Cryptococcus neoformans*	Add pyrimethamine + sulfadiazine; consider isoniazid, rifampin, pyrazinamide, and ethambutol for possible tuberculosis
Transplantation	*Aspergillus* sp, *Candida* sp, Mucorales, *Scedosporium* sp, Enterobacteriaceae, *Listeria monocytogenes*, *Nocardia* sp, *Toxoplasma gondii*, *Mycobacterium tuberculosis*	Add voriconazole + trimethoprim-sulfamethoxazole

[a]Treatment, namely use of targeted antimicrobials, may be modified based on isolation of specific microbes, sensitivities, and patient characteristics (i.e., allergies, risk factors).
[b]Cefotaxime or ceftriaxone.
[c]Additional agents should be added based on other likely microbiologic etiology.

Treatment

A suspected brain abscess requires urgent intervention. MRI or contrast CT should be performed to verify the presence of a brain abscess. Unless the surgical procedure poses a substantial risk, aspiration of the lesion is needed for microbial diagnosis. Corticosteroids should be administered to patients with significant edema, with mass effect causing increased intracranial pressure, or with a predisposition to transtentorial herniation. High-dose intravenous dexamethasone (16 to 24 mg/day in four divided doses) may be used for short periods until surgical intervention is possible. Corticosteroids may retard formation of a capsule around the brain abscess in its early stages and the immune response to infection. Seizures should be controlled because the tonic phase of a generalized seizure may increase intracranial pressure. In a patient with a large abscess, seizures may trigger a brain herniation. Seizure prophylaxis should be initiated in all patients with cortical or temporal lobe abscesses. Anticonvulsants that can be administered intravenously are preferred.

Successful treatment of brain abscesses relies on rapid verification of the abscess, identification of the responsible pathogen, timely surgical intervention, and appropriate antimicrobial therapy. Antibiotic management of brain abscess is based on knowledge of proven or suspected pathogens and antibiotic properties, such as CNS drug penetration capabilities and the spectrum of activity. Empirical antibiotic therapy without surgical intervention may be used if the primary source of infection outside of the CNS is identified, in patients with cerebritis without capsule formation, or in those with multiple, small abscesses or abscesses in basal ganglia or brain stem. If the organism is unknown, empirical therapy may include vancomycin, metronidazole, and a third- or fourth-generation cephalosporin. In brain stem abscesses, the possibility of *Listeria* infection should be considered, and treatment should include intravenous ampicillin. In HIV-infected patients with multiple ring-enhancing lesions, empirical therapy for toxoplasmosis should be initiated even if the patient is seronegative for *Toxoplasma*.

Voriconazole is the recommended antifungal therapy for patients with risk factors and imaging findings concerning for invasive aspergillosis. Recommendations for other causes of fungal brain abscess are shown in Table 5.6. Table 5.9 summarizes the predisposing conditions, microbiology, and recommended empiric treatment of brain abscesses.

Patients undergoing empirical therapy should be followed with repeat CT or MRI. Those who fail to respond should undergo surgical intervention. An important aspect of the management strategy is eradication of the predisposing condition or cause of the brain abscess, such as an oral, ear, cardiac, or pulmonary infection.

PARAMENINGEAL INFECTIONS

Parameningeal infections include infections that produce suppuration in potential spaces covering the brain and spinal cord (i.e., epidural abscess and subdural empyema) and those that produce occlusion of the contiguous venous sinuses and cerebral veins (i.e., cerebral venous sinus thrombosis).

Subdural Empyema
Definition

Subdural empyema refers to infection in the space separating the dura and arachnoid.

Pathology and Pathophysiology

Cranial subdural empyemas account for 15% to 20% of all localized intracranial infections. Two thirds of subdural empyemas result from frontal or ethmoid sinus infections, 20% from inner ear infections, and the remainder from trauma or neurosurgical procedures. The empyema is caused by direct or indirect extension from infected paranasal sinuses through a retrograde thrombophlebitis. Unilateral empyema is most common because the falx prevents passage across the midline,

表 5.9　脑脓肿的诱因、微生物学和经验疗法 [a]

诱因	常见病原体	抗菌治疗方案
中耳炎或乳突炎	链球菌（厌氧和需氧）、乳酸杆菌和前螺旋体、肠杆菌科	甲硝唑+第三代头孢菌素[b]
鼻窦炎	链球菌、拟杆菌属、肠杆菌科、金黄色葡萄球菌、嗜血杆菌	万古霉素+第三代头孢菌素[b]+甲硝唑
牙源性感染	梭杆菌属、普雷沃菌属、放线菌和拟杆菌属、链球菌	甲硝唑+第三代头孢菌素[b]
肺脓肿、脓胸、支气管扩张	梭杆菌属、放线菌属、拟杆菌属和普雷沃菌属、链球菌属、诺卡菌属	第三代头孢菌素[b]+甲硝唑+磺胺甲噁唑-甲氧苄啶
细菌性心内膜炎	金黄色葡萄球菌、链球菌	万古霉素[c]
先天性心脏病	链球菌、流感嗜血杆菌	第三代头孢菌素[b]
穿透性创伤或侵入性神经外科手术	金黄色葡萄球菌、链球菌、肠杆菌、梭状芽孢杆菌	万古霉素+第三代或第四代头孢菌素
中性粒细胞减少	需氧革兰氏阴性杆菌、曲霉菌属、毛霉菌属、念珠菌属、孢子菌属	万古霉素+头孢吡肟；考虑使用抗真菌药
HIV 感染	刚地弓形虫、诺卡菌属、分枝杆菌、单核细胞增生李斯特菌、新生隐球菌	乙胺嘧啶+磺胺嘧啶；考虑使用异烟肼、利福平、吡嗪酰胺和乙胺丁醇治疗可能的结核病
移植	曲霉菌属、念珠菌属、毛霉菌属、孢子菌属、肠杆菌科、单核细胞增生李斯特菌、球孢子菌属、诺卡菌、刚地弓形虫、结核分枝杆菌	伏立康唑+磺胺甲噁唑-甲氧苄啶

[a] 可根据分离到的特定微生物、敏感性和患者特征（如过敏、危险因素）对治疗方法（即有针对性地使用抗菌药物）进行调整。
[b] 头孢噻肟或头孢曲松。
[c] 应根据其他可能的微生物病因添加其他药物。

治疗

疑似脑脓肿需要紧急干预。应进行 MRI 或增强 CT 检查，以确认是否存在脑脓肿。除非手术风险很大，否则需要抽吸病灶以进行微生物诊断。对于水肿严重、占位效应导致颅内压增高或易发生脑疝的患者，应使用皮质类固醇。大剂量地塞米松（每天 16～24 mg，分 4 次服用）可短期静脉注射，直到可以进行手术治疗。皮质类固醇可能会延缓脑脓肿早期周围包囊的形成以及对感染的免疫反应。控制癫痫发作，因为癫痫发作的强直期可能会增加颅内压。对于大脓肿患者，癫痫发作可能会引发脑疝。所有皮质或颞叶脓肿患者都应开始预防癫痫发作。首选可静脉注射的抗惊厥药物。

脑脓肿的成功治疗有赖于快速核实脓肿、确定病原体、及时手术干预和适当的抗菌治疗。脑脓肿的抗生素治疗基于对已证实或可疑病原体和抗生素特性（如药物中枢神经系统渗透能力和抗菌谱）的了解。如果发现中枢神经系统以外的主要感染源，或脑脓肿囊腔未形成，或有多个小脓肿或基底节或脑干脓肿的患者，可采用经验性抗生素治疗，无须手术干预。如果病原体不明，经验性疗法可包括万古霉素、甲硝唑和第三代或第四代头孢菌素。对于脑干脓肿，应考虑李斯特菌感染的可能性，治疗应包括静脉注射氨苄西林。对于有多个环状强化病灶的 AIDS 患者，即使患者的弓形虫血清阴性，也应开始弓形虫病的经验性治疗。对于具有侵袭性曲霉菌病危险因素和影像学检查结果的患者，推荐使用伏立康唑进行抗真菌治疗。表 5.6 列出了针对其他原因引起的真菌性脑脓肿的建议。表 5.9 总结了脑脓肿的诱发条件、微生物学和推荐的经验性疗法。

接受经验性疗法的患者应复查 CT 或 MRI。无效者应接受手术治疗。根除脑脓肿的诱发条件或病因十分重要，如口腔、耳部、心脏或肺部感染。

脑膜周围感染

脑膜周围感染包括在覆盖大脑和脊髓的潜在空间中产生化脓的感染（即硬膜外脓肿和硬膜下积脓），以及在毗连静脉窦和脑静脉中产生闭塞的感染（即脑静脉窦血栓形成）。

硬膜下积脓

定义

硬膜下积脓指的是硬脑膜和蛛网膜之间的间隙发生感染。

病理学和病理生理学

头颅硬膜下积脓占所有颅内感染的 15%～20%。2/3 的硬膜下积脓由额窦或乙状窦感染引起，20% 由内耳感染引起，其余由外伤或神经外科手术引起。硬膜下腔积脓是由受感染的鼻旁窦通过逆行血栓性静脉炎直接或间接扩散引起的。单侧积脓最常见，因为大

but bilateral or multiple empyemas can occur. Cortical venous thrombosis or brain abscess develops in about 25% of patients. The infection is metastatic in about 5% of patients, primarily from a pulmonary source. In some patients, the subdural empyema may be associated with an epidural abscess or meningitis. These associations occur more often in children than in adults.

Clinical Presentation

The clinical presentation of cranial subdural empyema can be rapidly progressive with signs and symptoms resulting from increased intracranial pressure, meningeal irritation, or focal cortical inflammation. These include fever, intractable headache, vomiting, nuchal rigidity, focal neurologic deficits (e.g., hemiparesis, ocular palsies, dysphasia, dilated pupils, cerebellar signs, or seizures), and varying levels of altered consciousness. If untreated, mental status may decline to obtundation, and the septic mass and swollen underlying brain can lead to venous thrombosis or death from herniation. The clinical presentation of spinal subdural empyema may consist of radicular pain and symptoms of spinal cord compression including saddle anesthesia, lower extremity weakness, and bowel or bladder incontinence. The infection may occur at multiple levels. The presentation can be difficult to differentiate from spinal epidural abscess.

The major differential diagnosis is meningitis. Nuchal rigidity and obtundation occur in meningitis and cranial subdural empyema, but papilledema and lateralizing deficits are more common in cranial subdural empyema.

Diagnosis

Lumbar puncture should be avoided in patients with cranial subdural empyema to prevent cerebral herniation. Contrast-enhanced CT or MRI can be diagnostic of empyema, showing an extra-axial, crescent-shaped mass with an enhancing rim lying just below the inner table of the skull over the cerebral convexities or in the interhemispheric fissures. On MRI, subdural empyema has decreased signal intensity on T1-weighted imaging and increased signal intensity on T2-weighted scans. Similar to brain abscess, subdural empyema has high signal intensity on diffusion-weighted images and low signal intensity on ADC maps.

Treatment

Treatment requires prompt surgical drainage of the empyema cavity and prompt administration of intravenous antibiotics directed at organisms found at the time of craniotomy. Concomitant use of corticosteroids to reduce edema and increased intracranial pressure, as well as anticonvulsants to control seizures, are also important to reduce morbidity and mortality.

SPINAL EPIDURAL ABSCESS

Definition and Epidemiology

A *spinal epidural abscess* is an infection in the epidural space between the dura and the bones of the spine around the spinal cord. It can cause paralysis and death. The incidence is 0.5 to 1.0 cases per 10,000 hospital admissions in the United States, and the frequency is increased among injection drug users.

Pathology and Pathophysiology

Infections of the spinal epidural space originate from contiguous spread or through hematogenous routes from a distant source. Cutaneous infection, particularly in the back, is the most common remote source, especially among injection drug users. Abdominal, respiratory tract, and urinary sources are also common. As the use of epidural catheters has increased for pain management, epidural abscess and hematoma have been increasingly reported.

The anatomy of the epidural space dictates the location of the abscess. Because the size of the intravertebral canal remains relatively constant but the circumference of the spinal cord changes, abscess formation is maximal in the thoracic and lumbar regions and minimal at the cervical spine. Due to the loose connections between the dura and the bones of the spine, the abscess can extend to multiple levels, causing severe and extensive neurologic manifestations.

Causative organisms can be identified by culture or Gram stain from pus obtained at exploration (90% of patients), blood cultures (60% to 90%), or CSF (20%). *S. aureus* is the most common pathogen, followed by streptococci and gram-negative organisms. Tuberculous abscesses may occur in as many as 25% of patients in high-risk populations. In a previous epidemic, iatrogenic infection occurred with rare fungi after epidural injections of corticosteroids that were contaminated with a plant pathogen, *Exserohilum rostratum,* which rarely infects humans.

Clinical Presentation

The classic triad of fever, back pain, and neurologic deficits may not be identified in all patients, leading to a delay in diagnosis. Patients are usually febrile and have acute or subacute neck or back pain. An important physical finding is focal tenderness over the affected spinous processes. Stiff neck and headache are common. The pain can be mistaken for sciatica, a visceral abdominal process, chest wall pain, or cervical disk disease. If it goes unrecognized at this stage, the symptoms can evolve over a few hours to a few days to weakness, loss of lower extremity reflexes, and paralysis distal to the spinal level of the infection. In this clinical setting, urgent neuroradiologic imaging should be pursued followed by empiric antibiotics with concurrent corticosteroids, and surgical evaluation.

Diagnosis

The diagnosis is made by CT or MRI (Fig. 5.3). The differential diagnosis includes transverse myelitis, intervertebral disk herniation, epidural hemorrhage, and metastatic tumor. These conditions can usually be differentiated by MRI. Epidural abscess is often accompanied by diskitis or osteomyelitis of the vertebral bodies.

Treatment

Unless culture and sensitivities dictate otherwise, a penicillinase-resistant penicillin should be started empirically as antistaphylococcal treatment for presumed bacterial infection. If methicillin resistance is suspected, vancomycin should be used. Considering the severity of the disease, additional gram-negative coverage with a third- or fourth-generation cephalosporin or a fluoroquinolone may be needed. Other empiric agents, including antifungals, can be considered based on clinical suspicion and patient risk factors.

Surgical decompression was previously considered mandatory, but early diagnosis by MRI may allow for effective medical therapy if started before the occurrence of neurologic complications. These patients should be monitored closely, and if signs of neurologic deterioration emerge, surgical intervention may be necessary.

SINUS THROMBOSIS

Septic Cavernous Sinus Thrombosis

Septic cavernous sinus thrombosis usually results from spread of infection from paranasal sinusitis (especially of the sphenoid or ethmoid sinuses) or less commonly from spread of infection from the face and mouth. Symptoms include headache or lateralized facial pain, followed

脑镰阻碍了感染穿过中线，但也可能出现双侧或多发性脓肿。约 25% 的患者会出现皮质静脉血栓形成或脑脓肿。约 5% 的患者会发生远处感染转移而来，主要来自肺部。有些患者的硬膜下积脓可能伴有硬膜外脓肿或脑膜炎。与成人相比，这些并发症更常发生在儿童身上。

临床表现

颅内硬膜下积脓的临床表现可急剧进展，出现颅内压增高、脑膜刺激征或局灶性皮质炎症引起的体征和症状。这些症状包括发热、顽固性头痛、呕吐、颈强直、局灶性神经功能缺损（如偏瘫、眼肌麻痹、失语、瞳孔散大、小脑病变表现或癫痫发作）以及不同程度的意识改变。如果不及时治疗，患者可逐渐昏迷，化脓性肿块和脑组织肿胀可能导致静脉血栓或脑疝死亡。硬脊膜下脓肿的临床表现可能是根性疼痛和脊髓受压症状，包括鞍部感觉障碍、下肢无力和大小便失禁。感染可能发生在多个层面。这种表现很难与硬脊膜外脓肿相鉴别。

鉴别诊断主要是脑膜炎。脑膜炎和硬膜下积脓会出现颈强硬和昏迷，颅内硬膜下积脓则更常见视乳头水肿和偏侧障碍。

诊断

颅内硬膜下积脓患者应避免腰椎穿刺，以防脑疝。增强 CT 或 MRI 可诊断积脓，显示轴外、新月形肿块，边缘强化，位于脑凸上方的颅骨内下方或大脑半球间裂内。MRI 硬膜下积脓在 T1 加权成像上信号强度减弱，而在 T2 加权扫描上信号强度增强。与脑脓肿类似，硬膜下积脓在弥散加权成像上信号强度高，而在 ADC 图上信号强度低。

治疗

治疗需要及时手术引流脓液，并针对引流时明确的细菌及时静脉应用抗生素。同时使用类固醇激素减轻水肿和降低颅内压，以及抗惊厥药控制癫痫发作，对于降低发病率和死亡率也很重要。

硬脊膜外脓肿

定义和流行病学

硬脊膜外脓肿是脊髓周围硬膜外腔和脊柱骨骼之间的感染。它可导致瘫痪和死亡。在美国，其发病率为每 10 000 例住院患者中有 0.5～1.0 例，注射毒品者的发病率更高。

病理学和病理生理学

脊柱硬膜外腔感染源于毗连传播或来自远处的血源性途径。皮肤感染（尤其是背部）是最常见的远处感染源，尤其是在注射毒品者中。腹部、呼吸道、尿路感染来源也很常见。随着硬膜外导管在疼痛治疗中的使用增多，硬膜外脓肿和血肿的病例也越来越多。

硬膜外腔的解剖结构决定了脓肿的位置。由于椎管内的大小相对恒定，但脊髓的周径会发生变化，因此胸椎和腰椎部位的脓肿形成最多，而颈椎部位的脓肿形成最少。由于硬脊膜和脊柱骨骼之间的连接松散，脓肿可扩展到多个层面，导致严重和广泛的神经系统表现。

可通过从探查时获得的脓液（90% 的患者）、血液培养（60%～90%）或脑脊液（20%）培养或革兰氏染色确定致病菌。金黄色葡萄球菌是最常见的病原体，其次是链球菌和革兰氏阴性菌。在高危人群中，多达 25% 的患者可能会出现结核性脓肿。由于之前硬膜外注射皮质类固醇可继发一种罕见的真菌医源性感染，这是一种污染的，很少感染人类的植物病原体钩型突脐孢菌。

临床表现

典型的三联征包括发热、背痛和神经功能缺损的典型三联征，但并非所有患者都出现，不具备三联征的患者可导致诊断延误。患者通常会发热，并伴有急性或亚急性颈部或背部疼痛。一个重要的体格检查结果是受累棘突压痛。颈强直和头痛很常见。疼痛可被误以为是坐骨神经痛、内脏腹部病变、胸壁疼痛或颈椎间盘疾病。如果在这一阶段没有被发现，症状可能会在数小时至数天内发展为肌无力、下肢反射消失以及感染脊柱平面远端瘫痪。在这种临床情况下，应紧急进行神经影像学检查，经验性抗生素治疗，同时服用皮质类固醇，并考虑手术。

诊断

通过 CT 或 MRI 可以确诊（图 5.3）。鉴别诊断包括横贯性脊髓炎、椎间盘突出、硬膜外出血和转移瘤。这些疾病通常可以通过 MRI 进行鉴别。硬膜外脓肿通常伴有椎间盘炎或椎骨骨髓炎。

治疗

除非有明确的培养和药敏结果，否应根据经验使用耐青霉素酶的青霉素类药物针对金黄色葡萄球菌治疗。如果怀疑甲氧西林耐药，则应使用万古霉素。考虑到病情严重性，可能需要使用第三代或第四代头孢菌素或氟喹诺酮类药物来覆盖革兰氏阴性菌。根据临床推测和患者的危险因素，可考虑使用其他经验性药物，包括抗真菌药物。

以前认为必须进行手术减压，但如果能在出现神经系统并发症之前通过 MRI 进行早期诊断，就可以进行有效的药物治疗。应对这些患者进行密切监测，如果出现神经系统恶化的迹象，需要进行手术治疗。

窦血栓形成

感染中毒性（脓毒性）海绵窦血栓形成

感染中毒性海绵窦血栓通常是由副鼻窦炎（尤其是蝶窦或乙状窦）的感染扩散引起的，其次是由面部和口腔的感染扩散引起的，但并不常见。症状包括头

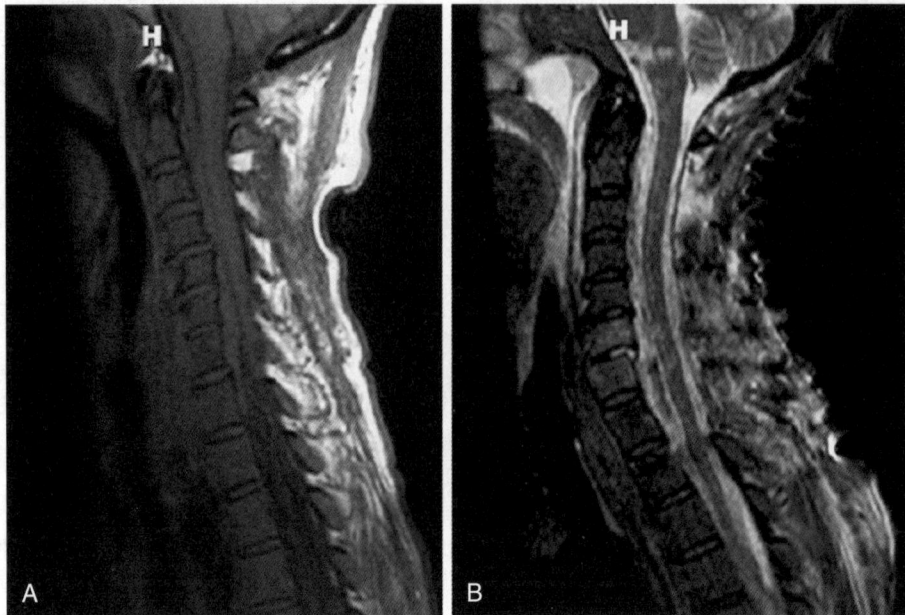

Fig. 5.3 Magnetic resonance imaging shows an epidural abscess due to *Staphylococcus* in the cervical spine of a patient with human immunodeficiency virus infection. (A) Noncontrast T1-weighted image shows an extensive lesion in the epidural space that extends from C2 to C7. Notice straightening of the cervical spine. (B) After a laminectomy from C2 to T1 and fusion, the short tau inversion recovery (STIR) image shows fluid collection in the epidural space as a high-signal-intensity lesion. Normal curvature of the spine is seen.

in a few days to weeks by fever and involvement of the orbit (i.e., proptosis and chemosis due to obstruction of the ophthalmic vein). Paralysis of oculomotor nerves follows rapidly. In some instances, sensory dysfunction occurs in the first and second divisions of the trigeminal nerve along with a decrease in the corneal reflex. Further involvement of the contiguous orbital contents follows, with mild papilledema and decreased visual acuity that sometimes progresses to blindness.

Extension to the opposite cavernous sinus or to other intracranial sinuses with cerebral infarction or increased intracranial pressure due to impaired venous drainage can result in stupor, coma, and death. The CSF is abnormal if there is accompanying meningitis or parameningeal infection. The most common causative organism is *S. aureus*, followed by streptococci and pneumococci; anaerobes and gram-negative bacilli may also be etiologic agents.

Diagnosis of cavernous sinus thrombosis is usually made by MRI with MR venogram. Radiologic evaluation includes imaging of the sphenoidal and ethmoidal sinuses, which may require drainage if infected. Empirical antimicrobial therapy should include an antistaphylococcal agent. An empirical combination therapy with parenteral metronidazole, vancomycin, and a third- or fourth-generation cephalosporin can achieve reasonable CSF and brain penetration and is likely to be active against *S. aureus* and the usual sinus pathogens.

Lateral Sinus Thrombosis

Septic thrombosis of the lateral sinus results from acute or chronic infections of the middle ear, including otitis media and mastoiditis. The infection spreads through emissary veins that connect the mastoid with the lateral venous sinus. It may spread to involve the sigmoid sinus. The symptoms include ear pain followed over several weeks by fever, headache, nausea, vomiting, and vertigo. Mastoid swelling may be seen. Sixth cranial nerve palsies and papilledema can occur, but other focal neurologic signs are rare.

The diagnosis can be established by MRI. Common pathogens of lateral sinus thrombosis include *S. aureus*, streptococci, and *E. coli*; rarely, *Fusobacterium necrophorum* and *Bacteriodes fragilis* have also been reported. Treatment includes an empirical regimen of broad-spectrum intravenous antibiotics to cover staphylococci, gram-negative bacilli, and anaerobes (i.e., vancomycin with metronidazole and a third- or fourth generation cephalosporin). Surgical drainage (i.e., mastoidectomy) may be required.

Septic Sagittal Sinus Thrombosis

Septic sagittal sinus thrombosis is uncommon and occurs as a consequence of purulent meningitis, infections of the ethmoidal or maxillary sinuses spreading through venous channels, face, scalp, subdural space, compound skull fractures, or neurosurgical wound infections (rare). Symptoms include manifestations of elevated intracranial pressure (e.g., headache, nausea, and vomiting) that evolve rapidly to stupor and coma. Motor deficits, nuchal rigidity, and papilledema may be seen. Seizures occur in more than half of these patients. Similar to other sinus thromboses, the likely microorganisms depend on the associated primary condition. Diagnosis and treatment are similar to the lateral venous sinus thrombosis described earlier.

NEUROLOGIC COMPLICATIONS OF INFECTIVE ENDOCARDITIS

Epidemiology

Neurologic complications are among the most common extra-cardiac complications of infective endocarditis and occur in one third of patients with bacterial endocarditis. They are associated with significant morbidity and triple the mortality rate of the disease. Cerebral (but not systemic) emboli from mitral valve endocarditis are increasingly common. Most emboli, regardless of the bacterial cause of the infection, occur before or early in the course of treatment. By 2 weeks

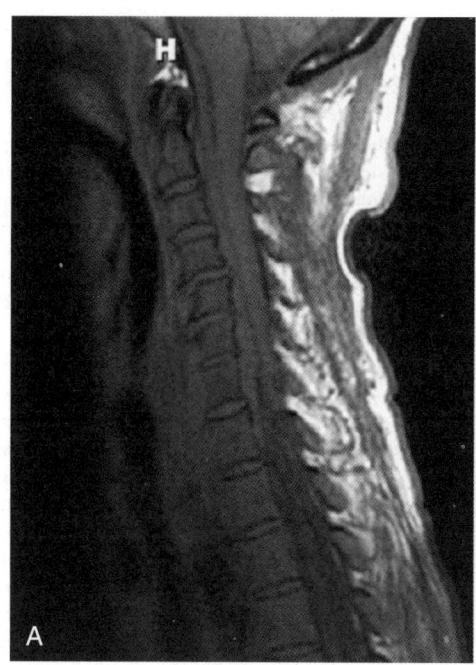 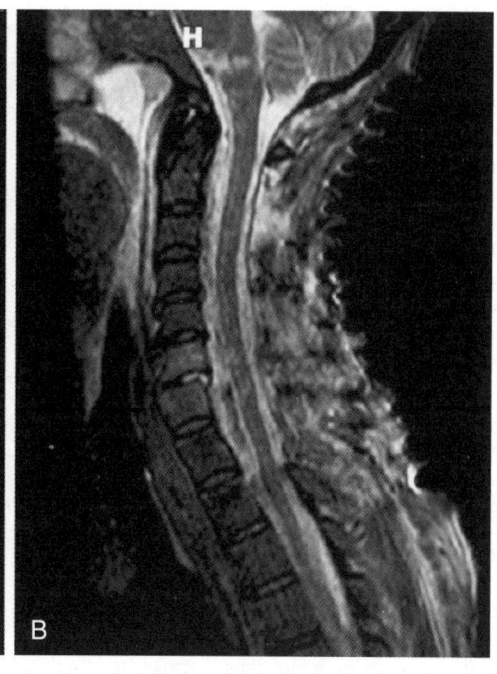

图 5.3 磁共振成像显示一名 HIV 感染患者由葡萄球菌引起的颈椎硬膜外脓肿。（A）非对比 T1 加权图像显示硬膜外腔有广泛病变，从 C2 一直延伸到 C7。（B）从 C2 到 T1 进行椎板切除和融合术后，短 tau 反转恢复（STIR）图像显示硬膜外间隙的液体聚集为高信号强度病变。（B）从 C2 到 T1 进行椎板切除和融合术后，反转恢复（STIR）图像显示硬膜外间隙的液体聚集为高信号强度病变。脊柱曲度正常

痛或面部偏侧疼痛，数天或数周后会出现发热和眼眶受累（即因眼静脉阻塞导致的突眼和球结膜水肿）。迅速出现动眼神经麻痹。在某些情况下，三叉神经的第一和第二分支出现感觉功能障碍，角膜反射也会减弱。随后，眼眶内容物会进一步受累，出现轻度乳头水肿和视力下降，有时会发展为失明。

病变扩展到对侧海绵窦或其他颅内海绵窦，继发脑梗死或静脉引流受阻导致颅内压增高，可导致昏睡、昏迷和死亡。如并发脑膜炎或脑膜周围感染，CSF 则异常。最常见的致病菌是金黄色葡萄球菌，其次是链球菌和肺炎链球菌；厌氧菌和革兰氏阴性杆菌也可致病。

海绵窦血栓的诊断通常是通过磁共振成像和磁共振静脉造影。影像检查包括蝶窦和乙状窦的成像，这些部位感染可能需要引流。经验性抗感染治疗需要覆盖葡萄球菌。经验性联合疗法包括静脉应用甲硝唑、万古霉素和第三代或第四代头孢菌素，在脑脊液和脑中达到有效的药物浓度，并可能对金黄色葡萄球菌和常见的鼻窦病原体有效。

侧窦血栓形成

急性或慢性中耳感染可导致感染中毒性侧窦血栓形成，包括中耳炎和乳突炎。感染通过连接乳突和侧静脉窦的导静脉扩散，也可能扩散到乙状窦。症状包括耳痛，随后数周出现发热、头痛、恶心、呕吐和眩晕，也可能出现乳突肿胀，可出现第Ⅵ脑神经麻痹和视乳头水肿，但其他局灶性神经系统症状很少见。

可进行 MRI 明确诊断。常见的侧窦血栓病原体包括金黄色葡萄球菌、链球菌和大肠埃希菌；也有坏死梭杆菌和脆弱拟杆菌的罕见报道。治疗包括经验性静脉注射广谱抗生素，以覆盖葡萄球菌、革兰氏阴性杆菌和厌氧菌（如万古霉素联合甲硝唑和第三代或第四代头孢菌素）。可能需要手术引流（如乳突切开术）。

感染中毒性（脓毒性）矢状窦血栓形成

感染中毒性矢状窦血栓并不常见，是化脓性脑膜炎、经静脉通道扩散的乙状窦或上颌窦感染、面部、头皮、硬膜下间隙、复合性颅骨骨折或神经外科伤口感染（罕见）的后遗症。症状包括颅内压升高（如头痛、恶心和呕吐），并迅速发展为昏睡或昏迷。还可出现运动障碍，颈强直和视乳头水肿，半数以上的患者会出现癫痫发作。与其他静脉窦血栓类似，可能的微生物取决于原发疾病，诊断和治疗与前面描述的侧静脉窦血栓类似。

感染性心内膜炎的神经系统并发症

流行病学

神经系统并发症是感染性心内膜炎最常见的心外并发症之一，1/3 的细菌性心内膜炎患者会出现神经系统并发症。神经系统并发症的发病率很高，一旦出现死亡率增加至 3 倍。二尖瓣心内膜炎引起的脑栓塞（而非全身性栓塞）越来越常见，大多数栓塞都发生在治疗前或

of therapy, the risk of embolization decreases dramatically. Mycotic aneurysms in the brain complicate endocarditis in 2% to 10% of patients and are more common in acute than subacute disease.

Pathophysiology
The risk of developing neurologic complications from infective endocarditis depends on a number of characteristics, principally the size and location of the vegetation as well as the duration of antibiotic treatment. Larger, left-sided vegetations involving the mitral valve are more likely to embolize.

Cerebral emboli are distributed in the brain in proportion to cerebral blood flow. Most emboli lodge in the branches of the middle cerebral artery peripherally. Multiple microabscesses can result and cause diffuse encephalopathy. Mycotic aneurysms occur most commonly in the middle cerebral artery, with the aneurysms located distally in the vessel. This differentiates them from congenital berry aneurysms.

Clinical Manifestations
Neurologic complications may be the presenting symptoms of infective endocarditis. Patients may present with severe headache, focal neurologic deficits, altered consciousness, mononeuropathy, or seizures. Embolic stroke is the most common complication. Other complications include ischemic or hemorrhagic stroke, meningitis, brain abscess, spinal epidural abscess, and infected intracranial aneurysm.

Diagnosis
The diagnosis of neurologic involvement from endocarditis is best made with CT or MRI. MRI findings in endocarditis include ischemic lesions, hemorrhagic lesions, subarachnoid hemorrhage, brain abscess, mycotic aneurysm, and cerebral microbleeds. The CSF is abnormal in 70% of patients and simulates purulent meningitis (i.e., polymorphonuclear predominance, elevated protein level, and low glucose level) or a parameningeal infection (i.e., lymphocytic predominance, modest protein elevation, and normal glucose level). If concomitant bacteremia is present, positive blood cultures help identify the causative pathogen.

Multidetector CT angiography may be necessary to diagnose aneurysms. Small brain abscesses may complicate the course of endocarditis, but macroscopic abscesses are rare, with most occurring in the setting of acute rather than subacute endocarditis. Multiple microabscesses may escape detection on CT and are not amenable to surgical drainage.

Treatment
Antibiotic treatment of the primary disease is indicated. Stroke is usually treated conservatively. There are no controlled trials for the management of unruptured mycotic aneurysms, although they may be managed with antibiotics alone. Ruptured aneurysms should be managed with a combination of antibiotics with surgery or endovascular therapy because treatment-related mortality is higher in patients with ruptured aneurysms than unruptured aneurysms. Patients with infective endocarditis who do not respond to conservative medical therapy can have prompt valve replacement despite intracerebral hemorrhage. The balance of risks and benefits should be tailored to each individual patient when considering surgical intervention in the setting of neurologic complications, which can significantly increase the risk of surgical complications. In general, anticoagulation use is not recommended due to the potential risk for hemorrhagic complications and because it does not appear to reduce the risk of embolism in patients with infective endocarditis.

PRION DISEASES
Etiology
Several human diseases have been attributed to a unique infectious protein, the prion. The infectious form of the prion protein is rich in β-sheets, detergent insoluble, multimeric, and resistant to proteinase K treatment.

Prion illnesses (i.e., transmissible spongiform encephalopathies) can be classified as sporadic, hereditary, or acquired. The most common form is sporadic Creutzfeldt-Jakob disease (sCJD). Familial forms include Gerstmann-Sträussler-Scheinker syndrome and familial fatal insomnia.

Acquired forms are caused by the transmission of an abnormal prion protein (PrP) from human to human or from cattle to humans. Accidental transmission of CJD between humans appears to have occurred with cadaveric dura mater grafting, corneal transplantation, receipt of human growth hormone or pituitary gonadotropin, contaminated electroencephalogram electrodes, and contaminated surgical instruments. This form of CJD has been called iatrogenic CJD (iCJD).

The appearance of variant CJD (vCJD) in Great Britain, which was associated with the outbreak of bovine spongiform encephalopathy and the contamination of beef, greatly increased interest in this group of illnesses. Kuru is another transmissible spongiform encephalopathy that was spread in New Guinea by cannibalism, a practice that ceased in the 1950s. The disease is now almost extinct.

Sporadic Creutzfeldt-Jakob Disease
Epidemiology
Illness from sCJD is seen worldwide, with an incidence of 0.5 to 1.0 cases per 1 million people in the general population per year.

Pathology
The pathologic hallmarks of CJD are spongiform or vacuolar changes in the brain without cellular inflammatory infiltrates. The pathogenic isoform of the prion protein can be demonstrated in brain tissue by immunocytochemical staining and by Western blot analysis. The fundamental process involved in human prion propagation is intercellular induction of protein misfolding and seeded aggregation of misfolded prion protein.

Clinical Manifestations
CJD is frequently diagnosed incorrectly initially. Prodromal symptoms include altered sleep patterns and appetite, weight loss, changes in sexual drive, and impaired memory and concentration. Disorientation, hallucinations, depression, and emotional lability are early signs, followed by a rapidly progressive dementia associated with myoclonus (about 90% of patients). Myoclonus is usually provoked by tactile, auditory, or visual startle stimuli. CJD has an abrupt onset in 10% to 15% of patients.

Other distinctive features include seizures, autonomic dysfunction, and lower motor neuron disease, suggesting amyotrophic lateral sclerosis–like characteristics. Cerebellar ataxia occurs in one third of patients.

Diagnosis
The clinical tetrad supporting the diagnosis of CJD consists of a subacute progressive dementia, myoclonus, typical periodic sharp waves on electroencephalography, and normal CSF. FLAIR MRI sequences show extensive curvilinear hyperintensity along the neocortex, called *cortical ribboning*, which affects frontal, parietal, and temporal lobes (in decreasing order of frequency). Routine CSF study is usually normal. A CSF test for the protein 14-3-3, which is released into spinal

治疗初期，与感染的细菌原因无关。治疗 2 周后栓塞的风险就会大大降低。2%～10% 的心内膜炎患者会并发脑部真菌性动脉瘤，急性期比亚急性期更常见。

病理生理学

感染性心内膜炎引起神经系统并发症的风险取决于多种因素，主要是赘生物的大小和位置以及抗生素治疗的持续时间。较大、位于左侧涉及二尖瓣的赘生物更容易发生栓塞。

脑栓塞在大脑中的分布与脑血流量成正比。大多数栓子停留在大脑中动脉的分支周围。多处微脓肿可导致弥漫性脑病。霉菌性动脉瘤最常发生在大脑中动脉，动脉瘤位于血管远端。这使其有别于先天性浆液性动脉瘤。

临床表现

神经系统并发症可能是感染性心内膜炎的主要症状。患者可能表现为剧烈头痛、局灶性神经功能缺损、意识障碍、单神经病变或癫痫发作。栓塞性卒中是最常见的并发症。其他并发症包括缺血性或出血性卒中、脑膜炎、脑脓肿、脊髓硬膜外脓肿和感染性颅内动脉瘤。

诊断

心内膜炎累及神经系统的诊断最好通过 CT 或 MRI 进行。心内膜炎的 MRI 检查结果包括缺血性病变、出血性病变、蛛网膜下腔出血、脑脓肿、真菌性动脉瘤和大脑微出血。70% 的患者脑脊液异常，类似化脓性脑膜炎（即多形核细胞为主、蛋白水平升高、葡萄糖水平较低）或脑膜周围感染（即淋巴细胞为主、蛋白水平中度升高、葡萄糖水平正常）。如果同时出现菌血症，血液培养阳性有助于确定致病病原体。

多层 CT 血管造影术可能是诊断动脉瘤的必要手段。小的脑脓肿可能继发于心内膜炎，大的脓肿很少见，大多数发生在急性而非亚急性心内膜炎。多发性微小脓肿可能无法在 CT 上发现，也不适合手术引流。

治疗

对原发疾病应进行抗生素治疗。卒中通常采用保守治疗。对于未破裂的真菌性动脉瘤，没有对照试验来指导治疗，尽管它们可能仅用抗生素管理。破裂的动脉瘤应在抗生素治疗同时评估手术或血管内治疗，破裂动脉瘤患者中治疗相关死亡风险高于未破裂动脉瘤。对保守治疗无效的感染性心内膜炎患者，尽管有脑内出血，也应及时进行瓣膜置换术。出现神经系统并发症会显著增加手术并发症的风险，因此在考虑对神经系统并发症患者进行手术治疗时，应根据每位患者的具体情况权衡风险与获益。一般来说，由于存在出血性并发症的风险，而且抗凝似乎并不能降低感染性心内膜炎患者发生栓塞的风险，因此不建议使用抗凝治疗。

朊病毒病

病原学

有几种人类疾病是由一种独特的传染性蛋白质——朊病毒引起的。朊病毒蛋白的感染形式富含 β 折叠，不溶于洗涤剂，呈多聚体，对蛋白酶 K 有抵抗力。

朊病毒病（即传染性海绵状脑病）可分为散发性、遗传性和获得性。最常见的是散发性克-雅病（sCJD）。家族性疾病包格斯特曼-施特劳斯勒尔-沙因克尔综合征和家族性致死性失眠。

获得性 CJD 是由异常朊病毒蛋白（PrP）在人与人之间或牛与人之间的传播引起的。CJD 在人与人之间的意外传播似乎发生在硬脑膜移植、角膜移植、接受人类生长激素或垂体促性腺激素、污染的脑电图电极和受污染的手术器械上。称为医源性 CJD（iCJD）。

变异型 CJD（vCJD）在英国的出现与牛海绵状脑病的暴发和牛肉污染有关，这大大提高了人们对这类疾病的关注。库鲁病是另一种可传播的海绵状脑病，在新几内亚通过食人的方式传播，这种做法在 20 世纪 50 年代已经停止。这种疾病现在几乎已经绝迹。

散发克-雅病

流行病学

sCJD 疾病遍布全球，普通人群中每年每 100 万人中有 0.5～1.0 例发病。

病理学

CJD 的病理特征是大脑出现海绵状或空泡状变化，但无炎症细胞浸润。通过免疫细胞化学染色和 Western 印迹分析，可在脑组织中发现朊病毒蛋白的致病异构体。人类朊病毒的传播过程是细胞间诱导蛋白质错误折叠和错误折叠的朊病毒蛋白感染其他脑组织。

临床表现

CJD 最初的往往被误诊。前驱症状有睡眠模式和食欲改变、体重减轻、性欲改变、记忆力和注意力减退。定向力下降、幻觉、抑郁和情绪不稳定是早期症状，随后是伴有肌阵挛的快速进展性痴呆（约 90% 的患者）。肌阵挛通常由触觉、听觉或视觉惊吓刺激引起。10%～15% 的患者会突然发病。

其他显著特点包括癫痫发作、自主神经功能障碍和下运动神经元病，显示出类似肌萎缩侧索硬化症的特征。1/3 的患者会出现小脑共济失调。

诊断

临床四联征包括亚急性进行性痴呆、肌阵挛、典型的周期性脑电图尖波和脑脊液正常，支持 CJD 诊断。FLAIR MRI 序列沿着新皮层呈现长曲线状高强度信号，称为皮质带，累及额叶、顶叶和颞叶（频率依次递减）。常规的脑脊液检查通常是正常的。CSF 检测蛋白 14-3-3，脑细胞死亡时这种蛋白会释放到脊髓液中，结

fluid when brain cells die, in the appropriate clinical context, is supportive for CJD.

Treatment

No effective therapy exits. The disease is inexorably progressive. The median time to death from onset is 5 months, and 90% of patients with sporadic CJD die within 1 year.

Although the illness is not communicable in the conventional sense, a risk exists in handling material contaminated with the prion protein. Gloves should be worn when handling blood, CSF, and other body fluids. Instruments must be disinfected and sterilized appropriately.

❖ For a deeper discussion of these topics, please see Chapter 384, "Meningitis: Bacterial, Viral, and Other"; Chapter 385, "Brain Abscess and Parameningeal Infections"; Chapter 386, "Acute Viral Encephalitis"; and Chapter 387, "Prion Diseases," in *Goldman-Cecil Medicine*, 26th Edition.

SUGGESTED READINGS

Brouwer MC, Thwaites GE, Tunkel AR, et al: Dilemmas in the diagnosis of acute community-acquired bacterial meningitis, Lancet 380:1684–1692, 2012.

Brouwer MC, Tunkel AR, McKhann II GM, van de Beek D: Brain abscess, N Engl J Med 371:447–456, 2014.

Colby DW, Prusiner SB: Prions, Cold Spring Harb Perspect Biol 3: a006833,2011

Dalmau J, Graus F: Antibody-mediated encephalitis, N Engl J Med 378:840–851, 2018.

Darouiche RO: Spinal epidural abscess, N Engl J Med 355:2012–2020, 2006.

Glaser CS, Honarmand S, Anderson LJ, et al: Beyond viruses: clinical profiles and etiologies associated with encephalitis, Clin Infect Dis 43:1565–1577, 2006.

Greenlee JE: Suppurative intracranial thrombophlebitis. In Roos KL, Tunkel AR, editors: Bacterial infections of the central nervous system, Edinburgh, 2010, Elsevier, pp 101–123.

McGill F, Heyderman RS, Panagiotou S, et al: Acute bacterial meningitis in adults, Lancet 388:306–3047, 2016.

Solomon T, Michael BD, Smith PE, et al: Management of suspected viral encephalitis in adults—association of British neurologists and British infection association national guidelines, J Infect 64:347–373, 2012.

Thigpen MC, Whitney CG, Messonnier NE, et al: Bacterial meningitis in the United States, 1998-2007, N Engl J Med 364:2016–2025, 2011.

Tunkel AR, Glaser CA, Block KC, et al: The management of encephalitis: clinical practice guidelines by the Infectious Diseases Society of America, Clin Infect Dis 47:303–327, 2008.

Tunkel AR, Hartman BJ, Kaplan SL, et al: Practice guidelines for the management of bacterial meningitis, Clin Infect Dis 39:1267–1284, 2004.

Tunkel AR, Hasbun R, Bhimraj A, et al: 2017 Infectious Diseases Society of America's clinical practice guidelines for healthcare-associated ventriculitis and meningitis, Clin Infect Dis 64:e34-e65, 2017.

Tyler KL: Acute viral encephalitis, N Engl J Med 379:557–566, 2018.

van de Beek D, Brouwer MC, Thwaites GE, et al: Advances in treatment of bacterial meningitis, Lancet 380:1693–1702, 2012.

Venkatesan A, Michael BD, Probasco JC, et al: Acute encephalitis in immunocompetent adults, Lancet 393:702–716, 2019.

Venkatesan A, Tunkel AR, Bloch KC, et al: Case definitions, diagnostic algorithms, and priorities in encephalitis; consensus statement of the International Encephalitis Consortium, Clin Infect Dis 57:1114–1128, 2013.

合相应的临床症状，支持 CJD 诊断。

治疗

目前没有有效的治疗方法。这种疾病的进展过程不可阻挡。从发病到死亡的中位时间为 5 个月，90% 的 sCJD 患者在 1 年内死亡。

尽管这种疾病不具有传统意义上的传染性，但在处理被朊病毒蛋白污染的物质时仍存在风险。处理血液、脑脊液和其他体液时应戴手套。器械必须进行严格的消毒和灭菌。

❖ 有关此专题的深入讨论，请参阅 *Goldman-Cecil Medicine* 第 26 版第 384 章"脑膜炎：细菌、病毒和其他"；第 385 章"脑脓肿和脑膜周围感染"；第 386 章"急性病毒性脑炎"；以及第 387 章"朊病毒病"。

推荐阅读

Brouwer MC, Thwaites GE, Tunkel AR, et al: Dilemmas in the diagnosis of acute community-acquired bacterial meningitis, Lancet 380:1684–1692, 2012.

Brouwer MC, Tunkel AR, McKhann II GM, van de Beek D: Brain abscess, N Engl J Med 371:447–456, 2014.

Colby DW, Prusiner SB: Prions, Cold Spring Harb Perspect Biol 3: a006833, 2011

Dalmau J, Graus F: Antibody-mediated encephalitis, N Engl J Med 378:840–851, 2018.

Darouiche RO: Spinal epidural abscess, N Engl J Med 355:2012–2020, 2006.

Glaser CS, Honarmand S, Anderson LJ, et al: Beyond viruses: clinical profiles and etiologies associated with encephalitis, Clin Infect Dis 43:1565–1577, 2006.

Greenlee JE: Suppurative intracranial thrombophlebitis. In Roos KL, Tunkel AR, editors: Bacterial infections of the central nervous system, Edinburgh, 2010, Elsevier, pp 101–123.

McGill F, Heyderman RS, Panagiotou S, et al: Acute bacterial meningitis in adults, Lancet 388:306–3047, 2016.

Solomon T, Michael BD, Smith PE, et al: Management of suspected viral encephalitis in adults—association of British neurologists and British infection association national guidelines, J Infect 64:347–373, 2012.

Thigpen MC, Whitney CG, Messonnier NE, et al: Bacterial meningitis in the United States, 1998-2007, N Engl J Med 364:2016–2025, 2011.

Tunkel AR, Glaser CA, Block KC, et al: The management of encephalitis: clinical practice guidelines by the Infectious Diseases Society of America, Clin Infect Dis 47:303–327, 2008.

Tunkel AR, Hartman BJ, Kaplan SL, et al: Practice guidelines for the management of bacterial meningitis, Clin Infect Dis 39:1267–1284, 2004.

Tunkel AR, Hasbun R, Bhimraj A, et al: 2017 Infectious Diseases Society of America's clinical practice guidelines for healthcare-associated ventriculitis and meningitis, Clin Infect Dis 64:e34-e65, 2017.

Tyler KL: Acute viral encephalitis, N Engl J Med 379:557–566, 2018.

van de Beek D, Brouwer MC, Thwaites GE, et al: Advances in treatment of bacterial meningitis, Lancet 380:1693–1702, 2012.

Venkatesan A, Michael BD, Probasco JC, et al: Acute encephalitis in immunocompetent adults, Lancet 393:702–716, 2019.

Venkatesan A, Tunkel AR, Bloch KC, et al: Case definitions, diagnostic algorithms, and priorities in encephalitis; consensus statement of the International Encephalitis Consortium, Clin Infect Dis 57:1114–1128, 2013.

6

Infections of the Head and Neck

David Kim, Roberto Cortez, Tareq Kheirbek

COMMON COLD

Definition and Epidemiology

The common cold is an acute viral syndrome involving the upper respiratory tract with symptoms of sore throat, rhinorrhea, and nasal congestion. It has a considerable economic burden, accounting for over 100 million physician visits annually with approximately 20 million lost workdays and costing $7 billion per year in sick days and lost productivity. The incidence of the common cold decreases with age with children having six to eight colds on average annually, whereas adults have two to three colds per year.

Pathogenesis and Microbiology

Rhinoviruses are the most common pathogen implicated in the common cold and are associated with more than 50% of all colds. However, the syndrome may be caused by over 200 viruses including influenza virus, coronavirus, adenovirus, respiratory syncytial virus, parainfluenza virus, metapneumovirus, and enterovirus. These viruses are transmitted either by direct contact or by aerosols through which they infect the nasal epithelium, thereby stimulating a nonspecific inflammatory response accounting for the associated symptoms.

Clinical Presentation

Onset of symptoms occurs 1 to 3 days following viral infection. The common cold typically manifests with an initial sore throat followed by rhinorrhea, nasal congestion, and sneezing by the third day. Patients may develop a cough later lasting for several days. Symptoms peak between day 3 and 6 and persist for approximately 7 to 10 days. Clinical findings are limited to the upper respiratory tract with increased nasal secretions. Additionally, patients may demonstrate mild oropharyngeal erythema, injected conjunctiva, edematous nasal mucosa, and anterior cervical lymphadenopathy.

Treatment

Treatment is largely symptomatic with rest, oral hydration, and over-the-counter medications including nasal decongestants, nonsteroidal anti-inflammatory drugs, lozenges, and cough suppressants. Antibiotics are not indicated.

ACUTE BACTERIAL RHINOSINUSITIS

Definition and Epidemiology

Acute rhinosinusitis is a common illness with one out of eight adults reporting receiving a diagnosis each year, resulting in more than 30 million patient visits annually. Acute bacterial rhinosinusitis is inflammation secondary to bacterial infection of the nasal cavity and paranasal sinuses lasting less than 4 weeks. Approximately 0.5% to 2% of acute viral rhinosinusitis cases are complicated by bacterial rhinosinusitis.

Pathogenesis and Microbiology

Following an upper respiratory infection, viral inoculation of the nasal cavity and the paranasal sinuses produces an acute viral rhinosinusitis leading to mucosal thickening, edema, and inflammation. Contaminated nasal secretions then enter the typically sterile paranasal sinuses that are normally cleared. However, mucosal inflammation and edema can obstruct sinus drainage and impair mucociliary clearance of bacteria, perpetuating bacterial infection. The most common bacteria associated with acute bacterial rhinosinusitis are *Streptococcus pneumoniae* and *Haemophilus influenzae*.

Clinical Presentation

Symptoms of acute rhinosinusitis may include purulent anterior or posterior nasal discharge, nasal congestion or obstruction, facial congestion or fullness, facial pain or pressure, hyposmia or anosmia, and fever. Patients may complain of headache, ear pain, maxillary tooth pain, cough, and fatigue. Clinical findings may include erythema and swelling of the nasal mucosa, purulent nasal discharge, and sinus tenderness. Clinical history, patterns, and duration of symptoms are helpful in the diagnosis of acute bacterial rhinosinusitis. These include symptoms of nasal congestion, rhinorrhea, and cough persisting greater than 10 days; severe symptoms including fever with purulent nasal discharge for greater than 3 days; or recurrence and worsening of common cold symptoms following a period of initial improvement or "double-sickening." Imaging is not routinely recommended in patients with uncomplicated acute rhinosinusitis.

Treatment

Acute bacterial rhinosinusitis typically resolves with symptomatic management within 2 weeks. Intranasal sterile saline irrigation has been shown to provide symptomatic relief. If symptoms persist in an otherwise immunocompetent patient or if reliable follow-up is unavailable, antibiotics are indicated and should be initiated for a duration of 5 to 7 days. First-line antibiotics are amoxicillin or amoxicillin-clavulanate. Azithromycin and trimethoprim-sulfamethoxazole are not recommended due to high prevalence of antibiotic resistance. Patients should respond to antibiotic therapy within 72 hours with improvement of symptoms. Failure to respond to initial therapy may require high-dose amoxicillin-clavulanate for a duration of 7 to 10 days.

Complications

Patients with acute bacterial rhinosinusitis who fail to respond to high-dose antibiotics warrant a referral to an otolaryngologist for further evaluation. Intracranial and orbital complications may arise from progressing infection (Fig. 6.1). Orbital complications include periorbital cellulitis, orbital cellulitis, and abscess, secondary to acute bacterial ethmoiditis. Intracranial complications include epidural abscess,

头颈部感染

韩红 译　朱华栋 彭俊平 审校　刘海鹰 通审

普通感冒

定义和流行病学

普通感冒是一种累及上呼吸道的急性病毒综合征，症状为咽痛、流涕和鼻塞。它造成巨大的经济负担，每年有超过1亿次就诊看病，损失约2000万个工作日，每年因病假和生产力丢失造成的损失达70亿美元。普通感冒的发病率随着年龄的增长而下降，儿童平均每年感冒6～8次，而成年人每年感冒2～3次。

发病机制和微生物学

鼻病毒是普通感冒中最常见的病原体，与50%以上的感冒有关。感冒可由流感病毒、冠状病毒、腺病毒、呼吸道合胞病毒、副流感病毒、偏肺病毒、肠道病毒等200多种病毒引起。这些病毒通过直接接触或者通过气溶胶传播感染鼻上皮细胞，从而刺激其产生非特异性炎症反应，导致相关症状。

临床表现

病毒感染后1～3天出现症状。普通感冒的典型症状是先出现咽痛，随后在第3天左右出现流涕、鼻塞和打喷嚏的症状。患者随后可能出现持续数天的咳嗽。症状在第3～6天达到高峰，并持续7～10天。临床表现仅限于上呼吸道，鼻分泌物增多。此外，患者可能表现为轻度口咽红肿、结膜充血、鼻黏膜水肿和颈前淋巴结肿大。

治疗

治疗主要是对症治疗，包括休息、口服补液和非处方药物，包括鼻腔减充血剂、非甾体抗炎药、含片和止咳药。不建议使用抗生素。

急性细菌性鼻窦炎

定义和流行病学

急性鼻窦炎是一种常见疾病，据报道每年有1/8的成年人诊断为急性鼻窦炎，每年有超过3000万患者就诊。急性细菌性鼻窦炎是继发于鼻腔和鼻旁窦细菌感染的炎症，持续时间不超过4周。0.5%～2%的急性病毒性鼻窦炎病例并发细菌性鼻窦炎。

发病机制和微生物学

随着上呼吸道感染，病毒定植于鼻腔和鼻旁窦后引起急性病毒性鼻窦炎，导致黏膜增厚、水肿和炎症。受污染的鼻分泌物进入通常是无菌鼻旁窦，正常情况下，分泌物会被清理。然而，黏膜炎症和水肿可阻碍窦口引流，减弱黏膜纤毛的细菌清除能力，使细菌感染难以清除。最常见的引起急性细菌性鼻窦炎的细菌是肺炎链球菌和流感嗜血杆菌。

临床表现

急性鼻窦炎的症状包括化脓性前鼻或后鼻分泌物、鼻塞或鼻堵、面部充血或肿胀、面部疼痛或压迫感、嗅觉减退或丧失以及发热。患者可主诉头痛、耳痛、上颌牙痛、咳嗽和疲劳。临床表现可能包括鼻黏膜充血和肿胀，脓鼻涕和鼻窦压痛。根据病史、临床类型和症状持续时间有助于诊断急性细菌性鼻窦炎。这些症状包括持续10天以上的鼻塞、流涕和咳嗽；严重症状包括超过3天的发热伴脓鼻涕，或在症状最初改善又恶化和复发或"双侧发病"。对于单纯的急性鼻窦炎患者，不推荐常规影像学检查。

治疗

急性细菌性鼻窦炎通常在两周内通过对症治疗而痊愈。鼻腔内无菌盐水冲洗已被证明可以缓解症状。如果在其他免疫功能正常的患者中症状持续存在，或者无法获得可靠的随访，则需要开始使用抗生素，并使用5～7天。一线抗生素是阿莫西林或阿莫西林-克拉维酸。由于抗生素耐药性高，不建议使用阿奇霉素和甲氧苄啶-磺胺甲噁唑。患者应在72 h内对抗生素治疗有反应，症状有改善。对初始治疗无效可能需要高剂量阿莫西林-克拉维酸治疗持续7～10天。

并发症

大剂量抗生素治疗无效的细菌性鼻窦炎患者，需要转诊耳鼻喉科医生作进一步评估。感染进展可引起颅内和眼眶并发症（图6.1）。眼眶并发症继发于急性细菌性筛窦炎，包括眶周蜂窝织炎、眼眶蜂窝织炎和

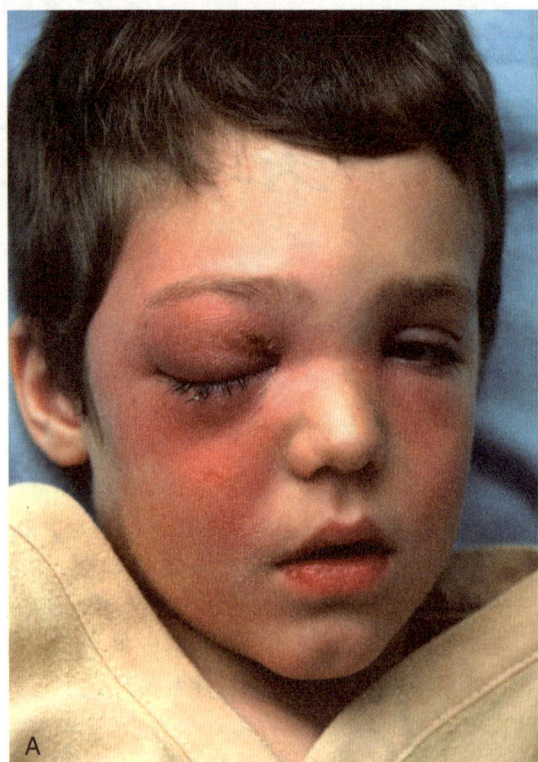
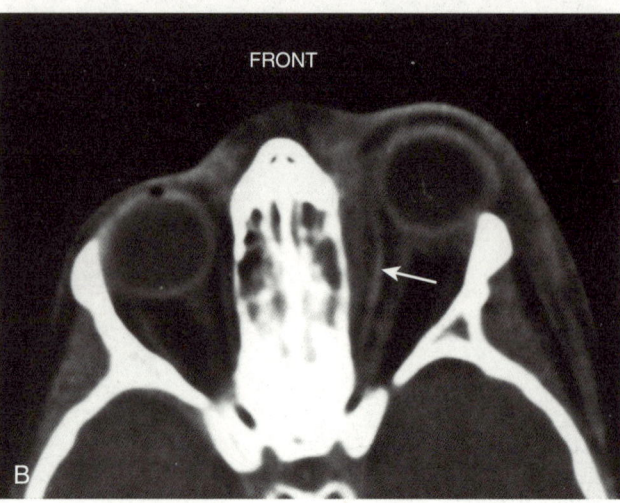

Fig. 6.1 (A) A child has an orbital abscess as a complication of ethmoid sinusitis. Note the marked edema and proptosis. (B) Computed tomography scan of the orbit demonstrates a subperiosteal abscess *(arrow)*. (A, Courtesy Gary Williams, MD; B, From DeMuri GP, Wald ER: Sinusitis. In Bennett JE, Dolin R, Blaser M, editors: Mandell, Douglas, and Bennett's principles and practice of infectious diseases, ed 8, Philadelphia, 2015, Saunders.)

meningitis, cavernous sinus thrombosis, subdural empyema, and brain abscess. In cases of complicated acute rhinosinusitis, evaluation should include computed tomography (CT) or magnetic resonance imaging with appropriate consultations with otolaryngology and/or ophthalmology. Oftentimes, management involves initiating broad-spectrum intravenous antibiotics and urgent surgical intervention in the setting of abscesses.

PHARYNGITIS AND TONSILLITIS

Definition and Epidemiology

Pharyngitis or sore throat is characterized by inflammation of the pharynx from environmental and chemical exposures or from infectious disease. In the United States, more than 10 million patients are diagnosed annually with acute pharyngitis, with incidence peaking in children and in the winter.

Tonsillitis is an inflammatory condition affecting the palatine tonsils, which, in addition to the pharyngeal, tubal, and lingual tonsils, comprise the Waldeyer ring. Tonsillitis refers to infections primarily involving the palatine tonsils, while pharyngitis affects the oropharynx, although they are frequently used interchangeably. Tonsillitis accounts for 1.3% of all outpatient primary care clinic visits with patients aged 5 to 15 years affected most commonly. Early spring and winter months demonstrate a notable up-tick in reported cases. Those afflicted can range from asymptomatic streptococcal carriers to a quinsy or peritonsillar abscess requiring emergent drainage.

Using a combination of history, clinical presentation, and several immediately available laboratory tests, the health care provider may readily distinguish patients with self-limited, viral illnesses from those requiring antibiotic treatment or procedural interventions.

Pathogenesis and Microbiology

Viral causes of pharyngitis account for greater than 70% of cases with common pathogens being rhinovirus, adenovirus, Epstein-Barr virus (EBV), and influenza viruses. The most commonly encountered bacterial pathogen is Group A Streptococcus (GAS), accounting for up to 30% of pharyngitis cases in children and 10% in adults.

The palatine tonsils are pharyngeal lymphoid organs surrounded by overlying respiratory epithelium that invaginate into crypts. These crypts may harbor bacteria and lead to acute or recurrent infections. Most cases of acute tonsillitis represent benign, self-limited episodes of viral origin. Pathogens responsible for the common cold frequently result in self-limited, benign cases of tonsillitis and include rhinovirus, coronavirus, respiratory syncytial virus, and adenovirus. More severe viral cases are less frequent but should raise suspicion for EBV, cytomegalovirus, rubella, and human immunodeficiency virus (HIV).

Difficulty in distinguishing viral from bacterial etiologies frequently results in unnecessary antibiotic therapy. While GAS infections are by far the most common bacterial source requiring antimicrobial therapy, infections yielding *S. aureus*, *S. pneumoniae*, and *H. influenzae* are also possible. Unvaccinated individuals may harbor infections with diphtheria-causing *Corynebacterium species*. A social and sexual history may yield prior or active infections with chlamydia, gonorrhea, HIV, and syphilis, which can also be observed in cases of acute or recurrent episodes of tonsillitis. Tuberculosis should be considered in patients

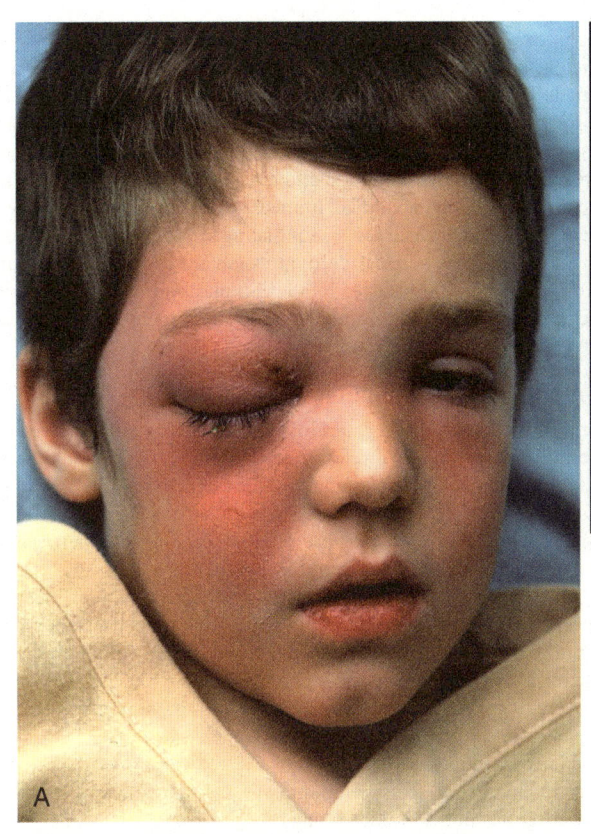
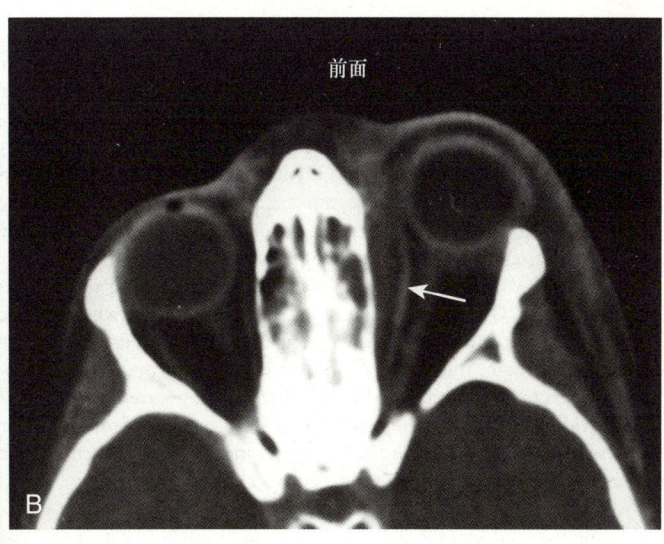

图 6.1 （A）患儿筛窦炎继发眶周脓肿，注意眼部肿胀和突出。（B）眼眶 CT 扫描表明骨膜下脓肿（箭头）（A，Courtesy Gary Williams，MD；B，From DeMuri GP，Wald ER：Sinusitis. In Bennett JE，Dolin R，Blaser M，editors：Mandell, Douglas, and Bennett's principles and practice of infectious diseases，ed 8，Philadelphia，2015，Saunders.）

脓肿。颅内并发症包括硬膜外脓肿、脑膜炎、海绵窦血栓形成、硬膜下脓肿、脑脓肿。在复杂的急性鼻窦炎病例中，应采用计算机断层成像（CT）或磁共振成像评估，并适当咨询耳鼻喉科和（或）眼科。通常，治疗方案包括应用广谱静脉抗生素和对脓肿的及时手术干预。

咽炎和扁桃体炎

定义和流行病学

咽炎或咽痛是由于环境和化学物质暴露或感染性疾病引起的咽部炎症为临床特征。在美国，每年有超过 1000 万患者被诊断为急性咽炎，儿童和冬季发病率最高。

扁桃体炎是腭扁桃体的炎症状态，腭扁桃体除了咽扁桃体、咽鼓管扁桃体和舌扁桃体外，还包括咽淋巴环。扁桃体炎是指主要涉及腭扁桃体的感染，而咽炎影响口咽部，尽管它们经常互换说法。扁桃体炎占所有初级保健门诊就诊量的 1.3%，年龄在 5～15 岁的患者最常见。早春和冬季报告的病例明显增加。患者可能是无症状链球菌携带者，也可能有需要紧急引流的扁桃体周脓肿或咽旁脓肿。

结合病史、临床表现和能立即获得的实验室检查，医务人员可以容易区分自限性病毒性疾病患者与需要抗生素治疗或操作干预的患者。

发病机制和微生物学

70% 以上的咽炎是病毒性的，常见的病原体是鼻病毒、腺病毒、EB 病毒（EBV）和流感病毒。最常见的细菌病原体是 A 组链球菌（GAS），占儿童咽炎病例的 30% 和成人咽炎病例的 10%。

腭扁桃体是咽部淋巴器官，被覆呼吸道上皮细胞，并内陷形成隐窝。这些隐窝可能藏匿细菌，导致急性或复发性感染。大多数急性病毒性扁桃体炎的病例预后良好，呈自限性发作。引起普通感冒的病原体经常导致自限性、良性扁桃体炎，包括鼻病毒、冠状病毒、呼吸道合胞病毒和腺病毒。严重的病毒性扁桃体炎病例较少发生，除非是 EB 病毒、巨细胞病毒、风疹和人类免疫缺陷病毒（HIV）的感染。

区分病毒和细菌病因的困难经常导致不必要的抗生素治疗。虽然 GAS 感染是迄今为止最常见的需要抗菌治疗的细菌感染，但由金黄色葡萄球菌、肺炎链球菌和流感嗜血杆菌引起感染也是可能的。未接种疫苗的人可能会感染引起白喉的棒状杆菌。社交和性生活史可能揭示了沙眼衣原体、淋病、HIV 和梅毒的潜伏或活动性感染，这些也可以在扁桃体炎的急性或复发性病例中观察到。对于居住在公共生活区、监禁设施

residing in common living quarters, incarcerated facilities, and homeless shelters.

Clinical Presentation

Common presentations include malaise, fever, sore throat, and tender anterior cervical lymphadenopathy. Odynophagia and/or dysphagia warrant further investigation for significant tonsillar swelling and the potential for airway compromise. A thorough history and physical should include onset of symptoms, sick contacts, medical comorbidities, living conditions, prior episodes of tonsillitis, as well as sexual and vaccination history. One must consider the spectrum of illness when navigating diagnostic and management strategies, as this differs greatly when handling benign, minimally symptomatic patients from those demonstrating a toxic appearance with difficulty handling secretions.

The provider should assess the patient's vital signs, paying attention to the presence of a fever, tachycardia, tachypnea, and marginal oxygen saturation levels. Next, a thorough head and neck examination may reveal tonsillar enlargement and exudates, tender cervical lymphadenopathy, and uvular deviation. Both the Infectious Diseases Society of America and the American Society of Internal Medicine recommend the use of scoring systems (i.e., Centor Score), which considers presence of fever, tonsillar exudates and/or enlargement, absence of cough, and tender cervical lymphadenopathy, each of which warrants one point. It has since been modified for age, where patients within age 3 to 15 are given an additional point, and patients 45 years or older have one point subtracted from the overall score. With scores of 0 or 1, no further testing is necessary. With 2 to 3 points, a rapid strep test and throat culture are feasible options. In patients scoring 4 or more points, clinicians should consider testing and beginning empiric antibiotics.

Treatment

Treatment of viral pharyngitis is encouraging symptom control with nonsteroidal anti-inflammatory drugs (NSAIDs) and hydration. First-line treatment of GAS pharyngitis is amoxicillin and penicillin V. For penicillin-allergic patients, first-generation cephalosporins, clindamycin or macrolides are reasonable alternatives. Of note, GAS antibiotic resistance to azithromycin and clindamycin are increasingly common. The recommended duration of treatment using β-lactam antibiotics is 10 days.

Complications include peritonsillar abscess, in which patients may appear ill with muffled speech, foul-smelling breath, uvula displacement, and drooling. Less common complications include contiguous neck space infections or rarely rheumatic fever.

DEEP NECK SPACE INFECTIONS

Definition and Epidemiology

Deep neck space infections most commonly arise from oral cavity or odontogenic origin, and knowledge of cervical anatomy (Fig. 6.2) and the fascial planes is paramount in understanding the infectious etiology and their potential for spread. In addition, the deep cervical fascia creates clinically relevant fascial spaces into which infections can spread rapidly with devastating consequences. Risk factors for developing deep neck space infections include uncontrolled or untreated dental infection, spread of infection from other local structures such as the tonsils, intravenous drug use, diabetes, HIV infection, and local trauma.

Submandibular Space Infection

The submandibular space is defined by the mandible anteriorly and laterally; the hyoid bone posteriorly; the mucosa of the floor of the mouth superiorly; and the superficial layer of the deep cervical fascia inferiorly. Ludwig angina is a severe infection of the submandibular space, typically caused by an infected lower molar tooth. Patients will oftentimes present acutely ill with mouth pain, a swollen, elevated tongue, dysphagia, drooling, stiff neck, and febrile (Fig. 6.3). If left untreated, the infection may spread to the lateral pharyngeal space, resulting in trismus. On exam, the submandibular tissues will appear swollen with woody induration and are generally not fluctuant. Once the disease has been identified, immediate medical and surgical treatment is necessary, which involves initiating broad-spectrum antibiotic therapy as well as surgical decompression through a neck incision and extraction of the infected tooth. Complications of Ludwig angina include death from airway obstruction, aspiration pneumonia, carotid artery erosion, and tongue necrosis.

Retropharyngeal Infection

Defined by the alar fascia anteriorly and the buccopharyngeal layer of the middle layer of cervical fascia covering the pharynx and esophagus posteriorly, the retropharyngeal space extends from the base of the skull to level of T2 approximately, where the two fascial layers fuse. Additionally, there is a distinct prevertebral space that is in between the prevertebral fascia and the vertebral column.

Of note, there is a "danger space" that lies in between the prevertebral space posteriorly and the retropharyngeal space anteriorly, extending from the base of the skull to the diaphragm. This area is of clinical importance because it is continuous with the mediastinum, allowing for infection to spread directly into the thorax and causing mediastinitis.

Many infections can spread into the retropharyngeal space and may develop into abscesses without appropriate treatment. For example, infections in the Waldeyer ring can spread to the retropharyngeal lymph nodes and into this space. Additionally, odontogenic infections that spread to the lateral pharyngeal space can also travel into the retropharyngeal space. Patients will present acutely ill with fever, sore throat, dysphagia, neck stiffness, and dyspnea. Airway obstruction can occur from bulging of the posterior pharyngeal wall anteriorly with supraglottic compression. Definitive treatment requires administration of broad-spectrum antibiotics and oftentimes, surgical drainage of abscess.

Lateral Pharyngeal Space Infection

The lateral pharyngeal space or the parapharyngeal space is located on the lateral aspect of the pharynx, continuous with the retropharyngeal space posteriorly and the submandibular space anteriorly. This space communicates with the submandibular, retropharyngeal, and peritonsillar spaces and is therefore susceptible to both oral cavity and odontogenic infections. Interestingly, *Fusobacterium necrophorum* can cause a rare syndrome called postangina septicemia or Lemierre syndrome, which manifests with severe sore throat and fever. In this syndrome, the lateral pharyngeal space becomes infected with resulting septic thrombophlebitis of the internal jugular vein. The mortality rate can be as high as 50%. Treatment requires prompt initiation of intravenous penicillin and emergent drainage of any abscess.

Bacterial Epiglottitis
Definition and Epidemiology

Epiglottitis is an inflammatory affliction of the epiglottis and nearby structures, which include the arytenoids, aryepiglottic folds, and vallecula. Widespread usage of the *H. influenzae* type b vaccine in children has worked to decrease the incidence of pediatric bacterial epiglottitis by nearly 99%. Prior to widespread vaccination, *H. influenzae* was the leading cause of bacterial meningitis in children and a frequent cause of pneumonia, epiglottitis, and septic arthritis. Health care providers should counsel parents regarding the dangers of *H. influenzae* and

和避难所的人群要考虑结核感染的可能。

临床表现

常见的症状包括不适、发热、咽痛和颈前淋巴结触痛。吞咽痛和（或）吞咽困难需要进一步检查是否有明显的扁桃体肿胀和气道受累的可能性。全面的病史和体检应包括初始症状、接触史、合并症、生活条件、扁桃体炎发作史以及性生活史和疫苗接种史。在指导诊断和管理策略时，必须考虑疾病谱，因为在处理良性的、症状轻微的患者和那些出现中毒症状和处理分泌物困难的患者时有很大的不同。

医生应首先评估患者的生命体征，关注是否有发热、心动过速、呼吸急促和外周血氧饱和度水平。其次，全面的头颈部检查可能会发现扁桃体肿大和渗出，触痛的颈部肿大淋巴结和悬雍垂偏斜。美国传染病学会和美国内科学会都推荐使用评分系统（即 Centor 评分），该评分系统考虑了发热、扁桃体渗出和（或）肿大、缺少咳嗽和痛性颈部肿大淋巴结，每一项都应得 1 分。对年龄进行了修正，年龄在 3～15 岁的患者加 1 分，45 岁或以上的患者从总得分中减去 1 分。如果得分为 0 或 1，则不需要进一步的检测。2～3 分，可行快速链球菌检测和咽拭子培养。住院患者得分为 4 分或以上，临床医生应考虑检测并开始经验性抗生素治疗。

治疗

病毒性咽炎的治疗是鼓励用非甾体抗炎药（NSAID）和水化控制症状。链球菌咽炎的一线治疗是阿莫西林和青霉素 V。对于青霉素过敏患者，第一代头孢菌素、克林霉素或大环内酯类药物是合理的选择。值得注意的是，对阿奇霉素和克林霉素的耐药性越来越普遍。推荐使用 β-内酰胺类抗生素治疗 10 天。

并发症包括扁桃体周脓肿，患者可表现为言语不清、口臭、悬雍垂偏斜和流涎，少见的并发症包括邻近的颈间隙感染或罕见的风湿热。

颈深间隙感染

定义和流行病学

颈深间隙感染最常起源于口腔或牙源性感染，了解颈部解剖结构（图6.2）和筋膜平面对于了解感染病因及其潜在的扩散至关重要。此外，颈深筋膜形成的筋膜间隙，感染可迅速扩散并带来灾难性后果。发生颈深间隙感染的危险因素包括不受控制或未经治疗的牙源性感染、从其他局部（如扁桃体）扩散的感染、静脉药物滥用、糖尿病、HIV 感染和局部创伤。

下颌下间隙感染

下颌下间隙由前方和侧方的下颌骨、后方的舌骨、上方的口腔底部的黏膜以及颈深部筋膜的浅层界定。脓性颌下炎是一种严重的下颌下间隙感染，典型的是由下颌的臼齿感染引起，患者有时表现为剧烈的口腔疼痛，舌肿胀并抬高、吞咽困难、流涎、颈部僵硬、发热（图6.3）。如果未经治疗，感染可能扩散到咽旁间隙，导致牙关紧闭。检查时，颌下组织会出现肿胀，硬度如木质，一般没有波动。一旦此疾病被识别，应立即启动内科和外科治疗，包括开始广谱抗生素治疗以及通过颈部切开进行手术减压和拔掉感染的牙齿。脓性颌下炎并发症包括死于呼吸道阻塞、吸入性肺炎、颈动脉侵蚀、舌坏死。

咽后感染

咽后间隙位于翼状筋膜和覆盖咽和食管的颈筋膜中间层的颊咽层之间，从颅底一直延伸至第二胸椎水平，在这里两层筋膜融合。此外，在椎前筋膜和脊柱之间有一个明显的椎前间隙。

值得注意的是，在后方的椎前间隙和前方的咽后间隙之间有一个"危险间隙"，从颅底延伸到膈肌。这一区域具有重要的临床意义，因为它与纵隔相连，可导致感染直接扩散到胸腔并引起纵隔炎。

许多感染如不适当治疗可扩散到咽后间隙发展为脓肿。例如咽淋巴环的感染可以扩散到咽后淋巴结进入这个区域。此外，牙源性感染可以扩散到咽旁间隙也可以进入咽后间隙。患者会出现发热、咽痛、吞咽困难、颈部僵硬、呼吸困难等急性症状。由于咽后壁向前凸出并压迫声门上区，可能会发生气道阻塞。标准治疗需要给予广谱抗生素，通常还需要进行手术引流脓肿。

咽旁间隙感染

咽侧间隙或咽旁间隙位于咽的侧面，连着后面的咽后间隙和前面的下颌下间隙，这个空间与下颌下方、咽后和扁桃体周围间隙相通，因此易受口腔和牙齿感染的影响。有趣的是，坏死梭杆菌可以引起一种叫作咽峡炎后感染中毒症或 Lemierre 综合征的罕见综合征，表现为严重的咽痛和发热。在这种综合征中，咽旁间隙感染伴随颈内静脉感染中毒性血栓性静脉炎，死亡率可以高达 50%。治疗需要立刻开始静脉注射青霉素，对任何脓肿都要进行紧急引流。

细菌性会厌炎

定义和流行病学

会厌炎是会厌及其临近结构（包括杓状软骨、杓状会厌襞和会厌谷）的炎症反应。在儿童中的广泛应用流感嗜血杆菌 b 疫苗后，已将儿童细菌性会厌炎的发病率降低了将近 99%。在广泛接种疫苗之前，流感嗜血杆菌是儿童细菌性脑膜炎的主要病因，也是肺炎、会厌炎、化脓性关节炎的常见病因。医疗保健人员应

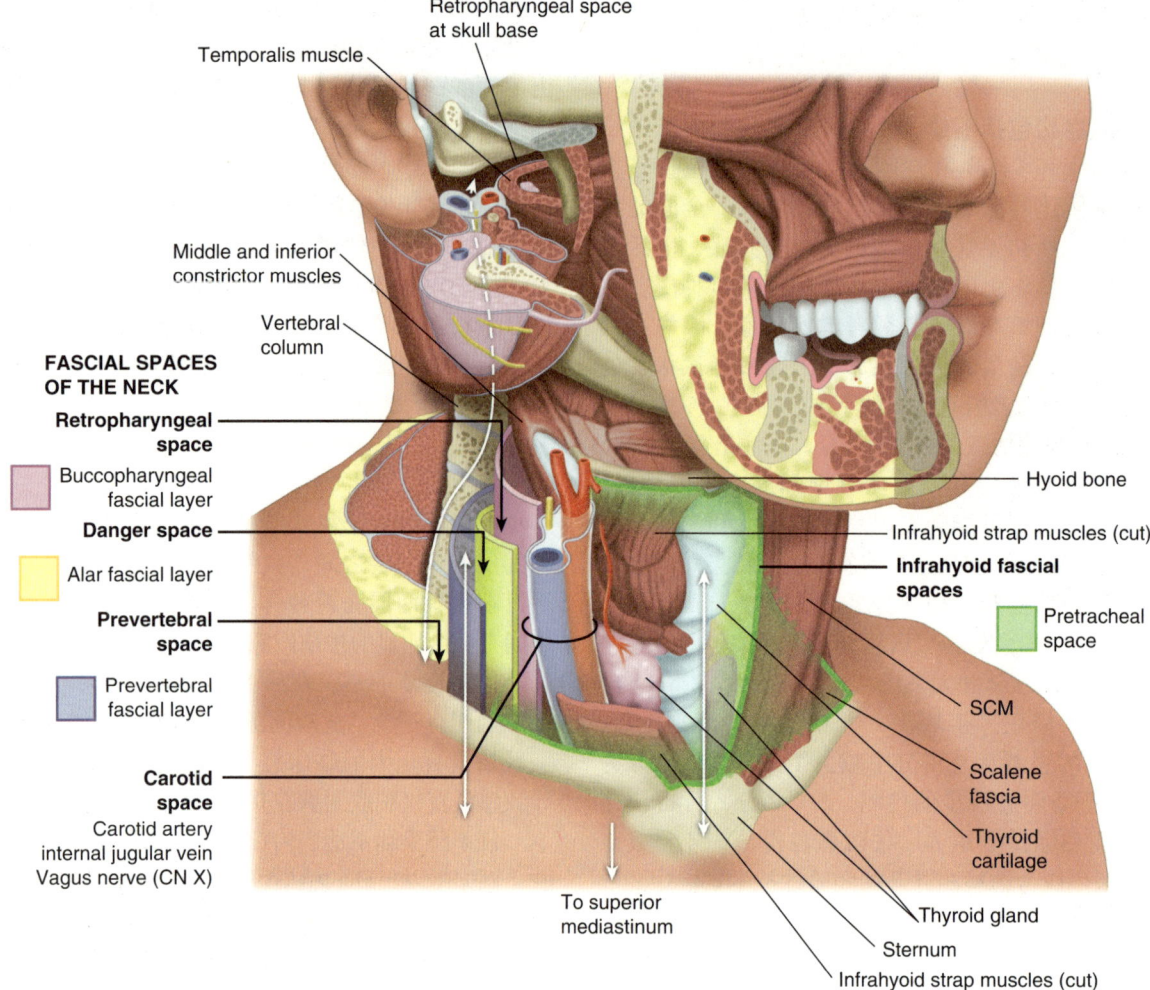

Fig. 6.2 Fascial spaces of the neck. (From Cillo JE: Atlas of oral and maxillofacial surgery, St. Louis, 2016, Elsevier Saunders, Fig. 8-1.)

recommend vaccination starting at 2 months of age. The incidence in adults has remained stable.

Pathogenesis and Microbiology

When compared to adults, the pediatric epiglottis demonstrates a more superoanterior position, more oblique angle, and less rigid structure, which account for increased risk of airway compromise in children compared to adults. Despite vaccination, *H. influenzae* remains the most common infectious cause of pediatric epiglottitis. *S. pyogenes*, *S. pneumoniae*, and *S. aureus* have also been implicated.

Clinical Presentation

Patients may present with fever, toxic appearance, drooling, dysphagia, tripod positioning, and neck hyperextension. Of importance is the sudden onset of symptoms, typically within the preceding 24 hours along with a frequently toxic, alarming appearance. The three D's refer classically to observable drooling, dysphagia, and distress. Inspiratory stridor due to turbulent flow through swollen upper airways represents severe upper airway obstruction and impending respiratory collapse, which should prompt immediate intervention.

Treatment

Airway management is paramount and frequently requires intubation by experienced providers. Edema may present significant challenges with a low threshold to utilize fiberoptic or camera-assisted intubation techniques. After securing the airway, the patient should be admitted to the intensive care unit. Broad-spectrum, empiric antibiotics are initiated and should be narrowed following culture sensitivity and susceptibility results. Although corticosteroids may shorten ICU length of stay, evidence supporting their widespread use is lacking.

Acute Bacterial Otitis Externa

Acute localized otitis externa is usually related to *S. aureus* and represents a localized, superficial infection of the outer ear canal. Oral agents against *Staphylococcus species* are adequate. Acute diffuse otitis externa, also known as swimmer's ear, is typically due to *Pseudomonas aeruginosa*. The infection is brought on by residual water left in the ear canal, which creates a moist environment that promotes bacterial growth. These patients may progress from seemingly benign itching to an erythematous and swollen outer ear canal with pain upon manipulation of the pinna or tragus. Treatment consists of topical antibiotics such as ciprofloxacin or neomycin plus polymyxin. Patients should be

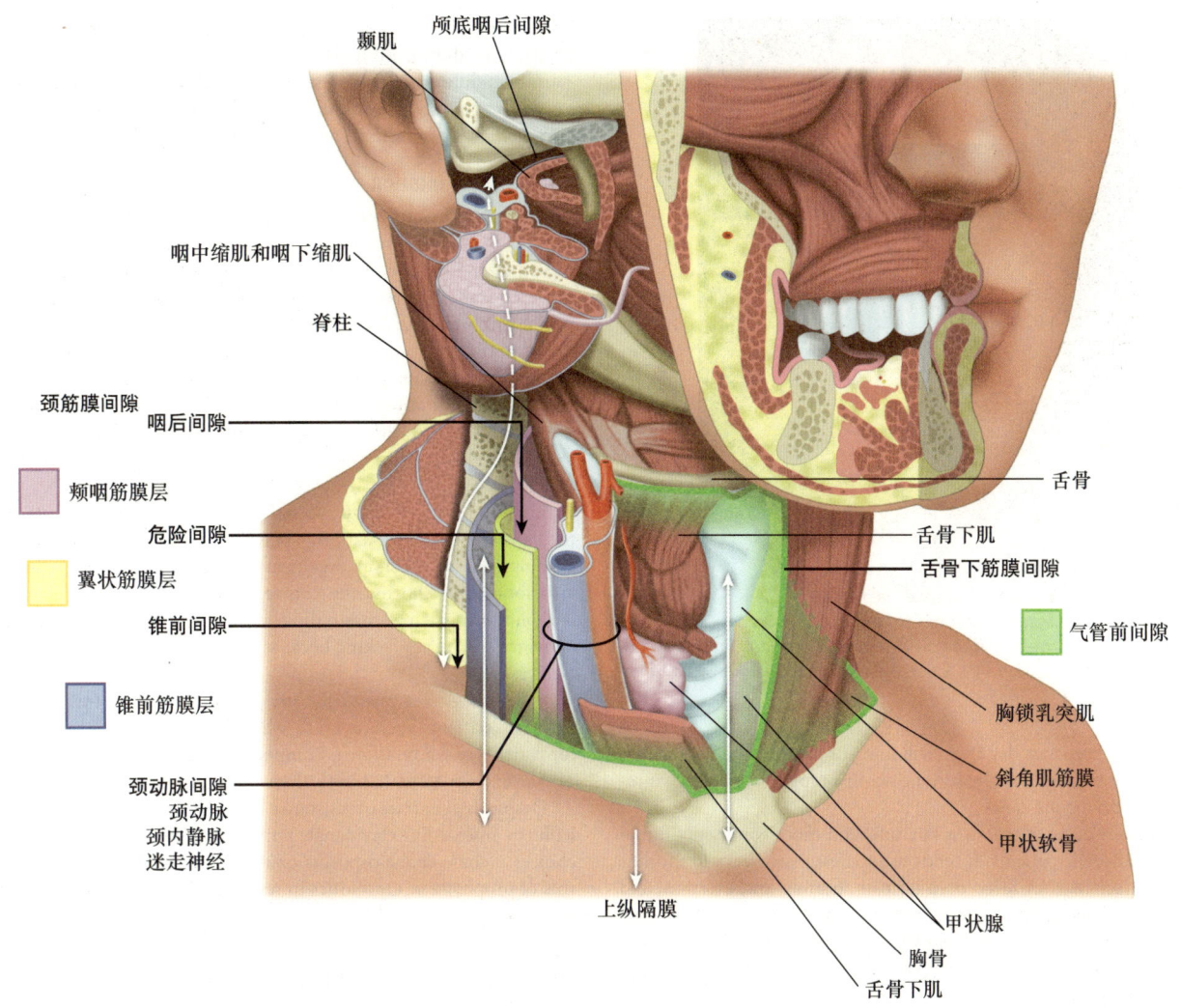

图 6.2　颈筋膜间隙（引自 Cillo JE: Atlas of oral and maxillofacial surgery, St. Louis, 2016, Elsevier Saunders, Fig. 8-1.）

该向家长说明流感嗜血杆菌的危害并建议在儿童 2 月龄时开始接种疫苗。成人的发病率保持稳定。

发病机制和微生物学

与成人相比，儿童会厌的位置更靠前，角度更斜，结构不僵硬，这导致儿童与成人相比气道受损的风险增加。尽管有疫苗接种，流感嗜血杆菌仍然是儿童会厌炎最常见的感染原因。化脓性链球菌、肺炎链球菌和金黄色葡萄球菌也是常见致病菌。

临床表现

患者可表现为发热、中毒面容、流涎、吞咽困难、三脚架征和颈部过伸。重要的是症状发作突然，通常在 24 h 内出现中毒和警示症状。典型的"3D"征指的是可观察到的流涎、吞咽困难和痛苦。由于气体湍流通过肿胀的上呼吸道引起的吸气相喘鸣代表严重的上呼吸道阻塞和即将发生的呼吸衰竭，应立即进行干预。

治疗

气道管理至关重要，经常需要由经验丰富的医护人员进行气管插管。水肿可能会带来巨大的挑战，应放低门槛地使用纤维光学或相机辅助的插管技术。在确保气道畅通后，应将患者送入重症监护室。应开始使用广谱、经验性抗生素治疗，然后根据培养和药敏结果进行调整。尽管皮质类固醇可以缩短 ICU 的住院时间，但缺乏支持其广泛使用的证据。

急性细菌性外耳炎

急性局部性外耳炎通常与金黄色葡萄球菌感染有关，表现为外耳道局部浅表感染，使用抗葡萄球菌的口服药物即可。急性弥漫性外耳炎，也称为游泳者耳，通常是由铜绿假单胞菌引起的感染。耳道内残留的水造成了潮湿的环境，促进了细菌的生长，从而引起了耳道感染。这些患者可能从看似良性的瘙痒发展为外耳道的红斑和肿胀，伴随牵拉耳郭或耳屏时产生疼痛。

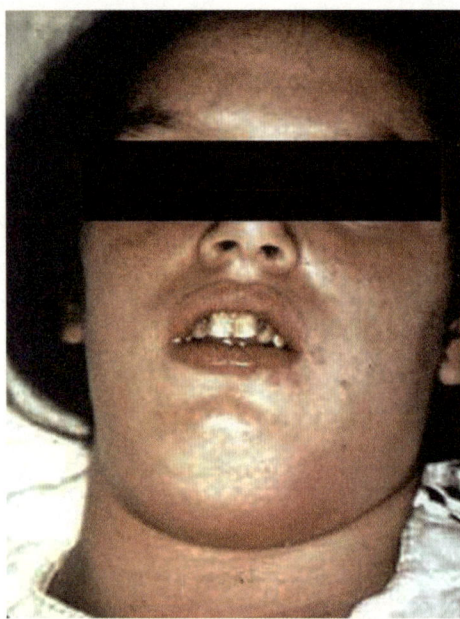

Fig. 6.3 Early appearance of a patient with Ludwig angina, who has a brawny, boardlike swelling in the submandibular spaces. (From Megran DW, Scehifele DW, Chow AW: Odontogenic Infections, Pediatric Infectious Diseases 3:262, 1984.)

counseled to keep ears dry after swimming or bathing and to consider preventative strategies such as acetic acid/isopropyl alcohol mixtures to assist in drying the canal.

Malignant otitis externa is a rare infection more commonly found in elderly diabetic patients. It tends to progress over weeks to months and is characterized by fever, deep ear pain, hearing loss, otorrhea, and granulation tissue on the posterior aspect of the external canal. Inciting agents are typical for the populations involved, which include the elderly, advanced diabetics, chemotherapy patients, and immunosuppressed or immunocompromised individuals. CT scan is the initial imaging modality of choice. The infection can progress to skull-based osteomyelitis and meningitis and has a significant mortality. Treatment consists of prompt surgical débridement and antipseudomonal systemic therapy.

Acute Bacterial Otitis Media
Definition and Epidemiology

Acute otitis media is a bacterial infection of the middle ear that commonly afflicts children with nearly all having at least one episode in the first 10 years of life. In fact, it is the most common pediatric bacterial infection, accounting for one fourth of all office visits, and is the second most common reason for surgery in children, only following circumcision.

Pathogenesis and Microbiology

Compared to adults, young children are more susceptible to otitis media because their eustachian tubes are shorter, wider, and more horizontal. This disease typically progresses from eustachian tube obstruction during or following a viral respiratory tract infection, causing middle ear effusion. Bacteria then colonize the middle ear and cannot be eliminated. The most common bacterial pathogens are *S. pneumoniae*, *H. influenzae*, and *Moraxella catarrhalis*.

Clinical Presentation

Acute bacterial otitis media presents with otalgia in the majority of patients as well as otorrhea and fever. The diagnosis can be difficult in young children because the history may be absent or inaccurate. Physical exam may reveal a middle ear effusion with a bulging tympanic membrane. Additionally, mobility of the tympanic membrane is imperceptible or absent by insufflation. Over time, perforation, drainage, fever, and decreased hearing may develop. Patients may also experience vertigo, tinnitus, and nystagmus. The course of otitis media is usually self-limited with most cases resolving within 1 week.

Treatment

Treatment has been controversial because for most patients otitis media is self-limiting. Inappropriate antibiotic use has resulted in the development of resistant organisms in the United States. Although antibiotics may shorten the course of the disease and may prevent complications such as mastoiditis, facial palsy, abscess, or meningitis, convincing data are lacking because the incidence of these complications is low.

Guidelines recommend the use of antibiotics in otitis media for high-risk patients such as those who are immunocompromised and for patients in whom there is complicated disease. If symptoms persist or worsen over 48 to 72 hours, then antibiotics should be initiated.

Despite higher rates of resistance to penicillin in recent years, amoxicillin or amoxicillin-clavulanate remains first-line therapy. Alternative choices include cephalosporins or macrolide antibiotics. There is no role of prophylactic antibiotics in reducing the frequency of recurrent acute otitis media.

SUGGESTED READINGS

Gallant J, Basem JI, Turner JH, Shannon CN, Virgin FW: Nasal saline irrigation in pediatric rhinosinusitis: a systematic review, Int J Pediatr Otorhinolaryngol 108:155–162, 2018.

Hindy J, Novoa R, Slovik Y, Puterman M, Joshua B: Epiglottic abscess as a complication of acute epiglottitis, Am J Otolaryngol Head Neck Med Surg 34(4):362–365, 2013.

Shulman ST, Bisno AL, Clegg HW, Gerber MA, Kaplan EL, et al: Clinical practice guideline for the diagnosis and management of group a streptococcal pharyngitis: 2012 update by the infectious diseases society of america, Clin Infect Dis 55(10):1279–1282, 2012.

Taub D, Yampolsky A, Diecidue R, Gold L: Controversies in the management of oral and maxillofacial infections, Oral Maxillofac Surg Clin 29(4):465–473, 2017.

Vandelaar LJ, Alava I: Cervical and craniofacial necrotizing fasciitis, Operat Tech Otolaryngol Head Neck Surg 28(4):238–243, 2017.

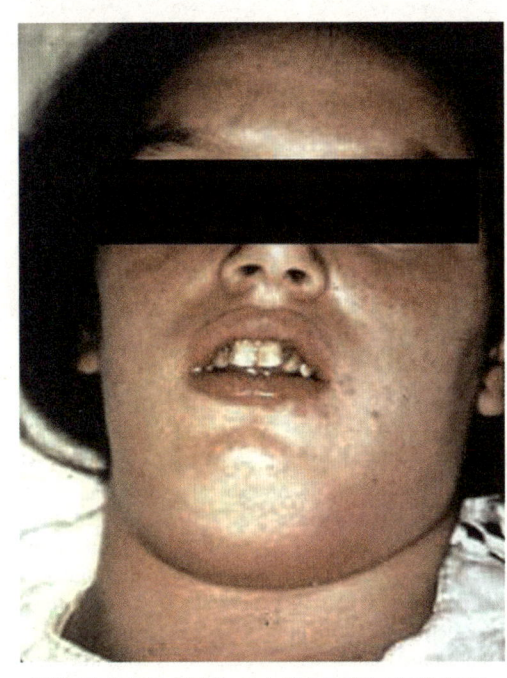

图 6.3 脓性颌下炎患者早期会出现在下颌下间隙坚实、木板样肿胀（引自 Megran DW, Scehifele DW, Chow AW: Odontogenic Infections, Pediatric Infectious Diseases 3: 262, 1984.）

治疗包括局部外用抗生素，如环丙沙星或新霉素加多黏菌素。应该建议患者在游泳或洗澡后保持耳朵干燥，并考虑采取预防措施，如醋酸/异丙醇混合物，以帮助干燥耳道。

恶性外耳炎是一种罕见的感染，多见于老年糖尿病患者。其病程通常为数周到数月，特征为发热、深部耳痛、听力丧失、耳漏和外耳道后部出现肉芽组织。诱发因素通常与所涉及的群体有关，包括老年人、晚期糖尿病患者、化疗患者和免疫抑制或免疫功能低下的个体。CT 扫描是首选的成像方式。感染可发展为颅底骨髓炎和脑膜炎，死亡率很高。治疗包括及时手术清创和抗假单胞菌全身治疗。

急性细菌性中耳炎

定义和流行病学

急性中耳炎是中耳细菌感染，几乎所有儿童在 10 岁前都至少经历过一次。事实上，它是最常见的儿科细菌感染，占所有就诊患者的 1/4，是儿童手术的第二大常见原因，仅次于包皮环切术。

发病机制和微生物学

与成年人相比，幼儿更容易患中耳炎，因为他们的咽鼓管更短，更宽，角度更平。这种疾病通常是病毒性呼吸道感染期间或之后导致咽鼓管阻塞发展而来，导致中耳积液。然后细菌在中耳定植并无法消除。最常见的细菌病原体是肺炎链球菌、流感嗜血杆菌和卡他莫拉菌。

临床表现

急性细菌性中耳炎在多数患者中表现为耳痛、耳漏和发热。由于病史可能缺失或不准确，对幼儿的诊断可能很困难。体格检查可发现中耳积液伴鼓膜膨出。此外，吹气法观察鼓膜的运动不明显或消失。随着时间的推移，可能出现鼓膜穿孔、耳漏、发热和听力下降。患者还可能出现眩晕、耳鸣和眼球震颤。中耳炎的病程通常是自限性的，大多数病例症状在 1 周内消退。

治疗

治疗一直存在争议，因为对大多数中耳炎患者来说，中耳炎是自限性的。在美国，不适当的抗生素使用导致了耐药菌的发展。虽然抗生素可缩短病程，并可预防诸如乳突炎、面瘫、脓肿或脑膜炎等并发症，但由于这些并发症的发生率较低，使用抗生素缺乏令人信服的数据。

指南建议对中耳炎高危患者使用抗生素，如免疫功能低下患者和有复杂疾病的患者。如果症状持续或恶化 48～72 h 或以上，则应开始使用抗生素。

尽管近年来青霉素的耐药性较高，阿莫西林或阿莫西林-克拉维酸仍然是一线治疗。其他的选择包括头孢菌素或大环内酯类抗生素。预防性使用抗生素在降低急性中耳炎复发率方面没有作用。

推荐阅读

Gallant J, Basem JI, Turner JH, Shannon CN, Virgin FW: Nasal saline irrigation in pediatric rhinosinusitis: a systematic review, Int J Pediatr Otorhinolaryngol 108:155–162, 2018.

Hindy J, Novoa R, Slovik Y, Puterman M, Joshua B: Epiglottic abscess as a complication of acute epiglottitis, Am J Otolaryngol Head Neck Med Surg 34(4):362–365, 2013.

Shulman ST, Bisno AL, Clegg HW, Gerber MA, Kaplan EL, et al: Clinical practice guideline for the diagnosis and management of group a streptococcal pharyngitis: 2012 update by the infectious diseases society of america, Clin Infect Dis 55(10):1279–1282, 2012.

Taub D, Yampolsky A, Diecidue R, Gold L: Controversies in the management of oral and maxillofacial infections, Oral Maxillofac Surg Clin 29(4):465–473, 2017.

Vandelaar LJ, Alava I: Cervical and craniofacial necrotizing fasciitis, Operat Tech Otolaryngol Head Neck Surg 28(4):238–243, 2017.

7

Infections of the Lower Respiratory Tract

John R. Lonks, Edward J. Wing

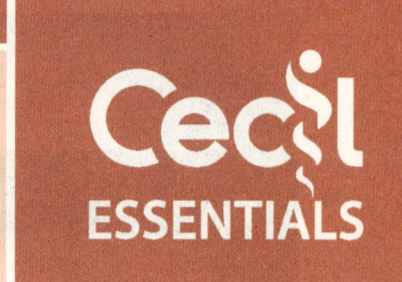

DEFINITION AND EPIDEMIOLOGY

Pneumonia, inflammation of the lung parenchyma, is usually caused by an acute infection. When the disease onset occurs outside of the hospital, it is referred to as community-acquired pneumonia (CAP). CAP ranges in severity from a mild self-limited disease to one that is fatal. CAP is common. Most patients with pneumonia are treated in the outpatient setting. Additionally, pneumonia is one of the most common reasons for hospitalization among all age groups and accounts for approximately 1 million hospitalizations per year. Each year approximately 50,000 people in the United States die from lower respiratory tract infections. Influenza and pneumonia are the leading cause of death due to infection and the eighth most common cause of death overall.

Numerous microorganisms cause pneumonia including bacteria, viruses, mycobacterium, and fungi. These infecting agents range from microorganisms that are part of the normal flora to exogenous microorganisms that are inhaled. Additionally, there are noninfectious diseases that can mimic pneumonia. The incidence of pneumonia is lowest during early adulthood and increases with each decade of life (Fig. 7.1).

PATHOLOGY

Bacterial pneumonia usually causes lobar pneumonia, consolidation of an entire lobe or a large portion of a lobe, or bronchopneumonia, patchy consolidation of the lung. Pneumococcal lobar pneumonia has 4 stages of the inflammatory response: consolidation, red hepatization, gray hepatization and resolution. The initial congestion is characterized by fluid, with some neutrophils and bacteria, filling the alveoli. Red hepatization is characterized by red blood cells along with numerous neutrophils and fibrin filling the alveoli. With gray hepatization there is breakdown of red blood cells and persistence of fibrin and neutrophils. Then the consolidated exudate within the alveolar spaces undergoes resolution.

Pathophysiology

The lower respiratory tract is virtually sterile. Normal host defenses that protect against pneumonia include mucous production and cilia; in combination these form the mucociliary escalator, which removes microorganisms from the lungs. Impairment of host defenses predisposes to the development of pneumonia. Loss or suppression of the cough reflex due to stroke and other neurologic diseases, drugs and alcohol, aging and associated medical illnesses, and environmental factors such as smoking and respiratory irritants impairs ciliary function and increases the likelihood of developing pneumonia. Mechanical obstruction of an airway such as by a tumor or foreign body leads to decreased clearance of microorganisms and may produce a postobstructive pneumonia. Those infected with HIV virus are at increased risk of developing pneumococcal pneumonia.

The two main mechanisms of entry of microorganisms into the lung are microaspiration of organisms that colonize the upper respiratory tract and inhalation of airborne particles that contain a pathogenic microorganism. When a sufficient inoculum enters the lung and normal host defenses are not able to clear the inoculum, subsequent bacterial replication leads to a lower respiratory tract infection.

Transmission of Respiratory Pathogens

Some pathogens are transmitted from person to person via droplet transmission. Droplets are created when a person coughs, sneezes or talks. Additionally, transmission can occur during medical procedures such as suctioning, endotracheal intubation, cardiopulmonary resuscitation or cough-producing procedures. The greatest distance of transmission is unresolved. Historically, a distance of less than or equal to 3 feet was used for person-to-person droplet transmission. Some data suggest that transmission may occur from as far as 6 feet. Respiratory droplets have also been defined by their size, usually greater than 5 μm in diameter. Pathogens that are transmitted via the droplet route include *S. pneumoniae, M. pneumoniae*, and influenza virus. Crowding such as occurs in prisons, barracks, and shelters is associated with increased spread. Infectious agents such as *Mycobacterium tuberculosis*, fungi, and anthrax spores are transmitted via airborne transmission. Microorganisms transmitted in this fashion can be spread over long distances (>6 feet) by air currents and normal airflow. The size of the droplet nucleoli particles that are transmitted via the airborne route are generally less than or equal to 5 μm in diameter.

Specific Etiologic Agents

Many bacteria and viruses cause pneumonia. *Streptococcus pneumoniae* (pneumococcus) is the most common cause of bacterial pneumonia. The classical description of pneumonia is based upon disease caused by *S. pneumoniae*. Hence, *S. pneumoniae* causes "classical" or "typical" pneumonia. Most cases of pneumococcal pneumonia occur between December and April. Pneumococci transiently colonize the upper respiratory tract. Microaspiration leads to entry into the lower respiratory tract. If aspirated in sufficient quantity so that normal host defenses do not clear the bacteria, the patient then develops pneumonia. Pneumococci have a polysaccharide capsule that prevents phagocytosis. Antibodies, acquired from prior exposure or vaccination, against the polysaccharide capsule opsonize pneumococci thus allowing phagocytosis. Other bacteria that can colonize the oropharynx and cause pneumonia when aspirated include *Haemophilus influenzae*, less commonly *Staphylococcus aureus*, and rarely *Streptococcus pyogenes* (group A streptococcus). Similarly, *Moraxella catarrhalis* in patients with chronic obstructive

下呼吸道感染

崔晓敬 译 刘智博 鲁炳怀 审校 曹彬 通审

定义和流行病学

肺炎是肺实质的炎症，通常由急性感染引起。肺炎在医院外起病时，称为社区获得性肺炎（CAP）。CAP 的严重程度从轻微的自限性疾病到致死性疾病不等。CAP 很常见，大多数患者在门诊接受治疗。此外，肺炎是所有年龄段人群住院的主要原因之一，每年约有 100 万人因肺炎住院治疗。美国每年约有 5 万人死于下呼吸道感染。流感和肺炎是感染致死的首要病因，也是第八大常见死因。

引起肺炎的微生物很多，包括细菌、病毒、分枝杆菌和真菌。这些病原体包括正常的呼吸道菌群和吸入的外源性致病菌。此外，还有一些非感染性疾病也会模仿肺炎。肺炎的发病率在成年早期最低，随着年龄的增长而逐年升高（图 7.1）。

病理学

细菌性肺炎通常会引起大叶性肺炎，即一个肺叶全部或大部分的实变，或引起支气管肺炎，表现为肺内的斑片状实变。肺炎球菌性大叶性肺炎的炎症反应分为 4 个阶段：实变期、红色肝变期、灰色肝变期、消退期。初期实变期的特点是肺泡内充满液体及一些中性粒细胞和细菌。红色肝变期的特点是肺泡内充满红细胞、大量中性粒细胞和纤维蛋白。在灰色肝变期，红细胞降解，纤维蛋白和中性粒细胞仍然存在。然后肺泡腔内的实变渗出物逐渐消解。

病理生理学

下呼吸道几乎无菌。正常的宿主防御系统包括分泌黏液和纤毛，它们共同组成了"黏膜纤毛电梯"，将微生物从肺部清除，可防止肺炎。宿主防御功能受损易引发肺炎。卒中和其他神经系统疾病、药物和酒精、衰老和相关的内科疾病可导致咳嗽反射丧失或抑制，吸烟和呼吸道刺激物等环境因素会损害纤毛功能，均增加患肺炎的可能性。肿瘤或异物等造成气道机械性阻塞会导致微生物清除减少，并可能引发梗阻后肺炎。HIV 病毒感染者罹患肺炎球菌性肺炎的风险增高。

微生物进入肺部的两种主要机制是上呼吸道定植微生物的微量吸入和含有病原微生物的空气颗粒的吸入。当足够的微生物进入肺部，而正常的宿主防御系统无法清除这些微生物时，随后的细菌复制就会导致下呼吸道感染。

呼吸道病原体的传播

一些病原体通过飞沫在人与人之间传播。人在咳嗽、打喷嚏或说话时会产生飞沫。此外，在吸痰、气管插管、心肺复苏或诱导咳嗽等医疗过程中也可能发生传播。传播的最大距离尚未确定。以往认为，人与人之间的飞沫传播距离小于或等于 3 英尺。一些数据表明，传播距离最远可达 6 英尺。也可以依据大小来定义呼吸道飞沫，其直径通常大于 5 μm。通过飞沫传播的病原体包括肺炎链球菌、肺炎支原体、流感病毒等。监狱、军营和避难所等场所的拥挤可增加传播。结核分枝杆菌、真菌和炭疽孢子等传染源通过空气传播。通过这种方式传播的微生物可以在气流的作用下传播很远（> 6 英尺）。通过空气传播的飞沫微粒核心直径一般小于或等于 5 μm。

特定病原体

许多细菌和病毒都会引起肺炎。肺炎链球菌（肺炎球菌）是细菌性肺炎最常见的病因。对肺炎的经典描述是基于肺炎链球菌引起的疾病。因此，肺炎链球菌会引起"经典"或"典型"肺炎。大多数肺炎球菌性肺炎病例发生在 12 月至次年 4 月之间。肺炎球菌可在上呼吸道暂时定植。微量吸入会导致细菌进入下呼吸道。如果吸入的数量足够多，以至于正常的宿主防御系统无法清除细菌，患者就会患上肺炎。肺炎球菌有多糖荚膜，可防止被吞噬。先前暴露或接种疫苗后获得的针对多糖荚膜的抗体，促使肺炎球菌被吞噬。其他可在口咽部定植并在吸入后引起肺炎的细菌包括流感嗜血杆菌、金黄色葡萄球菌（较少见）以及极少情况下的化脓性链球菌（A 组链球菌）。同样，慢性阻塞性肺疾病（COPD）患者和老年人口咽部定植的卡他莫拉菌以及酗酒者中口咽部定植的肺炎克雷伯菌也会引发肺

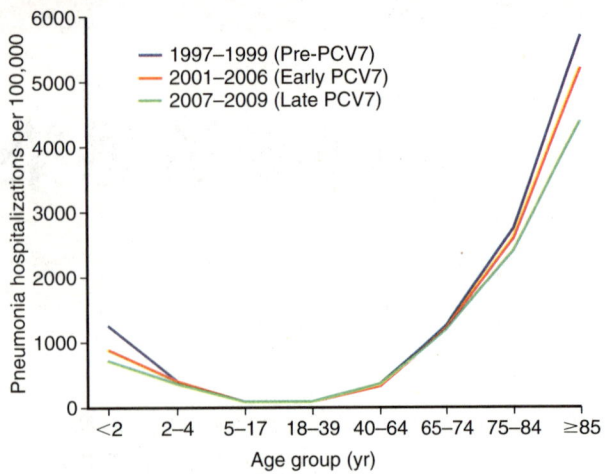

Fig. 7.1 Rate of hospitalization for pneumonia by age group. *PCV7*, Pneumococcus conjugate vaccine. (Data from New England Journal of Medicine 369: 155-63, 2013.)

pulmonary disease (COPD) and the elderly and *Klebsiella pneumoniae* in alcoholics colonize the oropharynx and can cause pneumonia. Most cases of community-acquired pneumonia are monomicrobial.

Patients with pneumococcal pneumonia can develop infections at other sites including empyema, pericarditis, meningitis, endocarditis, and septic arthritis. Approximately one out of five patients with pneumococcal pneumonia have bacteremia.

Mycoplasma pneumoniae usually causes milder disease. Its peak incidence is during the first two decades of life. Patients usually do not required hospitalization; however, some patients can develop severe disease.

Chlamydophila pneumoniae is a common cause of community-acquired pneumonia. It usually causes a milder disease and hence is seen more commonly among patients treated in the outpatient setting.

Legionella, an environmental organism, can cause pneumonia. *Legionella pneumophila* is the most common species to cause pneumonia. Other *Legionella* species such as *L. micdadei*, *L. bozemanii*, and others can also cause pneumonia. Most cases are sporadic. Outbreaks have occurred from contaminated point sources such as cooling towers and air conditioning units. Transmission is usually due to inhalation of aerosol particles; microaspiration of water containing *Legionella* has also occurred.

Staphylococcus aureus infrequently causes bacterial pneumonia, sometimes as a complication of influenza infection. More recently, community acquired methicillin-resistant strains (MRSA) have caused secondary bacterial pneumonias.

The etiology of CAP requiring hospitalization in adults is changing. More recently, the most commonly identified organisms, in order of decreasing frequency, are human rhinovirus followed by influenza, *Streptococcus pneumoniae*, human metapneumovirus, and respiratory syncytial virus. This change may be due in part to decreased invasive pneumococcal disease after the introduction of the conjugate vaccine, changes in the age distribution of patients and underlying illnesses of the adult population, as well as the ability to detect viral pathogens.

Rapid molecular techniques are now available for the detection of respiratory viral pathogens. The rapid identification of a virus can avoid the unnecessary use of antibiotics. A small subset (approximately 10%) of hospitalized patients with viral pneumonia are coinfected with a bacterium. This may occur because of damage to the respiratory epithelium caused by viral infection. Additionally, dysfunctional innate immune responses caused by a viral infection have been implicated to enhance susceptibility to secondary bacterial infection.

Fungi that cause pneumonia are not part of the normal flora. Certain dimorphic fungi (*Histoplasma capsulatum*, *Coccidioides immitis*, and *Blastomyces dermatitidis*) that reside in the soil cause pneumonia when inhaled. Dimorphic fungi form hyphae at ambient temperatures and yeasts at body temperature. The hyphal form and not the yeast form is the transmissible form of the fungus. The yeast form is not transmissible person to person. These fungi are limited to certain geographic areas: *Histoplasma capsulatum* in the Mississippi, Missouri, and Ohio river valleys; *Coccidioides immitis* in the southwestern United States; and *Blastomyces dermatitidis* in parts of the midwestern, south-central and southeastern regions of the United States. *H. capsulatum*, *C. immitis*, and *Blastomyces dermatitidis* cause disease in the normal host. *Aspergillus*, a mold ubiquitous in the environment, rarely if ever causes disease in the immunocompetent host. Patients that are immunocompromised or have abnormal airways are at risk of infection with *Aspergillus* and rarely other molds such as Zygomycetes (Mucorales). *Pneumocystis jirovecii*, an opportunistic fungus, causes pneumonia in immunocompromised patients such as those with lymphoma or HIV (see Chapter 16 for additional information).

Mycobacterium tuberculosis is not part of the normal flora. It is transmitted via small aerosol particles (<5 µm) that are inhaled directly into the alveolus. *M. tuberculosis* is a slow growing organism and usually causes chronic symptoms; however, it rarely can present acutely.

The normal flora of an acutely ill hospitalized patient is different from a healthy outpatient. Hospitalized patients are more frequently colonized with *S. aureus*, including methicillin-resistant strains, and gram-negative bacilli, including *Pseudomonas aeruginosa*. Hence, when a hospitalized patient aspirates their own oropharyngeal flora leading to hospital-acquired pneumonia (HaP) it may contain one of these organisms.

Some microorganisms almost never cause pneumonia; these include *Candida* species and enterococci.

CLINICAL PRESENTATION

Patients usually present with the acute onset of fever, chills, cough, sputum production, dyspnea, and sometimes pleuritic chest pain. Classically, patients may produce blood-tinged sputum that appears rust-colored specifically when infected with *S. pneumoniae*. Extrapulmonary signs and symptoms may include nausea, vomiting, diarrhea, abdominal pain, headache, confusion, arthralgia, myalgias, and change in mental status. Signs and symptoms can be blunted or absent in the elderly. Rales or rhonchi may be present on auscultation of the chest. Patients usually have a leukocytosis with left shift. Pulmonary signs and symptoms in combination with a new infiltrate on chest radiograph are used to diagnose pneumonia.

DIAGNOSIS

When pneumonia is suspected, the next step is to determine the etiologic diagnosis. Unfortunately, there is no single diagnostic test with a high sensitivity and high specificity. The sputum gram stain provides useful diagnostic information. Although epithelial cells from the upper respiratory tract and oropharyngeal flora may "contaminate" an expectorated sputum sample, careful examination of the sputum gram stain can reveal an area of the specimen that originated from the lower respiratory tract and examination for bacteria in that area can be helpful. Unfortunately, some patients do not produce sputum. Additionally, prior antibiotics can alter sputum results.

S. pneumoniae is a gram-positive coccus that forms pairs and chains; the cocci are sometimes pointed at one end ("lancet-shaped"). *H. influenzae* is a pleomorphic gram-negative rod. *S. aureus* is a gram-positive coccus that forms clusters. *M. catarrhalis* is a gram-negative diplococci. These distinct morphologic features allow for a presumptive diagnosis of a specific etiologic agent when seen on a gram stain of sputum (Fig. 7.2).

Mycoplasma, *Legionella*, *Mycobacterium*, and *Chlamydophila* are not seen on sputum gram stain. *Mycobacteria* are seen with special staining (acid fast).

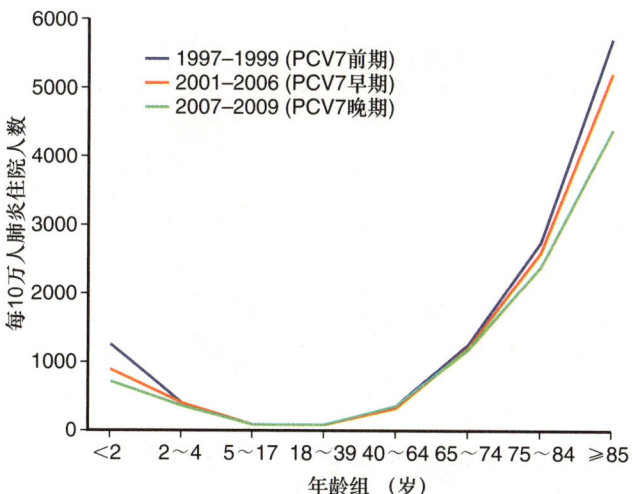

图 7.1 按年龄组划分的肺炎住院率。PCV7，肺炎球菌结合疫苗（数据引自 New England Journal of Medicine 369：155-63，2013.）

炎。大多数社区获得性肺炎病例都是单一病原体感染。

患肺炎球菌性肺炎的患者可能并发其他部位的感染，包括脓胸、心包炎、脑膜炎、心内膜炎和化脓性关节炎。大约 1/5 的肺炎球菌性肺炎患者会有菌血症。

肺炎支原体通常会引起较轻的疾病。发病高峰是在 20 岁以内。患者通常不需要住院治疗，但有些患者可能会发展成重症。

肺炎衣原体是社区获得性肺炎的常见病因。它通常引起较轻的疾病，因此在门诊治疗的患者中较为常见。

军团菌是一种环境微生物，可引发肺炎。嗜肺军团菌是最常见的引起肺炎的菌种。其他军团菌如麦氏军团菌、波兹曼军团菌等也可引起肺炎。大多数病例为散发。暴发性病例可能源于冷却塔和空调机组等污染点。传播通常是由于吸入气溶胶微粒；含军团菌的水的微量吸入也会造成传播。

金黄色葡萄球菌引起细菌性肺炎并不常见，有时作为流感感染的并发症。最近，社区获得的耐甲氧西林金黄色葡萄球菌（MRSA）已引起继发性细菌性肺炎。

需要住院治疗的成人 CAP 的病原正在发生变化。最近，最常发现的病原体依次为人鼻病毒、流感病毒、肺炎链球菌、人偏肺病毒和呼吸道合胞病毒。出现这种变化的部分原因可能是在引入结合疫苗后侵袭性肺炎球菌疾病减少、患者年龄分布和成人潜在疾病谱发生变化以及病毒病原体检测能力的提高。

现在已经有了检测呼吸道病毒病原体的快速分子技术。快速鉴定病毒可避免不必要地使用抗生素。一小部分（约 10%）病毒性肺炎住院患者会合并细菌感染。出现这种情况的原因可能是病毒感染导致呼吸道上皮受损。此外，病毒感染导致的天然免疫反应失调也会增加继发细菌感染的易感性。

引起肺炎的真菌不属于正常菌群。某些存在于土壤中的双相真菌（荚膜组织胞浆菌、粗球孢子菌和皮炎芽生菌）被吸入后会导致肺炎。双相真菌在环境温度下形成菌丝，在体温下形成孢子。真菌的传播形式是菌丝而非孢子。孢子相不会在人与人之间传播。这些真菌仅限于某些地理区域：荚膜组织胞浆菌分布在密西西比河、密苏里河和俄亥俄河流域；粗球孢子菌分布在美国西南部；皮炎芽生菌分布在美国中西部、中南部和东南部的部分地区。荚膜组织胞浆菌、粗球孢子菌和皮炎芽生菌在正常宿主中致病。曲霉菌是一种在环境中无处不在的霉菌，很少会在免疫功能正常的宿主中致病。免疫力低下或呼吸道结构异常的患者有感染曲霉菌的风险，其他霉菌罕见感染，如接合菌（毛霉菌目）。耶氏肺孢子菌是一种机会性真菌，在免疫力低下的患者如淋巴瘤患者或 HIV 感染者中会引发肺炎（更多信息见第 16 章）。

结核分枝杆菌不属于正常菌群。它通过直接吸入肺泡的小气溶胶颗粒（＜ 5 μm）传播。结核分枝杆菌是一种生长缓慢的微生物，通常会引起慢性症状；但也有极少数情况下会出现急性症状。

急性住院患者的正常菌群与健康门诊患者不同。住院患者更经常定植金黄色葡萄球菌（包括 MRSA）和革兰氏阴性杆菌（包括铜绿假单胞菌）。因此，当住院患者吸入自己的口咽菌群时，可能会含有其中一种微生物，从而导致医院获得性肺炎（HAP）。

有些微生物几乎不会引起肺炎，其中包括念珠菌和肠球菌。

临床表现

患者通常表现为急性发热、寒战、咳嗽、咳痰、呼吸困难，有时还会出现胸膜炎性胸痛。患者可能会产生带血的痰液，特别是感染肺炎链球菌后，痰呈现铁锈色。肺外症状和体征可能包括恶心、呕吐、腹泻、腹痛、头痛、意识障碍、关节痛、肌痛和精神状态改变。老年人的体征和症状会变得隐匿或消失。胸部听诊可出现啰音或哮鸣音。患者通常会出现白细胞增多伴核左移。肺部症状和体征结合胸部 X 线片上的新发浸润可诊断肺炎。

诊断

当怀疑肺炎时，下一步就是确定病因诊断。遗憾的是，目前还没有一种具有高敏感性和高特异性的诊断方法。虽然上呼吸道上皮细胞和口咽菌群可能会"污染"咳出痰样本，但仔细进行痰液革兰氏染色检查可以发现样本中来自下呼吸道的区域，检查该区域的细菌会有所帮助。遗憾的是，有些患者无痰。此外，之前使用过的抗生素也会改变痰液检查结果。

肺炎链球菌为革兰氏阳性球菌，成对或成链排列；其一端有时呈尖状（"柳叶刀状"）。流感嗜血杆菌为多形性革兰氏阴性杆菌。金黄色葡萄球菌为革兰氏阳性球菌，呈簇状。卡他莫拉菌是一种革兰氏阴性双球菌。如果在痰的革兰氏染色中看到这些明显的形态特征，就可以推定诊断出特定的病原体（图 7.2）。

支原体、军团菌、分枝杆菌和衣原体在痰液革兰氏染色中看不到。通过特殊染色（抗酸染色）可看到分枝杆菌。

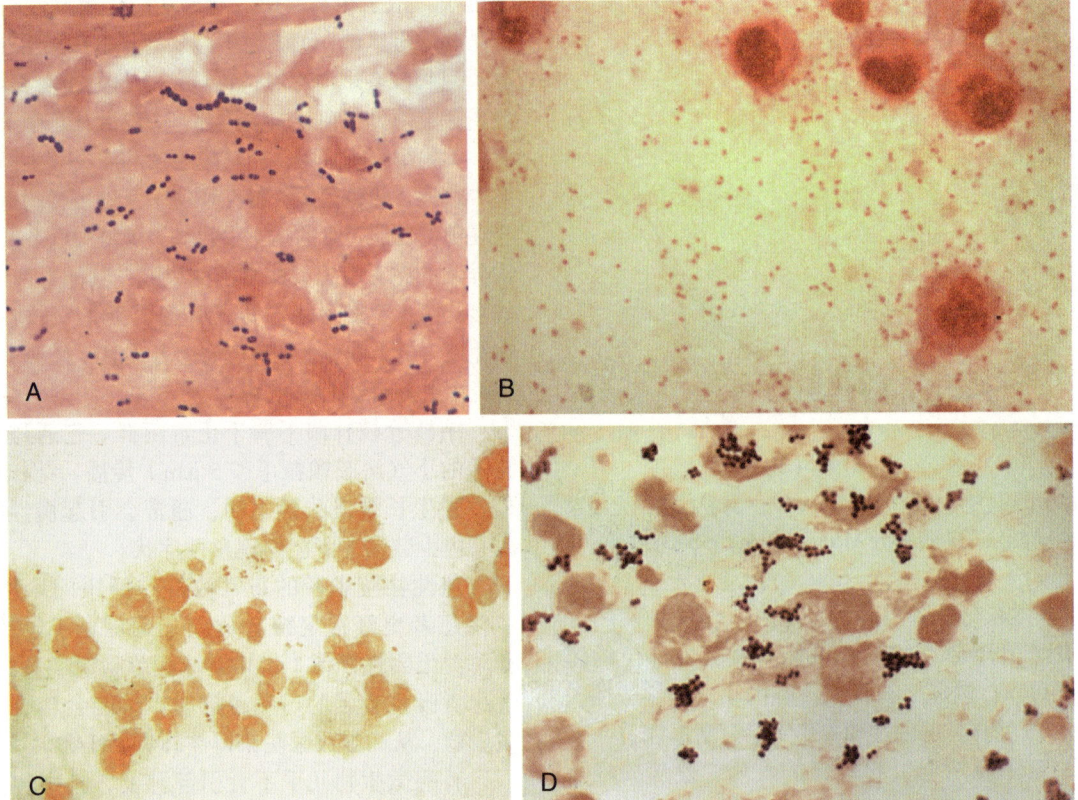

Fig. 7.2 Sputum Gram stain. (A) *Streptococcus pneumoniae*. (B) *Haemophilus influenzae*. (C) *Moraxella catarrhalis*. (D) *Staphylococcus aureus*.

Culture of sputum can reveal the etiologic diagnosis and should be correlated with findings on the sputum gram stain. However, pneumococci are fastidious. A study of patients with bacteremic pneumococcal pneumonia found that only 55% grew pneumococci from their sputum culture. *Mycoplasma*, *Legionella*, *Mycobacterium*, and *Chlamydophila* do not grow on routine agar. Special culture media are required for certain bacteria, such as Lowenstein-Jensen for *Mycobacteria* and buffered charcoal yeast extract (BCYE) for *Legionella*.

Blood cultures can be helpful. However, the ratio of bacteremic to nonbacteremic pneumococcal pneumonia is approximately 1:4. A positive blood culture is very helpful because the etiologic agent is definitely identified and susceptibility data are available to determine appropriate therapy.

Other diagnostic studies used to identify the causative organism include *Legionella* urinary antigen, histoplasmosis urinary antigen, and polymerase chain reaction (PCR) for respiratory viruses, *Mycoplasma*, and *Chlamydophila*.

Chest radiography of patients with pneumococcal pneumonia can show a consolidative lobar infiltrate, a bronchopneumonic (patchy) pattern or, less commonly, an interstitial pattern. A definitive etiologic diagnosis cannot be made based on chest radiograph appearance.

DIFFERENTIAL DIAGNOSIS

Not all patients with fever and a new pulmonary infiltrate have pneumonia. Noninfectious causes of pulmonary infiltrates and fever include pulmonary infarction, vasculitis (granulomatosis with polyangiitis), drug reaction, tumor, congestive heart failure, cryptogenic organizing pneumonia (COP), hypersensitivity pneumonitis, collagen vascular disease, aspiration (macroaspiration) of oropharyngeal or upper gastrointestinal contents, and acute respiratory distress syndrome (ARDS).

TREATMENT

The definitive treatment for pneumonia is to eradicate the infecting microorganism. Antibiotics are used to kill bacteria and hence decrease or stop the spread of infection in the lungs. Normal host responses are needed to repair the inflammatory process in the lungs. Penicillin therapy reduced the mortality rate of bacteremic pneumococcal pneumonia from 84% to 17%. However, antibiotics have little to no effect on mortality during the first 5 days of illness; those destined to die during the first 5 days of illness die whether or not they receive antibiotics.

When an etiologic agent is identified, then the appropriate antibiotic can be given (Table 7.1). When a specific etiologic diagnosis is not made, then empiric treatment with one of many different antimicrobial agents has been recommend. Guidelines are available (IDSA available at https://www.atsjournals.org/doi/full/10.1164/rccm.201908-1581ST).

The decision to admit a patient with pneumonia is based upon clinical prediction rules. These rules use mortality and sometimes other factors to stratify patients. The pneumonia severity index (PSI) stratifies patients into one of five risk groups. Those in a low risk group are treated as outpatients while those in a higher risk group are admitted to the hospital for treatment (see *The New England Journal of Medicine* 336: 243-250, 1997). The CURB-65 score (see *Thorax* 58: 377-382, 2003) is easier to calculate but has not been as rigorously validated as the PSI. Furthermore, psychosocial and other factors that impact the decision to admit a patient are not included by PSI or CURB-65.

Duration of therapy ranges from 3 to 28 days depending on the microorganism and clinical response. The shortest duration (3 days) has been given to patients with pneumococcal pneumonia while 28

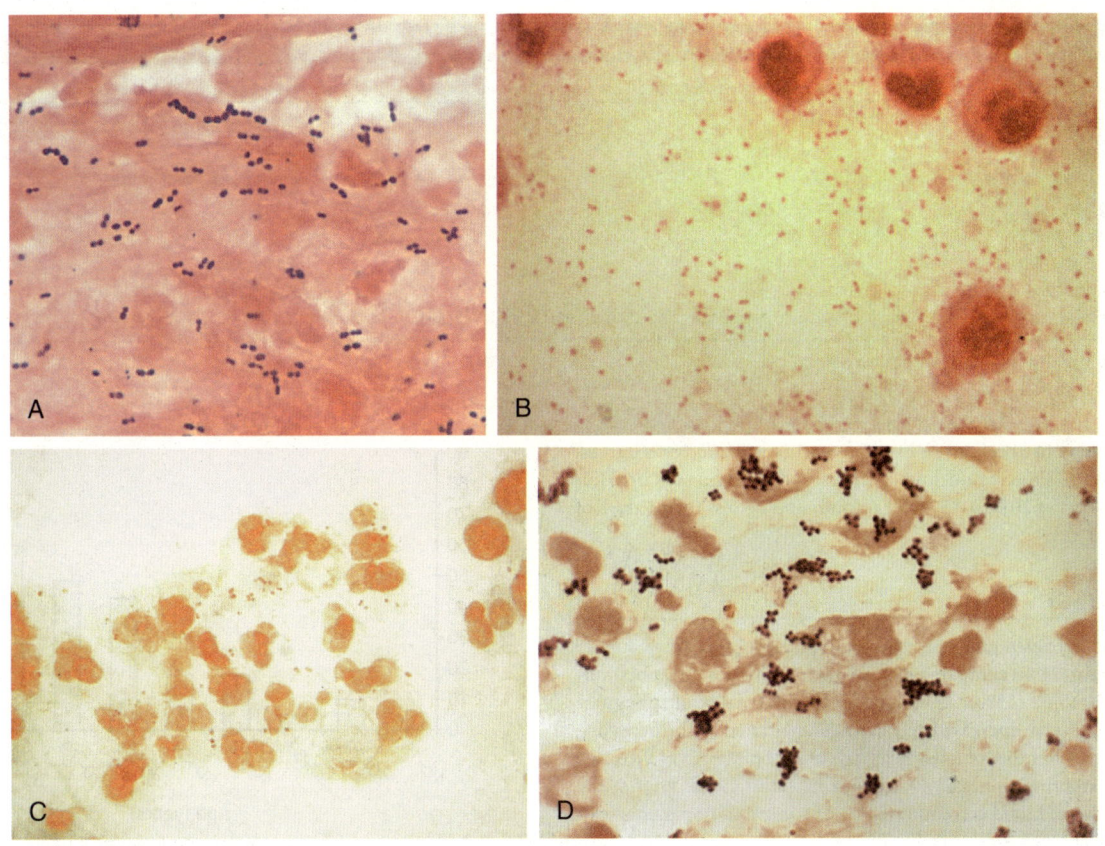

图 7.2 痰液革兰氏染色。（A）肺炎链球菌；（B）流感嗜血杆菌；（C）卡他莫拉菌；（D）金黄色葡萄球菌

痰培养可揭示病原学诊断，并应与痰革兰氏染色结果相关联。然而，肺炎球菌是苛养菌。一项针对菌血症性肺炎球菌性肺炎患者的研究发现，仅55%患者的痰培养肺炎球菌生长。支原体、军团菌、分枝杆菌和衣原体不能在常规琼脂培养基上生长。某些细菌需要使用特殊的培养基，如分枝杆菌使用罗氏培养基，军团菌使用缓冲炭酵母提取物（BCYE）培养基。

血培养可能会有所帮助。不过，肺炎球菌性肺炎伴发菌血症和不伴发菌血症的比例约为 1∶4。血培养阳性非常有帮助，可确定病原体，并获得药敏数据以确定适当的治疗方法。

用于确定致病菌的其他诊断方法包括军团菌尿抗原、组织胞浆菌尿抗原和针对呼吸道病毒、支原体和衣原体的聚合酶链反应（PCR）。

肺炎球菌性肺炎患者的胸部 X 线检查可显示大叶性浸润、支气管肺炎（斑片状）模式，或较少见的间质性模式。根据胸部 X 线片表现无法做出明确的病因诊断。

鉴别诊断

并非所有发热并伴有新的肺部浸润的患者都患有肺炎。导致肺部浸润和发热的非感染性原因包括肺梗死、血管炎（肉芽肿性多血管炎）、药物反应、肿瘤、充血性心力衰竭、隐源性机化性肺炎（COP）、过敏性肺炎、胶原血管病、口咽分泌物或上消化道内容物的大量吸入以及急性呼吸窘迫综合征（ARDS）。

治疗

肺炎的决定性治疗方法是根除感染的微生物。抗生素可杀死细菌，从而减少或阻止肺部感染的扩散。修复肺部炎症的过程需要正常的宿主反应。青霉素治疗可将肺炎球菌性肺炎伴发菌血症的死亡率从84%降至17%。然而，抗生素对发病最初5天内的死亡率影响很小或几乎没有影响；那些注定会在发病最初5天内死亡的患者无论是否接受抗生素治疗都会死亡。

一旦确定了病原体，就可以使用合适的抗生素（表7.1）。如无法做出具体的病原学诊断，则建议使用多种抗菌药物中的一种进行经验性治疗。可查阅相关指南（IDSA，网址：https://www.atsjournals.org/doi/full/10.1164/rccm.201908-1581ST）。

肺炎患者是否收治入院基于临床预测规则。这些规则利用死亡率，有时也利用其他因素对患者进行分层。肺炎严重程度指数（PSI）将患者分为五个风险组。低风险组的患者可在门诊接受治疗，而高风险组的患者则需住院接受治疗（见 the New England Journal of Medicine 336：243-250，1997）。CURB-65 评分（见 Thorax 58：377-382，2003）更容易计算，但没有 PSI 那样经过严格验证。此外，PSI 或 CURB-65 均不包括影响患者入院决定的心理社会因素和其他因素。

治疗疗程从3天到28天不等，取决于微生物和临床反应。肺炎球菌性肺炎患者的疗程最短（3天），而金黄色葡萄球菌患者的疗程为28天。最近的 ATS/IDSA 指南

TABLE 7.1 Treatment of Pneumonia by Specific Etiologic Agent

Etiologic Agent	Preferred Antimicrobial	Alternative Antimicrobial
Streptococcus pneumoniae	Penicillin	Cephalosporin, moxifloxacin, levofloxacin
Haemophilus influenzae	Cefuroxime, ceftriaxone	
Mycoplasma pneumoniae	Macrolide	Moxifloxacin, levofloxacin
Legionella	Macrolide or quinolone	
Staphylococcus aureus		
Methicillin-susceptible	Nafcillin	Cephalosporin
Methicillin-resistant	Vancomycin (IV)	Doxycycline or TMP/SMX (oral)
Moraxella catarrhalis	Amoxicillin/clavulanate, cefuroxime, ceftriaxone, TMP/SMX	

TMP/SMX, Trimethoprim/sulfamethoxazole

days of therapy has been given to patients with *Staphylococcus aureus*. Recent ATS/IDSA guidelines (https://www.atsjournals.org/doi/full/10.1164/rccm.201908-1581ST) recommend no less than 5 days of treatment.

PROGNOSIS

Patients with bacteremic pneumococcal pneumonia have a higher mortality rate (21%) compared to those with nonbacteremic pneumococcal pneumonia (13%). Among patients with bacteremic pneumococcal pneumonia, increased mortality is associated with increasing age (Fig. 7.3), number of lobes involved (one lobe 12% mortality, two lobes 24% and three lobes 63%), leukopenia (mortality 35%), normal peripheral white blood cell count (24%) as compared to patients with leukocytosis (14%). Additionally, mortality rates differ for each capsular type of pneumococcus. For example, the mortality rate among patients infected with type I capsular type is 3% compared to patients infected with capsular type III 22%. Patients who survive usually recover without sequelae.

PREVENTION

Influenza vaccine not only protects against influenza but also bacterial pneumonia since patients who do not have influenza are not at risk of developing secondary bacterial pneumonia. The 23-valent pneumococcal polysaccharide vaccine is recommended for adults 65 years and older (see *Morbidity and Mortality Weekly Report* Supplement/Vol. 62, pages 9-18, February 1, 2013 and *Morbidity and Mortality Weekly Report* Vol. 68, No. 46, pages 1069-1075, 2019). The conjugate pneumococcal vaccine has reduced invasive pneumococcal disease in both the recipients (children) as well as adults (Fig. 7.4). By decreasing carriage in children, there is a reduction in transmission to adults and subsequent adult disease. The pediatric conjugate vaccine has reduced the number of adult admissions for pneumonia (see Fig. 7.1). Additionally, the conjugate vaccine has decreased antibiotic resistance since the capsular types of pneumococci that are more likely to be antibiotic resistant are included in the vaccine.

TUBERCULOSIS

Definition

Tuberculosis (TB) is caused primarily by *Mycobacterium tuberculosis* (MTB), an acid-fast rod that has a slow generation time. Related species include *Mycobacterium bovis* that causes disease in cattle but can infect humans and *Mycobacterium africanum* that causes up to 50% of cases of tuberculosis in Africa. TB primarily causes pulmonary disease but can cause infection in almost any part of the body including

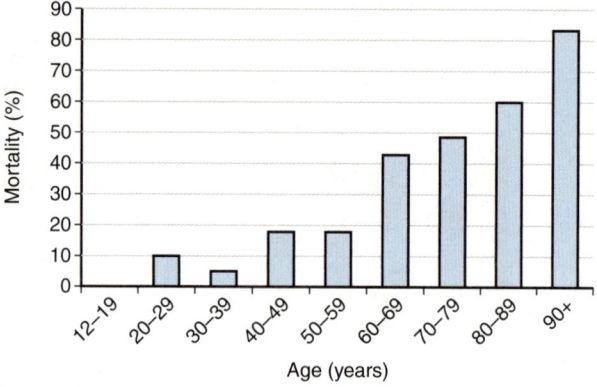

Fig. 7.3 Mortality from bacteremic pneumococcal pneumonia by age group. (Data from *Annals of Internal Medicine* 60: 760-776, 1964.)

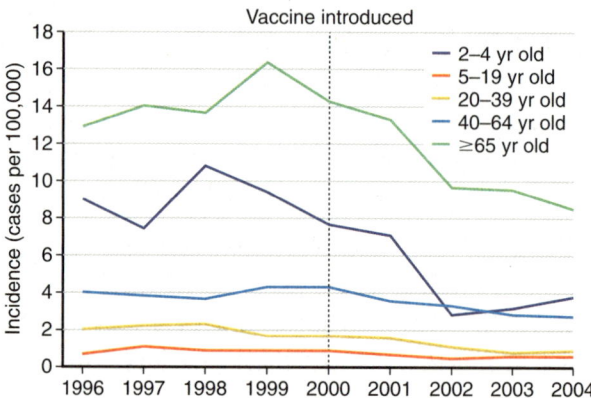

Fig. 7.4 Incidence of penicillin-resistant pneumococci by year for different age groups. (Data from *New England Journal of Medicine* 354: 1455-63, 2006.)

bone, the central nervous system, the gastrointestinal system, and the cardiovascular system. TB is characterized by asymptomatic, lifetime latency for up to 90% of infected individuals. Primary progressive infection typically occurs in 4% to 5% of patients up to 2 years after infection whereas reactivation disease occurs often decades after infection.

Epidemiology

MTB has caused infection in humans throughout history but became widespread during urbanization and industrialization in Europe in the 18th century, causing up to one quarter of all deaths. Rates of

表 7.1 基于特定病原体的肺炎治疗

病原体	首选抗菌药	替代抗菌药
肺炎链球菌	青霉素	头孢菌素、莫西沙星、左氧氟沙星
流感嗜血杆菌	头孢呋辛、头孢曲松	
肺炎支原体	大环内酯类	莫西沙星、左氧氟沙星
军团菌	大环内酯类或喹诺酮类	
甲氧西林敏感金黄色葡萄球菌	萘夫西林	头孢菌素
耐甲氧西林金黄色葡萄球菌	万古霉素（Ⅳ）	多西环素或 TMP/SMX（口服）
卡他莫拉菌	阿莫西林/克拉维酸、头孢呋辛、头孢曲松、TMP/SMX	

TMP/SMX，甲氧苄啶/磺胺甲噁唑

（https://www.atsjournals.org/doi/full/10.1164/rccm.201908-1581ST）建议治疗时间不少于 5 天。

预后

与无菌血症的肺炎球菌性肺炎患者的死亡率（13%）相比，伴菌血症的肺炎球菌性肺炎死亡率更高（21%）。在伴菌血症的肺炎球菌性肺炎患者中，死亡率的增加与年龄（图 7.3）、受累肺叶数量（一个肺叶受累死亡率为 12%，两个肺叶受累死亡率为 24%，三个肺叶受累死亡率为 63%）、白细胞减少（死亡率为 35%）、外周血白细胞计数正常（24%）等有关，而白细胞增多的患者的死亡率为 14%。此外，不同荚膜类型的肺炎球菌的死亡率也不同。例如，感染Ⅰ型荚膜型肺炎球菌的患者死亡率为 3%，而感染Ⅲ型荚膜型肺炎球菌死亡率为 22%。存活下来的患者通常会康复，不会留下后遗症。

预防

流感疫苗不仅能预防流感，还能预防细菌性肺炎，因为未患流感的患者不会有继发细菌性肺炎的风险。建议 65 岁及以上的成年人接种 23 价肺炎球菌多糖疫苗（见 *Morbidity and Mortality Weekly Report* Supplement/Vol. 62，pages 9-18，February 1，2013 和 *Morbidity and Mortality Weekly Report* Vol. 68，No. 46，pages 1069-1075，2019）。肺炎球菌结合疫苗降低了接种者（儿童）和成人的侵袭性肺炎球菌疾病的发病率（图 7.4）。通过减少儿童的带菌量，可以减少向成人的传播及随后的成人疾病。小儿结合疫苗减少了成人因肺炎入院的人数（图 7.1）。此外，由于疫苗中包含了更有可能产生抗生素耐药性的肺炎球菌荚膜型，因此结合疫苗降低了抗生素耐药性。

结核病

定义

结核病（TB）主要由结核分枝杆菌（MTB）引起，MTB 是抗酸杆菌，生长缓慢。相关菌种包括牛分枝杆菌和非洲分枝杆菌，牛分枝杆菌会导致牛患病，也会感染人类，在非洲，非洲分枝杆菌可导致高

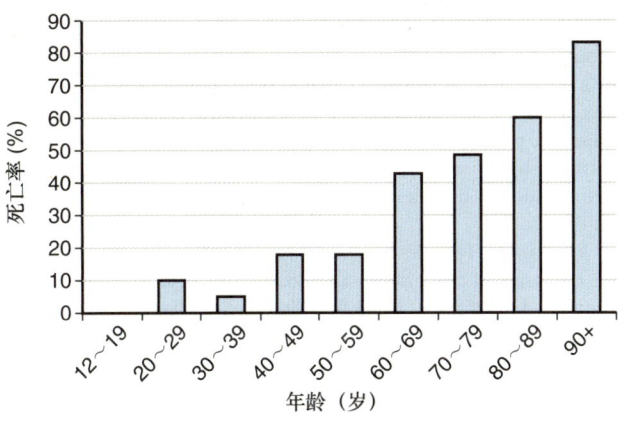

图 7.3 按年龄组划分的肺炎球菌性肺炎死亡率（数据引自 *Annals of Internal Medicine* 60：760-776，1964.）

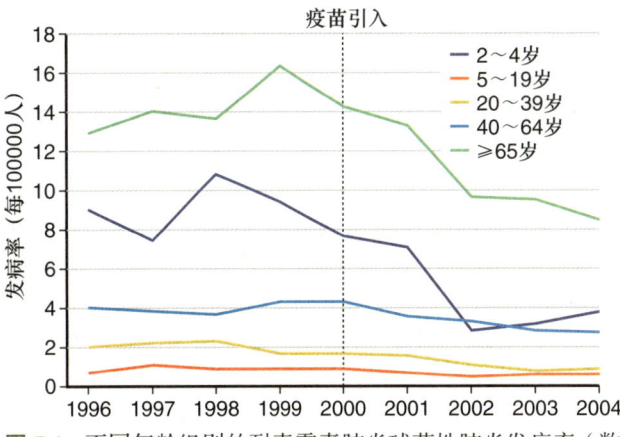

图 7.4 不同年龄组别的耐青霉素肺炎球菌性肺炎发病率（数据引自 *New England Journal of Medicine* 354：1455-63，2006.）

达 50% 的结核病病例。结核病主要为肺部疾病，但几乎可感染身体的任何部位，包括骨骼、中枢神经系统、消化系统和心血管系统。结核病的特点是高达 90% 的感染者无症状、终身潜伏。通常有 4%～5% 的患者会在感染后 2 年内出现原发感染进展，而感染后几十年还有可能会发生结核病再次激活。

流行病学

MTB 自古以来就曾引起人类感染，但在 18 世纪欧洲城市化和工业化过程中开始广泛传播，造成的死亡人数高达总死亡人数的 1/4。19 世纪末 20 世纪初，结核病发病率开始下降，有效抗生素的发现加速了结核病发病率的下降，1946 年首先发现了链霉素，1952 年发现了异

tuberculosis began falling in the late 19th and early 20th century and the fall was accelerated by the discovery of effective antibiotics, first streptomycin in 1946, and then isoniazid in 1952. Rates in the United States fell until the 1980s when they increased due to HIV and increased intravenous substance use. With effective antiretroviral therapy, the downward trend returned. For example, the incidence in the United States fell from 25,000 cases in 1993 to 9025 cases in 2018. Seventy percent of cases occurred in non-US-born people and approximately half were diagnosed 10 or more years after arriving in the United States, consistent with reactivation of previously acquired tuberculosis. There is a preponderance of cases in ethnic and racial minorities including Hispanic, American Indian/Alaska native, Asian, and Black individuals. Risk factors include diabetes mellitus, alcohol and substance abuse, HIV, homelessness, and incarceration.

Infection occurs when MTB is aerosolized by coughing, sneezing, shouting or singing from a patient with pulmonary disease and inhaled by a susceptible individual. Small infectious particles 1 to 5 μm in size can persist in the air, particularly in enclosed spaces, and very few infectious particles are required for infection. Household contacts are particularly at risk, with up to 50% becoming infected. Group home settings such as homeless shelters and prisons have been the sites of outbreaks.

Worldwide, TB is among the top ten causes of death and the number one cause of death due to an infection. In 2018, 10 million people contracted tuberculosis and 1.5 million died, including 251 thousand with HIV. Encouragingly, the TB mortality rate fell by 42% from 2000 to 2018. Four hundred eighty four thousand fell ill with drug-resistant tuberculosis (multidrug resistant or MDR defined as resistant to the two most effective drugs, INH and rifampin), and 6.2% of those had XDR-TB (defined as resistant to INH, rifampin, a fluoroquinolone, and second-line injectable drugs). Sixty-six percent of new cases occurred in India, China, Indonesia, the Philippines, Pakistan, Nigeria, Bangladesh, and South Africa. Rapid diagnostic tests (e.g., Xpert MTB/RIF) assays are in widespread use, and the global treatment success in 2017 of newly diagnosed cases was 85%. Newer drugs such as bedaquiline are coming into use for resistant TB. Furthermore, there are currently 14 vaccines in clinical trial.

Microbiology

MTB is an aerobic, nonmotile mycobacteria in the family Mycobacteriaceae with a cell wall content high in high-molecular-weight lipids. It has a slow multiplication time, between 15 to 20 hours, compared to most bacteria, which multiply in less than 1 hour. Humans are the only host. The organism can be identified in sputum by acid-fast staining (Ziehl-Neelsen or Kinyoun) or nucleic acid amplification, which is more common. Xpert MTB/RIF is an automated test that identifies MTB and whether the organism is resistant to rifampin, one of the most commonly used and effective anti-TB drugs. Growth on solid media occurs in 3 to 8 weeks whereas growth in liquid media takes up to 20 days. Culture of the organism is necessary to identify the full susceptibility of an isolate.

Pathobiology

Infection occurs when infectious particles reach the alveoli and are ingested by macrophages. MTB can resist destruction by macrophages and neutrophils and persist within phagosomes and multiply intracellularly, in part due to protective mechanisms such as the production of superoxide dismutase, which can neutralize the production of the bactericidal molecule superoxide anion. In addition, the mycobacteria appear to delay antigen presentation and the onset of immune cell responses mediated by $CD4^+$ T lymphocytes for 4 to 8 weeks. Infected macrophages produce cytokines that attract monocytes, other alveolar macrophages, and neutrophils. Eventually, delayed hypersensitivity as a measure of specific T cell immunity can be detected. Macrophages activated by T cell–produced cytokines such as gamma interferon result in a tuberculous granuloma containing Langhans giant cells—fused macrophages forming around tuberculous antigen. A form of incomplete necrosis can occur termed "caseous necrosis." If the bacterial replication is not controlled initially at the site of infection, the bacilli enter local draining lymph nodes. This leads to lymphadenopathy, a characteristic manifestation of primary TB. The lesion produced at the initial site of lung infection and lymph node involvement is called the Ghon complex (Fig. 7.5). Further dissemination may occur through the bloodstream.

In 90% of individuals the infection will be contained for their lifetime, although viable organisms persist, and the infection will be labelled latent TB or LTBI (Fig. 7.6). In 4% to 5% of individuals, mycobacteria will continue to multiply and spread within the lung and through the bloodstream to other sites, resulting in symptomatic infection usually within 1 year of infection. This is termed primary infection. In another 5% of people who have LTBI, reactivation will occur years later, sometimes triggered by the development of an immunocompromised state such as HIV or older age. A typical site is the posterior apical region of the lungs. Patients with LTBI have a very low number of organisms and do not transmit to other people.

Diagnosis

The diagnosis of LTBI depends on a positive QuantiFERON-TB Gold test (IGRA), which is an in vitro ELISA interferon release assay to MTB antigens, or a positive tuberculin skin test. The Mantoux skin test is an intradermal injection of 0.1 mL of purified protein derivative (PPD) tuberculin into the forearm. The diameter of induration at the injection site is measured 48 to 72 hours later. Both tests have a high sensitivity to previous infection (approximately 90%), but both may be negative in active disease. The IGRA test has the advantages of not requiring a second visit, not being reactive in individuals who had previously received bacillus Calmette-Guérin (BCG) vaccine, and not being dependent on the subjectivity of measurement.

The diagnosis of active TB depends on the identification of the organism in sputum, other body fluids such as cerebrospinal fluid (CSF) or urine, or in tissue as well as growth of MTB in culture. The mycobacteria can be identified as small, beaded rods that are acid fast by Ziehl-Neelsen or Kinyoun stain. Nucleic acid amplification testing (NAAT) is superseding older staining techniques because of its ease of testing and accuracy. One example is Xpert MTB/Rif testing, which can also give information on resistance. Other helpful clinical information for making the diagnosis includes history (e.g., chronic cough, fever and night sweats, weight loss), potential exposures (e.g., household contact or country of origin), imaging (e.g., chest radiograph showing posterior upper lobe infiltrates with or without cavitation), and laboratory data (e.g., anemia of chronic disease).

Neither tuberculin skin testing nor IGRA distinguish between active disease and latent infection. Additionally, patients with primary infection or reactivation may be anergic and have a negative test. Patients who are latently infected have a positive test but do not have active disease (no signs or symptoms).

Clinical Manifestations
Primary Infection

Primary infection with MTB is usually asymptomatic, although mild symptoms with fever, cough, and mid-lung field infiltrates may occur. With the onset of specific immunity as indicated by conversion of TB skin test or IGRA test, symptoms resolve and the patient may be left with a small parenchymal scar.

烟肼。美国的肺结核发病率一直在下降，直到20世纪80年代，由于HIV感染和静脉注射毒品的增加，发病率有所上升。随着抗逆转录病毒治疗的有效实施，发病率又呈下降趋势。例如，美国的发病人数从1993年的约25 000例降至2018年的9025例。70%的病例为非美国出生的人，大约一半的病例是在抵达美国10年或10年以上后确诊的，这与之前获得的结核感染再次激活的情况一致。病例主要集中在少数种族，包括西班牙裔、美国印第安人/阿拉斯加原住民、亚裔和黑人。危险因素包括糖尿病、酒精和药物滥用、HIV感染、无家可归和监禁。

患有肺部疾病的患者通过咳嗽、打喷嚏、大声喊叫或唱歌将MTB气溶胶化，随后被易感个体吸入，则发生感染。直径1~5 μm的小型传染性颗粒可以在空气中持续存在，尤其是在封闭空间内，而且只需极少量的传染性颗粒就能造成感染。家庭接触者尤其处于高风险之中，高达50%的家庭接触者可能被感染。无家可归者、收容所和监狱等集体居住环境曾发生过疫情暴发。

全球范围内，结核病是十大死因之一，也是由感染导致的头号死因。2018年，有1000万人患结核病，150万人死于结核病，25.1万人同时感染了HIV。令人鼓舞的是，从2000年到2018年，结核病的死亡率下降了42%。48.4万人患耐药结核病（多耐药结核病或MDR，定义为对异烟肼和利福平两种最有效的药物耐药），其中6.2%的人患广泛耐药结核病（XDRTB，定义为对异烟肼、利福平、氟喹诺酮类药物以及二线注射药物都耐药）。新病例中有66%发生在印度、中国、印度尼西亚、菲律宾、巴基斯坦、尼日利亚、孟加拉国和南非。快速诊断测试（如Xpert MTB/RIF）已广泛使用，2017年新确诊病例的全球治疗成功率达到了85%。对于耐药结核，新型药物如贝达喹啉开始投入使用。目前，有14种疫苗正在临床试验中。

微生物学

MTB是一种需氧的、无动力的分枝杆菌，属于分枝杆菌科，其细胞壁富含高分子量的脂质。其增殖缓慢，需15~20 h，而大多数细菌的增殖时间少于1 h。人类是唯一的宿主。在痰液中，通过抗酸染色（如齐-内染色或冷染色）或更常见的核酸扩增可以鉴定出这种病原体。Xpert MTB/RIF是一种自动化测试，可以鉴定MTB并检测该菌是否对利福平产生抗药性，利福平是最常用且有效的抗结核药物之一。MTB在固体培养基上生长需要3~8周，而在液体培养基上则需要20天。为了确定分离株的完整敏感性，需要进行菌体培养。

病理学

当传染性微粒到达肺泡并被巨噬细胞吞噬时，就会发生感染。MTB能够抵抗巨噬细胞和中性粒细胞的破坏，在吞噬体内存活并进行胞内增殖，部分原因是其产生超氧化物歧化酶等保护机制，这种酶可以中和杀菌分子超氧阴离子。此外，结核杆菌似乎会将抗原提呈和由$CD4^+$ T细胞介导的免疫细胞反应延迟4~8周的时间。受感染的巨噬细胞会释放吸引单核细胞、其他肺泡巨噬细胞和中性粒细胞的细胞因子。最终，可以检测到作为特异性T细胞免疫指标的迟发型超敏反应。由T细胞产生的细胞因子如γ干扰素激活的巨噬细胞会导致含有朗汉斯巨细胞的结核性肉芽肿形成——这些巨噬细胞围绕结核抗原融合，病变出现一种不完全坏死，称为干酪样坏死。如果最初感染部位的细菌复制未得到控制，结核杆菌会进入局部引流的淋巴结，导致淋巴结肿大，这是原发性结核病的一个特征表现。在肺部感染原发病灶和淋巴结受累处形成的病变称为冈氏综合征（图7.5）。还可以通过血液进一步播散。

虽然病原体仍存活，但90%个体感染终身都能得到控制，这种感染被称为潜伏结核或LTBI（图7.6）。在4%~5%的个体中，分枝杆菌会继续繁殖，并在肺部和血液中扩散到其他部位，通常在感染后一年内导致有症状的感染，这称为原发性感染。另外5%具有LTBI的个体可能会在几年后发生再激活，有时是由于免疫缺陷状态（如HIV感染）或年龄增大而引发的。典型的病变部位位于肺部的尖后叶。LTBI患者体内的细菌数量极低，不会传染给其他人。

诊断

LTBI的诊断依据为QuantiFERON-TB Gold测试（IGRA）结果阳性，或者结核菌素皮肤试验阳性，前者是一种体外ELISA方法，检测由MTB抗原刺激的干扰素释放水平。结核菌素皮肤试验是在前臂皮下注射0.1 ml结核菌素纯蛋白质衍生物（PPD）。48~72 h后测量注射部位的硬结直径。这两种测试对先前感染的敏感性都很高（约90%），但在活动性疾病中都可能呈阴性。IGRA测试的优点是不需要第二次就诊，不会对之前接种过的卡介苗（BCG）产生反应，且不依赖于测量者的主观性。

活动性结核病的诊断取决于在痰液、脑脊液（CSF）或尿液等其他体液或组织中鉴定或培养出MTB。通过齐-内染色或冷染色可显示分枝杆菌为具有抗酸性的串珠状小杆菌。核酸扩增试验（NAAT）因其检测简便、准确性高，正在取代旧的染色技术。Xpert MTB/Rif检测就是一个例子，还可提供耐药性信息。其他有助于诊断的临床信息包括病史（如慢性咳嗽、发热和盗汗、体重减轻）、潜在接触史（如家庭接触或原籍国）、影像学（如胸部X线片显示后上叶浸润伴或不伴空洞）和实验室检查数据（如慢性病贫血）。

结核菌素皮肤试验和IGRA都不能区分活动性疾病和潜伏感染。此外，先前感染或再激活的患者可能会是无变态反应性的，检测结果为阴性。潜伏感染的患者为上述检测呈阳性，但没有活动性疾病证据（无体征或症状）。

临床表现

原发感染

MTB的原发感染通常无症状，也可能出现轻微的症状，如发热、咳嗽和肺中野的浸润。当结核菌素皮肤试验或IGRA测试显示出特异性免疫形成时，患者症状会缓解，可能会留下小的肺实质瘢痕。

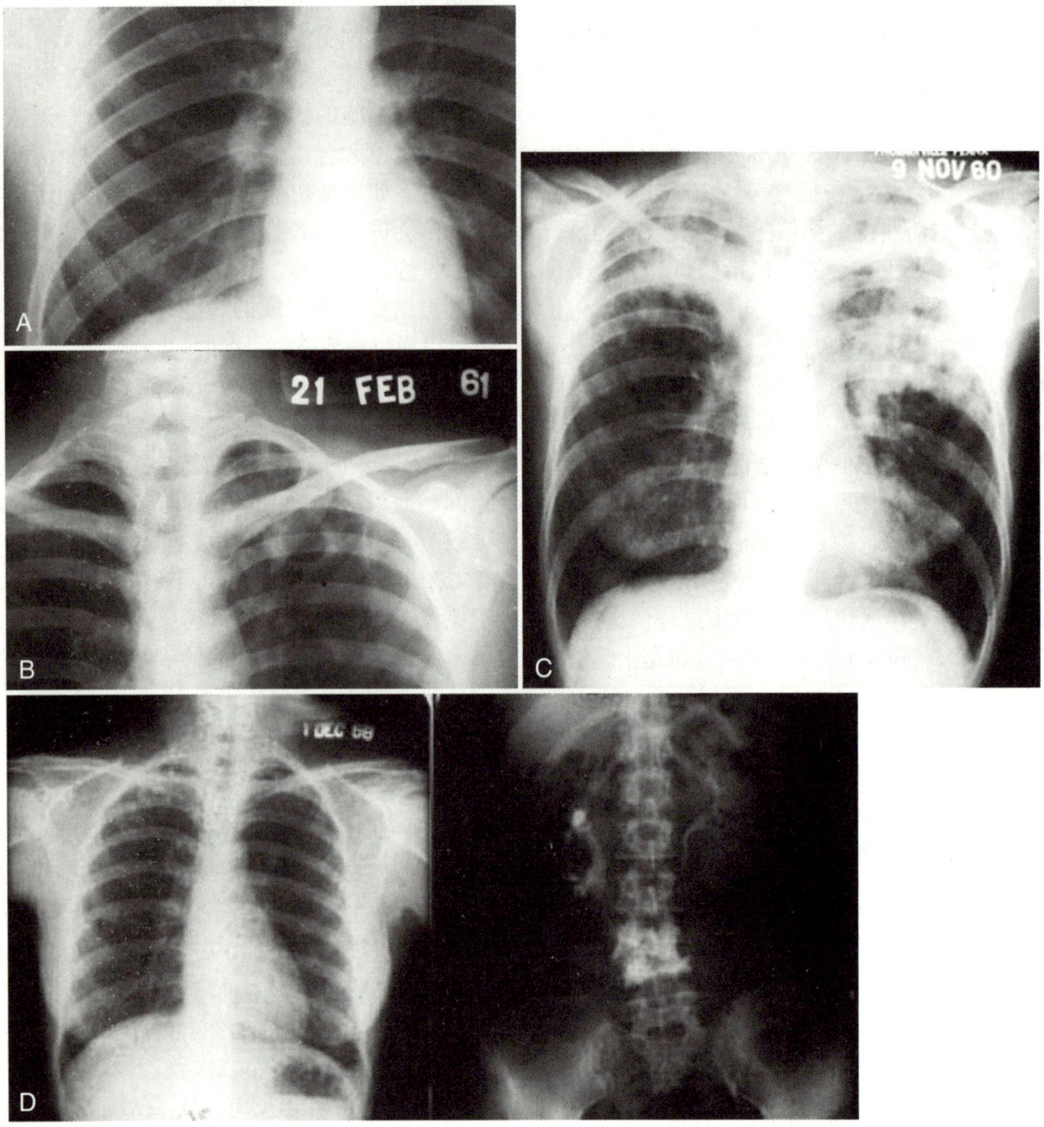

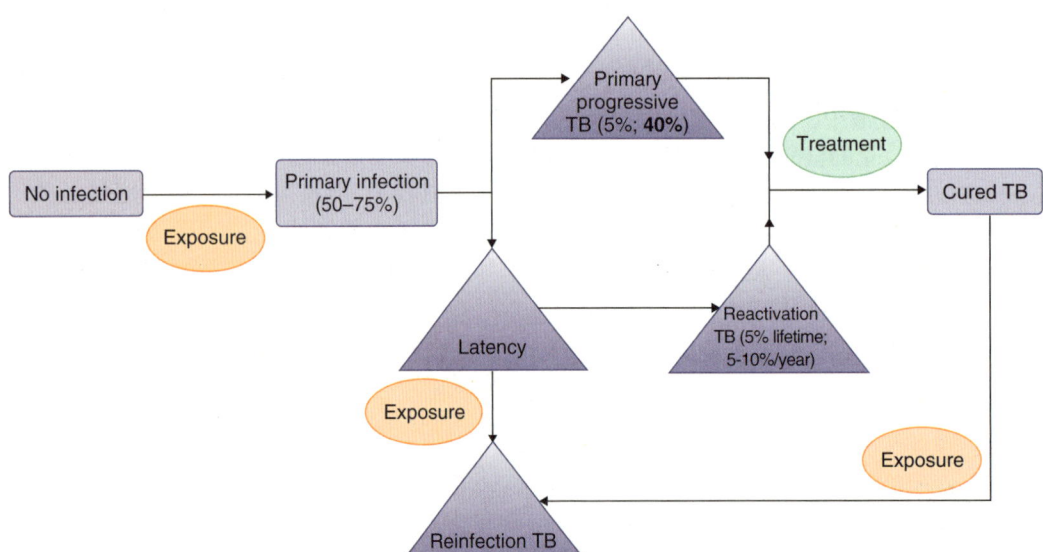

Fig. 7.5 (A) Ghon complex. (B) Moderately advanced pulmonary tuberculosis (TB). (C) Far advanced pulmonary TB. (D) Pulmonary *(left)* and extrapulmonary *(right)* TB.

Fig. 7.6 Natural history of TB. The proportion of individuals affected is shown in parentheses. Bolded figures are for HIV infection with severe immunosuppression. A number of medical risk factors besides HIV promote progression from *Mycobacterium tuberculosis* infection to disease.

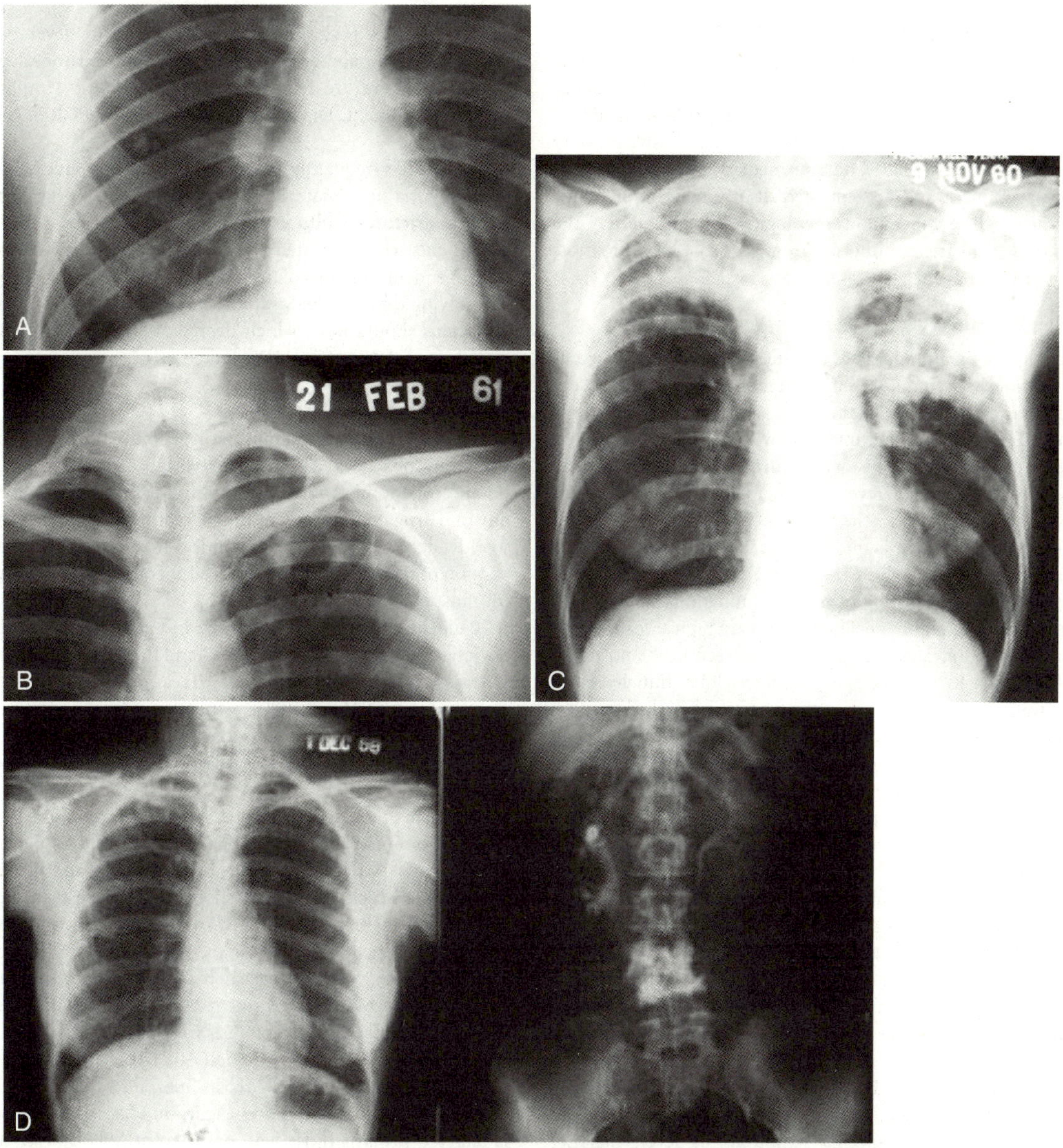

图 7.5 （A）冈氏综合征；（B）中度肺结核；（C）晚期肺结核；（D）肺结核（左）和肺外结核（右）

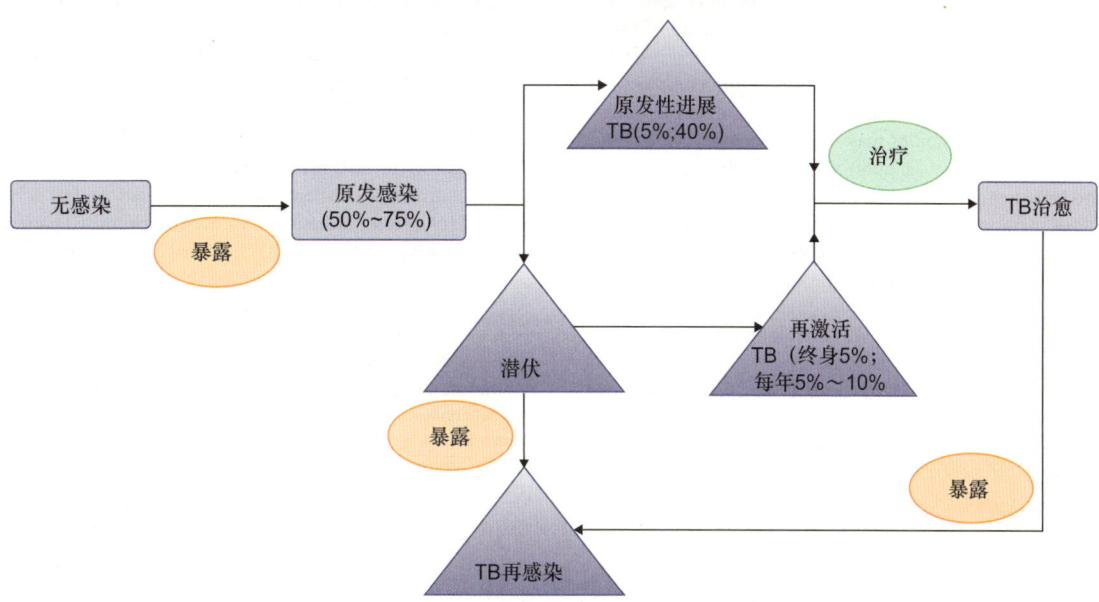

图 7.6 结核病的自然病史。括号内为患病人数比例。加粗部分为 HIV 感染并伴有严重免疫抑制。除 HIV 外，还有一些医疗风险因素会促进结核分枝杆菌感染发展为疾病

In approximately 4% to 5% of cases, the infection progresses within 1 to 2 years, manifesting as pulmonary infection either at the original site of infection or in the upper lobe as infiltrates with eventual cavitation. It is termed progressive primary tuberculosis. In high-incidence countries, most cases of pulmonary TB stem from progressive primary infection. In children particularly, hilar or mediastinal lymphadenopathy may be prominent and disseminated disease may occur manifesting as miliary TB or tuberculous meningitis. Young children, the elderly, and those who are immunocompromised (e.g., HIV) are most at risk for progressive primary disease.

Reactivation Infection

After 2 years, but often after decades, despite specific immunity, reactivation of previously latent foci of infection may occur, usually occurring as pulmonary disease. Patients may be asymptomatic with only radiograph findings of upper lobe infiltrates with or without cavitation (see Fig. 7.5) Patients give a history of chronic symptoms, usually greater than 3 weeks, of cough, fever, fatigue, night sweats, and weight loss. Hemoptysis and pleuritic chest pain occur in more advanced disease. Physical examination is often unrevealing. Fine, post-tussive rales may be heard at the apices. Chest radiograph findings are often more extensive than indicated by physical examination. Normocytic, normochromic anemia and hypoalbuminemia are typical for chronic disease. Classically, infiltrates and cavitation are seen in the posterior segment of an upper lobe or the apex of a lower lobe. Initially, cavities are thin walled without fluid but progress to thick-walled cavities. Patients who are immunocompromised, such as those with HIV, may have atypical findings with prominent lymphadenopathy or pulmonary infiltrates throughout the lungs. Patients with TB and cavities are highly infectious and should be placed in isolation immediately.

Extrapulmonary TB

Extrapulmonary TB usually results from a focus of organisms that have spread to extrapulmonary sites by either the bloodstream or lymphatics during initial phases of infection.

Pleural TB usually occurs 3 to 6 months after primary infection when a pleural-based nodule ruptures into the pleural space, producing pleuritic chest pain and a pleural effusion. There are few organisms in the pleural fluid. Pleural TB usually resolves spontaneously within months but is associated with a higher rate of subsequent active TB.

Miliary TB occurs when MTB disseminates widely in the bloodstream, often with nonspecific symptoms of fever, malaise, weight loss, and night sweats without localizing signs. Chest radiograph or CT scan, which has greater sensitivity, may show many small opacities up to 1 mm in size, resembling millet seeds—hence the name miliary—throughout all lung fields. Risk for dissemination is greatest in the very young, very old, and those who are immunocompromised. Physical examination may reveal lymphadenopathy and hepatosplenomegaly. Laboratory abnormalities may include anemia, a leukemoid reaction, and abnormal liver function tests. Mortality is high if the diagnosis and treatment are delayed.

Tuberculous meningitis typically presents over the space of several weeks with fever, stiff neck and headache. Cranial nerve abnormalities such as a VI nerve palsy may be seen. The CSF is characterized by a lymphocytic cell response, low sugar, and high albumin. Mortality is high, particularly if patients present with a prolonged course and have altered consciousness and neurologic findings.

Vertebral TB (also known as Pott disease) involves two adjacent vertebrae with destruction of the intervening disc in the lower thoracic or lumbar spine (see Fig. 7.5). Paraspinal abscess develops frequently. The differential diagnosis includes staphylococcal vertebral osteomyelitis. Bone biopsy may be necessary to establish the diagnosis.

Tuberculous peritonitis is characterized by fever, weight loss, and abdominal pain, either chronic or acute. Peritoneal fluid is exudative but there are few organisms. Mesenteric lymphadenopathy may be prominent. Diagnosis may be made by PCR or biopsy of the peritoneum.

Renal TB is frequently asymptomatic, the only clue being persistent sterile pyuria or hematuria. CT imaging shows cortical scarring and ureteral strictures. Cultures of the urine are positive.

Patients with untreated HIV and low CD4 T cell counts, particularly in endemic regions of the world, are at high risk for acquiring HIV and having disseminated, rapidly advancing TB with high mortality. Clinicians should have a high degree of suspicion for TB and other mycobacterial disease in AIDS patients.

Treatment and Prevention

TB requires prolonged therapy because of the slow multiplication rate of the mycobacteria. Also, multiple drugs are used to treat active TB because of the high rate of resistance each MTB population has to any one drug and because of the increasing rate of resistance of MTB worldwide. Since adherence is critical to successful therapy and prevention of resistance, direct observed therapy (DOT) is recommended for most patients.

Guidelines for treatment can be found at the American Thoracic Society/Centers for Disease Control and Prevention and the Infectious Diseases Society of America: Treatment of Drug-Susceptible Tuberculosis (2016). Initial treatment for most forms of TB in the United States includes isoniazid, rifampin, pyrazinamide, and ethambutol for 2 months and then isoniazid and rifampin for 4 to 6 months longer.

Regimens need to be adjusted for resistance and if there is resistance, it is important to never add one drug to a failing regimen. Treatment of MDR TB is much more difficult and usually includes five drugs to which the isolate is susceptible. This usually includes first-line drugs to which the organism is susceptible, a fluoroquinolone, an injectable such as amikacin, and second-line drugs such as ethionamide or PAS. Newer drugs such as bedaquiline, an ATP inhibitor, have been approved for treatment of MDR-TB. Guidelines for treatment of drug-resistant tuberculosis were published in 2019. Treatment of extensively drug resistant TB (XDR-TB) is based on resistant-based testing and often uses drugs such as linezolid and clofazimine.

Treatment of LTBI requires exclusion of active disease. Prevention is targeted towards those who have recent MTB infection and those with a significant risk factor or comorbidities such as HIV or diabetes. LTBI is treated with a single drug because there are so few organisms within the body that it is unlikely that there is a preexisting spontaneous drug-resistant mutant. Standard regimens include isoniazid alone for 6 or 9 months or rifampin alone for 4 months.

Prognosis

The prognosis for early primary and reactive pulmonary TB with appropriate treatment is excellent. Advanced disease, central nervous system and miliary disease, disease in immunocompromised patients, and disease in those with MDR and XDR-TB have a more guarded prognosis.

SUGGESTED READINGS

American Thoracic Society/Centers for Disease Control and Prevention and the Infectious Diseases Society of America: Treatment of Drug-Resistant Tuberculosis, 2019.

American Thoracic Society/Centers for Disease Control and Prevention and the Infectious Diseases Society of America: Treatment of Drug-Susceptible Tuberculosis, 2016.

4%～5% 的病例在 1～2 年内感染进展，表现为肺部感染，可能在原发感染部位或上叶出现浸润并最终形成空洞。这被称为进展性原发性结核病。在高发病率国家，大多数肺结核病例源于进展性原发性感染。尤其是儿童，可能会出现明显的支气管旁或纵隔淋巴结肿大，而播散性病变可能表现为粟粒性结核或结核性脑膜炎。幼儿、老年人以及免疫缺陷者（如 HIV 感染者）最易患进展性原发性结核病。

再激活感染

2 年后，但多在几十年后，尽管特异性免疫仍存在，此前潜伏的感染灶可能会再激活，感染部位多在肺部。患者可能没有任何症状，仅有上叶浸润的影像学表现，伴或不伴有空洞（图 7.5）。患者可有咳嗽、发热、乏力、盗汗和体重减轻的慢性症状，通常超过 3 周。进展期患者会出现咯血和胸膜炎性胸痛。体格检查通常没有异常发现。肺尖处可听到细微的叩诊后啰音。胸部 X 线片检查往往比体格检查所显示的病变更为广泛。正细胞正色素性贫血和低白蛋白血症是慢性疾病的典型表现。典型的浸润和空洞见于上叶的后段或下叶背端。最初为薄壁空洞，不伴液平，后来发展为厚壁空洞。免疫力低下的患者，如 HIV 感染者，可能会出现淋巴结肿大或整个肺部的浸润。空洞性肺核的患者具有高度传染性，应立即隔离治疗。

肺外结核

肺外结核通常是由于感染初期病原体通过血液或淋巴管扩散到肺外部位形成的病灶。

胸膜结核通常发生于原发感染后的 3～6 个月，胸膜结节破裂入胸膜腔，产生胸膜炎性胸痛和胸腔积液。胸腔积液中的微生物很少。胸膜结核常会在数月内自行消退，但随后活动性结核的发病率较高。

当 MTB 在血液中广泛传播时，会发生粟粒性肺结核，常伴有发热、乏力、体重减轻和盗汗等非特异症状，无局部体征。胸部放射影像或 CT 扫描的敏感性较高，可在所有肺野见到许多 1 mm 大小的不透明病灶，形似粟粒，因此被称为"粟粒性"。年幼、年老和免疫力低下者发生播散的风险最大。体格检查可发现淋巴结肿大和肝、脾大。实验室异常包括贫血、类白血病反应和肝功能检测异常。如果延误诊断和治疗，死亡率很高。

结核性脑膜炎通常表现为持续数周的发热、颈部僵硬和头痛。可能会出现脑神经异常，如第六脑神经麻痹。脑脊液呈现淋巴细胞增多、低糖和高白蛋白的特点。死亡率很高，尤其是在病程较长、出现意识改变和神经系统症状时。

脊柱结核（又称 Pott 病）会累及两个相邻的椎体，出现下胸椎或腰椎的椎间盘破坏（图 7.5）。经常发生脊柱旁脓肿。鉴别诊断包括葡萄球菌性脊椎骨髓炎。可能需要行骨活检以确定诊断。

结核性腹膜炎的特点是发热、体重减轻和腹痛，可呈慢性或急性。腹腔积液为渗出液，但菌体很少。肠系膜淋巴结病变可能很显著。可通过 PCR 或腹膜活检进行诊断。

肾结核常常没有症状，唯一的线索是持续无菌性脓尿或血尿。CT 显示皮质瘢痕和输尿管狭窄。尿液培养呈阳性。

未经治疗的 HIV 感染者和 $CD4^+$ T 细胞计数较低的患者，尤其是在流行地区，感染 HIV 的风险很高，极有可能患上播散性、进展迅速、高死亡率的结核病。临床医生应高度警惕 ADIS 患者患结核病和其他分枝杆菌疾病的可能。

治疗和预防

TB 需要长期治疗，因为分枝杆菌的繁殖速度很慢。此外，由于每群 MTB 对任何一种药物的耐药率都很高，且全球 MTB 的耐药率也在不断上升，因此需要使用多种药物来治疗活动性结核病。坚持治疗是成功治疗和预防耐药的关键，因此建议大多数患者采用直接面视下督导化疗（DOT）。

可在美国胸科学会/疾病控制与预防中心以及美国传染病学会找到治疗指南：《药物敏感性结核病的治疗（2016）》。在美国，大多数结核病的初始治疗包括异烟肼、利福平、吡嗪酰胺和乙胺丁醇治疗 2 个月，然后异烟肼和利福平治疗 4～6 个月。

治疗方案需要根据细菌耐药性进行调整，如果已存在耐药性，重要的是永远不要在失败的治疗方案中只添加一种药物。治疗 MDR-TB 更为复杂，通常需要使用对分离株敏感的五种药物。这通常包括对细菌敏感的一线药物、氟喹诺酮类药物、注射剂如阿米卡星以及二线药物，如乙胺丁醇或 PAS。新型药物如贝达喹啉（一种 ATP 抑制剂）已被批准用于治疗 MDR-TB。2019 年发布了治疗耐药结核病的指南。广泛耐药结核病（XDRTB）的治疗方案应基于耐药检测结果，通常会使用利奈唑胺和氯法齐明等药物。

治疗 LTBI 需要排除活动性结核病。预防目标主要是近期感染了 MTB 的人群以及有显著危险因素或共病的个体，如 HIV 感染者或糖尿病患者。由于体内结核菌数量很少，不太可能出现自发的耐药突变体，所以 LTBI 通常采用单药治疗。标准治疗方案包括单药异烟肼 6 个月或 9 个月，或者单药利福平 4 个月。

预后

早期的原发性和再激活肺结核经适当治疗后，预后良好。晚期结核、中枢神经系统结核、粟粒性结核、免疫力低下患者的结核，以及 MDR 和 XDRTB 患者的预后较差。

推荐阅读

American Thoracic Society/Centers for Disease Control and Prevention and the Infectious Diseases Society of America: Treatment of Drug-Resistant Tuberculosis, 2019.

American Thoracic Society/Centers for Disease Control and Prevention and the Infectious Diseases Society of America: Treatment of Drug-Susceptible Tuberculosis, 2016.

Austrian R, Gold J: Pneumococcal bacteremia with especial reference to bacteremic pneumococcal pneumonia, Ann Intern Med 60:760–776, 1964.

Fine M, Auble T, Yealy D: A prediction rule to identify low-risk patients with community acquired pneumonia, N Engl J Med 336:243–250, 1997.

Griffin M, Zhu Y, Moore M: U.S. Hospitalizations for pneumonia after a decade of pneumococcal vaccination, N Engl J Med 369:155–163, 2013.

Kyaw M, Lynfield R, Schaffner W: Effect of introduction of the pneumococcal conjugate vaccine on drug-resistant streptococcus pneumonia, N Engl J Med 354:1455–1463, 2006.

Lim WS, Van der Eerden MM, Laing R: Defining community acquired pneumonia severity on presentation to hospital: an international derivation and validation study, Thorax 58:377–382, 2003.

Austrian R, Gold J: Pneumococcal bacteremia with especial reference to bacteremic pneumococcal pneumonia, Ann Intern Med 60:760–776, 1964.

Fine M, Auble T, Yealy D: A prediction rule to identify low-risk patients with community acquired pneumonia, N Engl J Med 336:243–250, 1997.

Griffin M, Zhu Y, Moore M: U.S. Hospitalizations for pneumonia after a decade of pneumococcal vaccination, N Engl J Med 369:155–163, 2013.

Kyaw M, Lynfield R, Schaffner W: Effect of introduction of the pneumococcal conjugate vaccine on drug-resistant streptococcus pneumonia, N Engl J Med 354:1455–1463, 2006.

Lim WS, Van der Eerden MM, Laing R: Defining community acquired pneumonia severity on presentation to hospital: an international derivation and validation study, Thorax 58:377–382, 2003.

8

Infections of the Heart and Blood Vessels

Raul Macias Gil, Cheston B. Cunha

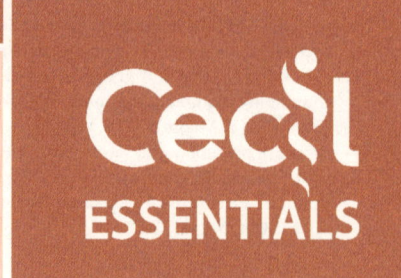

INFECTIVE ENDOCARDITIS

Definition

Infective endocarditis (IE) is an infection of the endocardium involving one or more cardiac valves or, less commonly, the mural endocardium. The pathologic lesion of IE is the vegetation (infected platelet and fibrin thrombus). The pathologic findings of IE were first described in 1646 by Lazare Rivière, a French physician at the University of Montpellier. At autopsy, Rivière described "small round outgrowths resembling the lungs in texture, the largest of which was about the size of a hazelnut, which blocked the aortic valve." The term *endocarditis* was first used in 1835 by the French physician Jean-Baptiste Bouillaud, but it was not until the 1880s that Sir William Osler was able to synthesize many of the prior clinical, pathologic, and microbiologic findings into a unified description of the disease.

Over the past 6 decades, the epidemiology, risk factors, and treatment of endocarditis have changed significantly. In the pre-antibiotic era, IE was uniformly fatal. Since the advent of antibiotics and valve replacement surgery, IE can be effectively treated and mortality can be significantly reduced, provided the diagnosis is made early. Despite progress, new challenges continue to arise in diagnosis and treatment. As more patients undergo intravascular manipulation, have intracardiac or intravascular devices placed, and harbor more resistant organisms, effective therapy for IE remains a challenge.

Traditionally, IE has been classified, based on the acuteness of onset, as subacute bacterial endocarditis (SBE) or acute bacterial endocarditis (ABE). This classification reflects the virulence of the causative agent: *Staphylococcus aureus* is a common cause of ABE, whereas low-virulence organisms such as viridans streptococci are more likely to be the cause of SBE. IE may also be subdivided according to the nature of the involved valve, as native valve endocarditis (NVE) or prosthetic valve endocarditis (PVE), or by the number of valves involved (multivalvular IE). IE from invasive procedures is classified as health care–associated IE or nosocomial IE. Endocarditis may be further divided according to the causative organism. These categories are often combined (e.g., *S. aureus* tricuspid valve nosocomial ABE).

Epidemiology

SBE is most common in older adults, and over the last 50 years, the average age of patients diagnosed with IE has gradually increased. More than one half of all cases of IE occur in patients older than 50 years of age. Rheumatic heart disease has decreased in the modern era and is now a less common predisposing factor.

While the incidence of IE can have geographic variations in the United States, the overall annual incidence is approximately 12.7 cases per 100,000 persons. A significant increase from prior years has been seen in the elderly, but also in younger patients. Multiple studies have shown that this increase in the incidence of IE could be explained by the alarming numbers of intravenous drug users from the current opioid epidemic in the United States. The age-adjusted hospital admission rate has increased by 2.4% annually, mirroring this increase in incidence. SBE usually involves the mitral valve or, less commonly, the aortic valve. IE of the pulmonic valve is relatively rare, and right-sided ABE occurs primarily in intravenous drug abusers. Individuals with congenital heart disease may be predisposed to IE, depending on the lesion.

Pathogenesis

Normal cardiac endothelium is relatively resistant to bacterial invasion. If the cardiac endothelium is damaged, an uninfected platelet and fibrin thrombus may form. This nonbacterial thrombotic endocarditis may become infected due to bacteremia, forming a vegetation. Endothelial damage may result from degenerative valvular disease, rheumatic heart disease, congenital heart disease, or intracardiac instrumentation or devices.

Predisposing Cardiac Factors

Approximately 15% of patients diagnosed with NVE have underlying congenital heart disease. Of these diseases, tetralogy of Fallot has the highest IE potential. Other lesions that predispose to IE include ventricular septal defect, bicuspid valves, and coarctation of the aorta. Significant mitral valve regurgitation is the most important predisposing factor for IE, with mitral valve prolapse accounting for 20% of NVE cases. Degenerative valvular disease predisposes to SBE in the elderly, and the mitral valve is most frequently involved. Aortic valve IE is rare in hypertrophic cardiomyopathy or asymmetric septal hypertrophy.

Noncardiac Predisposing Factors

Some hosts, particularly intravenous drug abusers, are predisposed to IE. Illicit intravenous drug use can lead to valvular or endothelial damage. Bacteremia with skin, oral flora, or with other organisms contaminating the substance(s) to be injected can develop from the act of injecting the drug(s). Central venous catheters and intracardiac devices can cause endocardial injury, predisposing to IE. The most frequent nosocomial IE pathogens are *S. aureus*, coagulase-negative staphylococci, group D enterococci, and aerobic gram-negative bacilli. Infections with these organisms usually occur less than 1 month after the procedure. Nosocomial IE may affect normal or abnormal valves. Because ABE pathogens are more virulent, nosocomial IE is associated with a high mortality rate.

Low-virulence and noninvasive organisms (e.g., viridans streptococci) are the most common SBE pathogens. The SBE potential of

心脏和血管的感染

宁永忠　张利军　译　康梅　路明　审校　曹彬　通审

感染性心内膜炎

定义

感染性心内膜炎（IE）是一种涉及一个或多个心脏瓣膜的心脏内膜感染，或者不太常见的心室壁感染。IE 的病理损害是赘生物（感染的血小板和纤维蛋白血栓）。1646 年，法国蒙彼利埃大学医生 Lazare Rivière 首次描述了 IE 的病理结果。在尸检中，Rivière 描述了"质地类似肺的圆形小突起，其中最大的约榛子大小，堵塞了主动脉瓣"。心内膜炎一词于 1835 年由法国医生 Jean-Baptiste Bouillaud 首次使用，但直到 19 世纪 80 年代，William 奥斯勒爵士才将之前的许多临床、病理和微生物学结果综合成对该疾病的统一描述。

在过去 60 年里，心内膜炎的流行病学、危险因素和治疗方法发生了重大变化。在前抗生素时代，IE 是致命的。自从抗生素和瓣膜置换术问世以来，只要及早诊断，IE 可以得到有效治疗，死亡率显著降低。尽管我们在 IE 的诊断和治疗方面取得了很多进展，但仍不断面临新的挑战。尤其是随着越来越多的患者接受血管内操作，放置心脏内或血管内装置，并携带更加耐药的微生物，使得 IE 的有效治疗仍然是挑战。

传统上，根据发病的缓急程度，IE 分为亚急性细菌性心内膜炎（SBE）或急性细菌性心内膜炎（ABE）。这种分类方法反映了病原体的毒力：金黄色葡萄球菌是 ABE 的常见原因，而毒力较低的微生物，如草绿色链球菌，更有可能是 SBE 的原因。IE 也可以根据累及瓣膜的性质进一步分为自体瓣膜心内膜炎（NVE）或人工瓣膜心内膜炎（PVE），或根据累及的瓣膜数量细分（多瓣膜 IE）。侵入性手术引起的 IE 可分为医疗照护相关 IE 或医院获得性 IE。心内膜炎也可根据病因进一步划分。这些通常是综合性分类（例如，金黄色葡萄球菌三尖瓣医院获得性 ABE）。

流行病学

SBE 在老年患者最常见。在过去 50 年中，诊断为 IE 的患者平均年龄逐渐增加。超过一半的 IE 病例年龄在 50 岁以上。风湿性心脏病如今已经减少，不再是 IE 常见的易感因素。

IE 的发病率在美国存在地域差异，每年的总发病率约为 12.7 例 /10 万人。与前几年相比，老年患者的发病率明显增加，但年轻患者的发病率也有所增加。多项研究表明，IE 发病率增加与美国当前阿片类药物流行导致的数量惊人的静脉吸毒相关。经年龄调整后的住院率，每年增加 2.4%，也反映了发病率的增加。SBE 通常累及二尖瓣，或者不太常见的主动脉瓣。肺动脉瓣 IE 相对罕见，右心的 ABE 主要发生在静脉吸毒者。先天性心脏病患者可能容易患 IE，具体取决于病变情况。

发病机制

正常的心脏内皮对细菌入侵具有相对的抵抗力。如果心脏内皮受损，可形成未感染的无微生物的血小板和纤维蛋白血栓。这种非细菌性血栓性心内膜炎可能因菌血症而感染，形成赘生物。内皮损伤可能由退行性瓣膜病、风湿性心脏病、先天性心脏病或心内植入物或装置引起。

心脏诱发因素

诊断为自体瓣膜心内膜炎（NVE）的患者中，约 15% 有潜在的先天性心脏病。在这些疾病中以法洛四联症最为常见。其他易患 IE 的病变包括室间隔缺损、二尖瓣疾病和主动脉缩窄。严重的二尖瓣反流是 IE 最重要的诱发因素，二尖瓣脱垂占 NVE 病例的 20%。老年患者退行性瓣膜病变易发生 SBE，并且最常累及二尖瓣。主动脉瓣 IE 在肥厚型心肌病或非对称性室间隔肥厚中很少见。

非心脏诱发因素

还有些人群也易患 IE，特别是静脉吸毒者。非法静脉吸毒会导致瓣膜或内皮损伤。静脉吸毒可导致菌血症，细菌自来于皮肤、口腔，或污染的注射器。中心静脉导管和心内装置可导致心内膜损伤，此类患者也易患 IE。最常见的院内 IE 病原体是金黄色葡萄球菌、凝固酶阴性葡萄球菌、D 组肠球菌和需氧革兰氏阴性杆菌。这些微生物所致的感染通常发生在手术后 1 个月内。医院获得性 IE 可累及正常或异常的瓣膜。由于 ABE 的病原体毒性更强，因此医院获得性 IE 会导致更高的死亡率。

低毒力和非侵入性微生物（如草绿色链球菌）是 SBE 最常见的病原体。草绿色链球菌的荚膜有助于其黏附在受损的心脏瓣膜上，因此草绿色链球菌所致 SBE 的致病力与其荚膜的厚度直接相关。草绿色链球菌是口腔和胃肠道的正常定植菌。侵入性牙科手术经常引起一过性菌血症，可能导致不正常的受损心瓣膜

viridans streptococci is directly related to the thickness of the capsule, which permits adherence to damaged cardiac valves. Viridans streptococci are normal inhabitants of the mouth and gastrointestinal tract. Invasive dental procedures frequently cause transient bacteremias that may result in SBE on damaged but not normal cardiac valves. Transient bacteremias of viridans streptococci may form a vegetation in the sterile platelet and fibrin thrombus covering an area of damaged endothelium or intracardiac devices. The gastrointestinal or genitourinary tract is the usual source of bacteremia in cases of native valve SBE due to group D enterococci.

Diagnosis

The clinical diagnosis of IE relies on a combination of clinical, laboratory, and echocardiographic findings. Epidemiologic clues to the potential IE pathogens are outlined in Table 8.1. The most important finding in IE is the demonstration of continuous bacteremia, usually by multiple positive blood cultures. Table 8.2 contains the modified Duke criteria that are frequently used to predict the likelihood that a patient has IE.

Clinical Features

The cardinal clinical features of IE are fever (90% of cases) and heart murmur (85%). In the antibiotic era, fever may not be present if the patient has been taking antibiotics for another reason. Acute versus subacute presentation is determined by the virulence of the IE pathogen. SBE often manifests with sweats, malaise, and anorexia. The course of SBE tends to be more indolent and may be accompanied by back pain, joint pains (>50% of patients), or embolic stroke. As SBE progresses, circulating immune complexes may deposit in the kidney, causing interstitial nephritis, glomerulonephritis, and even renal failure. Osler nodes (painful, subcutaneous nodules on the distal pads of the fingers or toes), Janeway lesions (hemorrhagic, nonpainful macules on the palms and soles), and Roth spots (retinal hemorrhages with small central clearing) are classic findings related to microemboli and SBE immune-mediated vasculitis.

Patients with ABE tend to have a more fulminant course because of the greater virulence of the pathogen. The fever of ABE is usually high (>102° F) and is often accompanied by rigors. If there is mechanical dysfunction of the valve, symptoms of congestive heart failure will predominate. Often, a presenting feature of right-sided ABE is septic pulmonary emboli with pleuritic chest pain. The clinical findings of SBE and ABE are presented in Table 8.3.

Clinically, PVE may be considered as early (<2 months) or late (>2 months) following implantation of the prosthetic valve. Early PVE is caused by virulent pathogens (e.g., *S. aureus*) that infect the prosthetic valve before endothelialization is complete. Endothelialization of a mechanical valve is partially protective against transient bacteremias in late PVE. Over time, bioprosthetic valves have the same IE potential as mechanical ones.

Early PVE pathogens such as *S. aureus* and *Pseudomonas aeruginosa* are typically highly virulent and invasive. Late PVE more closely resembles SBE, is caused by less virulent pathogens, and has a more indolent course. The most common etiologic agents are coagulase-negative staphylococci, but viridans streptococci also cause late PVE.

Nosocomial IE results from invasive intravascular or intracardiac procedures that damage the endothelium or the valves; it can also be caused by direct extension of infection, such as from ABE associated with a pacemaker wire. The organisms causing nosocomial IE originate from the skin (e.g., *S. aureus*, coagulase-negative staphylococci), from gastrointestinal or genitourinary procedures (e.g., group D enterococci), or from central venous catheters, ports, or hemodialysis catheters (e.g., *Candida* spp, aerobic gram-negative bacilli). IE related to total parenteral nutrition (TPN) is most often caused by *Candida* spp; other TPN-associated fungemias cause IE less frequently. In intravenous drug abusers, tricuspid valve ABE is usually caused by *S. aureus* or *P. aeruginosa* (depending on the geography and drug-related materials).

An otherwise unexplained high-grade or continuous bacteremia and murmur should suggest IE. If blood cultures are negative but a murmur, vegetation, and peripheral manifestations of IE are present, a diagnosis of infectious culture-negative endocarditis (CNE) should be considered. Infectious CNE is caused by organisms that are difficult to culture, such as *Legionella* spp, *Brucella* spp, *Tropheryma whipplei*, and *Coxiella burnetii* (which produces Q fever). Legionnaires disease may cause NVE or PVE. CNE due to *Brucella* spp can be a difficult diagnosis, but an antecedent history of contact with livestock or consumption of unpasteurized dairy products should suggest the diagnosis, and echocardiography often reveals large vegetations. A difficult infectious CNE diagnosis is Q fever. Q fever SBE may be suggested by a history of animal contact. Clinical findings of Q fever are often present, but the diagnosis can be missed because Q fever vegetations are not easily visualized.

Laboratory Findings

The isolation of a microorganism(s) in blood cultures is crucial for the diagnosis and management of IE. At least two sets of blood cultures from two different peripheral veins should be obtained in patients with high suspicion for IE, especially those at high risk (e.g., PVE, intracardiac devices, prior history of IE, etc.). The likelihood of isolating a causative pathogen is higher in patients who are not actively taking or have not received antibiotics 2 weeks prior to collection of blood cultures. Most bacterial and even some fungal organisms can be isolated in standard blood cultures, except for pathogens known to cause CNE.

Diagnosis of *Legionella*-related IE is based on an antecedent pneumonia and elevated titers of urinary antigen. *Brucella*-related IE is confirmed by titers or by polymerase chain reaction or both. A clue to Q fever CNE is enhanced valve uptake on positron-emission tomography (PET) or computed tomography (CT), and such a result should prompt testing for Q fever.

With the advent of sophisticated microbiologic testing, HACEK organisms (*Haemophilus* spp, *Aggregatibacter actinomycetemcomitans* [formerly called *Actinobacillus actinomycetemcomitans*], *Cardiobacterium hominis*, *Eikenella corrodens*, and *Kingella kingae*) grow relatively rapidly and no longer manifest as CNE. Newer molecular-based tests using microbial cell-free DNA sequencing may allow improved diagnosis, and implementation of prompt targeted therapy.

With IE, many nonspecific laboratory abnormalities may occur (Table 8.4); when placed in the appropriate context, these can be a significant aid to diagnosis.

Imaging Studies

Echocardiography is an important element in diagnosis and management; it should be performed for all patients with suspected IE. In those with a low likelihood of having IE or small body habitus, a transthoracic echocardiogram (TTE) may be sufficient. Although TTE is often sufficient to screen for NVE, the "gold standard" remains transesophageal echocardiogram (TEE), which is more sensitive at detecting smaller vegetations, paravalvular abscess, and PVE. If the TTE or TEE demonstrates a vegetation but blood cultures remain negative, the diagnosis of infectious CNE should be considered. A tiered diagnostic approach to such cases is presented in Table 8.5.

Radiologic testing in IE is primarily focused on identifying complications of IE. Although echocardiography is still the preferred method for detecting vegetations, improvements in multislice CT scans have

发生 SBE。草绿色链球菌的一过性菌血症可使覆盖于受损内皮或心内装置表面的无菌性血小板和纤维蛋白血栓形成细菌性赘生物。由 D 组肠球菌引起的自体瓣膜 SBE，胃肠道或泌尿生殖道是菌血症的常见来源。

诊断

IE 的临床诊断依赖于临床、实验室和超声心动图的综合判断。表 8.1 概述了 IE 可能的病原体的流行病学线索。IE 中最重要的表现是持续性菌血症，通常由多次血培养阳性来确定。表 8.2 包含了修改后的杜克标准，该标准常用于预测 IE 的可能性。

临床特征

IE 的主要临床特征是发热（90%）和心脏杂音（85%）。在抗生素时代，如果患者因其他原因服用抗生素，可能会不发热。急性和亚急性表现由 IE 病原体的毒力决定。SBE 通常表现为多汗、全身不适和食欲减退。SBE 的病程往往更为缓慢，可能伴有背痛、关节疼痛（>50% 的患者）或栓塞性卒中。随着 SBE 的进展，循环免疫复合物可能沉积在肾，导致间质性肾炎、肾小球肾炎，甚至肾衰竭。奥斯勒结节（远端指腹或远端趾腹疼痛性皮下结节）、詹韦损害（手掌和足底无痛性出血性红斑）和罗特斑（视网膜上的出血斑，中心呈白色）是与微血栓栓子和 SBE 免疫介导的血管炎相关的典型表现。

如果病原体毒力强，ABE 患者往往呈暴发性病程。常有高热（>102℉），常伴寒战。如果瓣膜出现机械功能障碍，可主要表现为充血性心力衰竭的症状。右心 ABE 常见的特征是感染中毒性（脓毒性）肺栓塞伴胸膜炎性胸痛。SBE 和 ABE 的临床结果如表 8.3 所示。

临床上，PVE 可分为人工瓣膜植入后早期（<2 个月）或晚期（>2 个月以上）。早期 PVE 是在内皮化完成之前由毒力较强的病原（如金黄色葡萄球菌）感染人工瓣膜引起。机械瓣膜的内皮化对晚期 PVE 中的一过性菌血症具有部分保护作用。随着时间的推移，生物瓣膜与机械瓣膜具有相同的发生 IE 可能性。

早期 PVE 的病原，如金黄色葡萄球菌和铜绿假单胞菌，通常具有高毒力和侵袭性。晚期 PVE 更像 SBE，是由毒性较弱的微生物引起，并且具有更隐匿的过程。最常见病原是凝固酶阴性葡萄球菌，但草绿色链球菌也可引起晚期 PVE。

医院获得性 IE 是由损伤内皮或瓣膜的侵入性血管内或心脏内手术引起的；它也可能是由感染的直接扩散所致，例如起搏器导线相关的 ABE。引起医院获得性 IE 的微生物，可来源于皮肤（如金黄色葡萄球菌、凝固酶阴性葡萄球菌）、胃肠道或泌尿生殖道操作（如 D 组肠球菌）或中心静脉导管、输液港或血液透析导管（如念珠菌属、需氧革兰氏阴性杆菌）。与全胃肠外营养（TPN）相关的 IE 最常由念珠菌引起；TPN 相关的其他真菌血症导致则 IE 则并不常见。静脉吸毒者三尖瓣 ABE 通常由金黄色葡萄球菌或铜绿假单胞菌引起（取决于具体部位和注射药物的相关器材）。

不能用其他原因解释的高级别或持续性菌血症伴心脏杂音提示有 IE［译者注：high-grade bacteremia 译作高级别菌血症。指血液定量培养显示浓度超过 100 CFU/ml 的菌血症。见文献 J Clin Microbiol. 2009，47（10）：3255-3260. J Clin Microbiol. 1987，25（2）：207-210. 国内不做定量培养，这个词用得少］。如果血液培养阴性，但存在心脏杂音、赘生物和 IE 的外周表现，则应考虑诊断为感染性培养阴性心内膜炎（CNE）。感染性 CNE 是由难以培养的微生物引起，如军团菌属、布鲁菌属、惠普尔养障体和贝纳柯克斯体（可引起 Q 热）。军团病可引起 NVE 或 PVE。布鲁菌引起的 CNE 可能是一种很难诊断的疾病，但先前与牲畜接触或食用未经巴氏消毒的乳制品的病史，可提示诊断，超声心动图通常显示大片赘生物。一种难以诊断的感染性 CNE 是 Q 热。Q 热 SBE 可能有动物接触史的提示。Q 热患者经常有相应临床症状，但由于不易看到 Q 热赘生物，因此可能会漏诊。

实验室检查

血培养中微生物的分离对 IE 的诊断和处理至关重要。对于高度怀疑 IE 的患者，尤其是高风险患者（如 PVE、心内装置、既往 IE 病史等），应至少从两个不同的外周静脉位点采集两套血培养。没有正在应用或在采集血培养前 2 周没有用过抗生素治疗的患者，分离到病原的可能性更高。除了已知导致 CNE 的病原外，大多数细菌甚至一些真菌都可以在标准血培养中分离培养出来。

军团菌相关 IE 的诊断，一般基于先前的肺炎和尿抗原滴度升高。布鲁菌相关 IE 可通过血清抗体滴度或聚合酶链反应或两者结合来确定。Q 热 CNE 的一个线索是正电子发射体层成像（PET）的瓣膜摄取增高或 CT 上的瓣膜强化，如果出现上述结果，提示需要进行 Q 热相关检查。

随着复杂的微生物学检查的出现，HACEK 群微生物［嗜血杆菌属、伴放线凝聚杆菌（以前称为伴放线杆菌）、人心杆菌、啮蚀艾肯菌和金氏杆菌］生长相对较快，不再表现为 CNE。使用新的基于微生物游离 DNA 测序的分子检测方法，可以改善诊断，实施及时的靶向治疗［译者注：HACEK 群的菌种范围目前已经扩展。见 Expert Rev Anti Infect Ther. 2016，14（5）：523-530. 增加的菌种包括：嗜沫凝聚杆菌、副嗜沫凝聚杆菌、惰性聚集杆菌、瓣膜心杆菌、反硝化金菌］。

IE 可能会有许多非特异的实验室异常表现（表 8.4）；在适当的场景中，这些异常表现可对诊断有重大帮助。

影像学研究

超声心动图是诊断和处理的重要组成部分；对所有疑似 IE 的患者均应进行超声心动图检查。对于那些 IE 可能性较低或体型小的患者，可进行经胸超声心动图（TTE）检查。尽管经胸超声心动通常足以筛查 NVE，但"金标准"仍然是经食管超声心动图（TEE），它在检测较小的赘生物、瓣周脓肿和 PVE 时更敏感。如果 TTE 或 TEE 显示有赘生物，但血液培养仍呈阴性，则应考虑诊断为感染性 CNE。表 8.5 列出了此类病例的分层诊断方法。

TABLE 8.1 Clues to the Likely Pathogen in Infective Endocarditis

Epidemiologic Features	Pathogens	Epidemiologic Features	Pathogens
Intravenous drug abuse	Staphylococcus aureus Pseudomonas aeruginosa β-Hemolytic streptococci Aerobic GNB Polymicrobial Fungi	Diabetes mellitus	S. aureus β-Hemolytic streptococci S. pneumoniae
		Early PVE	S. aureus Aerobic GNB Fungi Corynebacterium spp
Indwelling cardiovascular device	S. aureus CoNS Aerobic GNB Corynebacterium spp	Late PVE	CoNS S. aureus Viridans streptococci Enterococcus spp Corynebacterium spp Legionella spp
Genitourinary disorders, infection, manipulation	Enterococcus spp Group B streptococci (Streptococcus agalactia) Aerobic GNB		
Chronic skin disorders	S. aureus β-Hemolytic streptococci	Dog or cat exposure	Bartonella spp Pasteurella spp Capnocytophaga spp
Poor dentition, dental procedures	Viridans streptococci Nutritionally variant streptococci (Abiotrophia spp, Granulicatella spp) Gemella spp HACEK organisms[a]	Contact with contaminated milk or infected farm animals	Brucella spp Coxiella burnetii (Q fever) Erysipelothrix rhusiopathiae
		Homelessness	Bartonella spp
		Human immunodeficiency virus infection	S. pneumoniae Salmonella spp S. aureus
Alcoholic cirrhosis	Streptococcus pneumoniae Bartonella spp L. monocytogenes β-Hemolytic streptococci	Pneumonia and meningitis[b]	S. pneumoniae
		Solid organ transplants	S. aureus Aspergillus fumigatus Enterococcus spp Candida spp
Burns	S. aureus Aerobic GNB P. aeruginosa Fungi	Gastrointestinal lesions	Streptococcus bovis Enterococcus spp

Modified from Baddour LM, Wilson WR, Bayer AS, et al: Infective endocarditis: diagnosis, antimicrobial therapy, and management of complications: a statement for healthcare professionals from the Committee on Rheumatic Fever, Endocarditis, and Kawasaki Disease, Council on Cardiovascular Disease in the Young, and the Councils on Clinical Cardiology, Stroke, and Cardiovascular Surgery and Anesthesia, American Heart Association; endorsed by the Infectious Diseases Society of America, Circulation 111:e394-e433, 2005.
CoNS, Coagulase-negative staphylococci; GNB, gram-negative bacilli; PVE, prosthetic valve endocarditis.
[a]HACEK organisms: Haemophilus spp, Aggregatibacter actinomycetemcomitans, Cardiobacterium hominis, Eikenella corrodens, and Kingella kingae.
[b]With alcoholic cirrhosis.

allowed chest CT to detect vegetations and valvular abnormalities in addition to the septic emboli seen in right-sided IE. Magnetic resonance imaging (MRI) of the spine is useful in patients with IE who report back pain; it is the preferred method to detect the presence of vertebral osteomyelitis caused by IE. Mental status changes or new focal neurologic signs should prompt CT or MRI imaging of the head to assess for septic emboli to the brain. Although it is less invasive than TEE, cardiac MRI often lacks the special resolution to detect smaller vegetations; however, it may be helpful in identifying aortic root pseudoaneurysms, sinus of Valsalva aneurysms, and embolic vascular lesions.

Differential Diagnosis and Mimics

The diagnosis of SBE is based an otherwise unexplained high-grade or continuous bacteremia caused by a known endocarditis pathogen plus a cardiac vegetation. Depending on the duration before presentation (usually 1 to 3 months), IE may be accompanied by peripheral manifestations such as Osler nodes, Janeway lesions, splinter hemorrhages, or conjunctival hemorrhages. Splenomegaly or embolic phenomena may also accompany SBE. However, peripheral manifestations that are seen in SBE may also be present in other disorders. Before ascribing peripheral manifestations to SBE, physicians need to rule out other systemic disorders and confirm the diagnosis of SBE.

Clinically, the disorders most likely to mimic SBE are Libman-Sacks endocarditis (associated with systemic lupus erythematosus [SLE]), marantic endocarditis (caused by a malignancy, usually lymphoma, lung cancer, or pancreatic cancer), and atrial myxoma. Myocarditis of any etiology may mimic SBE with fever, murmur, and peripheral embolic phenomena. Cardiomegaly, which is usually present with myocarditis, is typically absent with SBE. Leukopenia and thrombocytopenia may be clues to viral myocarditis, and either finding argues against a diagnosis of SBE. Cardiac echocardiography shows myocarditis but no vegetations, and bacteremia is not present.

SLE, particularly between flares, may mimic SBE with low-grade fevers, murmur, peripheral manifestations, and splenomegaly. Laboratory findings in SLE include the anemia of chronic disease and a mildly to moderately elevated erythrocyte sedimentation rate (ESR). Even if Libman-Sacks vegetations are present, SBE is rare in

表8.1 感染性心内膜炎可能病原的线索

流行病学因素	病原体	流行病学因素	病原体
静脉吸毒	金黄色葡萄球菌 铜绿假单胞菌 乙型溶血性链球菌 需氧GNB 多种微生物的混合感染 真菌	糖尿病	金黄色葡萄球菌 乙型溶血性链球菌 肺炎链球菌
		早期PVE	金黄色葡萄球菌 需氧GNB 真菌 棒状杆菌属
心血管植入物	金黄色葡萄球菌 CoNS 需氧GNB 棒状杆菌属	晚期PVE	CoNS 金黄色葡萄球菌 草绿色链球菌 肠球菌属 棒状杆菌属 军团菌属
泌尿生殖道疾病，感染，医疗操作	肠球菌属 B组链球菌（无乳链球菌） 需氧GNB		
慢性皮肤疾病	金黄色葡萄球菌 乙型溶血性链球菌	狗或猫暴露接触	巴尔通体属 巴斯德菌属 二氧化碳嗜纤维菌属
口腔卫生状态差，牙科操作	草绿色链球菌 营养变异链球菌（乏养菌属、颗粒链菌属） 孪生球菌属 HACEK群微生物[a]	与污染的牛奶或感染的农场动物相接触	布鲁菌属 贝纳柯克斯体（Q热） 猪红斑丹毒丝菌
		无家可归的流浪者	巴尔通体属
酒精性肝硬化	肺炎链球菌 巴尔通体属 单核细胞增生李斯特菌 乙型溶血性链球菌	HIV感染	肺炎链球菌 沙门菌属 金黄色葡萄球菌
		肺炎和脑膜炎[b]	肺炎链球菌
烧伤	金黄色葡萄球菌 需氧GNB 铜绿假单胞菌 真菌	实体器官移植	金黄色葡萄球菌 烟曲霉 肠球菌属 念珠菌属
		胃肠道损伤	牛链球菌 肠球菌属

改编自 Baddour LM, Wilson WR, Bayer AS, et al: Infective endocarditis: diagnosis, antimicrobial therapy, and management of complications: a statement for healthcare professionals from the Committee on Rheumatic Fever, Endocarditis, and Kawasaki Disease, Council on Cardiovascular Disease in the Young, and the Councils on Clinical Cardiology, Stroke, and Cardiovascular Surgery and Anesthesia, American Heart Association; endorsed by the Infectious Diseases Society of America, Circulation 111: e394-e433, 2005.
CoNS，凝固酶阴性葡萄球菌；GNB，革兰氏阴性杆菌；PVE，人工瓣膜心内膜炎。
[a] HACEK群细菌包括：嗜血杆菌属、伴放线凝聚杆菌、人心杆菌、啮蚀艾肯菌和金氏杆菌。
[b] 伴酒精性肝硬化。

IE 的影像学检查，主要聚焦在识别 IE 的并发症。尽管超声心动图仍然是检查赘生物的首选方法，但随着多层螺旋 CT 扫描技术的进步，使胸部 CT 能够检查到赘生物和瓣膜异常，以及右心 IE 中出现的感染中毒性（脓毒性）栓塞。脊柱磁共振成像（MRI）对主诉背痛的 IE 患者很有价值；这是用来检测 IE 引起的脊椎骨髓炎的推荐方法。当出现意识状态变化或新发局灶性神经系统体征时，应进行头部 CT 或 MRI 检查，以评估是否有感染中毒性（脓毒性）脑栓塞。虽然心脏 MRI 比经食管超声心动图的创伤要小，但它对检测较小赘生物缺乏特殊分辨率；然而，它可能有助于识别主动脉根部假性动脉瘤、瓦尔萨尔瓦窦动脉瘤（译者注：即主动脉窦瘤）和栓塞性血管病变。

鉴别诊断与容易混淆的情况

SBE 的诊断是基于已知心内膜炎病原体引起的无法解释的高级别或持续性菌血症和心脏赘生物。根据发病前的持续时间（通常为 1～3 个月），IE 可能伴有外周表现，如奥斯勒结节、詹韦损害、视网膜裂片样出血或结膜出血。脾大或栓塞现象也可能伴随 SBE。然而，SBE 的外周表现也可见于其他疾病。在将外周表现归因于 SBE 之前，医生需要排除其他系统性疾病，并确诊 SBE。

临床上，最有可能与 SBE 混淆的疾病是 Libman-Sacks 心内膜炎（与系统性红斑狼疮相关）、消耗性心内膜炎（由恶性肿瘤引起，通常是淋巴瘤、肺癌或胰腺癌）和心房黏液瘤。任何病因的心肌炎都可能有发热、心脏杂音和外周栓塞现象等类似 SBE 的临床表现。心肌炎通常表现为心脏肥大，但 SBE 通常没有心脏肥大。白细胞减少和血小板减少可能是病毒性心肌炎的线索，这两种情况都不支持 SBE 的诊断。心脏超声心动图显示心肌炎，但没有赘生物，也没有菌血症。

SLE，尤其是两次发作之间，可能与 SBE 的症状相同，如低热、心脏杂音、外周表现和脾大。SLE 的实验室检查结果包括慢性疾病引起的贫血和轻中度的红细胞沉降率（ESR）升高。即使存在 Libman-Sacks 赘生物，SBE 在 SLE 中也是罕见的。狼疮发作时可有类

TABLE 8.2 Modified Duke Criteria for Diagnosis of Infective Endocarditis

Diagnostic Criteria

Definite IE (any of the following):
  Positive findings for IE in the pathology or microbiology of the vegetation
  Two major criteria
  One major and three minor criteria
  Five minor criteria
Possible IE (any of the following):
  One major and one minor criteria
  Three minor criteria
Not IE (any of the following):
  Definite alternative diagnosis or resolution with <4 days of antibiotic therapy
  Does not meet the criteria of possible IE

Major Criteria

Positive blood cultures for IE (any of the following):
  Typical microorganism for IE from two separate blood cultures:
  - Viridans streptococci, Streptococcus gallolyticus (formerly Streptococcus bovis biotype I), or the nutritional variant strains (Granulicatella spp and Abiotrophia defectiva)
  - HACEK group: Haemophilus spp, Aggregatibacter actinomycetemcomitans), Cardiobacterium hominis, Eikenella corrodens, and Kingella kingae
  - Staphylococcus aureus
  Community-acquired enterococci, in the absence of a primary focus
Persistently positive blood culture, defined as recovery of a microorganism consistent with IE from any of the following:
  Blood cultures drawn more than 12 hr apart
  All three or a majority of four or more separate blood cultures, with first and last drawn at least 1 hr apart
  [a]Single positive blood culture for Coxiella burnetii or antiphase I IgG antibody titer >1:800
Evidence of endocardial involvement
Positive echocardiogram for IE:
  [a]TEE is recommended in patients with prosthetic valves rated at least "possible IE" by clinical criteria, or with complicated IE (paravalvular abscess); TTE as first test in other patients
  Definition of positive echocardiogram (any of the following):
  - Oscillating intracardiac mass, on valve or supporting structures, or in the path of regurgitant jets, or on implanted material, in the absence of an alternative anatomic explanation
  - Abscess
  - New partial dehiscence of prosthetic valve
  New valvular regurgitation (increase in or change in preexisting murmur is not sufficient)

Minor Criteria ([a]Echocardiographic minor criteria have been eliminated)

Predisposition: predisposing heart condition or intravenous drug use
Fever: 38.0° C (100.4° F)
Vascular phenomena: major arterial emboli, septic pulmonary infarcts, mycotic aneurysm, intracranial hemorrhage, conjunctival hemorrhages, Janeway lesions
Immunologic phenomena: glomerulonephritis, Osler nodes, Roth spots, rheumatoid factor
Microbiologic evidence: positive blood culture but not meeting major criterion (excluding single positive cultures for coagulase-negative staphylococci and organisms that do not cause endocarditis) or serologic evidence of active infection with organism consistent with IE

Modified from Li JS, Sexton DJ, Mick N, et al: Proposed modifications to the Duke criteria for the diagnosis of infective endocarditis, Clin Infect Dis 30:633-638, 2000.
IE, Infective endocarditis; IgG, immunoglobulin G; TEE, transesophageal echocardiography; TTE, transthoracic echocardiography.
[a]Represents a change from the previously published Duke criteria.

SLE. A lupus flare may resemble ABE with high fevers (>102° F), tender fingertips (mimicking Osler nodes), and funduscopic findings of cotton-wool spots or Roth spots. Conjunctival and splinter hemorrhages are rare in SLE but common in SBE. Microscopic hematuria is the usual renal manifestation of SBE (i.e., focal glomerulonephritis), but full-blown nephritis with proteinuria and hematuria are typical of SLE renal involvement. Although clinical findings of SLE and SBE may overlap, SBE is ruled out by the absence of high-grade or continuous bacteremia.

Atrial myxomas may mimic SBE with fever, murmurs, and embolic phenomena (e.g., splinter hemorrhages). Highly elevated ESR levels are common with atrial myxomas, but biologically false-positive results on Venereal Disease Research Laboratory (VDRL) testing, elevated rheumatoid factors, and renal involvement are not seen. On TTE or TEE, atrial myxomas appear as masses or vegetations on the atrial surface rather than on a valve as in IE. SBE is ruled out by the absence of bacteremia.

Besides clinical mimics of SBE, there are also echocardiographic mimics, including papillary fibromas, thrombi, calcified valves, myxomatous degeneration, and marantic endocarditis. These disorders are usually unaccompanied by fever or bacteremia. The term *marantic endocarditis* refers to uninfected vegetations with a murmur and negative blood cultures that occur secondary to malignancy. Patients with marantic endocarditis are afebrile unless fever is caused by the underlying malignancy (e.g., lymphoma). The patient with marantic endocarditis due to lymphoma may have fever, splenomegaly, and other manifestations of SBE. Negative blood cultures effectively rule out IE. Infectious CNE (e.g., Q fever) may show little or no visible vegetations. Infectious CNE should be considered if fever, murmur, and vegetation are present along with peripheral manifestations of IE.

Treatment

Effective treatment of IE depends on the antibiotic susceptibility of the pathogen, the penetration of the antibiotic into the vegetation, and the appropriate duration of antibiotic therapy. Antibiotics selected for IE preferably should be bactericidal. In IE, the organisms are deeply embedded in the vegetation, and prolonged therapy is necessary for penetration and sterilization of the vegetation. Early in IE therapy, blood cultures rapidly become negative, but treatment is continued because infection in the vegetation has not been eradicated. Multiplication of bacteria, which is required for bactericidal activity of antibiotics, is reduced within vegetations and is one reason for the requirement for prolonged antibiotics. It is important to note that in cases of *Staphylococcus aureus* endocarditis, blood cultures may not clear rapidly and may remain positive for days despite appropriate antibiotic therapy. Penetration into the vegetation is critical; for example, viridans streptococci are highly susceptible to β-lactam antibiotics but require a prolonged course of antimicrobial therapy to eradicate the pathogens in the vegetation.

Whereas some cases of uncomplicated IE may be treated with 2 weeks of antimicrobial therapy, the usual duration of monotherapy or combination therapy is 4 to 6 weeks, depending on the pathogen.

Current guidelines for the treatment for IE recommend intravenous (IV) antibiotics. However, the POET trial has confirmed what prior evidence had shown, that transition from IV to oral antibiotics showed no inferiority compared to IV antibiotics alone in patients with left-sided IE in patients with *Streptococcus* spp, *Enterococcus faecalis*, *Staphylococcus aureus*, and coagulase-negative *Staphylococcus*. This adds to the significant studies already available, demonstrating the effectiveness of PO therapy for serious systemic infections. As safety and efficacy of oral antibiotic therapy for the treatment of IE is

表 8.2 感染性心内膜炎诊断的改良杜克标准
诊断标准
确诊 IE（以下任意一种）：
赘生物病理学或微生物学检查，有 IE 阳性结果
2 项主要标准
1 项主要标准加 3 项次要标准
5 项次要标准
拟诊 IE（以下任意一种）：
1 项主要标准和 1 项次要标准
3 项次要标准
非 IE（以下任何一种）：
抗生素治疗 < 4 天时，明确了其他诊断或治疗方案
不符合拟诊 IE 的标准
主要标准
血培养阳性提示 IE（以下任何一种）：
2 套不同的血培养均检出 IE 典型微生物：
• 草绿色链球菌、解没食子酸链球菌（以前为牛链球菌生物型 I）或营养变异菌株（颗粒链菌属和毗邻贫养菌）
• HACEK 组：嗜血杆菌属、伴放线凝聚杆菌、人心杆菌、啮蚀艾肯菌和金氏杆菌
• 金黄色葡萄球菌
社区获得性肠球菌，没有原发感染灶
血培养持续阳性：定义为以下任何一种情况有符合 IE 的微生物生长：
血培养采样时间相隔 12 h 以上
3 套全部阳性，或 4 套或更多套不同的血培养中的大多数阳性，第一次和最后一次采样时间至少间隔 1 h
[a] 贝纳柯克斯体血培养单一阳性，或抗 I 相 IgG 抗体滴度 > 1：800（译者注：须注意，第 13 版《临床微生物学手册》提到的阈值是 1：512。数值的不同，部分显然是实验室稀释方式的影响。该手册还提到，这个阈值需要由实验室自己确定）
心内膜受累的证据
超声心动图提示 IE：
[a] 根据临床标准，人工瓣膜至少为"拟诊 IE"，或复杂 IE（瓣周脓肿）的患者，建议使用 TEE；TTE 作为其他患者的首选检查
超声心动图阳性的定义（以下任何一种）：
• 在没有其他解剖解释的情况下，心内肿块、瓣膜或支撑结构上、反流射流路径上或植入材料上的振荡
• 脓肿
• 人工瓣膜新出现的部分裂开
新的瓣膜反流（先前存在的杂音没有增加或改变）
次要标准（[a] 已取消超声心动图次要标准）
易感因素：存在易感的心脏病或静脉吸毒
发热：体温 ≥ 38.0℃（100.4℉）
血管相关表现：大动脉栓塞、感染中毒性肺梗死、真菌性动脉瘤、颅内出血、结膜出血、詹韦损害
免疫相关表现：肾小球肾炎、奥斯勒结节、罗特斑、类风湿因子
微生物学证据：血培养阳性，但不满足主要标准（排除单瓶凝固酶阴性葡萄球菌阳性和不会引起心内膜炎的微生物单瓶阳性）或与 IE 一致的微生物活动性感染的血清学证据

改编自 Li JS, Sexton DJ, Mick N, et al: Proposed modifications to the Duke criteria for the diagnosis of infective endocarditis, Clin Infect Dis 30: 633-638, 2000.

IE, 感染性心内膜炎；IgG, 免疫球蛋白 G；TEE, 经食管超声心动图；TTE, 经胸超声心动图。

[a] 表示对先前发布的杜克标准的改良。

似于 ABE 的表现，如高热（> 102℉）；指尖红斑伴触痛（类似奥斯勒结节）；眼底镜检查发现棉绒斑或罗特斑。结膜出血和裂片状出血在 SLE 中很少见，但在 SBE 中常见。镜下尿血是 SBE（即局灶性肾小球肾炎）的常见肾表现，如伴有蛋白尿和血尿的典型的肾炎则是 SLE 肾受累的典型表现。SLE 和 SBE 的临床表现可能重叠，如果没有高级别或持续性菌血症，则可以排除 SBE。

心房黏液瘤，可有与 SBE 相似的表现，如发热、心脏杂音和栓塞现象（如裂片样出血）。ESR 增快在心房黏液瘤中很常见，但并无梅毒血清学性病研究实验室（VDRL）试验的生物学假阳性、类风湿因子升高和肾受累。在经胸超声心动图或经食管超声心动图上，心房黏液瘤表现为心房表面的肿块或赘生物，而不是 IE 的瓣膜表现。没有菌血症，则可以排除 SBE。

乳头状纤维瘤、血栓、钙化瓣膜、黏液瘤变性和非细菌性栓塞性心内膜炎等疾病除了临床表现与 SBE 相似，超声心动图也有相似表现。这些疾病通常不伴有发热或菌血症。非细菌性栓塞性心内膜炎是指继发于恶性肿瘤的伴有杂音和血培养阴性的非感染性的赘生物。非细菌性栓塞性心内膜炎的患者通常无发热，除非发热是由潜在的恶性肿瘤（如淋巴瘤）引起的。淋巴瘤引起的非细菌性栓塞性心内膜炎，可能有发热、脾大和 SBE 的其他表现。阴性血培养可有效排除 IE。感染性 CNE（如 Q 热）可能很少或没有可见的赘生物。如果出现发热、杂音和赘生物伴随 IE 的外周表现，则应考虑感染性 CNE。

治疗

IE 的有效治疗取决于病原体的抗生素敏感性、抗生素对赘生物的渗透以及抗生素治疗的适当持续时间。治疗 IE 选择的抗生素最好是杀菌性的。在 IE 中，病原菌深度包裹在赘生物中，需要长期治疗才能穿透赘生物并起到杀菌作用。在 IE 治疗的早期，血液培养很快呈阴性，但由于赘生物中的感染尚未根除，治疗仍需要继续。抗生素的杀菌活性导致赘生物中细菌繁殖减少，这也是需要延长抗生素治疗的原因之一。值得注意的是，在金黄色葡萄球菌心内膜炎的病例中，尽管进行了适当的抗生素治疗，但血培养可能不会表现为迅速清除，并可能在数天内保持阳性。药物在赘生物中的渗透力至关重要；例如，草绿色链球菌对 β-内酰胺类抗生素高度敏感，但需要长期的抗微生物治疗才能根除赘生物中的病原菌。

尽管一些无并发症的 IE 病例可以接受 2 周的抗微生物治疗，但根据病原体的不同，单药治疗或联合治疗的持续时间通常为 4～6 周。

目前 IE 的治疗指南建议静脉注射（IV）抗生素。然而，POET 试验证实了先前的证据，即在链球菌属、粪肠球菌、金黄色葡萄球菌和凝固酶阴性葡萄球菌的左心 IE 患者中，从静脉输注到口服抗生素的序贯治疗与单独静脉输注抗生素相比没有劣效性。这和现有重要研究相结合，证明了口服治疗严重的系统性感染的

TABLE 8.3 Clinical Findings for Subacute Bacterial Endocarditis (SBE) and Acute Bacterial Endocarditis (ABE)

Symptoms and Findings[a]	ABE	SBE
Anorexia	−	+
Weight loss	−	±
Myalgias or arthralgias	+	±
Fatigue	−	+
Dyspnea	+	−
Pleuritic chest pain[b]	+	−
Low back pain	+	+
Headache	+	±
Mental status changes	+	±
Acute confusion	+	−
Cerebrovascular accident	−	+
Sudden unilateral blindness	−	+
Left upper quadrant pain	Splenic abscess	Splenic infarct
Fever	>102° F[c]	<102° F
New or changing heart murmur	±	±
Splenomegaly	−	+
Petechiae	+	+
Osler nodes	−	+
Janeway lesions	+	−
Splinter hemorrhages	±	+
Roth spots	−	+
Congestive heart failure (LVF)	+	−

Modified from Cunha BA, Gill MV, Lazar JM: Acute infective endocarditis: diagnostic and therapeutic approach, Infect Dis Clin North Am 10:811-834, 1996.
LVF, Left ventricular fibrillation; +, present; −, absent; ±, present or absent.
[a]Otherwise unexplained.
[b]With septic pulmonary emboli from tricuspid valve ABE.
[c]Fever may be <102° F in intravenous drug abusers with ABE.

TABLE 8.4 Nonspecific Laboratory Tests for Infective Endocarditis

Laboratory Findings	Percentage
Anemia	70–90[a]
Leukocytosis	20–30
Elevated ESR	90–100
C-reactive protein (CRP)	100
Histiocytes in blood smear	25
Positive rheumatoid factor (RF)	50[a]
Circulating immune complexes	65–100[a]
Microscopic hematuria	30–50

Data from Brusch JL: Clinical manifestations of endocarditis. In Brusch JL, editor: Infective endocarditis, New York, 2007, Informa Healthcare, pp 143-166.
ESR, Erythrocyte sedimentation rate.
[a]Most consistent with SBE

TABLE 8.5 Diagnostic Approach to Culture-Negative Endocarditis

Valvular Biopsy Unavailable
1. Q fever and *Bartonella* serology: If negative, then use lysis-centrifugation system for blood cultures and inform microbiology laboratory of concern for fastidious organisms to allow use of special media and culture techniques: thioglycolate-, pyridoxal hydrochloride–, or L-cystine–enriched media for *Abiotrophia*; buffered charcoal yeast extract (BCYE) agar for *Legionella*; prolonged incubation for HACEK organisms[a]
2. Rheumatoid factor (RF), antinuclear antibodies (ANA)
3. PCR for *Bartonella* spp and *Tropheryma whipplei*
4. Nested PCR for fungi, tissue for *Cryptococcus neoformans* capsular antigen, and urine for *Histoplasma capsulatum* antigen: If negative, then obtain serum serology studies for *Mycoplasma pneumoniae*, *Legionella pneumophila*, *Brucella melitensis*, and *Bartonella* spp by Western blot

Valvular Biopsy Available
1. Broad-range PCR for bacteria (16S rRNA) and fungi (18S rRNA)
2. Histologic examination with direct staining for *Chlamydia* spp, *Coxiella burnetii*, *Legionella* spp, fungi, and *T. whipplei*
3. Primer extension enrichment reaction (PEER) or autoimmunohistochemistry (AIHC)

Modified from Fournier PE, Thuny F, Richet H, et al: Comprehensive diagnostic strategy for blood culture-negative endocarditis: a prospective study of 819 new cases, Clin Infect Dis 51:131-140, 2010; and Mylonakis E, Calderwood SB: Infective endocarditis in adults, N Engl J Med 345:1320, 2001.
PCR, Polymerase chain reaction; rRNA, ribosomal RNA.
[a]HACEK organisms: *Haemophilus* spp, *Aggregatibacter actinomycetemcomitans*, *Cardiobacterium hominis*, *Eikenella corrodens*, and *Kingella kingae*.

continued to be proven in future trials, not only would this reduce the morbidity associated with long-term IV catheters, but it would also be ideal for patients who are otherwise not eligible for long-term IV antibiotics. Long-acting lipoglycopeptides (dalbavancin, oritavancin) have been used in a very small number of retrospective studies showing potential promises for treating IE. However, we should be cautious as failures have been documented, and potential for increasing resistance to standard therapy remains.

Effective antimicrobial therapy does not eliminate suppurative or embolic complications of endocarditis. Therapeutic failure is usually related to valvular destruction, a complication that may require valve replacement. Suppurative intracardiac or extracardiac complications usually require drainage for cure of IE. The overarching principles of IE therapy are presented in Table 8.6 , and Table 8.7 provides an outline of specific antibiotic regimens that may be used to treat IE.

Complications of endocarditis may be intracardiac or extracardiac, and they may also be classified by damage mechanism (i.e., immunologic vs. infectious). The infectious intracardiac complications of IE include purulent pericarditis and paravalvular abscess; they manifest clinically with persistent fever or persistent bacteremia despite appropriate antibiotic therapy. Complications may be septic or immunologic; for example, splenic involvement may be immunologic (splenic infarct) or septic (splenic abscess). Embolic events are related to vegetation size. Bland central nervous system emboli (e.g., aseptic meningitis) may complicate SBE, whereas septic emboli (e.g., acute bacterial meningitis) may complicate ABE. Particularly with ABE, there may be valvular perforation or destruction resulting in acute congestive heart failure. It is often these complications that dictate whether and when surgery will occur. The indications for surgical intervention are shown in Table 8.8 . As a general principle, paravalvular abscess or intractable congestive heart failure requires urgent surgical intervention. Persistent vegetations or embolic disease that occurs after 1 week of appropriate antibiotic therapy should also prompt surgical consideration.

表8.3 亚急性细菌性心内膜炎（SBE）和急性细菌性心内膜炎（ABE）的临床表现

症状和体征[a]	ABE	SBE
食欲减退	−	+
体重减轻	−	±
肌痛或关节痛	+	±
疲劳	−	+
呼吸困难	+	−
胸膜炎性胸痛[b]	+	−
腰痛	+	+
头痛	−	+
意识状态变化	+	±
急性意识障碍	+	−
脑血管意外	−	+
突然单侧失明	−	+
左上腹疼痛	脾脓肿	脾梗死
发热	>102°F[c]	<102°F
新发或变化的心脏杂音	±	±
脾大	−	+
出血点	+	+
奥斯勒结节	−	+
詹韦损害	+	−
裂片样出血	±	+
罗特斑	−	+
充血性心力衰竭（LVF）	+	−

改编自 Cunha BA, Gill MV, Lazar JM: Acute infective endocarditis: diagnostic and therapeutic approach, Infect Dis Clin North Am 10: 811-834, 1996.
LVF，左心室颤动；+，存在；−，不存在；±，可能存在或不存在。
[a] 其他原因无法解释。
[b] 三尖瓣感染中毒性（脓毒性）肺栓塞。
[c] ABE 静脉注射吸毒者，发热体温可能低于 102°F。

表8.4 感染性心内膜炎的非特异性实验室检查

实验室检查发现	百分比
贫血	70～90[a]
白细胞升高	20～30
ESR 升高	90～100
C 反应蛋白（CRP）升高	100
血液涂片查见组织细胞	25
类风湿因子（RF）阳性	50[a]
循环免疫复合物	65～100[a]
镜下血尿	30～50

数据引自 Brusch JL: Clinical manifestations of endocarditis. In Brusch JL, editor: Infective endocarditis, New York, 2007, Informa Healthcare, pp 143-166.
ESR，红细胞沉降率。
[a] 和 SBE 最符合。

表8.5 培养阴性的心内膜炎的诊断方法

不可做瓣膜活检
1. Q 热和巴尔通体血清学：如果阴性，则使用裂解离心系统进行血液培养，并告知微生物学实验室关注苛养菌，以便使用特殊的培养基和培养技术：巯基乙酸盐、盐酸吡哆醛或 l-胱氨酸富集培养基用于乏养菌属；活性炭酵母提取物（BCYE）琼脂用于军团菌；HACEK 群微生物需要延长孵育时间
2. 类风湿因子（RF）、抗核抗体（ANA）
3. 采用 PCR 检测巴尔通体和惠普尔养障体
4. 采用巢式 PCR 检测真菌，组织标本检测新型隐球菌荚膜抗原，尿液标本检测荚膜组织胞浆菌抗原；如果阴性，则采用蛋白印迹技术进行肺炎支原体、嗜肺军团菌、布鲁菌和巴尔通体的血清学检测

可做瓣膜活检
1. 细菌（16S rRNA）和真菌（18S rRNA）广谱 PCR
2. 直接染色进行组织学检查：衣原体属、贝纳柯克斯体、军团菌属、真菌和惠普尔养障体
3. 引物延伸富集反应（PEER）或自身免疫组织化学（AIHC）

改编自 Fournier PE, Thuny F, Richet H, et al: Comprehensive diagnostic strategy for blood culture-negative endocarditis: a prospective study of 819 new cases, Clin Infect Dis 51: 131-140, 2010; and Mylonakis E, Calderwood SB: Infective endocarditis in adults, N Engl J Med 345: 1320, 2001.
PCR，聚合酶链反应；rRNA，核糖体 RNA。
[a] HACEK 群微生物：嗜血杆菌属、伴放线凝聚杆菌、人心杆菌、啮蚀艾肯菌和金氏杆菌。

性研究中有使用，显示出治疗 IE 的潜在前景。然而，我们对此应该谨慎，因为也有失败的记录，而对标准治疗的耐药性也有可能增加。

有效的抗微生物治疗不能消除心内膜炎的化脓性或栓塞性并发症。治疗失败通常与瓣膜破坏有关，这种并发症可能需要行瓣膜置换。化脓性心内并发症或心外并发症通常需要引流来治疗 IE。IE 治疗的总体原则如表 8.6 所示，表 8.7 概述了可用于治疗 IE 的特定抗生素方案。

心内膜炎的并发症可能是心内的并发症或心外的并发症，也可以根据损伤机制（如免疫性 vs. 感染性）进行分类。IE 的感染性心内并发症包括化脓性心包炎和瓣周脓肿；临床表现为在适当的抗生素治疗的情况下依然持续发热或持续菌血症。并发症可能是感染中毒性或免疫性的；例如，脾受累可能是免疫性的（脾梗死）或感染中毒性的（脾脓肿）。栓塞事件与赘生物大小有关。Bland 中枢神经系统栓塞（如无菌性脑膜炎）可能使 SBE 复杂化，而感染中毒性栓塞（如急性细菌性脑膜炎）则可能使 ABE 复杂化。特别是 ABE，可能会出现瓣膜穿孔或破坏，导致急性充血性心力衰竭。通常正是这些并发症决定了是否以及何时进行手术。手术干预的适应证如表 8.8 所示。一般来说，瓣周脓肿或顽固性充血性心力衰竭需要紧急手术干预。在适当的抗生素治疗 1 周后出现的持续性赘生物或栓塞性疾病，也应立即考虑手术治疗。

有效性。 随着口服抗生素治疗 IE 的安全性和有效性在未来的试验中不断得到证明，这不仅可以降低与长期静脉导管相关的发病率，而且对于那些不太可能进行长期静脉输注抗生素的患者来说也是理想的。长效脂糖肽类药物（达巴万星，奥利万星）在极少数的回顾

Prognosis

The prognosis of all forms of IE depends directly on any complications related to the infection. Consequently, early diagnosis and initiation of appropriate antibiotic therapy is the key to limiting mortality. Recent studies have supported the role of early surgical intervention, when appropriate, as a significant aid to decreasing morbidity and mortality, specifically in relation to having fewer embolic events. If treated in a timely fashion and with appropriate antibiotics, the cure rate for viridans streptococci and *S. bovis* is estimated to be 98% in NVE and up to 88% in PVE. Right-sided endocarditis in intravenous drug abusers is usually caused by *S. aureus* and typically has a cure rate of 90% in NVE and 75% to 80% in PVE. However, among non–intravenous drug abusers, cure rates in IE involving *S. aureus* are far lower: 60% to 70% in NVE and 50% in PVE. When gram-negative bacilli or fungal organisms are the causative agent, cure rates are significantly lower (40% to 60%). Increased age, diabetes, aortic valve involvement, and developing complications of IE including congestive heart failure and emboli to the central nervous system are all highly predictive of increased mortality and morbidity.

Infective Endocarditis Prophylaxis

The most recent American Heart Association guidelines state that not all patients require antibiotic prophylaxis and that prophylaxis should be considered only for a specific subset of patients. Antibiotic prophylaxis is indicated for patients with prosthetic heart valves, cardiac transplant recipients with valvular disease, patients with a history of IE, and patients with certain forms of congenital heart disease. Among patients with congenital heart disease, only those with unrepaired or partially repaired lesions and those with prosthetic material should receive prophylactic antibiotics (grade IIa recommendation).

Typically, antibiotic regimens used for prophylaxis against IE prior to invasive procedures above the waist are directed against viridans streptococci. For invasive dental procedures, the recommended prophylactic agent is amoxicillin, 2 g PO as a single dose 30 to 60 minutes before the procedure. In patients with penicillin allergy, clindamycin or a macrolide may be substituted.

ENDARTERITIS AND SUPPURATIVE PHLEBITIS

The term *infectious endarteritis* refers to an intravascular infection of the arteries that affects coarctation of the aorta, aortic valve shunts, or a patent ductus arteriosus, analogous to IE at other sites. As with IE, continuous or high-grade bacteremia in the absence of an intracardiac vegetation should suggest the diagnosis. Imaging studies (e.g., PET scans) delineate the extent of arterial involvement. Treatment is the same as for IE.

The term *suppurative thrombophlebitis* refers to an intravenous infection that is characterized by an intravenular abscess; it is a complication of the use of central venous catheters. Patients have phlebitis with high fevers (>102° F, compared with <102° F in uncomplicated phlebitis with fevers), bacteremia due to a skin organism (e.g., *S. aureus*) and often expressible pus from the catheter site. Treatment consists of a combination of antibiotic therapy and resection of the involved venous segment.

CENTRAL VENOUS CATHETER–RELATED BLOODSTREAM INFECTIONS

Central venous catheter–related bloodstream infections are relatively common, with an annual incidence of approximately 200,000 in the United States. Central venous catheter infection should be suspected if the patient develops fevers, chills, or hypotension without another obvious source of infection. The likelihood of infection increases with the length of time the catheter is in place. In addition to the clinical signs, blood cultures, drawn from the periphery as well as the line, should demonstrate growth of the causative organism. If the culture drawn from the catheter shows growth of bacteria at least 2 hours earlier than the peripheral blood cultures do, infection associated with the central line, rather than bacteremia in the setting of a catheter, should be strongly suspected.

Treatment of catheter-related infections varies depending on what action will be taken with the catheter (i.e., removal, exchange, or salvage). In any case, empirical antibiotic therapy should be initiated against the most likely pathogens. Empirical therapy should cover *S. aureus* and nosocomial gram-negative bacilli. Therapy may then be modified based on the results of blood cultures or catheter tip culture. If a catheter-related bloodstream infection is suspected, immediate removal of the catheter should occur if the infection has led to septic shock or IE. The line also should be removed if blood cultures remain positive for the causative organism for 72 hours longer or if evidence of septic thrombophlebitis develops.

Salvage therapy may be considered in hemodynamically stable patients except when the infection is caused by *S. aureus*, *P. aeruginosa*, *Bacillus* spp, *Micrococcus* spp, *Propionibacterium acnes* or other propionibacteria, fungi, or mycobacteria. Salvage therapy relies on concurrent use of systemic antimicrobial agents and antibiotic or ethanol locks.

Guidewire exchange should be reserved for cases in which there is a high risk for complications if the original catheter were to be removed. Guidewire exchange has a lower chance of eliminating the infection than does removal of the catheter.

For a deeper discussion of these topics, please see Chapter 67, "Infective Endocarditis," in *Goldman-Cecil Medicine*, 26th Edition.

TABLE 8.6 Principles of Therapy for Infective Endocarditis

1. Antibiotic selection initially is made empirically on the basis of physical examination and clinical history.
2. Bactericidal antibiotics are prescribed.
3. The MIC and MBC are measured to ensure adequate dosing of the agent.
4. Intermittent dosing provides superior penetration into the thrombus compared with continuous infusion; penetration is directly related to peak serum level.
5. The patient should be treated in a health care facility for the first 1–2 wk.
6. The usual duration of therapy is 4–6 wk.
7. A 4-wk course is appropriate for an uncomplicated case of NVE (a shorter course of 2 wk may be appropriate in some cases); a 6-wk course is required for the treatment of PVE and those infections with large vegetations (i.e., infection by HACEK organisms[a]).

Modified from Brusch JL: Diagnosis of infective endocarditis. In Brusch JL, editor: Infective endocarditis, New York, 2007, Informa Healthcare, pp 241-254.
MBC, Minimal bactericidal concentration; *MIC*, minimal inhibitory concentration.
[a]HACEK organisms: *Haemophilus* spp, *Aggregatibacter actinomycetemcomitans*, *Cardiobacterium hominis*, *Eikenella corrodens*, and *Kingella kingae*.

预后

所有类型 IE 的预后，都直接取决于与感染相关的任何并发症。因此，早期诊断和开始适当的抗生素治疗是控制死亡率的关键。最近的研究支持在适当的情况下进行早期手术干预，作为降低发病率和死亡率的重要帮助，特别是与减少栓塞事件有关。如果及时治疗并使用适当的抗生素，NVE 中的草绿色链球菌和牛链球菌的治愈率估计为 98%，PVE 中的治愈率为 88%。静脉吸毒者的右侧心内膜炎通常由金黄色葡萄球菌引起，NVE 的治愈率通常为 90%，PVE 为 75%～80%。然而，在非静脉注射的吸毒者，涉及金黄色葡萄球菌的 IE 的治愈率要低得多：NVE 为 60%～70%，PVE 为 50%。当革兰氏阴性杆菌或真菌是病原体时，治愈率明显较低（40%～60%）。高龄、糖尿病、主动脉瓣受累以及进展为 IE 并发症，包括充血性心力衰竭和中枢神经系统栓塞，都是死亡率和发病率增加的高风险预测因素。

感染性心内膜炎的预防

美国心脏协会最新的指南指出，并非所有患者都需要抗生素预防，预防应仅考虑在特定的患者群体。抗生素预防适用于人工心脏瓣膜患者、患有瓣膜病的心脏移植受者、有 IE 病史的患者和某些类型的先天性心脏病患者。在先天性心脏病患者中，只有病变未修复或部分修复的患者以及使用假体材料的患者才应接受预防性抗生素治疗（推荐 II a 级）。

通常，在腰部以上的侵入性手术之前用于预防 IE 的抗生素方案是针对草绿色链球菌的。对于侵入性牙科手术，推荐的预防药物是阿莫西林 2 g 口服，手术前 30～60 min，单次给药。对于青霉素过敏的患者，可以用克林霉素或大环内酯类代替。

动脉内膜炎和化脓性血栓性静脉炎

术语感染性动脉内膜炎是指影响主动脉缩窄、主动脉瓣分流或动脉导管未闭的动脉血管内感染，类似于其他部位的 IE。与 IE 一样，在没有心内赘生物的情况下出现持续性或高级别菌血症，可以提示诊断。影像学研究（如 PET 扫描）呈现了动脉受累的程度。治疗与 IE 相同。

术语化脓性血栓性静脉炎是指以静脉内脓肿为特征的静脉感染；这是使用中心静脉导管的并发症。患者有伴高热的静脉炎（＞102℉，相比较而言，无并发症的静脉炎发热一般＜102℉）、由皮肤微生物引起的菌血症（如金黄色葡萄球菌）以及导管部位常见脓性渗出。治疗包括抗生素治疗和切除受累静脉段。

表 8.6　感染性心内膜炎的治疗原则

1. 抗生素的选择，最初是基于体格检查和临床病史凭经验进行的。
2. 使用杀菌剂。
3. 测定 MIC 和 MBC 以确保给药剂量的充足（译者注：国内常规微生物学工作不测 MBC。本书后文也没有 MBC 对应信息）。
4. 与连续输注相比，间歇给药具有更好的血栓渗透性；渗透性与血清峰值水平直接相关。
5. 在治疗的第 1～2 周，患者应在医疗机构住院接受治疗。
6. 一般治疗时间为 4～6 周。
7. 4 周疗程适用于无并发症的 NVE 病例（在某些情况下，2 周的较短疗程也可能适用）；需要 6 周的疗程来治疗 PVE 和那些具有体积大的赘生物感染（如 HACEK 群感染[a]）。

改编自 Brusch JL: Diagnosis of infective endocarditis. In Brusch JL, editor: Infective endocarditis, New York, 2007, Informa Healthcare, pp 241-254.
MBC，最小杀菌浓度；MIC，最小抑菌浓度。
[a] HACEK 群微生物：嗜血杆菌属、伴放线凝聚杆菌、人心杆菌、啮蚀艾肯菌和金氏杆菌。

中心静脉导管相关血流感染

中心静脉导管相关血流感染相对常见，在美国每年的发病例数约为 20 万。如果患者在没有其他明显感染源的情况下出现发热、寒战或低血压，应怀疑中心静脉导管感染。感染的可能性随着导管放置时间的延长而增加。除了临床症状外，从外周和经导管采集的血液培养可以显示致病微生物生长。如果导管血采集比外周血采集的培养提前至少 2 h 显示细菌生长，则强烈怀疑中央管路相关感染，而不仅仅是置管状态下的（单纯的）菌血症。

导管相关感染的治疗因对导管采取的措施（即拔除、更换或补救）而异。在任何情况下，应针对最可能的病原体开始经验性抗生素治疗。经验性治疗应包括金黄色葡萄球菌和院内获得性革兰氏阴性杆菌。然后可以基于血液培养或导管尖端培养的结果来调整治疗。如果怀疑导管相关的血流感染，一旦感染已导致感染中毒性休克或 IE，则应立即拔除导管。如果血液培养阳性持续 72 h 以上，或出现感染中毒性血栓性静脉炎的迹象，也应拔除导管。

血流动力学稳定的患者可考虑进行补救治疗，但由金黄色葡萄球菌、铜绿假单胞菌、芽孢杆菌属、微球菌属、痤疮丙酸杆菌或其他丙酸杆菌、真菌或分枝杆菌引起的感染除外。补救治疗依赖于同时使用全身抗微生物药物，以及抗生素封闭或乙醇封闭。

导丝更换应限于如果拔除原导管则并发症风险较高的情况。与拔除导管相比，更换导丝消除感染的可能性更低。

有关此专题的深入讨论，请参阅 *Goldman-Cecil Medicine* 第 26 版第 67 章"感染性心内膜炎"。

TABLE 8.7 Antimicrobial Treatment of Infective Endocarditis

Causative Organism	NATIVE VALVE		PROSTHETIC VALVE	
	Antibiotic Therapy	Comments	Antibiotic Therapy	Comments
Penicillin-susceptible viridans streptococci, *Streptococcus bovis*, and other streptococci with MIC of penicillin ≤0.1 μg/mL	Penicillin G or ceftriaxone for 4 wk[a]	A 2-wk regimen of penicillin G or ceftriaxone combined with gentamicin may be considered in patients with right-sided NVE without evidence of embolic disease (excluding pulmonary emboli) or other complications.	Penicillin G for 6 wk and gentamicin for 2 wk[a]	Shorter duration of treatment with an aminoglycoside (2 wk) is usually appropriate for PVE due to penicillin-susceptible viridans streptococci, *S. bovis*, or other streptococci with MIC of penicillin ≤0.1 μg/mL.
Relatively penicillin-resistant streptococci (MIC of penicillin >0.1 to 0.5 μg/mL)	Penicillin G for 4 wk and gentamicin for 2 wk[a]		Penicillin G for 6 wk and gentamicin for 4 wk[a]	
Streptococcus species with MIC of penicillin >0.5 μg/mL, *Enterococcus* species, or *Abiotrophia* species	Penicillin G or ampicillin and gentamicin for 4–6 wk[a]	6 wk of therapy is recommended for patients with symptoms lasting >3 mo, myocardial abscess, or selected other complications.	Penicillin G or ampicillin and gentamicin for 6 wk[a]	A study by Fernando-Hidalgo et al. showed that the combination of ampicillin and ceftriaxone is as effective as the combination of ampicillin and gentamicin for treating *Enterococcus faecalis* IE.
Methicillin-susceptible staphylococci	Nafcillin or oxacillin for 4–6 wk, with or without addition of gentamicin for the first 3–5 days of therapy[b]	In the few patients infected with a penicillin-susceptible staphylococcus, penicillin G may be substituted for nafcillin or oxacillin.	Nafcillin or oxacillin with rifampin for 6 wk and gentamicin for 2 wk[b]	It may be prudent to delay initiation of rifampin for 1 or 2 days, until therapy with two other effective antistaphylococcal drugs has been initiated.
Methicillin-resistant staphylococci	Vancomycin, with or without addition of gentamicin, for the first 3–5 days of therapy		Vancomycin with rifampin for 6 wk and gentamicin for 2 wk	If the staphylococcus is resistant to gentamicin, an alternative third agent should be chosen on the basis of in vitro susceptibility testing.
Right-sided staphylococcal NVE in selected patients	Nafcillin or oxacillin with gentamicin for 2 wk	This 2-wk regimen has been studied for infections caused by an oxacillin- and aminoglycoside-susceptible isolate. Exclusions to short-course therapy include any cardiac or extracardiac complications associated with IE, persistence of fever for ≥7 days, and infection with HIV. Patients with vegetations >1–2 cm should probably be excluded from short-course therapy.		
HACEK organisms[c]	Ceftriaxone for 4 wk	Ampicillin and gentamicin for 4 wk is an alternative regimen, but some isolates may produce β-lactamase, thereby reducing the efficacy of this regimen.	Ceftriaxone for 6 wk	Ampicillin and gentamicin for 6 wk is an alternative regimen, but some isolates may produce β-lactamase, thereby reducing the efficacy of this regimen.

Modified from Mylonakis E, Calderwood SB: Infective endocarditis in adults, N Engl J Med 345:1318-1330, 2001.
HIV, Human immunodeficiency virus; *IE*, infective endocarditis; *NVE*, native valve endocarditis; *PVE*, prosthetic valve endocarditis.
[a]Vancomycin therapy is indicated for patients with confirmed immediate hypersensitivity reactions to β-lactam antibiotics.
[b]For patients who have IE due to methicillin-susceptible staphylococci and are allergic to penicillin, a first-generation cephalosporin or vancomycin may be substituted for nafcillin or oxacillin. Cephalosporins should be avoided in patients with confirmed immediate-type hypersensitivity reactions to β-lactam antibiotics.
[c]HACEK organisms: *Haemophilus* spp, *Aggregatibacter actinomycetemcomitans*, *Cardiobacterium hominis*, *Eikenella corrodens*, and *Kingella kingae*.

表 8.7　感染性心内膜炎的抗菌治疗

致病微生物	自体瓣膜		人工瓣膜	
	抗生素治疗方案	治疗评价	抗生素治疗方案	治疗评价
青霉素敏感的草绿色链球菌、牛链球菌和其他链球菌，青霉素 MIC ≤ 0.1 µg/ml	青霉素 G 或头孢曲松，4 周[a]	对没有栓塞性疾病（不包括肺栓塞）或其他并发症证据的右侧 NVE 患者，可以考虑使用青霉素 G 或头孢曲松联合庆大霉素 2 周方案	青霉素 G 6 周，庆大霉素 2 周	氨基糖苷类治疗时间较短（2 周）通常适用于下列病原所致 PVE，包括青霉素敏感草绿色链球菌、牛链球菌或对青霉素 MIC ≤ 0.1 µg/ml 的其他链球菌
对青霉素相对耐药的链球菌（青霉素 MIC > 0.1 至 0.5 µg/ml）	青霉素 G 4 周，庆大霉素 2 周[a]		青霉素 G 6 周，庆大霉素 4 周[a]	
青霉素 MIC > 0.5 µg/ml 的链球菌属、肠球菌属或乏养菌属	青霉素 G 或氨苄西林联合庆大霉素 4~6 周[a]	对于症状持续 > 3 个月、心肌脓肿或有其他特定并发症的患者，推荐进行 6 周的治疗	青霉素 G 或氨苄西林和庆大霉素 4~6 周[a]	Fernando Hidalgo 等的一项研究表明，氨苄西林和头孢曲松联合治疗类肠球菌 IE，与氨苄西林与庆大霉素联合治疗等效
甲氧西林敏感葡萄球菌	萘夫西林或苯唑西林 4~6 周，在治疗的前 3~5 天联合或不联合庆大霉素[b]	对极少数感染青霉素敏感的葡萄球菌的患者，青霉素 G 可以代替萘夫西林或苯唑西林	萘夫西林或苯唑西林联合利福平 6 周，庆大霉素 2 周[b]	谨慎的做法是，在使用了另外两种有效的抗葡萄球菌药物后，延迟 1~2 天再启用利福平
耐甲氧西林葡萄球菌	万古霉素，在治疗开始的 3~5 天选择联合或不联合庆大霉素		万古霉素与利福平联合用药 6 周，庆大霉素联合用药 2 周	如果葡萄球菌对庆大霉素耐药，则应在体外药敏试验的基础上选择替代的第三种药物
右心葡萄球菌 NVE 的特定患者	萘夫西林或苯唑西林联合庆大霉素 2 周	这种 2 周方案经过研究可用于由苯唑西林和氨基糖苷类敏感株引起的感染。短期治疗的例外情况包括与 IE 相关的任何心脏或心外并发症、持续发热 ≥ 7 天以及感染 HIV。赘生物 > 1~2 cm 的患者应很可能不适合短期治疗		
HACEK 群微生物[c]	头孢曲松 4 周	氨苄西林和庆大霉素 4 周是一种替代方案，但一些分离株可能产生 β-内酰胺酶，从而降低了该方案的疗效	头孢曲松 6 周	氨苄西林和庆大霉素 6 周是一种替代方案，但一些分离株可能产生 β-内酰胺酶，从而降低了该方案的疗效

改编自 Mylonakis E，Calderwood SB：Infective endocarditis in adults, N Engl J Med 345：1318-1330，2001.
HIV，人体免疫缺陷病毒；IE，感染性心内膜炎；NVE，自体瓣膜心内膜炎；PVE，人工瓣膜心内膜炎。
[a] 万古霉素治疗适用于对 β-内酰胺类抗生素有明确的超敏反应的患者。
[b] 对于因甲氧西林敏感葡萄球菌引起 IE 并对青霉素过敏的患者，可以用第一代头孢菌素或万古霉素代替萘夫西林或苯唑西林。对 β-内酰胺类抗生素有速发型超敏反应的患者应避免使用头孢菌素类药物。
[c] HACEK 生物：嗜血杆菌属、伴放线凝聚杆菌、人心杆菌、啮蚀艾肯菌和金氏杆菌。
译者注：上表提及，对青霉素相对耐药的链球菌指其青霉素 MIC > 0.1 至 0.5 µg/ml。2024 版 CLSI M100 文件草绿色链球菌青霉素折点：敏感是 ≤ 0.125，耐药是 ≥ 4。而上表和《热病》都是以 0.5 为阈值，推测是针对自体瓣膜赘生物的特殊选择。

TABLE 8.8 Echocardiographic Indications for Surgical Intervention in Infective Endocarditis

Vegetation
Persistent vegetation after systemic embolization
Anterior mitral valve leaflet vegetation (particularly if ≥1 embolic events occur during the first 2 wk of antimicrobial therapy)[a]
Increase in vegetation size despite appropriate antimicrobial therapy[a,b]

Valvular Dysfunction
Acute aortic or mitral insufficiency with signs of ventricular failure[b]
Heart failure unresponsive to medical therapy[b]
Valve perforation or rupture[b]
Large abscess or extension of abscess despite appropriate antimicrobial therapy[b]

Paravalvular Extension
Valvular dehiscence, rupture, or fistula[b]
New heart block[b]
Large abscess or extension of abscess despite appropriate antimicrobial therapy[b]

Modified from Baddour LM, Wilson WR, Bayer AS, et al: Infective endocarditis: diagnosis, antimicrobial therapy, and management of complications: a statement for healthcare professionals from the Committee on Rheumatic Fever, Endocarditis, and Kawasaki Disease, Council on Cardiovascular Disease in the Young, and the Councils on Clinical Cardiology, Stroke, and Cardiovascular Surgery and Anesthesia, American Heart Association; endorsed by the Infectious Diseases Society of America, Circulation 111:e394-e433, 2005.
[a]Surgery may be required because of risk of embolization.
[b]Surgery may be required because of failure of medical therapy or heart failure.

SUGGESTED READINGS

Baddour LM, Cha YM, Wilson WR: Clinical practice: infections of cardiovascular implantable electronic devices, N Engl J Med 367:842–849, 2012.

Blauwkamp TA, Thair S, Rosen MJ, et al: Analytical and clinical validation of a microbial cell-free DNA sequencing test for infectious disease, Nat Microbiol 4:663–674, 2019.

Bor DH, Woolhandler S, Nardin R, et al: Infective endocarditis in the U.S., 1998–2009: a nationwide study, PloS One 8(e60033):2013.

Brouqt P, Raoult D: Endocarditis due to rare and fastidious bacteria, Clin Microbiol Rev 14:177–207, 2001.

Fernández-Hidalgo N, Almirante B, Gavaldà J, et al: Ampicillin plus ceftriaxone is as effective as ampicillin plus gentamicin for treating Enterococcus faecalis infective endocarditis, Clin Infect Dis 56:1261–1268, 2013.

Fournier PE, Thuny F, Richet H, et al: Comprehensive diagnostic strategy for blood culture-negative endocarditis: a prospective study of 819 new cases, Clin Infect Dis 51:131–140, 2010.

Garcia-Cabera E, Fernandez-Hidalgo N, Almirante B, et al: Neurological complications of infective endocarditis: risk factors, outcome, and impact of cardiac surgery: a multicenter observational study, Circulation 127:2272–2284, 2013.

Iversen K1, Ihlemann N1, Gill SU1, et al: Partial oral versus intravenous antibiotic treatment of endocarditis, N Engl J Med 380(5):415–424, 2019.

Kadri AN, Wilner B, Hernandez AV, et al: Geographic trends, patient characteristics, and outcomes of infective endocarditis associated with drug abuse in the United States from 2002 to 2016, JAHA 8:e12969, 2019.

Kang DH, Kim YJ, Kim SH, et al: Early surgery versus conventional treatment for infective endocarditis, N Engl J Med 366:2466–2473, 2012.

Kiefer T, Park L, Tribouilloy C, et al: Association between valvular surgery and mortality among patients with infective endocarditis complicated by heart failure, J Am Med Assoc 306:2239–2247, 2011.

Li JS, Sexton DJ, Mick N, et al: Proposed modifications to the Duke criteria for the diagnosis of infective endocarditis, Clin Infect Dis 30:633–638, 2000.

Mermel LA, Allon M, Bouza E, et al: Clinical practice guidelines for the diagnosis and management of intravascular catheter-related infection: 2009 Update by the Infectious Disease Society of America, Clin Infect Dis 49:1–45, 2009.

Morrisette T, Miller MA, Montague BT, et al: Long-acting lipoglycopeptides: "Lineless Antibiotics" for serious infections in persons who use drugs, Open Forum Infect Dis 6(7):ofz274, 2019, Published 2019 Jun 5.

Mylonakis E, Calderwood SB: Infective endocarditis in adults, N Engl J Med 345:1318–1330, 2001.

Steele JM, Seabury RW, Hale CM, et al: Unsuccessful treatment of methicillin-resistant Staphylococcus aureus endocarditis with dalbavancin, J Clin Pharm Ther 43:101–103, 2018.

Wilson W, Taubert KA, Gewitz M, et al: Prevention of infective endocarditis: guidelines from the American Heart Association: a guideline from the American Heart Association Rheumatic Fever, Endocarditis, and Kawasaki Disease Committee, Council on Cardiovascular Disease in the Young, and the Council on Clinical Cardiology, Council on Cardiovascular Surgery and Anesthesia, and the Quality of Care and Outcomes Research Interdisciplinary Working Group, Circulation 116:1736–1754, 2007.

表 8.8　感染性心内膜炎手术干预的超声心动图适应证

赘生物
- 系统性栓塞后的持续性赘生物
- 二尖瓣前叶赘生物（尤其是在抗微生物治疗的前 2 周发生 ≥ 1 次栓塞事件的情况下）[a]
- 尽管进行了适当的抗微生物治疗，赘生物体积仍在增加[b]

瓣膜功能障碍
- 急性主动脉或二尖瓣关闭不全伴心室衰竭[b]
- 心力衰竭对药物治疗无反应[b]
- 瓣膜穿孔或破裂[b]
- 尽管进行了适当的抗微生物治疗，但仍存在大脓肿或脓肿扩展[b]

瓣膜旁扩展
- 瓣膜开裂、破裂或瘘管[b]
- 新出现的心脏传导阻滞[b]
- 尽管进行了适当的抗微生物治疗，但仍存在大脓肿或脓肿扩展[b]

改编自 Baddour LM, Wilson WR, Bayer AS, et al: Infective endocarditis: diagnosis, antimicrobial therapy, and management of complications: a statement for healthcare professionals from the Committee on Rheumatic Fever, Endocarditis, and Kawasaki Disease, Council on Cardiovascular Disease in the Young, and the Councils on Clinical Cardiology, Stroke, and Cardiovascular Surgery and Anesthesia, American Heart Association; endorsed by the Infectious Diseases Society of America, Circulation 111: e394-e433, 2005.

[a] 由于存在栓塞风险，可能需要手术治疗。
[b] 由于药物治疗失败或心力衰竭，可能需要进行手术。

推荐阅读

Baddour LM, Cha YM, Wilson WR: Clinical practice: infections of cardiovascular implantable electronic devices, N Engl J Med 367:842–849, 2012.

Blauwkamp TA, Thair S, Rosen MJ, et al: Analytical and clinical validation of a microbial cell-free DNA sequencing test for infectious disease, Nat Microbiol 4:663–674, 2019.

Bor DH, Woolhandler S, Nardin R, et al: Infective endocarditis in the U.S., 1998–2009: a nationwide study, PloS One 8(e60033):2013.

Brouqt P, Raoult D: Endocarditis due to rare and fastidious bacteria, Clin Microbiol Rev 14:177–207, 2001.

Fernández-Hidalgo N, Almirante B, Gavaldà J, et al: Ampicillin plus ceftriaxone is as effective as ampicillin plus gentamicin for treating Enterococcus faecalis infective endocarditis, Clin Infect Dis 56:1261–1268, 2013.

Fournier PE, Thuny F, Richet H, et al: Comprehensive diagnostic strategy for blood culture-negative endocarditis: a prospective study of 819 new cases, Clin Infect Dis 51:131–140, 2010.

Garcia-Cabera E, Fernandez-Hidalgo N, Almirante B, et al: Neurological complications of infective endocarditis: risk factors, outcome, and impact of cardiac surgery: a multicenter observational study, Circulation 127:2272–2284, 2013.

Iversen K1, Ihlemann N1, Gill SU1, et al: Partial oral versus intravenous antibiotic treatment of endocarditis, N Engl J Med 380(5):415–424, 2019.

Kadri AN, Wilner B, Hernandez AV, et al: Geographic trends, patient characteristics, and outcomes of infective endocarditis associated with drug abuse in the United States from 2002 to 2016, JAHA 8:e12969, 2019.

Kang DH, Kim YJ, Kim SH, et al: Early surgery versus conventional treatment for infective endocarditis, N Engl J Med 366:2466–2473, 2012.

Kiefer T, Park L, Tribouilloy C, et al: Association between valvular surgery and mortality among patients with infective endocarditis complicated by heart failure, J Am Med Assoc 306:2239–2247, 2011.

Li JS, Sexton DJ, Mick N, et al: Proposed modifications to the Duke criteria for the diagnosis of infective endocarditis, Clin Infect Dis 30:633–638, 2000.

Mermel LA, Allon M, Bouza E, et al: Clinical practice guidelines for the diagnosis and management of intravascular catheter-related infection: 2009 Update by the Infectious Disease Society of America, Clin Infect Dis 49:1–45, 2009.

Morrisette T, Miller MA, Montague BT, et al: Long-acting lipoglycopeptides: "Lineless Antibiotics" for serious infections in persons who use drugs, Open Forum Infect Dis 6(7):ofz274, 2019, Published 2019 Jun 5.

Mylonakis E, Calderwood SB: Infective endocarditis in adults, N Engl J Med 345:1318–1330, 2001.

Steele JM, Seabury RW, Hale CM, et al: Unsuccessful treatment of methicillin-resistant Staphylococcus aureus endocarditis with dalbavancin, J Clin Pharm Ther 43:101–103, 2018.

Wilson W, Taubert KA, Gewitz M, et al: Prevention of infective endocarditis: guidelines from the American Heart Association: a guideline from the American Heart Association Rheumatic Fever, Endocarditis, and Kawasaki Disease Committee, Council on Cardiovascular Disease in the Young, and the Council on Clinical Cardiology, Council on Cardiovascular Surgery and Anesthesia, and the Quality of Care and Outcomes Research Interdisciplinary Working Group, Circulation 116:1736–1754, 2007.

9

Acute Bacterial Skin and Skin Structure Infections

Sajeev Handa

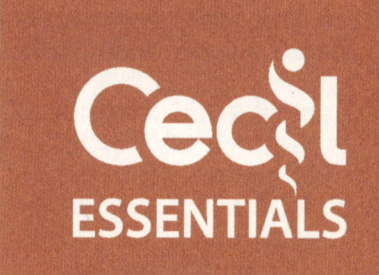

DEFINITION

Acute bacterial skin and skin structure infections (ABSSSIs) comprise infections of the skin, subcutaneous tissue, fascia, and muscle by a multitude of organisms. The focus of this chapter is on bacterial causes; however, references will be made to select viruses and fungi.

EPIDEMIOLOGY

ABSSSIs are among the most common infections found in all age groups. Although the exact incidence is unknown, several factors predispose to development of ABSSSIs:
- Epidermal breaks caused by trauma, surgical wounds, human or animal bites, or dry and irritated skin with concomitant tinea infection
- Immunosuppressed states caused by malnutrition, diabetes mellitus, or acquired immunodeficiency syndrome (AIDS)
- Chronic venous or lymphatic insufficiency

PATHOLOGY

Infectious Mechanisms

Microbes penetrate the integument after entering through a cut, bite, or hair follicle. Components of the host's defense system, including oxygen radicals, complement, immunoglobulins, macrophages, lymphocytes, and granulocytes, are recruited to the site of invasion through a vast plexus of dermal capillaries.

Bacteria contain proteins whose *N*-terminal amino acid sequence begins with an *N*-formyl-methionine group that is chemoattractive to phagocytes, including macrophages and granulocytes. Other microbial cell wall components, such as the zymosan of yeast, endotoxins of gram-negative bacteria, and the peptidoglycans of gram-positive bacteria, activate the alternative complement pathways, producing serum-derived chemotactic factors. Efflux of phagocytes occurs from the capillary through endothelial cell interstices and follows the gradient of chemotactic factors derived from bacteria and serum to the site of active infection.

Activated endothelial cells also produce chemotactic cytokines such as interleukin-8 (IL-8). Activated granulocytes synthesize leukotriene B_4 from arachidonic acid, a potent chemoattractant for leukocytes. Production of proinflammatory cytokines such as IL-1, IL-6, and tumor necrosis factor augments immune function, inducing fever, priming neutrophils, and increasing antibody production and synthesis of acute phase reactants such as C-reactive protein.

Cytokine-driven stimulation of endothelial cells generates nitric oxide and prostaglandins, both of which cause vasodilatation. The net physiologic effect is greater blood flow to the tissue, causing acute inflammation. As described by Celsus (30 BC to 38 AD), acute inflammation is characterized by rubor (i.e., redness), calor (i.e., increased heat), tumor (i.e., swelling), dolor (i.e., pain), and, as added by Virchow in the 19th century, function laesa (i.e., loss of function). Chapter 88 discusses host defenses against infection in more depth.

Pathologic Manifestations

Impetigo is characterized by thick, crusted lesions with rounded or irregular margins that typically occur on the face. Most cases are caused by *Staphylococcus aureus*, including methicillin-resistant *S. aureus* (MRSA), or by group A streptococci (e.g., *Streptococcus pyogenes*). Certain strains of streptococci causing impetigo have been implicated in the development of poststreptococcal glomerulonephritis.

Folliculitis is a superficial bacterial infection of the hair follicles. Purulent material is found in the epidermis. It manifests as clusters of multiple, small, raised, pruritic, erythematous lesions that are typically less than 5 mm in diameter.

Furuncles (i.e., boils) are infections of the hair follicle. Purulent material extends through the dermis into the subcutaneous tissue, where small abscesses may form. A carbuncle is coalescence of several inflamed follicles into a single inflammatory mass. Purulent drainage exudes from multiple follicles.

Cellulitis is superficial inflammation of the skin and underlying tissues. It is characterized by erythema, warmth, and tenderness of the involved area (Fig. 9.1). Erysipelas ("red skin") is a variant of cellulitis that is predominantly caused by toxin-producing *S. pyogenes*. It manifests as a superficial, spreading, warm, erythematous (fiery red) lesion distinguished by its indurated and elevated margin. Lymphatic involvement and vesicle formation are common. Groups B, C, and D streptococci may also be implicated (Fig. 9.2).

Necrotizing fasciitis is a progressive and rapidly spreading inflammatory reaction deep in the fascia associated with secondary necrosis of the subcutaneous tissues. Thrombosis of the dermal vessels is responsible for tissue necrosis. Necrotizing fasciitis may be polymicrobial (type I), involving aerobic microbes (e.g., streptococci, staphylococci, gram-negative bacilli) and anaerobes (e.g., *Peptostreptococcus, Bacteroides, Clostridioides* spp), or it may be monomicrobial (type II) and caused by *S. pyogenes* (Fig. 9.3). When involving the scrotum and perineal area, it is known as *Fournier gangrene*.

Pyomyositis is a less serious infection involving the musculature that results from direct inoculation of bacteria. For example, infection can result from injection drug use or from secondary seeding by *S. aureus* or group A β-hemolytic streptococci from an incidental bacteremia or a hematoma caused by non-penetrating trauma.

Ecthyma is an ulcerative pyoderma of the skin that extends into the dermis (unlike impetigo). It is caused by group A streptococci and *Pseudomonas* species.

急性细菌性皮肤和皮肤结构感染

张碧莹　路明　译　宁永忠　黄磊　审校　曹彬　通审

定义

急性细菌性皮肤和皮肤结构感染（ABSSSI）包括多种微生物引起的皮肤、皮下组织、筋膜和肌肉的感染。本章节重点关注细菌感染，在参考信息中也会提及特定的病毒和真菌内容。

流行病学

ABSSSI 在不同年龄的人群中都是最常见的感染之一，其具体的发病率尚不清楚，通常有几个常见的诱发因素：

- 外伤、手术切口、人或动物咬伤，或皮肤干燥并伴有足癣感染引起的表皮破损
- 营养不良、糖尿病或获得性免疫缺陷综合征（AIDS）引起的免疫抑制状态
- 慢性静脉或淋巴管功能不全

病理学

感染机制

微生物可通过皮肤切口、叮咬或毛囊进入并穿透表皮。宿主的防御系统成员，包括氧自由基、补体系统、免疫球蛋白、巨噬细胞、淋巴细胞和粒细胞等，可通过庞大的真皮毛细血管网被募集到微生物入侵部位。

以 N-甲酰蛋氨酸基起始的 N 末端氨基酸序列的细菌蛋白质对巨噬细胞和粒细胞等吞噬细胞具有趋化性。其他微生物的细胞壁组分，包括酵母的酵母聚糖、革兰氏阴性菌的内毒素和革兰氏阳性菌的肽聚糖，也可激活补体系统旁路途径，产生血清源性趋化因子。吞噬细胞穿过毛细血管内皮细胞间隙，并沿着细菌和血清的趋化因子梯度变化到达活动性的感染部位。

活化的内皮细胞也会产生白细胞介素-8 等趋化因子。活化的粒细胞可催化花生四烯酸合成另外一种强效的白细胞趋化因子白三烯 B_4。白细胞介素-1、白细胞介素-6 和肿瘤坏死因子等促炎细胞因子的产生可增强机体免疫功能，导致发热、中性粒细胞增多、抗体产生增加和急性相反应物如 C 反应蛋白的合成增加。

受到细胞因子刺激的内皮细胞可产生一氧化氮和前列腺素，引起血管舒张，使得更多的血液流向病变组织，从而导致急性炎症反应。正如古罗马时期医学家 Celsus（公元前 30 年—公元 38 年）所描述，急性炎症的特征是红（皮肤表面发红）、热（皮温升高）、肿（局部肿胀）、痛（疼痛）。到了 19 世纪，德国病理学家 Virchow 新增加了一个特征，即功能不全。第 88 章更深入地讨论了宿主对感染的防御作用。

病理表现

脓疱病的特征是皮肤变厚变硬，边缘呈圆形或不规则，通常发生在面部。大多数病例是由金黄色葡萄球菌（包括耐甲氧西林金黄色葡萄球菌，MRSA）或 A 组链球菌（即化脓性链球菌）所引起。导致脓疱病的某些链球菌可并发链球菌后肾小球肾炎。

毛囊炎是累及毛囊的浅表皮肤细菌感染，在表皮中可见化脓性物质，表现为多发、小的、隆起皮面的伴瘙痒的红斑，直径通常小于 5 mm。

疖是毛囊的感染。化脓性物质可通过真皮扩散到皮下组织，形成小的脓肿。痈是相邻的多个发炎毛囊融合汇聚成的一个炎症包块。脓液可从多个毛囊中渗出。

蜂窝织炎是皮肤和皮下组织的浅表炎症，其特征是受累区域出现皮肤发红、皮温升高和触痛（图 9.1）。丹毒（"红皮肤"）是蜂窝织炎的一种变体，主要由产毒素的化脓性链球菌引起。临床表现为浅表性、蔓延性、皮温升高的红斑（火红色），特征为皮肤发硬和边缘隆起，常可见淋巴受累和水疱形成。B 组、C 组和 D 组链球菌也可引起本病（图 9.2）。

坏死性筋膜炎是由细菌入侵筋膜深处引起的进展性和快速扩散的炎症反应，并伴有皮下组织的继发坏死。皮肤血管内血栓形成是导致皮肤组织坏死的主要原因。Ⅰ 型坏死性筋膜炎常由多种细菌混合感染所致，包括需氧菌（如链球菌、葡萄球菌、革兰氏阴性杆菌）和厌氧菌（如消化链球菌、拟杆菌、梭状芽孢杆菌属）等。而 Ⅱ 型坏死性筋膜炎常由单一细菌（如化脓性链球菌）感染所致（图 9.3）。当病变累及阴囊和会阴区时，称为富尼埃坏疽。

化脓性肌炎是细菌直接入侵肌肉组织的感染，通常病情并不严重。感染可由吸毒注射药物所致，也可由金黄色葡萄球菌或 A 组乙型溶血性链球菌等引起的偶发菌血症导致的细菌定植继发，还可由非穿透性创伤引起的血肿所致。

臁疮，是由 A 组链球菌和假单胞菌属的某些菌种所引起的一种延伸至真皮的溃疡性脓皮病，与脓疱病有明显差异。

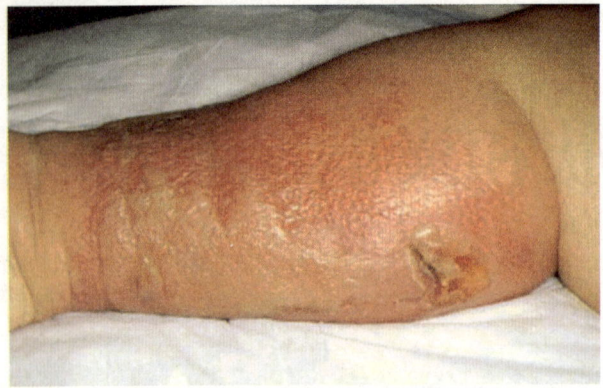

Fig. 9.1 Ill-defined erythema and edema with bullae formation is characteristic of lower extremity cellulitis. (From Pride HB: Cellulitis and erysipelas. In Zaoutis LB, Chiang VW, editors: Comprehensive pediatric hospital medicine, Philadelphia, 2007, Mosby, Fig. 156-1.)

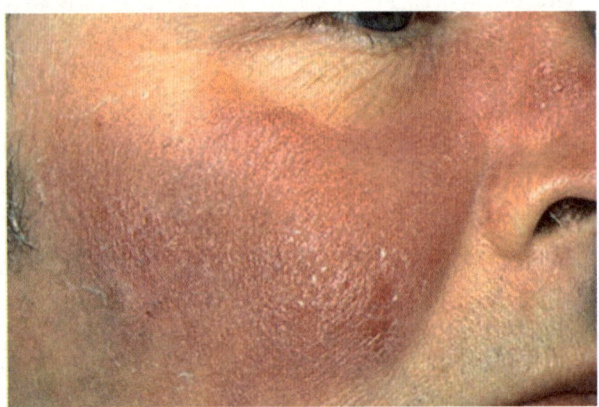

Fig. 9.2 Sharply defined erythema and edema is characteristic of erysipelas. (From Pride HB: Cellulitis and erysipelas. In Zaoutis LB, Chiang VW, editors: Comprehensive pediatric hospital medicine, Philadelphia, 2007, Mosby, Fig. 156-2.)

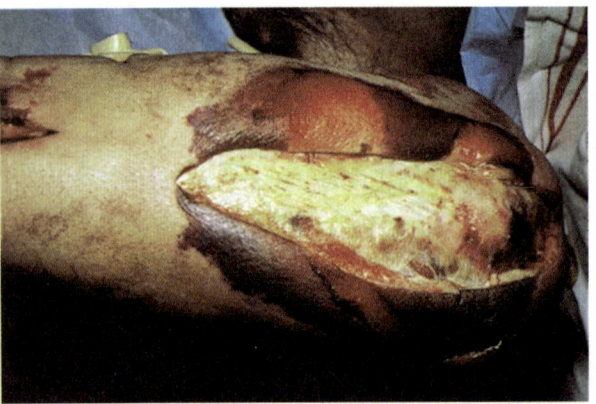

Fig. 9.3 Spontaneous necrotizing fasciitis due to *Clostridioides septicum*. The patient developed sudden onset of severe pain in the forearm. Swelling rapidly ensued, and he sought medical treatment. Crepitus was found on physical examination, and gas in the soft tissue was verified with routine radiographs. Immediate surgical débridement revealed necrotizing fasciitis but sparing of the muscle. Notice the purple-violaceous appearance of the skin. (From Stevens DL, Aldape MJ, Bryant AE. Necrotizing fasciitis, gas gangrene, myositis and myonecrosis. In Cohen J, Powderly WG, Opal SM, editors: Infectious diseases, ed 3, London, 2010, Mosby, Fig. 10-11.)

ETIOLOGY AND CLINICAL PRESENTATION

Causative Organisms

A multitude of organisms can cause ABSSSIs. However, three are most common: *S. pyogenes*, *S. aureus*, and *Streptococcus agalactiae*.

S. pyogenes (i.e., group A β-hemolytic streptococci) is a gram-positive coccus that may cause erysipelas, streptococcal cellulitis, necrotizing fasciitis, myositis, myonecrosis, and streptococcal toxic shock syndrome. Streptococcal cellulitis arises from infection of wounds, burns, or surgical incisions and may progress to involve large areas. Injection drug users and individuals with impaired lymphatic drainage are at high risk. Systemic manifestations include fever, chills, malaise with or without associated lymphangitis, and bacteremia. In contrast to erysipelas, the affected area is not raised, and the demarcation between involved skin and uninvolved skin is indistinct. The lesions tend to be more pink than fiery red.

Streptococcal toxic shock syndrome manifests with hypotension and is associated with acute kidney injury, elevated aminotransferases, rash or soft tissue necrosis, and coagulopathy. It may be complicated by the acute respiratory distress syndrome. Isolation of the organism from a sterile site provides a definite diagnosis.

S. aureus is a gram-positive coccus that is found in the anterior nares of up to 30% of healthy people. It is responsible for a variety of invasive and suppurative infections. Localized ABSSSIs include furuncles, carbuncles, bullous and nonbullous impetigo, mastitis, ecthyma, cellulitis, and wound and foreign body infections. Bacteremia may be complicated by septicemia, endocarditis, pericarditis, pneumonia, empyema, osteomyelitis, and abscesses of the soft tissue, muscle, and viscera.

Staphylococcal toxic shock syndrome is typically associated with tampon use but may occur after childbirth or surgery and can be associated with cutaneous lesions. It manifests with the acute onset of fever, erythroderma, hypotension, and multisystem involvement (e.g., acute kidney injury, elevated levels of aminotransferases, coagulopathy, nausea, vomiting, diarrhea).

Community-associated MRSA is the most common identifiable cause of ABSSSIs in the emergency department. Isolates contain genes encoding for multiple toxins, including cytotoxins that result in leukocyte destruction and tissue necrosis.

S. agalactiae (a group B streptococcus) is a gram-positive diplococcus. It may account for up to one third of ABSSSIs among adults. Cellulitis, foot ulcers, and infection of decubitus ulcers are common manifestations. Cellulitis has been associated with foreign bodies such as breast or penile implants. Less commonly, polymyositis, blistering dactylitis, and necrotizing fasciitis may occur.

Other Organisms

Aeromonas hydrophila, *Aeromonas veronii*, and *Aeromonas schubertii* are gram-negative rods found in salt and fresh water. They may cause mild to severe wound infections after injury, producing cellulitis, myonecrosis, and rhabdomyolysis. Necrotizing fasciitis has been reported with *A. veronii* and *A. schubertii* infections. *Aeromonas* wound infections have also been reported as a result of the medicinal use of leeches.

Arcanobacterium haemolyticum is a gram-positive, weakly acid-fast bacillus. It has been isolated from soft tissue infections, including chronic ulcers, cellulitis, and paronychia.

Bacillus anthracis is a gram-positive bacillus that forms spores. Transdermal inoculation of the spores from even incidental trauma can result in cutaneous anthrax. It manifests initially as a small, pruritic papule that becomes surrounded by painless, nonpurulent vesicles that easily rupture, leaving a black eschar at the base of the ulceration.

第 9 章 急性细菌性皮肤和皮肤结构感染

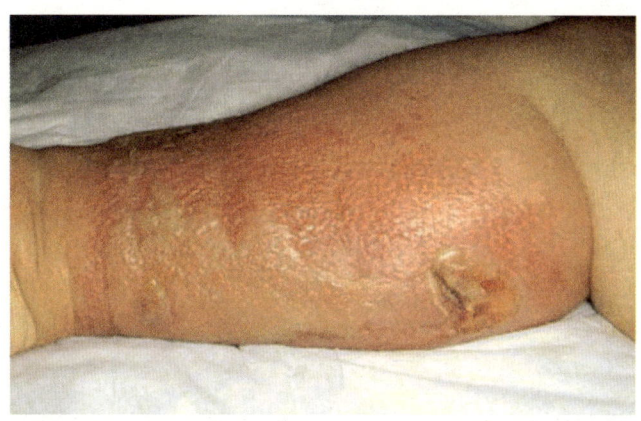

图 9.1 边界不清的红斑和水肿以及水疱形成是下肢蜂窝织炎的特征性表现（引自 Pride HB：Cellulitis and erysipelas. In Zaoutis LB, Chiang VW, editors: Comprehensive pediatric hospital medicine, Philadelphia, 2007, Mosby, Fig. 156-1.）

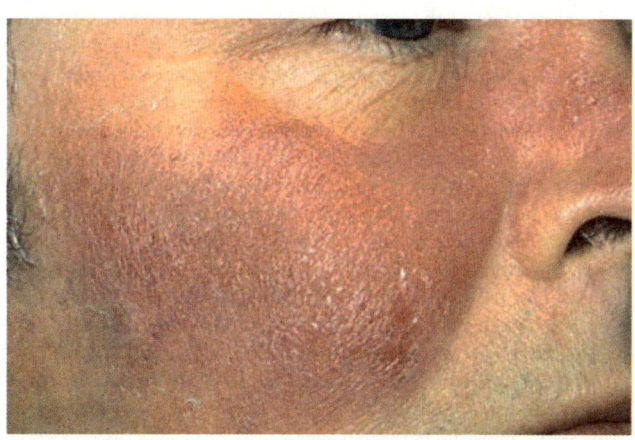

图 9.2 边界清晰的红斑和水肿是丹毒的特征性表现（引自 Pride HB：Cellulitis and erysipelas. In Zaoutis LB, Chiang VW, editors: Comprehensive pediatric hospital medicine, Philadelphia, 2007, Mosby, Fig. 156-2.）

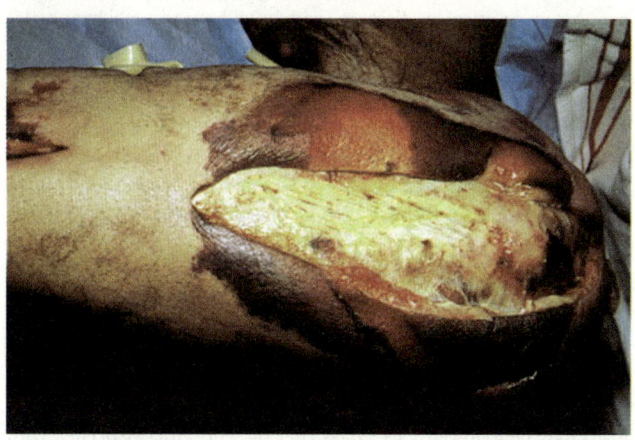

图 9.3 由梭状芽孢杆菌属引起的自发性坏死性筋膜炎。该患者因突发前臂严重疼痛，随后迅速肿胀而就诊。体格检查发现皮肤握雪感，X线片证实软组织内存在气体。立即行手术清创证实为坏死性筋膜炎，但肌肉未受累。注意皮肤外观呈紫色（引自 Stevens DL, Aldape MJ, Bryant AE. Necrotizing fasciitis, gas gangrene, myositis and myonecrosis. In Cohen J, Powderly WG, Opal SM, editors: Infectious diseases, ed 3, London, 2010, Mosby, Fig. 10-11.）

病因和临床表现

致病微生物

许多微生物都可以引起 ABSSSI。其中最常见的三个致病菌为化脓性链球菌、金黄色葡萄球菌和无乳链球菌。

化脓性链球菌（即 A 组乙型溶血性链球菌）是一种革兰氏阳性球菌，可引起丹毒、链球菌蜂窝织炎、坏死性筋膜炎、肌炎、肌坏死和链球菌中毒性休克综合征。链球菌性蜂窝织炎由伤口、烧伤或手术切口感染引起，可逐渐进展累及大面积皮肤区域。静脉吸毒者和淋巴引流功能受损者是高风险人群。全身表现包括发热、寒战、乏力，伴或不伴有淋巴管炎和菌血症。与丹毒相比，受累皮肤不隆起于皮面，受累皮肤和未受累皮肤之间的界线不清楚。病变更多呈粉红色，而不是火红色。

链球菌中毒性休克综合征表现为低血压伴有急性肾损伤、转氨酶升高、皮疹或软组织坏死，以及凝血功能障碍，也可能会并发急性呼吸窘迫综合征。从无菌部位分离到微生物可确诊。

金黄色葡萄球菌是一种革兰氏阳性球菌，从高达 30% 的健康人群的前鼻孔可检出该菌，可导致多种侵袭性和化脓性感染。局限性 ABSSSI 包括疖、痈、大疱性和非大疱性脓疱病、乳腺炎、臁疮、蜂窝织炎、伤口和异物继发感染等。菌血症可并发感染中毒症、心内膜炎、心包炎、肺炎、脓胸、骨髓炎，以及软组织、肌肉和内脏脓肿。

葡萄球菌中毒性休克综合征通常与卫生棉条的使用有关，但也会发生在分娩或手术后，与皮肤病变相关。通常表现为急性发热、皮肤发红、低血压和多系统受累（如急性肾损伤、转氨酶升高、凝血功能障碍、恶心、呕吐、腹泻）。

社区相关性 MRSA 是急诊科 ABSSSI 最常见的可识别的病因。分离的致病菌中常含有编码导致白细胞破坏和组织坏死等多种毒素的基因。

无乳链球菌（B 组链球菌）是一种革兰氏阳性双球菌，约占成人 ABSSSI 的 1/3。

蜂窝织炎、足部溃疡和压疮感染是常见的表现。蜂窝织炎往往与乳房或阴茎假体植入物等异物有关。而多发性肌炎、水疱性指（趾）炎和坏死性筋膜炎则并不常见。

其他微生物

嗜水气单胞菌，维氏气单胞菌和舒伯特气单胞菌是在盐水和淡水中发现的革兰氏阴性杆菌。这些细菌可导致损伤后的伤口感染，从轻微到严重的感染，包括蜂窝织炎、肌坏死和横纹肌溶解。有研究报道，维氏气单胞菌和舒伯特气单胞菌可导致坏死性筋膜炎，医用水蛭也可引起气单胞菌伤口感染。

溶血性隐秘杆菌是一种革兰氏染色阳性、抗酸染色弱阳性的杆菌，可从慢性溃疡、蜂窝织炎和甲沟炎等感染的软组织中分离到。

炭疽杆菌是能够形成芽孢的革兰氏阳性杆菌。即使是很偶然的创伤，该菌芽孢也可经皮肤进入，导致皮肤炭疽。它最初表现为很小的化脓性丘疹，之后周围出现无痛性的非脓性小疱，小疱很容易破裂，在溃

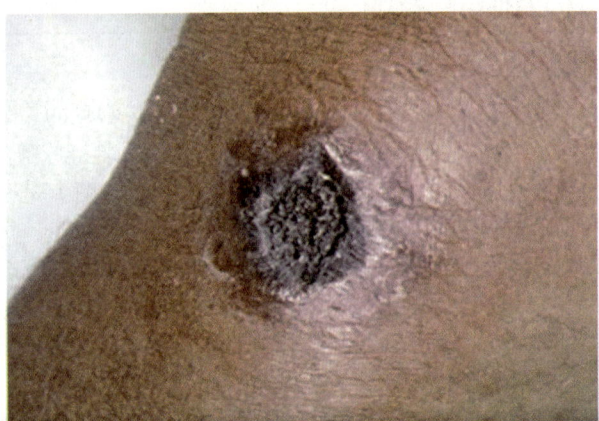

Fig. 9.4 Cutaneous anthrax lesion on the skin of the forearm caused by the bacterium *Bacillus anthracis*. (From Centers for Disease Control and Prevention: Public health image library. Available at http://phil.cdc.gov/Phil/home.asp. Accessed October 31, 2014.)

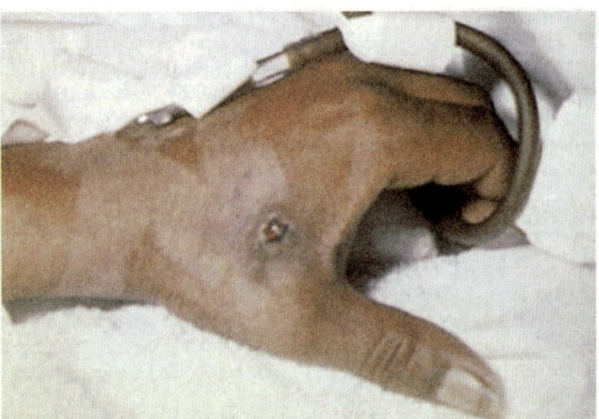

Fig. 9.5 Tularemic ulcer with eschar formation after percutaneous inoculation of *Francisella tularensis*. (From Beard CB, Dennis DT: Tularemia. In Cohen J, Powderly WG, Opal SM, editors: Infectious diseases, ed 3, London, 2010, Mosby.)

Uncomplicated disease heals without scar formation in 1 to 3 weeks. Serious cutaneous disease is marked by extensive edema, worsening inflammation, and toxemia (Fig. 9.4).

Bartonella henselae is a gram-negative bacillus that causes cat-scratch disease. Between 3 and 10 days after a bite or scratch from a cat or other vector, a tender, erythematous papule appears. Lymphadenopathy ipsilateral to the site of inoculation occurs 1 to 3 weeks later, and the patient typically experiences constitutional symptoms. The lymphadenopathy may take months to resolve.

Capnocytophaga canimorsus is a thin, gram-negative bacillus with tapered ends. It is strongly associated with dog (primarily) and cat bites and scratches. Asplenic patients are at particular risk for sepsis due to this organism.

Clostridioides perfringens is an anaerobic, large, gram-positive rod. It can cause cellulitis or life-threatening necrotizing infections of skin, muscle, and other soft tissues. The latter is characterized by rapidly progressive tissue destruction, gas in tissues, shock, and death. Conditions such as trauma or illicit drug injection produce anaerobic tissue conditions that favor the organism. The condition can also develop in patients with bowel carcinoma or neutropenia. Gram stain of tissue or exudate reveals large, gram-positive rods and no inflammatory cells.

Edwardsiella tarda is a gram-negative rod found in fresh water environments. It is associated with wound infections, abscesses, and bacteremia. The mortality rate is high among patients with liver disease and iron overload.

Eikenella corrodens is a gram-negative bacillus that is part of the normal human oral flora. It is an important pathogen in human bite wounds, closed-fist injuries, and infections seen in chronic finger or nail biters. Severe soft tissue infection may occur, leading to septic arthritis and osteomyelitis.

Erysipelothrix rhusiopathiae is a gram-positive rod, but it may appear as gram-negative because of rapid decolorization. Its major reservoir is in domestic swine, and infection occurs by direct cutaneous contact through a cut or abrasion. Disease is characterized as erysipeloid (i.e., subacute cellulitis with vesiculation), as a diffuse cutaneous eruption with systemic symptoms, or as bacteremia that is often associated with endocarditis.

Francisella tularensis is a gram-negative coccobacillus found in rabbits, hares, hamsters, and rodents. Ulceroglandular tularemia occurs 3 to 5 days after humans are inoculated cutaneously during contact with any of these species. A papule is formed initially, followed by ulceration with enlargement of the regional lymph nodes. Vesicles may be seen. If left untreated, the ulcer remains for weeks before healing, leaving a residual scar. Suppuration of the affected lymph nodes is the most common complication, occurring despite appropriate treatment (Fig. 9.5). *B. anthracis* and *F. tularensis* have been used as agents in bioterrorism.

Mycobacterium marinum is an atypical, acid-fast bacillus; it is the most common atypical mycobacterium that causes infection in humans. After inoculation of a skin abrasion or puncture wound in salt or fresh water (nonchlorinated), lesions appear as papules on an extremity. Lesions progress to shallow ulcers and form scars. Typically, lesions are solitary, but they may take on the appearance of ascending, sporotrichoid-like, nodular lymphangitis that may involve the local joint or tendons.

Mycobacterium leprae is a slow-growing, acid-fast bacillus that cannot be grown in vitro. It is the cause of leprosy (Hansen disease). It is primarily transmitted by the airborne route and causes chronic disfiguring skin lesions and nerve damage.

For a deeper discussion of this topic, please see Chapter 310, "Leprosy (Hansen Disease)" in *Goldman-Cecil Medicine*, 26th Edition.

Pasteurella multocida is a gram-negative coccobacillus that may occur at the site of a scratch or bite from a dog or cat. Cellulitis results within 24 hours of the injury, producing swelling, erythema, tenderness, serous or purulent discharge with or without regional lymphadenopathy, chills, and fever.

Pseudomonas aeruginosa is a gram-negative rod and primarily a nosocomial pathogen. In the community, serogroup 0:11 may cause folliculitis related to the use of hot tubs, whirlpools, and swimming pools. Typically, the eruption occurs 48 hours after exposure and consists of tender, pruritic papules, papulopustules, or nodules. It is an important pathogen in burn wound infections, which may progress to sepsis.

Vibrio vulnificus is a gram-negative bacillus that is spread by contamination of a superficial wound with warm seawater. It can cause rapidly developing and intense cellulitis, necrotizing fasciitis, and ulcer formation. Aggressive soft tissue infection may occur with necrosis, fever, sepsis, and bullae formation. Ingestion of raw oysters, particularly by immunocompromised patients (e.g., liver cirrhosis, iron overload) may be followed 1 to 3 days later by septicemia associated with necrotizing cutaneous lesions.

Select Fungi and Viruses

Cryptococcus neoformans, Candida albicans, Histoplasma capsulatum, Blastomyces dermatitidis, Coccidioides immitis, and

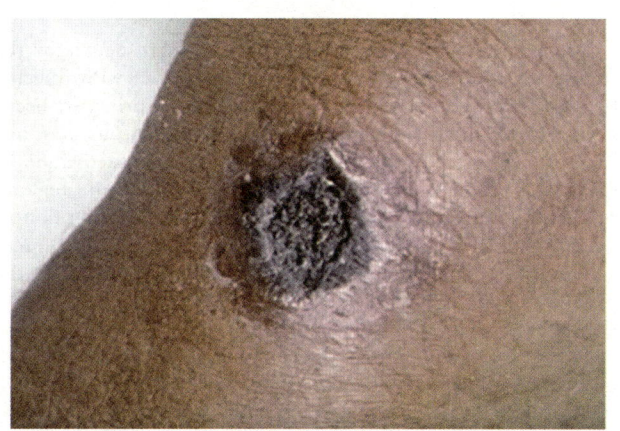

图 9.4 炭疽杆菌引起的前臂皮肤炭疽（引自 Centers for Disease Control and Prevention: Public health image library. Available at http://phil.cdc.gov/Phil/home.asp. Accessed October 31, 2014.）

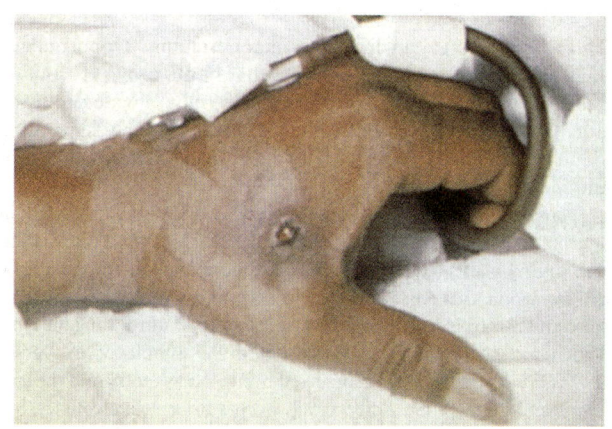

图 9.5 土拉热弗朗西丝菌经皮肤入侵后感染形成焦痂的兔热病溃疡（引自 Beard CB, Dennis DT: Tularemia. In Cohen J, Powderly WG, Opal SM, editors: Infectious diseases, ed 3, London, 2010, Mosby.）

疡底部留下黑色焦痂。非复杂性疾病通常在 1～3 周愈合，不留疤痕。严重的皮肤病变可表现为广泛水肿、进行性恶化的炎症和毒血症（图 9.4）。

汉赛巴尔通体是革兰氏阴性杆菌，可导致猫抓病。在猫或其他宿主动物咬或抓之后的 3～10 天，局部皮肤会出现有触痛的红色斑丘疹。随后的 1～3 周，可出现患侧淋巴结肿大和全身症状。肿大的淋巴结可能需要数月才能消退。

犬咬二氧化碳嗜纤维菌是一种细长的革兰氏阴性杆菌，末端呈锥形，其感染与狗（最常见）、猫的咬伤和抓伤密切相关。无脾患者是该菌感染的高风险人群，感染后易导致感染中毒症。

产气荚膜梭菌是一种厌氧的、粗大的革兰氏阳性杆菌，可引起蜂窝织炎或危及生命的皮肤、肌肉和其他软组织的坏死性感染。后者的特征是快速进展的组织坏死、组织内气体产生、休克和死亡。创伤或静脉吸毒等情况可导致机体组织出现有利于该微生物生长的厌氧环境。也可发生于小肠癌或中性粒细胞缺乏的患者。组织或渗出物的革兰氏染色显示可见粗大的革兰氏阳性杆菌，而没有炎症细胞。

迟钝爱德华菌是在淡水环境中发现的革兰氏阴性杆菌，与伤口感染、脓肿和菌血症有关。有基础肝病和铁过载的患者的死亡率高。

啮蚀艾肯菌是一种革兰氏阴性杆菌，为正常人类口腔菌群的一部分。在人类咬伤伤口、闭合拳头伤（译者注：即一个人握紧的拳头打在另一个人的牙齿上导致的拳头损伤）和慢性啃手指或啃指甲的感染中，是非常重要的病原体。严重的软组织感染可导致化脓性关节炎和骨髓炎。

猪红斑丹毒丝菌是一种革兰氏阳性杆菌，但由于快速脱色，也可能呈现为革兰氏染色阴性。该菌的主要储存宿主是家猪，主要通过切口或磨损的皮肤直接接触引发感染。本病的临床特点是类丹毒样表现（即亚急性蜂窝织炎伴水疱形成），伴有全身症状的弥漫性皮肤红疹，或者常与心内膜炎相关的菌血症。

土拉热弗朗西丝菌是在家兔、野兔、仓鼠和啮齿动物中发现的革兰氏阴性球杆菌。溃疡性兔热病通常发生在人类皮肤直接接触该菌并入侵皮肤导致感染的 3～5 天。皮疹最初为丘疹，后形成溃疡并伴有局部淋巴结肿大。还可见水疱。如果治疗不及时，溃疡会持续数周才愈合，并会留疤。即使给予了合适的治疗，受累区域的淋巴结化脓也是最常见的并发症（图 9.5）。炭疽杆菌和土拉热弗朗西丝菌已用于生物恐怖袭击。

海分枝杆菌是一种非典型的抗酸杆菌，是导致人类感染最常见的非典型分枝杆菌。皮肤擦伤或穿刺伤后，在盐水或未氯化的淡水中接触该菌后可导致感染，病变表现为四肢的丘疹，继而发展为浅层溃疡并形成瘢痕。典型者呈孤立性病灶，但也可表现为逐渐进展的孢子丝菌病样的结节性淋巴管炎，可累及局部关节或肌腱。

麻风分枝杆菌是一种慢生长的抗酸杆菌，不能在体外生长。它是麻风病（Hansen 病）的病因，主要通过空气传播，可引起慢性毁容性皮肤损伤和神经损伤。

有关此专题的深入讨论，请参阅 Goldman-Cecil Medicine 第 26 版第 310 章"麻风病"。

多杀巴斯德菌是一种革兰氏阴性球杆菌，可发生于狗或猫的抓伤或咬伤的部位。在损伤后的 24 h 内可引起蜂窝织炎，产生肿胀、红斑、触痛、浆液性或脓性分泌物，伴或不伴局部淋巴性肿大、寒战和发热。

铜绿假单胞菌是一种革兰氏阴性杆菌，主要是医院感染的病原体。在社区中，血清型 0：11 可能会导致毛囊炎，与使用热水浴缸、漩涡池和游泳池相关。皮疹通常发生在暴露后 48 h，表现为压痛和瘙痒性丘疹、脓疱性丘疹或结节。铜绿假单胞菌是烧伤伤口感染的重要病原体，可发展为感染中毒症。

创伤弧菌是一种革兰氏阴性杆菌，通过温暖的海水污染浅表伤口而传播。它可引起迅速进展的严重的蜂窝织炎、坏死性筋膜炎和溃疡。侵袭性软组织感染可伴有坏死、发热、感染中毒症和大疱形成。食用生蚝的患者，特别是免疫抑制宿主（如肝硬化、铁过载），可能在 1～3 天后出现与皮肤坏死相关的感染中毒症。

特定的真菌和病毒

新型隐球菌、白念珠菌、荚膜组织胞浆菌、皮炎

opportunistic fungi can have skin manifestations. Opportunistic fungi, including *Aspergillus* species, fungi in the order Mucorales, and *Fusarium* species, can infect the skin of immunocompromised patients. Skin manifestations of fungal infections include papules, nodules, circumscribed erythematous lesions, ulcers, verrucous lesions, and eschars.

Sporothrix schenckii is a dimorphic fungus ubiquitous primarily in the tropical parts of North and South America. Cutaneous inoculation from thorny plants (e.g., rose bushes) is followed by development of a painless papule that enlarges slowly to become a nodular lesion with a violaceous hue or ulceration. Secondary lesions may form along the lymphatic drainage distribution. Exposure to herpes simplex virus types 1 and 2 (HSV-1 and HSV-2) at abraded skin sites allows entry into the epidermis and dermis. Infection typically occurs from sexual contact, but it occasionally occurs at extraoral or extragenital sites, such as the hands of health care workers, producing a painful erythema primarily at the junction of the nail bed and skin (i.e., whitlow). This progresses to a vesicopustular lesion that can mimic a bacterial infection (i.e., paronychia). Sexually transmitted diseases are discussed in Chapter 100.

Primary varicella-zoster virus (VZV) infection occurs by the respiratory route but may occur through contact with infected lesions. Viremia results in crops of papules that primarily occur on the trunk and progress to vesicles and then to pustules, followed by crusting. Zoster or shingles represents reactivation of the latent virus in the sensory neurons of the dorsal root ganglion, resulting in pain that proceeds to a rash in the distribution of the affected dermatome in a few days. The appearance of papules and vesicles in a unilateral dermatomal distribution confirms the diagnosis. Ramsay Hunt syndrome occurs when the VZV infection involves the geniculate ganglia and causes a painful eruption in the ear canal and tympanic membrane that is associated with ipsilateral seventh cranial nerve palsy. Vesicles that appear on the tip of the nose (i.e., Hutchinson sign) may be preceded by development of ophthalmic zoster and involvement of the cornea. Immunosuppressed individuals are at higher risk for disseminated disease.

Table 9.1 provides a classification for the spectrum of skin involvement by bacteria and fungi.

TABLE 9.1 Classification of Bacterial and Mycotic Infections of the Skin

Disease or Disorder	Microorganisms
Primary Pyodermas	
Impetigo	*Staphylococcus aureus*, group A streptococci
Folliculitis	*S. aureus, Candida* spp, *Pseudomonas aeruginosa* (diffuse folliculitis), *Malassezia furfur, Pityrosporum ovale*
Furuncles and carbuncles	*S. aureus*
Paronychia	*S. aureus*, group A streptococci, *Candida, P. aeruginosa*
Ecthyma	Group A streptococci, *Pseudomonas* spp
Erysipelas	Group A streptococci
Chancriform lesions	*Treponema pallidum, Haemophilus ducreyi, Sporothrix, Bacillus anthracis, Francisella tularensis, Mycobacterium ulcerans, Mycobacterium marinum*
Membranous ulcers	*Corynebacterium diphtheriae*
Cellulitis	Group A or other streptococci, *S. aureus*; rarely, various other organisms
Infectious Gangrene and Gangrenous Cellulitis	
Streptococcal gangrene and necrotizing fasciitis	Group A streptococci, mixed infections with Enterobacteriaceae and anaerobes
Progressive bacterial synergistic gangrene	Anaerobic streptococci plus a second organism (*S. aureus, Proteus* spp)
Gangrenous balanitis and perineal phlegmon	Group A streptococci, mixed infections with enteric bacteria (*Escherichia coli, Klebsiella* spp), anaerobes
Gas gangrene, crepitant cellulitis	*Clostridioides perfringens* and other clostridial species; *Bacteroides* spp, peptostreptococci, *Klebsiella* spp, *E. coli*
Gangrenous cellulitis in immunosuppressed patients	*Pseudomonas, Aspergillus* spp, agents of mucormycosis
Preexisting Skin Lesions With Secondary Bacterial Infections	
Burns	*P. aeruginosa, Enterobacter* spp, various other gram-negative bacilli, various streptococci, *S. aureus, Candida* spp, *Aspergillus* spp
Eczematous dermatitis and exfoliative erythrodermas	*S. aureus*, group A streptococci
Chronic ulcers (varicose, decubitus)	*S. aureus*, streptococci, coliform bacteria, *P. aeruginosa*, peptostreptococci, enterococci, *Bacteroides* spp., *C. perfringens*
Dermatophytosis	*S. aureus*, group A streptococci
Traumatic lesions (abrasions, animal bites, insect bites)	*Pasteurella multocida, C. diphtheriae, S. aureus*, group A streptococci
Vesicular or bullous eruptions (varicella, pemphigus)	*S. aureus*, group A streptococci
Acne conglobata	*Cutibacterium* (formerly *Propionibacterium*) *acnes*
Hidradenitis suppurativa	*S. aureus, Proteus* spp. and other coliforms, streptococci, peptostreptococci, *P. aeruginosa, Bacteroides* spp.
Intertrigo	*S. aureus*, coliforms, *Candida* spp
Pilonidal and sebaceous cysts	Peptostreptococci, *Bacteroides* sp, coliforms, *S. aureus*
Pyoderma gangrenosa	*S. aureus*, peptostreptococci, *Proteus* spp and other coliforms, *P. aeruginosa*

芽生菌、粗球孢子菌和机会性真菌也可引起皮肤病变。机会性真菌，包括曲霉菌属、毛霉菌目和镰刀菌属，可以导致免疫抑制患者的皮肤发生感染，表现包括丘疹、结节、局限性红斑、溃疡、疣状病变和焦痂。

申克孢子丝菌是一种双相真菌，主要普遍存在于北美和南美洲的热带地区。皮肤在接触多刺植物（如玫瑰丛）后感染，最初为无痛性丘疹，后慢慢扩大为紫色结节或溃疡。继发性病变的形成可沿淋巴管流向分布。

皮肤擦伤部位暴露于1型和2型单纯疱疹病毒（HSV-1和HSV-2）后，病毒可以进入表皮和真皮。感染通常发生在性接触后，但偶尔发生在口腔外或生殖器外的部位，如医护人员的手部，主要在甲床和皮肤的交界处，引起疼痛的红斑。这种情况可进展为脓疱样病变，类似细菌感染（即，甲沟炎）。性传播疾病的相关内容会在第100章进行讨论。

原发性水痘-带状疱疹病毒（VZV）感染通过呼吸道传播，也可能通过皮肤接触而传播。病毒血症导致主要发生于躯干部位的大量丘疹，后发展为小水疱，再发展为脓疱，然后结痂。带状疱疹反映了潜伏于背根神经节感觉神经元中病毒的重新激活，初始表现为疼痛，几天后在受累皮肤区域出现皮疹。表现为在单侧皮肤分布的丘疹和水疱，有助于确定诊断。当水痘-带状疱疹病毒感染累及膝状神经节，导致耳道和鼓膜疼痛性皮疹时，称为拉姆齐·亨特综合征，这与同侧第Ⅶ脑神经麻痹有关。出现在鼻尖上的水疱（即Hutchinson征）可先于眼带状疱疹和角膜的受累而出现。免疫抑制患者发生播散性疾病的风险更高。

表9.1提供了涉及皮肤的细菌和真菌感染的疾病谱分类。

表9.1 皮肤细菌和真菌感染的分类	
疾病	微生物
原发性脓皮病	
脓疱病	金黄色葡萄球菌，A组链球菌
毛囊炎	金黄色葡萄球菌，念珠菌属，铜绿假单胞菌（弥漫性毛囊炎），毛皮马拉色菌
疖、痈	金黄色葡萄球菌
甲沟炎	金黄色葡萄球菌，A组链球菌，念珠菌属，铜绿假单胞菌
臁疮	A组链球菌，假单胞菌属
丹毒	A组链球菌
下疳样病变	梅毒螺旋体，杜克雷嗜血杆菌，孢子丝菌，炭疽杆菌，土拉热弗朗西丝菌，溃疡分枝杆菌，海分枝杆菌
膜性溃疡	白喉棒状杆菌
蜂窝织炎	A组或其他组链球菌，金黄色葡萄球菌，罕见；其他微生物
感染性坏疽与坏疽性蜂窝织炎	
链球菌坏疽和坏死性筋膜炎	A组链球菌，混合感染肠杆菌科和厌氧菌
进行性细菌性协同性坏疽	厌氧链球菌＋另一种微生物（金黄色葡萄球菌，变形杆菌属）
坏疽性龟头炎和会阴蜂窝织炎	A组链球菌，混合感染肠杆菌科细菌（大肠埃希菌、克雷伯菌属），厌氧菌
气性坏疽，气肿性蜂窝织炎	产气荚膜梭菌和其他梭菌属；拟杆菌属，消化链球菌，克雷伯菌属，大肠埃希菌
免疫抑制患者的坏疽性蜂窝织炎	假单胞菌属，曲霉，毛霉
基础皮病病继发细菌感染	
烧伤	铜绿假单胞菌，肠杆菌属，多种其他革兰阴性杆菌，多种链球菌，金黄色葡萄球菌，念珠菌，曲霉菌
湿疹性皮炎和剥脱性红皮病	金黄色葡萄球菌，A组链球菌
慢性溃疡（静脉曲张、压疮）	金黄色葡萄球菌，链球菌，大肠埃希菌，铜绿假单胞菌，消化链球菌，肠菌属，拟杆菌属，产气荚膜梭菌
皮癣	金黄色葡萄球菌，A组链球菌
外伤（擦伤、动物咬伤、昆虫咬伤）	多杀巴斯德菌，白喉棒状杆菌，金黄色葡萄球菌，A组链球菌
水疱或大疱性皮疹（水痘、天疱疮）	金黄色葡萄球菌，A组链球菌
聚合型痤疮	痤疮皮肤杆菌（旧称痤疮丙酸杆菌）
化脓性汗腺炎	金黄色葡萄球菌，变形杆菌属和其他肠杆菌，链球菌和消化链球菌，铜绿假单胞菌，拟杆菌属
擦烂	金黄色葡萄球菌，肠杆菌属，念珠菌属
皮脂腺囊肿	消化链球菌，拟杆菌属，肠杆菌和金黄色葡萄球菌
坏疽性脓皮病	金黄色葡萄球菌，消化链球菌，变形杆菌属和其他肠杆菌，铜绿假单胞菌

TABLE 9.1 Classification of Bacterial and Mycotic Infections of the Skin—cont'd

Disease or Disorder	Microorganisms
Cutaneous Involvement in Systemic Infections	
Bacteremias	S. aureus, group A streptococci (and other groups such as D), Neisseria meningitidis, Neisseria gonorrhoeae, P. aeruginosa, Salmonella typhi, Haemophilus influenzae
Infective endocarditis	Viridans streptococci, S. aureus, group D streptococci, and others
Fungemias	Candida spp, Cryptococcus spp, Blastomyces dermatitidis, Fusarium
Listeriosis	Listeria monocytogenes
Leptospirosis (Weil disease and pretibial fever)	Leptospira interrogans serotypes
Rat-bite fever	Streptobacillus moniliformis, Spirillum minus
Melioidosis	Burkholderia pseudomallei
Glanders	Burkholderia mallei
Carrión's disease (verruga peruana)	Bartonella bacilliformis
Scarlet Fever Syndromes	
Scarlet fever	Group A streptococci, rarely S. aureus
Scalded skin syndrome	S. aureus (phage group II)
Toxic shock syndrome	Group A streptococci, S. aureus (pyrogenic toxin–producing strains)
Parainfectious and Postinfectious Nonsuppurative Complications	
Purpura fulminans (manifestation of disseminated intravascular coagulation)	Group A streptococci, N. meningitidis, S. aureus, pneumococcus
Erythema nodosum	Group A streptococci, Mycobacterium tuberculosis, Mycobacterium leprae, Coccidioides immitis, Leptospira autumnalis, Yersinia enterocolitica, Legionella pneumophila
Erythema multiforme–like lesions (rarely), guttate psoriasis	Group A streptococci
Other Lesions	
Erythrasma	Corynebacterium minutissimum
Nodular lesions	Candida, Sporothrix, S. aureus (botryomycosis), M. marinum, Leishmania brasiliensis; leprosy due to M. leprae can cause popular lesions, nodular, and ulcerative lesions
Hyperplastic (pseudoepitheliomatous) and proliferative lesions (e.g., mycetomas)	Nocardia spp, Scedosporium apiospermum (formerly Pseudallescheria boydii), Blastomyces dermatitidis, Paracoccidioides brasiliensis, Phialophora, Cladosporium
Vascular papules/nodules (bacillary angiomatosis, epithelioid angiomatosis)	Bartonella henselae, Bartonella quintana
Annular erythema (erythema chronicum migrans)	Borrelia burgdorferi

Modified from Mandell GL, Bennett JE, Dolin R, editors: Mandell, Douglas, and Bennett's principles and practice of infectious diseases, ed 9, Philadelphia, 2020, Elsevier.

DIAGNOSIS

A thorough medical history is critical; it should assess the specific risk factors, such as travel history, animal contacts, marine exposures, occupational and avocational hazards (e.g., farming, gardening), and immune status. If an animal bite has occurred, the timing of the bite, circumstances of injury, and health status of the animal should be determined. Human bites are classified as self-inflicted, occlusal (i.e., intentional), or closed-fist injuries.

In addition to wound assessment, evaluation for other transmissible pathogens, including human immunodeficiency virus (HIV), HSV, *Treponema pallidum* (the etiologic agent of syphilis), and hepatitis B and C viruses, should be pursued. A thorough clinical examination should follow. Initial antimicrobial management, if indicated, is directed by the history and physical examination findings.

Evaluation of hospitalized patients should include a complete blood count and a basic metabolic panel. The C-reactive protein level may be useful as a marker for inflammation and guidance for treatment. The creatine phosphokinase concentration may be helpful, but it is not specific for cases of compartment syndrome and necrotizing fasciitis involving the musculature. Cultures are not indicated for uncomplicated common forms of ABSSSIs managed in the outpatient setting. The benefit of blood cultures for cellulitis in hospitalized patients is uncertain because the yield is low. Cultures are indicated for patients who require incision and drainage because of the risk of deep structure and underlying tissue involvement.

The most sensitive and specific test for the diagnosis of HSV and VZV cutaneous lesions is nucleic acid amplification. A sample is scraped from the base of an active dermal lesion with a swab. Direct fluorescent antibody testing is less sensitive. Incision and drainage of these lesions is contraindicated.

Special Diagnostic Considerations
Animal Bites
Blood cultures, tissue biopsy, and aspirates for culture of aerobic or anaerobic organisms are preferred methods in cases of animal bites.

表 9.1 皮肤细菌和真菌感染的分类（续表）

疾病	微生物
系统性疾病皮肤受累	
菌血症	金黄色葡萄球菌，A 组链球菌（和其他组链球菌，如 D 组），脑膜炎奈瑟球菌，淋病奈瑟球菌，铜绿假单胞菌，伤寒沙门菌，流感嗜血杆菌
感染性心内膜炎	草绿色链球菌，金黄色葡萄球菌，D 组链球菌及其他
真菌血症	念珠菌属，隐球菌属，皮炎芽生菌，镰孢菌
李斯特菌病	单核细胞增生李斯特菌
钩端螺旋体病（威尔病和胫前热）	问号血清型钩端螺旋体
鼠咬热	念珠状链杆菌，小螺菌
类鼻疽	类鼻疽伯克霍尔德菌
鼻疽	鼻疽伯克霍尔德菌
卡里翁病（秘鲁疣）	杆菌状巴尔通体
猩红热综合征	
猩红热	A 组链球菌，金黄色葡萄球菌罕见
皮肤烫伤样综合征	金黄色葡萄球菌（Ⅱ组噬菌体）
中毒性休克综合征	A 组链球菌，金黄色葡萄球菌（致热产毒型菌株）
感染伴发和感染后非化脓性并发症	
暴发性紫癜（弥散性血管内凝血的表现）	A 组链球菌，脑膜炎奈瑟球菌，金黄色葡萄球菌，肺炎链球菌
结节性红斑	A 组链球菌，结核分枝杆菌，麻风分枝杆菌，粗球孢子菌，秋季钩端螺旋体，小肠结肠炎耶尔森菌，嗜肺军团菌
多形性红斑样病变（罕见），滴状银屑病	A 组链球菌
其他病变	
红癣	极小棒杆菌
结节样病变	念珠菌，孢子丝菌，金黄色葡萄球菌（肉毒杆菌病），海分枝杆菌，巴西利什曼原虫；麻风杆菌引起的麻风病可引起常见病变，结节和溃疡性病变
增生性（假上皮瘤样）和增殖性病变（如霉菌瘤）	诺卡菌属，尖端赛多孢子菌，皮炎芽生菌，巴西副球孢子菌，瓶霉，芽枝霉
血管丘疹/结节（细菌性血管瘤病、上皮样血管瘤病）	汉赛巴尔通体，五日热巴尔通体
环状红斑（慢性游走性红斑）	伯氏疏螺旋体

改编自 Mandell GL, Bennett JE, Dolin R, editors: Mandell, Douglas, and Bennett's principles and practice of infectious diseases, ed 9, Philadelphia, 2020, Elsevier.

诊断

全面的病史询问至关重要；应注意评估具体的危险因素，如旅行史、动物接触、海水接触、职业和业余爱好（如农业、园艺）以及免疫状态等。如果发生了动物咬伤，应确定咬伤的时间、受伤的环境以及动物的健康状况。人类咬伤分为自伤、咬合伤（即故意咬伤）或闭合拳头伤。

除了评估伤口之外，还应进行其他评估，包括人类免疫缺陷病毒（HIV）、单纯疱疹病毒（HSV）、苍白螺旋体（梅毒的病原体）以及乙型和丙型肝炎病毒。随后应进行彻底的临床检查。如果需要，根据病史和查体结果即可进行初步抗微生物药物治疗。

对住院患者的评估应包括血常规和生化。C 反应蛋白水平可作为炎症的标志物并用以指导治疗。肌酸激酶水平可能对临床有一定帮助，但对累及肌肉的肌间隔室综合征和坏死性筋膜炎病例缺乏特异性。在门诊，对于非复杂性的 ABSSSI，通常不需要病原学培养。由于血培养阳性率低，因此对住院蜂窝织炎患者进行血培养的益处尚不确定。对于那些深层结构和潜在组织受累需要切开和引流的患者，则需要进行病原学培养。

核酸扩增技术是诊断单纯疱疹病毒（HSV）和水痘-带状疱疹病毒（VZV）皮肤病变最敏感和最特异的检测，用棉签从活动性感染的皮肤损伤底部刮取样本即可。而直接荧光抗体检测的灵敏度较低。对于这些病变，禁忌行切开和引流。

特殊诊断注意事项

动物咬伤

在动物咬伤的情况下，血培养、组织活检和抽吸物均可用于需氧或厌氧微生物培养。

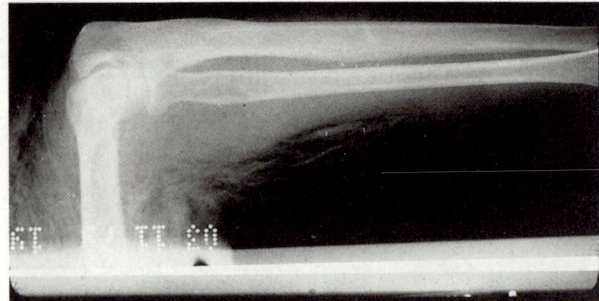

Fig. 9.6 Radiograph of patient with clostridial myonecrosis shows gas in the tissues. (Courtesy J.W. Tomford, MD.)

Human Bites

Wounds swabs may produce misleading information in cases of human bites. A Gram stain should be performed to assess organisms, neutrophils (i.e., inflammation), and squamous epithelial cells (i.e., superficial contamination). If feasible, tissue biopsy or aspiration of the infected site can provide specimens for aerobic and anaerobic culture.

Traumatic Wounds

The optimal time to acquire specimens for cultures is immediately after débridement of the wound site and not within the first 48 hours post-trauma. Analysis of initial cultures should focus on common pathogens, and additional testing should be reserved for uncommon or rare infections associated with unusual circumstances, such as *Vibrio* species after salt water exposure. Tissue biopsy and special stains may be required in certain situations, such as suspected infection with *M. marinum*.

Burn Wounds

Before sampling, the burn area must be clean and devoid of topical antimicrobial agents. Sampling of the burn wound by either surface swab or tissue biopsy for culture is recommended for monitoring the presence and extent of infection. Quantitative evaluation of swab or culture specimens is recommended twice weekly to monitor colonization. Evidence of systemic infection related to the wound should prompt blood cultures.

Diabetic Foot Infections

Superficial swab cultures of ulcerations can be misleading and should be avoided. If surgical débridement is performed, deep tissue specimens should be sent to the microbiology laboratory for evaluation.

Radiographs should be obtained if bone involvement is suspected, and they may also be useful in demonstrating soft tissue gas before crepitus is detected (Fig. 9.6). Magnetic resonance imaging is the most sensitive modality. Chapter 2 discusses the laboratory diagnosis of infectious diseases in more detail.

Differential Diagnosis

Many noninfectious conditions can mimic SSTIs:
- Brown recluse spider bite
- Contact dermatitis
- Gout
- Psoriatic arthritis with distal dactylitis
- Reactive arthritis
- Relapsing polychondritis
- Ruptured Baker cyst
- Mixed cryoglobulinemia due to immune complex disease from chronic hepatitis C or B infection (may have an erythematous rash)
- Pyoderma gangrenosum
- Sweet syndrome (acute febrile neutrophilic dermatosis)
- Venous stasis

TREATMENT

Pharmacologic and Supportive Care

Mild cases of cellulitis may be managed on an outpatient basis with penicillin VK, amoxicillin, or if the patient has a history of a penicillin skin rash and nothing to suggest an IgE-mediated reaction, cephalexin. If clinically unclear whether the infection is due to *S. pyogenes* or *S. aureus*, get cultures and start empiric therapy with amoxicillin or penicillin VK or cephalexin and trimethoprim-sulfamethoxazole (TMP-SMX).

Azithromycin, linezolid, tedizolid or delafloxacin may be used in patients with a past history of IgE-mediated allergic reaction to β-lactam antibiotics. Severe cellulitis should be managed with parenteral penicillin, cefazolin or ceftriaxone. Vancomycin may be used in patients with allergies to penicillin.

Concomitant tinea infection should be treated with a topical antifungal agent such as clotrimazole or terbinafine.

For suspected methicillin-susceptible *S. aureus* (MSSA) (fluctuance or positive Gram stain) dicloxacillin may be used as an outpatient, nafcillin or oxacillin as an inpatient. For MRSA, doxycycline or TMP-SMX may be used as an outpatient, vancomycin as an inpatient. Other inpatient options include daptomycin, telavancin, ceftaroline, clindamycin (watch for inducible resistance), or linezolid. Dalbavancin and oritavancin may be used as alternatives in ABSSSIs for those who are moderately ill and who refuse hospitalization.

Note that neither doxycycline nor TMP-SMX provides adequate streptococcal coverage. A β-lactam antibiotic may be considered for hospitalized patients with nonpurulent cellulitis, with modification to MRSA-active treatment if there is no clinical response. Cellulitis associated with an abscess requires surgical drainage.

In addition to supportive care, urgent surgical consultation should be obtained in the event that crepitus, bullae, rapidly evolving cellulitis, or pain disproportional to physical examination findings suggests necrotizing fasciitis. Initial parenteral therapy with vancomycin, daptomycin, or linezolid combined with piperacillin-tazobactam or a carbapenem (either meropenem or ertapenem) is appropriate. Type II necrotizing fasciitis due to *S. pyogenes* or clostridial myonecrosis should prompt combined therapy with parenteral penicillin and clindamycin. Clindamycin by virtue of its mechanism of action suppresses streptococcal toxin and cytokine production. The use of intravenous immune globulin in cases of necrotizing fasciitis remains controversial.

Compartment syndrome requires emergent surgical decompression to prevent muscle necrosis and irreversible neuronal damage.

Special Treatment Considerations
Animal Bites

Mild cases of animal bites (dog or cat) may be treated with amoxicillin-clavulanate. Inpatient parenteral agents including ampicillin-sulbactam or piperacillin-tazobactam may be used for those who require hospitalization.

For patients with a penicillin allergy, a fluoroquinolone plus clindamycin may be used in dog bites, doxycycline in cat bites. As with all animal bites, rabies postexposure prophylaxis and vaccination should be considered.

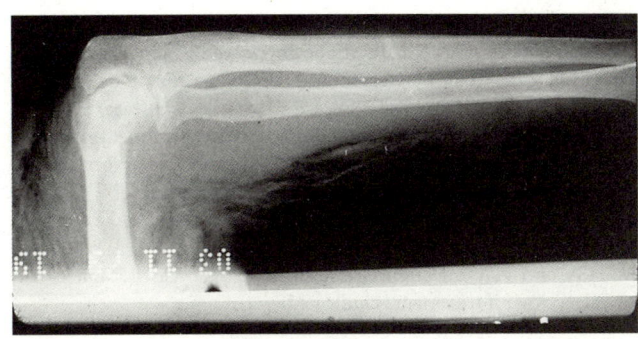

图 9.6 梭状芽孢杆菌性肌坏死患者的 X 线片显示组织中有气体（授权自 J.W. Tomford，MD.）

人咬伤

在人咬伤的情况下，伤口拭子可能会产生误导性信息。应对标本进行革兰氏染色以评估病原体、中性粒细胞（即炎症）和鳞状上皮细胞（即表面污染）。如果可行，对感染部位进行组织活检或抽吸物也可作为病原学（需氧和厌氧）培养样本。

外伤

获得用于培养标本的最佳时间是在伤口部位清创术后立即取材，而不是在创伤后的前 48 h 内。对培养物的初始分析应侧重于常见病原体，并为某些特殊情况下的罕见感染保留额外的检测准备，如接触盐水后的弧菌。同样，在某些情况下如果怀疑海分枝杆菌感染，则可能需要进行组织活检和特殊染色。

烧伤

烧伤部位取样前必须进行清创，且未使用局部抗微生物药物。对烧伤创面进行取样培养可用于监测感染的存在和程度，可采用表面拭子，也可通过组织活检获得标本。建议每周 2 次对拭子或培养标本进行定量评估，以监测细菌定植情况。如果出现与伤口有关的全身感染证据，则应立即抽取血培养。

糖尿病足感染

应避免进行溃疡表面拭子培养，因为可能会带来误导性。建议进行外科清创术，将深层组织标本送往微生物学实验室进行评估。

如果怀疑骨骼受累，应进行 X 线检查，并且在查体发现皮肤握雪感（皮下气肿）之前，X 线检查有助于发现软组织内气体影（图 9.6）。磁共振成像（MRI）是最敏感的检查手段。第 2 章更详细地讨论了感染病的实验室诊断。

鉴别诊断

许多非感染性疾病可以有类似皮肤软组织感染的表现：

- 棕色隐逸蜘蛛咬伤
- 接触性皮炎
- 痛风
- 银屑病关节炎伴远端指关节炎
- 反应性关节炎
- 复发性多软骨炎
- 腘窝囊肿破裂
- 慢性丙型肝炎或乙型肝炎感染所致的免疫复合物疾病引起的混合性冷球蛋白血症（可能有红斑皮疹）
- 坏疽性脓皮病
- Sweet 综合征（急性发热性嗜中性皮肤病）
- 静脉淤滞

治疗

药物治疗和支持治疗

轻度蜂窝织炎病例可以在门诊使用青霉素 VK、阿莫西林治疗，或者如果患者有使用青霉素后出现皮疹病史，但没有提示 IgE 介导的反应时，则可以使用头孢氨苄。如果临床上不确定感染是由化脓性链球菌还是金黄色葡萄球菌引起，可以进行细菌培养，并同时给予阿莫西林、青霉素 VK、头孢氨苄或甲氧苄啶-磺胺甲噁唑（TMP-SMX）的经验性治疗。

如果患者既往有 IgE 介导的对 β-内酰胺类抗生素过敏反应史，可使用阿奇霉素、利奈唑胺、特地唑胺或德拉沙星。严重的蜂窝织炎应使用青霉素、头孢唑林或头孢曲松静脉输液治疗。对青霉素过敏的患者，可使用万古霉素。

伴发的皮癣感染应局部使用抗真菌药物治疗，如克霉唑或阿莫罗芬。

对于疑似甲氧西林敏感金黄色葡萄球菌（MSSA）感染的患者，门诊可使用双氯西林，住院可使用萘夫西林或苯唑西林治疗。对于耐甲氧西林金黄色葡萄球菌（MRSA），多西环素或 TMP-SMX 可作为门诊治疗用药，万古霉素用于住院患者。住院患者的其他选择还包括达托霉素、特拉凡星、头孢洛林、克林霉素（注意诱导耐药）或利奈唑胺。达巴凡星和奥利万星可作为拒绝住院的中度 ABSSSI 患者的替代治疗。

需要注意的是，无论是多西环素还是 TMP-SMX 都不能提供足够的链球菌覆盖。β-内酰胺类抗生素可考虑用于非化脓性蜂窝织炎的住院患者，如果疗效不佳，可改为具有抗 MRSA 活性的药物治疗。伴有脓肿的蜂窝织炎需要手术引流。

如果出现皮肤握雪感、大疱、快速进展的蜂窝织炎或与体检结果不相称的疼痛，往往提示坏死性筋膜炎，除了支持性治疗外，还应请外科急会诊。初始治疗选择万古霉素、达托霉素或利奈唑胺联合哌拉西林-他唑巴坦或碳青霉烯类（美罗培南或厄他培南）静脉输液治疗是合理的。由化脓性链球菌引起的 II 型坏死性筋膜炎和梭状芽孢杆菌引起的肌坏死应及时给予青霉素联合克林霉素静脉输液治疗，其中克林霉素可抑制链球菌毒素和细胞因子的释放。静脉注射免疫球蛋白治疗坏死性筋膜炎尚有争议。

间隔综合征则需要紧急外科手术减压，以防止肌肉坏死和不可逆的神经元损伤。

Human Bites

Patients who have human bite wounds without evidence of infection should receive prophylactic treatment with amoxicillin-clavulanate for 3 to 5 days. Closed-fist injuries require radiographic evaluation and consultation with a hand surgeon for possible wound exploration. Parenteral treatment with ampicillin-sulbactam or moxifloxacin is recommended.

Burn Wounds

Systemic therapy with antibiotics and antifungals is reserved for burn patients demonstrating signs of sepsis or septic shock. Infection due to mucormycoses requires liposomal amphotericin B.

Diabetic Foot Infections

Simple infections such as cellulitis are most often caused by group A streptococci or *S. aureus* and should be managed accordingly. If ulcers do not have purulence or inflammation, antimicrobials are not indicated. Severe limb-threatening infections require surgical evaluation and broad-spectrum antibiotic coverage because infection tends to include aerobic and anaerobic organisms. Empirical therapy directed at *P. aeruginosa* is not usually necessary unless the patient has other risk factors. MRSA-active treatment is recommended for patients with a history of MRSA, when the local prevalence of MRSA is high in the community, or if the infection is severe. All wounds require adequate wound irrigation and débridement.

Marine Lacerations and Punctures

The treatment regimen for marine lacerations and punctures should include doxycycline and ceftazidime or a fluoroquinolone to provide adequate coverage for *V. vulnificus*. Treatment of fresh water injuries should also include a third- or fourth-generation cephalosporin (i.e., ceftazidime or cefepime) or a fluoroquinolone. If *M. marinum* is suspected, treatment with clarithromycin, minocycline, doxycycline, sulfamethoxazole-trimethoprim, or rifampin plus ethambutol is appropriate. Aeromonas wound infections may be treated with either ciprofloxacin or levofloxacin.

Others

Cellulitis or wound infections attributed to *A. hemolyticum* may be treated with clindamycin, erythromycin, vancomycin, or tetracycline.

Animal handlers with cutaneous anthrax infection (naturally acquired) require treatment with amoxicillin or penicillin. Cases of suspected bioterrorism, however, must be treated with ciprofloxacin or levofloxacin and must be reported immediately.

Tularemia is treated with streptomycin or gentamicin/tobramycin. Mild cases may be treated with ciprofloxacin or doxycycline. Azithromycin is the drug of choice for cat-scratch disease. For individuals at risk for *E. rhusiopathiae* infection, the treatment of choice is penicillin or amoxicillin for localized skin infection and parenteral penicillin or ceftriaxone for widespread skin infection.

Lymphocutaneous/cutaneous sporotrichosis *(S. schenkii)* may be treated with itraconazole.

HSV and VZV infections are susceptible to acyclovir, famciclovir, or valacyclovir if treatment is indicated.

PROGNOSIS

Full recovery is expected for patients with simple ABSSSIs provided they receive appropriate treatment. For those who develop complications such as necrotizing fasciitis, the estimated mortality rate is between 30% and 70%. The prognosis is guarded for patients with multiple comorbidities and those who are immunosuppressed.

SUGGESTED READINGS

Cohen J, Powderly WG, Opal SM, editors: Infectious diseases, ed 3, London, 2010, Mosby.

Golstein EJ: Bite wounds and infectious, Clin Infect Dis 14:633–640, 1992.

Herchline T: Cellulitis treatment and management. Available at http://emedicine.medscape.com/article/214222-overview. Accessed October 31, 2014.

Lipsky BA, Berendt AR, Cornia PB, et al: Infectious Diseases Society of America clinical practice guideline for the diagnosis and treatment of diabetic foot infections, Clin Infect Dis 54:132–173, 2012, 2012.

Liu C, Bayer A, Cosgrove SE, et al: Clinical practice guidelines by the Infectious Diseases Society of America for the treatment if methicillin-resistant *Staphylococcus aureus* infectious in adults and children, Clin Infect Dis 52:e18–e55, 2011.

Miller JM, Binnicker MJ, et al: A guide to utilization of the microbiology laboratory for diagnosis of infectious diseases: 2018 update by the Infectious Diseases Society of America (IDSA) and the American Society of Microbiology (ASM). Available at https://www.idsociety.org/practice-guideline/laboratory-diagnosis-of-infectious-diseases/.

Spelman D: Cellulitis and skin abscess: clinical manifestations and diagnosis. UpToDate. Available at http://www.uptodate.com/contents/cellulitis-and-skin-abscess-clinical-manifestations-and-diagnosis. Accessed September 16, 2019.

Stevens DL, Bisno AL, Chambers HF, et al: Practice guidelines for the diagnosis and management of skin and soft-tissue infections, Clin Infect Dis 59(2):e10–e52, 2014.

特殊处理时的注意事项

动物咬伤

轻度动物咬伤（狗或猫）可使用阿莫西林-克拉维酸治疗。需要住院治疗的患者可给予氨苄西林-舒巴坦或哌拉西林-他唑巴坦输液治疗

对于青霉素过敏的患者，氟喹诺酮联合克林霉素可用于狗咬伤，多西环素用于猫咬伤。与所有动物咬伤一样，应给予狂犬病预防和疫苗接种。

人咬伤

没有感染迹象的人类咬伤，应给予患者 3～5 天阿莫西林-克拉维酸预防性治疗。闭合拳头伤需要进行影像学检查评估，咨询手外科医生以进行可能的伤口探查。建议使用氨苄西林-舒巴坦或莫西沙星静脉输液治疗。

烧伤

抗生素和抗真菌药物的全身治疗仅适用于出现感染中毒症或感染中毒性休克的烧伤患者。毛霉引起的真菌感染需要两性霉素 B 脂质体。

糖尿病足感染

蜂窝织炎等简单感染最常由 A 组链球菌或金黄色葡萄球菌引起，应予以相应处理。如果溃疡没有化脓或炎症，则不需要使用抗微生物药物。严重的威胁肢体的感染则需要手术评估和广谱抗生素覆盖，因为此时的感染往往包括需氧菌和厌氧菌的混合感染。除非患者有其他危险因素，否则通常不需要针对铜绿假单胞菌的经验性覆盖治疗。当 MRSA 在当地社区中的局部流行率很高，或者如果感染很严重时，建议对有 MRSA 病史的患者进行积极的抗 MRSA 治疗。所有伤口均需要充分的伤口冲洗和清创修复。

海洋割伤和穿刺伤

海洋割伤和穿刺伤的治疗方案应包括多西环素和头孢他啶或氟喹诺酮类药物，以充分覆盖创伤弧菌。淡水相关损伤的治疗也应包括第三代或第四代头孢菌素（即头孢他啶或头孢吡肟）或氟喹诺酮类药物。如果怀疑海分枝杆菌，合适的治疗方案包括克拉霉素、米诺环素、多西环素、甲氧苄啶-磺胺甲噁唑或利福平联合乙胺丁醇。气单胞菌伤口感染可以使用环丙沙星或左氧氟沙星治疗。

其他

由 A 组溶血性链球菌引起的蜂窝织炎或伤口感染可以使用克林霉素、红霉素、万古霉素或四环素治疗。

患有皮肤炭疽感染（自然获得）的动物饲养员需要使用阿莫西林或青霉素进行治疗。但疑似生物恐怖事件的病例必须使用环丙沙星或左氧氟沙星治疗，并且必须立即报告。

兔热病的治疗使用链霉素或庆大霉素/妥布霉素。轻症病例可使用环丙沙星或多西环素治疗。阿奇霉素是治疗猫抓病的首选药物。对于有感染猪红斑丹毒丝菌风险的患者，可选择青霉素或阿莫西林治疗局部皮肤感染，或者选择青霉素或头孢曲松静脉输液治疗广泛皮肤感染。

淋巴皮肤/皮肤孢子丝菌病（申克孢子丝菌）可使用伊曲康唑治疗。

HSV 和 VZV 对阿昔洛韦、泛昔洛韦或伐昔洛韦敏感，如果有适应证，推荐应用。

预后

单纯 ABSSSI 患者，只要接受适当的治疗，足以完全康复。而对于那些出现坏死性筋膜炎等并发症的患者，估计死亡率在 30%～70%。对于患有多种合并症和免疫抑制的患者，预后往往不容乐观。

推荐阅读

Cohen J, Powderly WG, Opal SM, editors: Infectious diseases, ed 3, London, 2010, Mosby.

Golstein EJ: Bite wounds and infectious, Clin Infect Dis 14:633–640, 1992.

Herchline T: Cellulitis treatment and management. Available at http://emedicine.medscape.com/article/214222-overview. Accessed October 31, 2014.

Lipsky BA, Berendt AR, Cornia PB, et al: Infectious Diseases Society of America clinical practice guideline for the diagnosis and treatment of diabetic foot infections, Clin Infect Dis 54:132–173, 2012, 2012.

Liu C, Bayer A, Cosgrove SE, et al: Clinical practice guidelines by the Infectious Diseases Society of America for the treatment if methicillin-resistant *Staphylococcus aureus* infectious in adults and children, Clin Infect Dis 52:e18–e55, 2011.

Miller JM, Binnicker MJ, et al: A guide to utilization of the microbiology laboratory for diagnosis of infectious diseases: 2018 update by the Infectious Diseases Society of America (IDSA) and the American Society of Microbiology (ASM). Available at http://www.idsociety.org/practice-guideline/laboratory-diagnosis-of-infectious-diseases/.

Spelman D: Cellulitis and skin abscess: clinical manifestations and diagnosis. UpToDate. Available at http://www.uptodate.com/contents/cellulitis-and-skin-abscess-clinical-manifestations-and-diagnosis. Accessed September 16, 2019.

Stevens DL, Bisno AL, Chambers HF, et al: Practice guidelines for the diagnosis and management of skin and soft-tissue infections, Clin Infect Dis 59(2):e10–e52, 2014.

Intraabdominal Infections

Eric Benoit

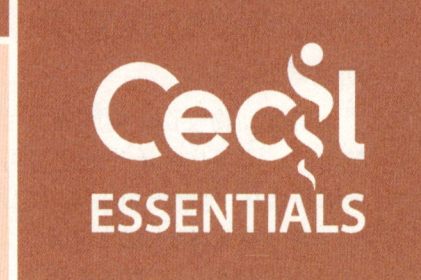

INTRODUCTION

Intraabdominal infections are common in hospitalized patients, both as a primary indication for admission and as a complication. Although antibiotics play a central role in treatment, many of these patients require source control and warrant surgical consultation to manage complications such as perforation and peritonitis. Intraabdominal infections are usually polymicrobial and are caused by components of bowel flora most commonly including aerobic *Escherichia coli* and other Enterobacteriaceae and anaerobic *Bacteroides fragilis* and streptococci.

SOURCE CONTROL AND TIMING OF ANTIBIOTICS

Early administration of broad-spectrum antibiotics has become standard of care in patients with suspected infection. Mortality increases with every hour delay to antibiotic therapy in septic patients. However, antibiotics alone are not sufficient for most intraabdominal infections, which require an intervention to control the source of infection. Purulence must be drained. This may be surgical removal of the infected tissue as in appendectomy, percutaneous drainage of an abscess by interventional radiology, or endoscopic retrograde cholangiopancreatography (ERCP) to remove obstructing stones in cases of cholangitis. Appropriate source control has been shown to be as important to outcomes as early antibiotics.

The Study to Optimize Peritoneal Infection Therapy (STOP-IT) trial demonstrated that most intraabdominal infections may be treated for 4 days after achieving source control, and this is true even for complicated intraabdominal infections. Furthermore, prolonged antibiotic administration in the setting of intraabdominal infection has been shown to increase the risk of further infections including bacteremia and *Clostridioides difficile* infections as well as increase the rate of in-hospital mortality. Source control and limited duration of antibiotic therapy, therefore, are critical considerations in management of intraabdominal infections.

PERITONITIS

Peritonitis is a disseminated infection of the peritoneal cavity and typically presents with diffuse, rather than localized, tenderness. Primary peritonitis is most often seen in patients with ascites from cirrhosis. It may be managed with antibiotics alone and after therapy may require suppressive antibiotics. Diagnosis is made by sampling peritoneal fluid; the diagnosis is likely if the number of neutrophils is greater than 250/microliter. Cultures may be negative.

Secondary peritonitis is due to an inciting event, such as hollow viscus perforation, ischemia, or a localized abscess that has spread, and is more common than primary peritonitis. Any intraabdominal infection may progress from localized to diffuse peritonitis. Patients with peritonitis are tachycardic, tachypneic, and acutely uncomfortable. They avoid movement, and merely jostling the bed exacerbates the pain. The patient's abdomen may be rigid due to involuntary tightening of the muscles of the abdominal wall (guarding). The onset of peritonitis is ominous as it may herald the progression to sepsis and septic shock. These cases mandate emergent surgical consultation prior to imaging and almost always require operative exploration. Elderly patients or those with diabetes or on steroids may have a blunted response to peritonitis, and they should therefore be approached with a high degree of suspicion regarding complications of intraabdominal infections.

APPENDICITIS

When the lumen of the appendix is occluded either by a lymphatic tissue or a fecalith, mucosal fluid secretion and bacterial overgrowth cause an increase in pressure within the appendix. This eventually leads to venous outflow obstruction and further increases in pressure until arterial inflow is compromised, and the resulting ischemia leads to perforation. The classic presentation is periumbilical pain that migrates to the right lower quadrant, frequently associated with anorexia and nausea. Patients in whom the appendix has perforated often describe a sudden relief of localized pain followed several hours later by the onset of diffuse peritonitis. Leukocytosis, if present, is often not severe.

CT scan of the abdomen has become the diagnostic tool of choice with both sensitivity and specificity over 90% for detection of acute appendicitis. Findings of dilated appendix, fecalith, and stranding of the fat around the appendix are suggestive of acute appendicitis. CT scan may also detect a phlegmon (inflamed infected tissue) or abscess associated with perforated appendicitis (Fig. 10.1). Ultrasound may be useful in children, and MRI is an alternative imaging modality in pregnant women. Clinical diagnosis of appendicitis can be challenging, but the prevalence of CT scanning has markedly decreased the negative appendectomy rate.

Management of appendicitis is appendectomy, most often performed laparoscopically. Although there is active research into antibiotic therapy alone for appendicitis, this is not standard of care. Those patients who do not undergo appendectomy at initial presentation are often brought back for an interval appendectomy 6 to 8 weeks later. More advanced appendicitis may present with a phlegmon. These patients may be treated with antibiotics until an abscess develops, at which time drainage by interventional radiology is appropriate. Patients who develop signs of physiologic compromise (tachycardia, tachypnea, peritonitis) should instead proceed urgently to the operating room. Patients with perforated appendicitis may require more extensive surgery (e.g., ileo-cecectomy) and have a higher risk of intraabdominal abscess. Appendicitis is a polymicrobial infection with colonic bacteria *E. coli* and *Bacteroides* species being common. Antibiotics should be

腹腔内感染

黄磊 译　路明 康梅 审校　曹彬 通审

引言

　　腹腔内感染在住院患者中很常见，其既是入院的主要指征，也是一种并发症。尽管抗生素在治疗中发挥着核心作用，但其中许多患者需要进行感染源控制和外科会诊，以处理穿孔和腹膜炎等并发症。腹腔内感染通常是由多种微生物所致的混合感染，这些微生物通常是肠道菌群的组成成分，其中最常见的是需氧的大肠埃希菌和其他肠杆菌，以及厌氧的脆弱拟杆菌和链球菌。

感染源控制和抗生素用药时机

　　早期使用广谱抗生素已成为疑似感染患者的标准治疗。对于感染中毒症患者，每小时的抗生素延迟使用都会增加死亡率。然而，对于大多数腹腔内感染，仅使用抗生素是不够的，还需要采取干预措施以控制感染源。脓液必须引流。可以手术去除感染组织，如阑尾切除术，或通过介入放射学方法经皮穿刺引流脓肿，或通过内镜逆行胰胆管造影（ERCP）清除胆管炎患者体内的梗阻结石等。有研究证实，合理的感染源控制对临床结局的影响与早期使用抗生素同等重要。

　　优化腹腔感染治疗的研究（STOP-IT）的结果显示，在实现感染源控制后，大多数腹腔内感染治疗4天即可达到治疗目标，即使对于复杂性腹腔内感染也是如此。此外，也有研究表明，在腹腔内感染的情况下延长抗生素的使用会进一步增加菌血症和艰难梭菌感染等的风险，并增加住院死亡率。因此，感染源控制和适当限制抗生素使用时间是腹腔内感染治疗中的关键。

腹膜炎

　　腹膜炎是一种腹膜腔的播散性感染，通常表现为弥漫而非局限性的压痛。原发性腹膜炎最常见于肝硬化腹水患者。它可以单独使用抗生素进行治疗，治疗结束后可能仍需使用抑制性抗生素预防复发。诊断依赖抽取腹水进行检查；如果腹水中性粒细胞数大于$250/\mu l$，则诊断可能成立。腹水细菌培养可以是阴性。

　　继发性腹膜炎比原发性腹膜炎更常见，常见继发原因包括空腔脏器穿孔、局部缺血或局部脓肿播散。任何腹腔内感染都可能从局限性腹膜炎进展为弥漫性腹膜炎。腹膜炎患者通常表现为心动过速，呼吸急促，急性不适，往往抗拒运动，仅仅推动床铺也可加剧疼痛。患者腹部可能因腹壁肌肉不自主地收紧（保护性）而僵硬。腹膜炎的发生预示着病情恶化的可能，继而进展为感染中毒症和感染中毒性休克。这些病例在进行影像学检查前常需外科急会诊，且几乎都需要手术探查。老年人、糖尿病患者或使用类固醇激素史的患者可能对腹膜炎的反应迟钝，因此应高度警惕腹腔内感染的并发症。

阑尾炎

　　当阑尾管腔被淋巴组织或粪石堵塞时，黏膜液分泌和细菌过度生长可导致阑尾内压力增加，最终导致静脉回流受阻，压力进一步升高，直至动脉流入受阻，导致缺血或穿孔。典型的症状为脐周疼痛转移至右下腹，常伴有厌食和恶心。阑尾穿孔的患者常描述为弥漫性腹膜炎发生数小时后局部疼痛突然缓解。可有白细胞增多，但往往并不严重。

　　腹部CT检查已成为急性阑尾炎首选的诊断方法，其敏感性和特异性均超过90%。阑尾增粗、粪石及阑尾周围脂肪条索状物的发现提示急性阑尾炎。CT扫描还可以检测到的蜂窝织炎（发炎的感染组织）或与穿孔性阑尾炎相关的脓肿（图10.1）。超声可用于儿童检查，而MRI是孕妇可选的影像检查方法。阑尾炎的临床诊断很有挑战性，但CT扫描的普及显著降低了阴性阑尾切除的发生率。

　　阑尾炎的治疗方法是阑尾切除术，最常用的是腹腔镜手术。虽然单用抗生素治疗阑尾炎并不是标准的治疗方法，但一直是研究热点。对于初次就诊时未行阑尾切除术的患者，往往要在6~8周后行间歇性阑尾切除术。更晚期的阑尾炎可表现为蜂窝织炎，此时合适的处理办法为使用抗生素治疗直至脓肿形成，随后使用介入放射学方法予以引流。如果患者出现生命体征不稳定的征象（心动过速、呼吸急促、腹膜炎），应行急诊手术。穿孔性阑尾炎患者可能需要更广泛的手术范围（例如，回肠-盲肠切除术），并有更高的腹腔脓肿形成风险。阑尾炎通常是多种细菌的混合感染，

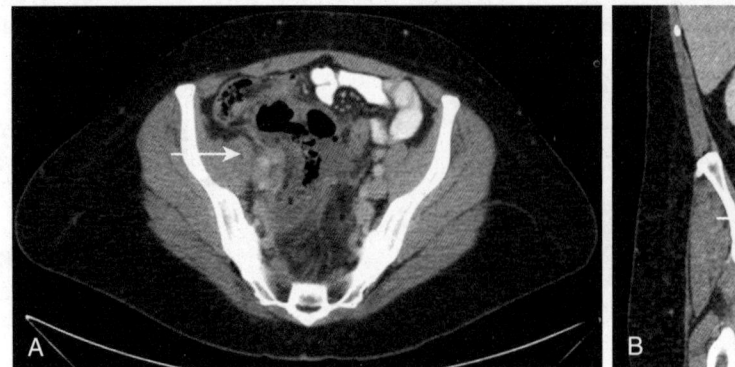 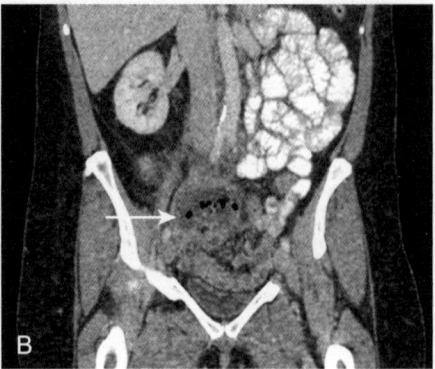

Fig. 10.1 CT scan may detect (A) a phlegmon (inflamed infected tissue) or (B) an abscess associated with perforated appendicitis.

administered until time of operation and may be stopped thereafter in uncomplicated cases. Perforated appendicitis should be treated with antibiotics for 4 days after surgery. Uncomplicated appendicitis has a mortality rate less than 1%, but perforation, particularly in pediatric or elderly patients, increases the risk significantly. Other complications after appendicitis include intraabdominal abscess and wound infection.

DIVERTICULITIS

Diverticula are herniations of the colonic mucosa through naturally occurring openings in the taenia coli through which vessels run (Fig. 10.2). They are most commonly found in the sigmoid colon but may also be present in the right colon. The presence of diverticula (diverticulosis) increases with age, and diet influences their development. Low dietary fiber present in the Western diet contributes to rates of diverticulosis as high as 50% in Americans over the age of 80. Dietary fiber is thought to protect against the development of diverticulosis as demonstrated by lower rates of disease in countries in Asia and Africa. While right-sided diverticular disease is prone to bleeding, sigmoid diverticulosis risks development of diverticulitis, the infection of diverticula. Approximately 10% to 25% of patients with diverticula will develop diverticulosis in their lifetime. The pathophysiology of diverticulitis is similar to appendicitis: occlusion of a diverticulum results in bacterial overgrowth, vascular compromise, ischemia, and perforation.

Diverticulitis can present with varying degrees of severity that are enumerated by the Hinchey classification (Table 10.1). Local infection and inflammation may be self-limited or managed by outpatient antibiotics. More severe cases result in microperforation of diverticula with contained air or abscess within the bowel wall. Complicated diverticulitis results in a distant abscess in the abdomen, pelvis, or retroperitoneum. The most severe cases present with free intraabdominal air and purulent or feculent peritonitis.

Patients with diverticulitis most often present with left lower quadrant pain and tenderness. More severe cases may develop fever and leukocytosis whereas the most critical cases have frank peritonitis and physiologic compromise such as acidosis, acute kidney injury, and hypotension.

Imaging with IV contrast CT scan is standard of care, both to diagnose the presence and severity of diverticulitis and to identify complications such as abscess. However, patients with peritonitis due to suspected diverticulitis should not undergo CT imaging but instead belong in the operating room. An upright chest radiograph may demonstrate free air under the diaphragm in cases of perforation.

Simple diverticulitis may be managed with outpatient antibiotics. More severe cases require admission for intravenous antibiotics, bowel rest, and IV hydration. As the pain and tenderness resolve, the diet may be advanced. Complicated diverticulitis with uncontained abscess requires source control, and these patients should be evaluated for drainage by interventional radiology or laparoscopic drainage by surgery. Patients with free perforation require urgent surgery for control of contamination and resection of perforated bowel. The most common procedure is sigmoid resection with colostomy, although there is increasing evidence to support primary anastomosis with or without a diverting loop ileostomy.

Delayed complications of diverticulitis include abscess, colonic stricture, and fistulae (colovesical, colovaginal or coloenteric). Patients should undergo colonoscopy 6 to 8 weeks after diverticulitis to assess for colorectal cancer. Diverticulitis may recur in up to 20% of patients over 10 years. Although recurrence does make patients more prone to future episodes, the risk of complications such as free perforation does not increase with recurrence. Recurrent diverticulitis does not mandate surgery, but for those patients who wish to avoid future episodes elective sigmoid resection removes the burden of left-sided diverticulosis, effectively eliminating the source of disease. Regardless of treatment plan, patients should be encouraged to pursue a high-fiber diet. Former teaching suggested eliminating such foods as seeds and nuts, but this has not been shown to influence the recurrence of diverticulitis.

Like appendicitis, diverticulitis is a polymicrobial infection with colonic flora such as *E. coli* and bacteroides predominating. Accordingly, broad-spectrum antibiotics such as piperacillin/tazobactam are appropriate, and the duration of therapy is 7 to 10 days. Patients who have resolution of pain while on IV antibiotics may be transitioned to oral agents (such as amoxicillin/clavunate) and complete their course as outpatients.

INFECTIOUS BOWEL DISEASE

Infectious Colitis

Infectious colitis is an infection of the bowel that may be caused by bacteria (*E. coli, Campylobacter, Shigella*), viruses (*norovirus, rotavirus, cytomegalovirus*) or parasites (*Entamoeba histolytica*) (see Chapter 11). These patients present with abdominal pain that is frequently crampy in nature and diarrhea. In older patients particularly, infectious colitis may be difficult to distinguish from ischemic colitis. CT scan with IV contrast demonstrates inflammation of the bowel wall, in contrast to the lack of enhancement seen in ischemic disease. The presence of free fluid is ominous. For many patients with infectious colitis either symptomatic relief or a course of antibiotics directed at potential bacterial

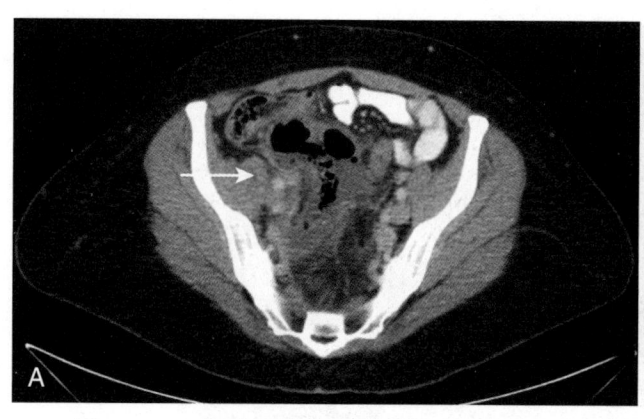 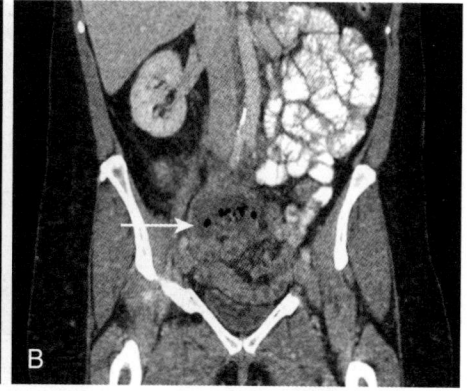

图 10.1　CT 扫描可见（A）蜂窝织炎（发炎的感染组织）或（B）与穿孔性阑尾炎相关的脓肿

以结肠内的大肠埃希菌和拟杆菌属最为常见。抗生素应该给药直至手术，对于无并发症患者此后可以停药。穿孔性阑尾炎术后应继续使用抗生素治疗 4 天。无并发症阑尾炎的死亡率低于 1%，但穿孔性阑尾炎，特别是儿童或老年患者的风险显著增加。阑尾炎的其他并发症包括腹腔脓肿、切口感染等。

憩室炎

憩室是结肠黏膜的突出物，其突出部位在结肠带，该处有血管穿过结肠带所自然形成的开口与肠壁深面相通（图 10.2）。最常见于乙状结肠，也可位于右半结肠。憩室（憩室病）的发生率随年龄增长而增加，其形成受饮食影响。西方的低膳食纤维饮食导致 80 岁以上美国人憩室病的发病率高达 50%。而亚洲和非洲国家的憩室病发病率则较低，这说明膳食纤维可预防憩室病的发生。右侧憩室易发生出血，而乙状结肠憩室易发展为憩室炎（憩室感染）。10%～25% 有憩室的患者在其一生中会发生憩室病。憩室炎的病理生理学与阑尾炎相似，即憩室管腔的阻塞导致细菌过度繁殖，继而发生血运受阻、缺血和穿孔。

根据 Hinchey 分类，不同严重程度的憩室炎可分为不同等级（表 10.1）。局部感染和炎症具有自限性，或者可在门诊接受抗生素治疗。严重者可导致憩室微穿孔，肠壁内可出现气体或脓肿。复杂的憩室炎可在腹腔、盆腔或腹膜后出现远处脓肿。最严重者可表现为腹腔内游离气体和化脓性或粪性腹膜炎。

憩室炎患者最常见的表现为左下腹疼痛和压痛，严重者可出现发热和白细胞增多，而最危重的病例则可出现明显的腹膜炎和生理损害，如酸中毒、急性肾损伤和低血压。

增强 CT 扫描是标准检查，既能有助于憩室炎的诊断和病情严重程度评估，又能识别脓肿等并发症。但怀疑为憩室炎引起腹膜炎的患者不应进行 CT 检查，而应行急诊手术。对于穿孔患者，立位 X 线片可以显示膈下游离气体。

单纯性憩室炎可予门诊抗生素治疗，严重者则需静脉应用抗生素、禁食和静脉补液等治疗。随着腹部疼痛和压痛逐渐缓解，饮食可适当增加。憩室炎并未控制的脓肿时，需要进行感染源控制，应进行介入放射学方法引流或腹腔镜手术引流予以评估。游离性穿孔患者需行紧急手术控制污染并切除穿孔的肠道。尽管越来越多的证据支持一期肠吻合术或联合或不联合回肠袢式造口术，但最常见的手术方式仍然是乙状结肠切除联合结肠造口术。

憩室炎的迟发并发症包括脓肿、结肠狭窄、瘘管（结肠膀胱瘘、结肠阴道瘘或结肠肠瘘）。患者应在憩室炎后 6～8 周接受结肠镜检查，以评估是否患有结肠直肠癌。10 年以上的随访发现，高达 20% 的憩室炎可能会复发。虽然患者未来确实容易复发，但并不会增加游离穿孔等并发症的风险。复发性憩室炎并不一定必须手术治疗，但对于那些希望避免复发的患者可选择行乙状结肠切除术以去除左侧憩室的负担，有效消除疾病根源。无论何种治疗方案，均应鼓励患者进行高纤维饮食。以前的教学建议患者尽量避免种子和坚果等食物，但这并没有被证明会影响憩室炎的复发。

和阑尾炎相似，憩室炎也是一种以大肠埃希菌和拟杆菌属等结肠菌群为主要致病原的多种细菌混合感染。因此，可选用哌拉西林/他唑巴坦等广谱抗生素，疗程为 7～10 天。疼痛缓解后，静脉抗生素可序贯为口服制剂（如阿莫西林/克拉维酸），在门诊完成疗程。

感染性肠病

感染性结肠炎

感染性结肠炎是由细菌（大肠埃希菌、弯曲菌、志贺菌）、病毒（诺如病毒、轮状病毒、巨细胞病毒）或寄生虫（溶组织内阿米巴）引起的肠道感染（见第 11 章）。患者通常会出现痉挛性腹痛和腹泻。感染性结肠炎很难与缺血性结肠炎相鉴别，尤其是在老年患者中。但增强 CT 扫描可显示肠壁有炎症，而缺血性疾病则没有强化。游离积液往往提示病情严重。对于许多

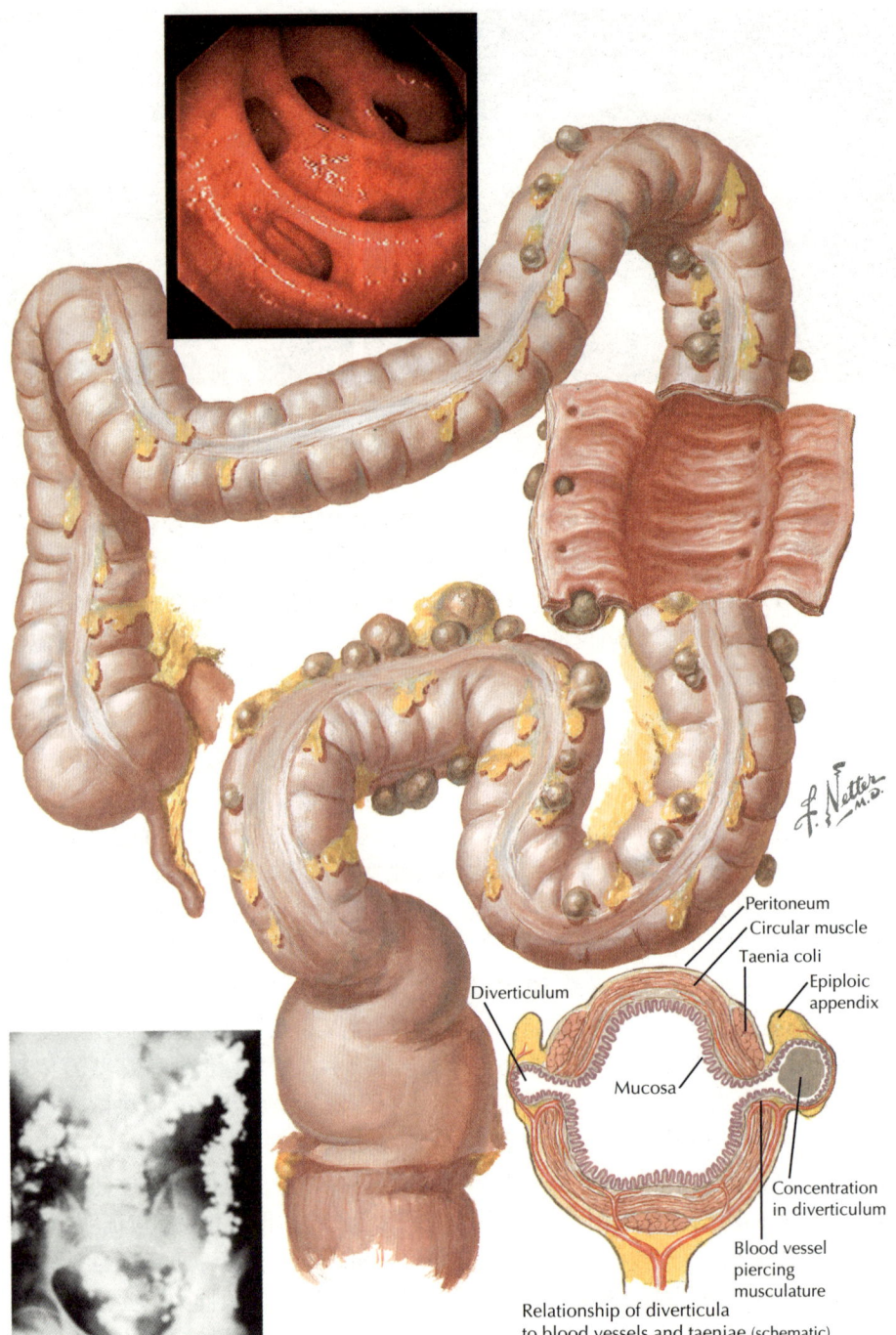

Fig. 10.2 Diverticulosis. (From the Netter Collection of Medical Illustrations. Available at www.netterimages.com. Accessed October 31, 2014.)

pathogens may be sufficient. Stool samples may aid in diagnosis and treatment of different pathogens. Regardless of etiology these patients require frequent abdominal exams, and in rare cases, should they progress to worsening pain, fever, tachycardia, hypotension or peritonitis, they belong in the operating room for colectomy.

Cytomegalovirus Colitis

Cytomegalovirus is a common, self-limited viral infection, but it may cause colitis in immunocompromised patients, such as transplant patients, those who undergo frequent steroid therapy for ulcerative colitis or as a complication of acquired immunodeficiency syndrome (AIDS). Diagnosis of CMV colitis requires a high degree of suspicion in the correct clinical context. Colonoscopy may demonstrate ulcerated lesions and CMV immunohistochemistry on biopsy specimens. Antimicrobial therapy is with an antiretroviral agent such as ganciclovir. Surgery is reserved for complications such as perforation.

Clostridioides difficile Colitis

Clostridioides difficile colitis is most often a complication of antibiotic therapy. It occurs when healthy intraluminal bacteria are depleted,

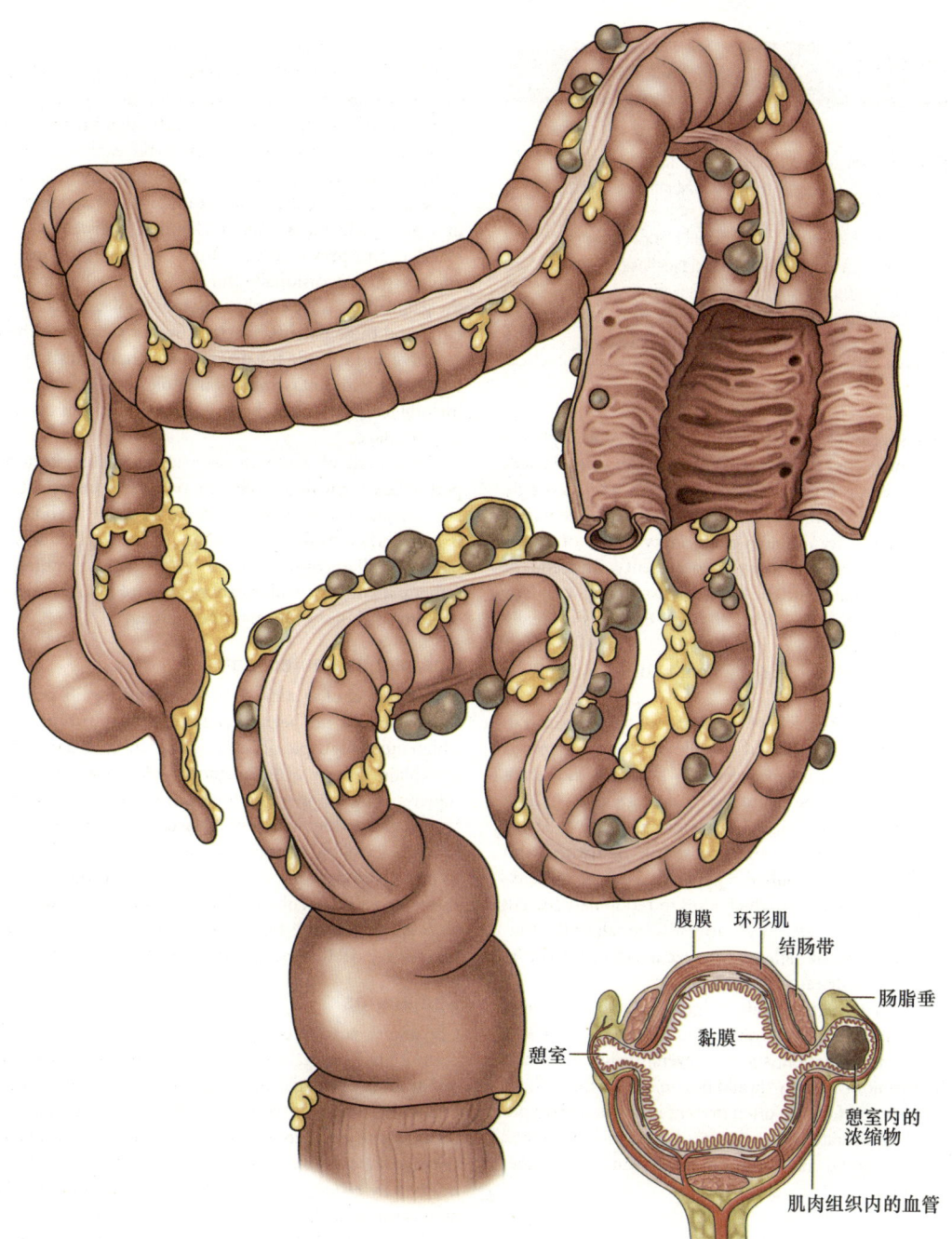

图 10.2　憩室病（原图引自 the Netter Collection of Medical Illustrations. Available at www.netterimages.com. Accessed October 31, 2014. 因版权限制，中译文本图已作修改。）

感染性结肠炎患者，缓解症状或针对潜在细菌使用一个疗程的抗生素可能就足够了。粪便标本有助于不同病原体的诊断和指导治疗。无论病因如何，这些患者都需要经常进行腹部检查，在极少数情况下，如果患者出现疼痛加剧、发热、心动过速、低血压或腹膜炎，则需要进行结肠切除术。

巨细胞病毒结肠炎

巨细胞病毒（CMV）感染是一种常见的、自限性的病毒感染，但可引起免疫缺陷患者的结肠炎，如移植患者、因溃疡性结肠炎频繁使用类固醇激素的患者，或作为获得性免疫缺陷综合征（AIDS）的并发症。诊断 CMV 结肠炎需要在一定的临床诊疗背景下保持高度警惕。结肠镜检查可获取活检标本，从而观察溃疡病变并进行 CMV 免疫组化检测。可使用更昔洛韦等抗病毒药物进行治疗。对于穿孔等并发症可进行手术治疗。

艰难梭菌结肠炎

艰难梭菌结肠炎是抗生素治疗最常见的并发症，常发生在健康的肠道内细菌被清除，而导致致病菌占

TABLE 10.1	Hinchey Classification of Diverticulitis	
Class	Description	Treatment
0	Mild clinical diverticulitis	Oral antibiotics
Ia	Contained pericolic inflammation or phlegmon	IV antibiotics, bowel rest
Ib	Contained pericolic abscess	IV antibiotics, bowel rest
II	Pelvic, distant intraabdominal or retroperitoneal abscess	Percutaneous drainage, IV antibiotics
III	Purulent peritonitis	Operative drainage/resection
IV	Feculent peritonitis	Operative drainage/resection

allowing pathogenic species to predominate. Agents such as cephalosporins, fluoroquinolones, and clindamycin are commonly implicated, but any antibiotic in the preceding several months—even a single dose—increases the risk of *C. difficile* colitis. Hospitalized patients are at greater risk due to exposure, although community strains of *C. difficile* have been identified. Patients most often present with frequent diarrhea as well as abdominal pain. The disease is associated with leukocytosis sometimes as high as 30,000 to 40,000. Diagnosis is ideally sought in those with greater than or equal to three unformed stools in 24 hours. The diagnosis is confirmed by stool studies with PCR for toxin.

Infectious Disease Society Guidelines recommend oral vancomycin or fidaxomicin for 10 days for an initial episode of *C. difficile* colitis. Metronidazole is an alternative if vancomycin or fidaxomicin are not available. Fulminant cases may be treated with oral vancomycin and, if ileus is present, vancomycin enema. Intravenous metronidazole should also be given. First recurrent infection should be treated with oral vancomycin as a tapered and pulsed regimen or a course of fidaxomicin. Fecal microbiota transplant, which aims to repopulate the gut with healthy bacteria, should be considered investigational; while studies have demonstrated utility in patients with recurrent or refractory disease, it carries the risk of disease transmission.

Patients with *C. difficile* colitis remain at high risk of bowel perforation as well as progression to toxic megacolon. Those patients with signs of unremitting inflammation, such as fevers, tachycardia, and tenderness despite antibiotic therapy should be considered for surgery. Patients who progress to perforation often present in shock with hypotension and altered mental state. These patients have a high mortality, and surgery mandates subtotal colectomy, often with vancomycin enemas to the rectal stump.

BILIARY INFECTIONS

Cholecystitis

The gallbladder, like the appendix, is an anatomic cul-de-sac, and the narrow neck of the cystic duct is prone to occlusion by gallstones or edema, preventing drainage of bile and leading to bacterial overgrowth. The undrained, infected fluid present in cholecystitis leads to an increase in pressure that may progress to ischemia of the gallbladder wall, gangrene, and perforation.

Cholecystitis may be distinguished from biliary colic by its duration; biliary colic typically resolves spontaneously and patients are able to eat. Cholecystitis, on the other hand, is marked by prolonged pain and tenderness and is frequently associated with leukocytosis. Patients report right-sided or epigastric pain, often associated with a recent meal. On examination, tenderness is usually localized to the right upper quadrant. However, in cases of gallbladder perforation, infected bile may flow down the right paracolic gutter, leading to right-sided abdominal or even pelvic tenderness. The classic finding of Murphy's sign is the abrupt cessation of inspiration when palpating the right upper quadrant; the excursion of the diaphragm during inspiration displaces the gallbladder inferiorly to the examiner's hand, resulting in sudden, exquisite pain that interrupts the patient's breathing.

Right upper quadrant ultrasound is the imaging modality of choice in which gallbladder wall thickening, a distended, fluid-filled gallbladder, and pericholecystic fluid are findings consistent with acute cholecystitis. Occasionally the ultrasound will demonstrate air within the gallbladder wall; emphysematous cholecystitis carries a high mortality and these patients warrant urgent surgery. Although CT scan is sensitive and specific for diagnosis of cholecystitis, it exposes patients to radiation and may miss non-cholesterol stones. Laboratory values include leukocytosis and elevated total bilirubin from the blockage of bile drainage.

Treatment of acute cholecystitis is cholecystectomy, most often performed laparoscopically. In patients who are too sick to tolerate operation, percutaneous drainage with a cholecystostomy tube is appropriate to decompress the infected gallbladder. Some of these patients will recover sufficiently to undergo surgery 6 weeks later. Other patients, particularly those who are elderly and frail, may require prolonged cholecystotomy tube drainage.

Acalculous Cholecystitis

Acalculous cholecystitis occurs in critically ill patients, particularly those who have not been receiving enteral nutrition. Diagnosis requires a high index of suspicion, especially in intubated patients. Patients with unexplained fever or leukocytosis without an obvious source should undergo a right upper quadrant ultrasound, which demonstrates a distended gallbladder with a thickened wall. These patients are frequently too sick to tolerate surgical cholecystectomy and instead are referred to interventional radiology for a cholecystostomy tube to decompress the infected bile. Tube drainage is often continued until the patient recovers sufficiently to tolerate cholecystectomy, although for some chronically debilitated patients tube drainage may suffice.

Cholangitis

Cholangitis is an infection due to the blockage of the bile ducts, most commonly from gallstones. These patients present with right upper quadrant or epigastric pain. The classic findings are right upper quadrant pain, fever and jaundice (Charcot's triad) that may progress to include altered mental status and shock (Reynold pentad). These patients have infected bile or pus within the biliary tree, and this is best drained by ERCP with sphincterotomy and stenting. Ascending cholangitis can be an aggressive infection, with patients rapidly progressing to septic shock. Antibiotics alone are not sufficient and source control is mandated. Suspicion of cholangitis should prompt urgent consultation with a gastroenterologist and a surgeon, and these patients often require fluid resuscitation and admission to a critical care unit.

Right upper quadrant ultrasound in cases of cholangitis may demonstrate cholelithiasis without findings of cholecystitis, but a dilated common bile duct as evidence of a stone that has passed out of the gallbladder. Important laboratory values include hyperbilirubinemia, leukocytosis, and an elevated alkaline phosphatase as evidence of bile duct irritation. Patients who undergo ERCP with sphincterotomy may have pneumobilia on subsequent imaging; this is due to retrograde passage of air from the duodenum into the biliary tree and may not indicate infection.

Bacteria associated with biliary infections include *E. coli*, *Klebsiella*, and *Pseudomonas* but may also include *Enterobacter* and *Bacteroides*. Biliary cultures are rarely used to guide therapy and therefore

表 10.1	憩室炎的 Hinchey 分类	
分类	描述	治疗
0	轻度临床憩室炎	口服抗生素
Ⅰa	周围局限性炎症或蜂窝织炎	静脉抗生素，禁食
Ⅰb	周围局限性脓肿	静脉抗生素，禁食
Ⅱ	盆腔、远处腹腔或腹膜后脓肿	经皮引流术，静脉抗生素
Ⅲ	化脓性腹膜炎	手术引流/切除
Ⅳ	粪性腹膜炎	手术引流/切除

优势时。头孢菌素类、氟喹诺酮类和克林霉素等药物通常与艰难梭菌感染有关，但其实在前几个月使用过任何抗生素，即使是仅一次剂量，也会增加艰难梭菌结肠炎的风险。尽管已经发现有社区来源的艰难梭菌，但住院患者因暴露于抗生素而面临更大的感染风险。患者最常见的临床表现为频繁的腹泻和腹痛。可伴有白细胞增多，有时可高达 3 万～4 万。如果 24 h 内有 3 次及以上不成形大便，理论上就该考虑此诊断。但最终确诊有赖于粪便毒素 PCR 检测。

感染病学会指南推荐初发艰难梭菌结肠炎患者口服万古霉素或非达霉素 10 天。如无法获取万古霉素或非达霉素，可用甲硝唑替代。对于暴发性病例可予口服万古霉素联合甲硝唑静脉输液治疗，如果存在肠梗阻，可用万古霉素灌肠。首次复发应以逐渐减量配合脉冲方案口服万古霉素，或给予一个疗程的非达霉素。粪菌移植的目的是用健康人的肠道细菌重建患者的肠道菌群，有研究表明这种方法对复发或难治性疾病有益，但也有传播疾病的风险，因此这种方法目前尚处进一步研究阶段。

艰难梭菌结肠炎患者有很高的肠穿孔及进展为中毒性巨结肠的风险。如果患者使用了抗生素仍有发热、心动过速和压痛等持续炎症征象，应考虑手术治疗。进展为穿孔的患者常出现休克伴低血压和精神状态改变。这些患者的死亡率很高，必须进行结肠次全切除术，常需要进行直肠残端万古霉素灌肠。

胆道感染

胆囊炎

胆囊与阑尾一样，是一个解剖上的盲囊，胆囊管狭窄的颈部容易被胆结石或水肿阻塞，阻碍胆汁引流，导致细菌过度生长。胆囊炎中不能排出的感染的液体导致胆囊内压力增加，可进展为胆囊壁缺血、坏疽和穿孔。

胆囊炎与胆绞痛可以根据病程长短相鉴别。胆绞痛一般可自行缓解，患者也可进食。而胆囊炎以长时间的疼痛和压痛为特征，并且常伴有白细胞增多，患者表现为右侧或上腹部疼痛，常与进餐有关。查体时，压痛点通常位于右上腹。但当胆囊穿孔时，感染的胆汁会向下流至右结肠旁沟，导致右侧腹部甚至盆腔压痛。墨菲征的典型表现是在触诊右上腹时患者会突然停止吸气，这是因为患者吸气时膈肌的下移会使胆囊向下靠近检查者的手指，从而导致突然的剧烈疼痛而中断呼吸。

右上腹超声是首选的影像学检查。急性胆囊炎超声表现为胆囊壁增厚、胆囊胀大、胆囊内和胆囊周围积液。偶尔超声会显示胆囊壁内的气体；气肿性胆囊炎的死亡率很高，这些患者往往需要紧急手术治疗。虽然 CT 扫描对胆囊炎诊断敏感性和特异性均很高，但有辐射，还可能会遗漏非胆固醇结石。实验室检查会有白细胞升高和胆汁引流受阻导致的总胆红素升高。

急性胆囊炎的治疗方法是胆囊切除术，多采用腹腔镜手术。对于病情严重不能耐受手术的患者，宜采用经皮胆囊造瘘管引流术对感染的胆囊进行减压，部分患者 6 周后足以恢复到可接受手术治疗的状态，但有些年老体弱的患者，可能需要更长时间的胆囊切开置管引流。

无结石胆囊炎

无结石胆囊炎好发于危重症患者，尤其是未接受肠内营养的患者。因此，尤其是对于气管插管的患者，我们要想到该病的可能性。对于不明原因发热或无明显原因白细胞增多的患者应行右上腹超声检查，可见胆囊扩张伴囊壁增厚。这些患者常因病情太重而不能耐受外科胆囊切除术，可转至介入放射科行胆囊造瘘减压，引流感染的胆汁。虽然对于一些慢性衰弱的患者而言，放置引流管可能就足够了，但通常引流维持直至患者情况可以承受胆囊切除术。

胆管炎

胆管炎是由于胆管阻塞引起的感染，最常见于胆结石。表现为右上腹或上腹疼痛。经典症状为右上腹痛、发热和黄疸（沙尔科三联征），可进一步出现精神状态改变和休克（雷诺五联征）。这些患者胆道树内有感染的胆汁或脓液，最好通过 ERCP 进行括约肌切开术和支架置入术引流。上行性胆管炎可以是一种侵袭性感染，患者迅速进展为感染中毒性休克。此时，仅使用抗生素是不够的，必须同时进行感染源控制。怀疑胆管炎时，应立即请消化科医生和外科医生紧急会诊，这些患者往往需要进行液体复苏并入住重症监护室。

右上腹超声可显示无胆囊炎的胆石症表现，而扩张的胆总管表明结石已从胆囊排出至胆总管。重要的实验室指标包括高胆红素血症、白细胞增多和碱性磷酸酶升高（提示胆管受到刺激）。接受 ERCP 并行括约肌切开术的患者在随后的造影检查中可能会出现胆道积气，这是由于空气从十二指肠逆行进入胆管，并不提示感染。

与胆道感染相关的细菌包括大肠埃希菌、克雷伯菌属和假单胞菌属，但也可能包括肠杆菌属和拟杆菌属。不过，我们很少进行胆汁培养用于指导治疗，因此抗菌

antimicrobial therapy uses broad-spectrum agents such as piperacillin/tazobactam. For patients with uncomplicated acute cholecystitis, antibiotics may be stopped after surgery. For those too sick to undergo surgery, antibiotics are continued for 7 to 10 days, depending on clinical improvement. Patients with cholangitis require broad-spectrum antibiotics and source control in addition to fluid resuscitation.

PANCREATITIS AND PANCREATIC INFECTION

Pancreatitis is usually a self-limited inflammation of the pancreas. A small percentage progress to pancreatic necrosis, which is a risk factor for infected pancreatitis. Percutaneous aspiration of pancreatic fluid collections is not advised due to the risk of seeding sterile collections. The question of prophylactic antibiotics in cases of pancreatic necrosis has been actively debated for decades. In the interest of limiting antibiotic exposure and selecting resistant organisms, we defer antibiotics until there is evidence of infected pancreatic necrosis such as air within the fluid collections. Antibiotic therapy consists of a carbapenem and the duration is dictated by clinical improvement. Patients with infected pancreatic necrosis may undergo percutaneous drainage, but the infected material is often too thick to allow drainage. However, drain placement may be preliminary to creating a tract for videoscopic-assisted retroperitoneal dissection (VARDS) of the necrotic pancreas. Patients with unremitting signs of infection and inflammation may require surgery for drain placement and lavage.

INTRAABDOMINAL ABSCESS

Solid Organ Abscesses

Solid organ abscesses may form in the liver, spleen, and less commonly, the kidneys. The most common causes of hepatic abscess in the United States are biliary tract infection and portal vein bacteremia from diverticulitis, appendicitis or inflammatory bowel disease. Colonic bacteria predominate, including *Klebsiella pneumoniae* as well as anaerobes such as *Bacteroides* spp, *Fusobacterium*, and streptococcal species. Hepatic abscesses present with fevers as well as right upper quadrant pain. Laboratory data may show leukocytosis and an elevated alkaline phosphatase. CT scan is the imaging modality of choice for solid organ abscesses. Hepatic abscesses may be multifocal. Multiple, small abscesses are best treated with antibiotics whereas large, persistent abscesses may require percutaneous drainage. An important but less common cause of liver abscess is due to *Entamoeba histolytica* found frequently in patients from developing countries (see Chapter 18).

Splenic abscesses are seen in patients with infected endocarditis resulting from septic emboli or those who have undergone splenic artery embolization. The resulting ischemia and necrosis of splenic parenchyma serves as a nidus of infection. The presence of a splenic abscess should prompt a search for the source, including an echocardiogram. Patients may be treated with antibiotics and percutaneous drainage. Splenic abscesses may prove difficult to eradicate, in which case splenectomy is an option.

Renal abscesses may occur with recurrent pyelonephritis, particularly in the setting of urinary tract obstruction such as staghorn renal calculi. Source control may require percutaneous nephrostomy tubes to drain infected urine that cannot drain distally, and nephrectomy is indicated in cases of recurrent, fistulizing disease.

Intraabdominal and Intrapelvic

Intraabdominal and intrapelvic abscesses may form as a result of other infections, such as perforated appendicitis or diverticulitis, or after surgery for perforation of the alimentary tract. The omentum may form adhesions around the site of infection, walling it off from the remainder of the peritoneal cavity and allowing an abscess to form. This appears as a rim-enhancing fluid collection on CT scan (with IV contrast). Small abscesses (≈2 cm) in an otherwise healthy patient with a functional immune system may be treated with antibiotics alone. Larger abscesses, however, may require drainage because antibiotics may not penetrate the infected area. Source control may be accomplished with percutaneous drainage, although this warrants a conversation with the interventional radiologist as the location may preclude safe drainage due to surrounding structures. Operative source control may be accomplished by laparoscopic washout and drain placement, although this carries the risk of bowel injury due to the friable nature of the inflamed bowel. Small bowel often forms the wall of deep abscesses and surgical source control often requires bowel resection in these cases.

CONCLUSIONS

Although early administration of broad-spectrum antibiotics remains a mainstay of treatment of intraabdominal infections, source control and early identification of complications such as peritonitis from free perforation or disseminated infection are critical concepts for the clinician to understand. CT scan with intravenous contrast is the imaging modality of choice for most intraabdominal infections. Elderly patients, those with diabetes, those taking steroids, or immunocompromised patients may not mount the same exuberant response of peritonitis, and therefore they must be approached with a high degree of suspicion regarding complications.

SUGGESTED READINGS

Ahmed M: Acute cholangitis—an update, World J Gastrointest Pathophysiol 9(1):1–7, 2018.

Broad JB, Wu Z, Ng J, et al: Diverticular disease management in primary care: how do estimates from community-dispensed antibiotics inform provision of care? PloS One 14(7):e0219818, 2019.

Eid AI, Mueller P, Thabet A, Castillo CF, Fagenholz P: A step-up approach to infected abdominal fluid collections: not just for pancreatitis, Surg Infect (Larchmt) 21(1):54–61, 2020.

Kumar A, Roberts D, Wood KE, et al: Duration of hypotension before initiation of effective antimicrobial therapy is the critical determinant of survival in human septic shock, Crit Care Med 34(6):1589–1596, 2006.

Kumar V, Fischer M: Expert opinion on fecal microbiota transplantation for the treatment of clostridioides difficile infection and beyond, Expert Opin Biol Ther 20(1):73–81, 2020.

Maconi G, Barbara G, Bosetti C, Cuomo R, Annibale B: Treatment of diverticular disease of the colon and prevention of acute diverticulitis: a systematic review, Dis Colon Rectum 54(10):1326–1338, 2011.

Martinez ML, Ferrer R, Torrents E, et al: Impact of source control in patients with severe sepsis and septic shock, Crit Care Med 45(1):11–19, 2017.

Mazuski JE, Tessier JM, May AK, et al: The surgical infection society revised Guidelines on the management of intra-abdominal infection, Surg Infect (Larchmt) 18(1):1–76, 2017.

McDonald LC, Gerding DN, Johnson S, et al: Clinical practice guidelines for clostridium difficile infection in adults and children: 2017 update by the Infectious Diseases Society of America (IDSA) and society for Healthcare Epidemiology of America (SHEA), Clin Infect Dis 66(7):987–994, 2018.

Mourad MM, Evans R, Kalidindi V, Navaratnam R, Dvorkin L, Bramhall SR: Prophylactic antibiotics in acute pancreatitis: endless debate, Ann R Coll Surg Engl 99(2):107–112, 2017.

Podda M, Cillara N, Di Saverio S, et al: Antibiotics-first strategy for uncomplicated acute appendicitis in adults is associated with increased rates of peritonitis at surgery. A systematic review with meta-analysis of randomized controlled trials comparing appendectomy and non-operative management with antibiotics, Surgeon 15(5):303–314, 2017.

治疗需使用广谱抗生素,如哌拉西林/他唑巴坦。对于无急性胆囊炎并发症的患者,术后即可停用抗生素。对于因病情严重而无法接受手术的患者,可根据临床症状的改善情况,抗生素连续使用7~10天。胆管炎患者,除了液体复苏外,还需使用广谱抗生素和进行感染源控制。

胰腺炎和胰腺感染

胰腺炎通常是一种自限性炎症。小部分进展为胰腺坏死,是感染性胰腺炎的危险因素。由于存在胰液渗漏的风险,因此不建议经皮抽吸。关于胰腺坏死患者预防性使用抗生素的问题,数十年来一直争论不休。为了减少抗生素暴露和微生物选择性耐药,我们会尽量推迟抗生素使用,直到出现积液中出现空气征等感染性胰腺坏死的证据。抗生素可选择碳青霉烯类药物,用药时间取决于临床症状的改善情况。感染性胰腺坏死的患者可以行经皮穿刺引流,但感染物往往太浓稠而不易引流。然而,引流管的放置可能是为坏死胰腺的视频辅助腹膜后剥离术(VARDS)建立通道的初步准备。有持续感染和炎症征象的患者可进行手术放置引流管和灌洗。

腹腔内脓肿

实质器官脓肿

实质器官脓肿形成可见于肝、脾,较少见的是肾。在美国肝脓肿最常见的病因是胆道感染、憩室炎、阑尾炎或炎症性肠病的门静脉菌血症。结肠来源细菌占主导地位,包括肺炎克雷伯菌以及拟杆菌属、梭杆菌属和消化链球菌等厌氧菌。肝脓肿表现为发热和右上腹疼痛。实验室检查可有白细胞和碱性磷酸酶升高。CT扫描是实质器官脓肿的首选影像学检查。肝脓肿可呈多灶性。多发的小脓肿最好采用抗生素治疗,而较大的持续存在的脓肿则可能需经皮穿刺引流。肝脓肿的一个重要但不常见的致病原是溶组织内阿米巴,其在发展中国家患者中较为常见(见第18章)。

脾脓肿可因感染性心内膜炎导致的感染中毒性(脓毒性)栓塞或脾动脉栓塞而引起。由此导致的脾实质缺血和坏死可成为感染灶。因此,对于脾脓肿应积极寻找感染来源,包括进行超声心动图检查。治疗包括抗生素和经皮穿刺引流。由于脾脓肿难以根除,因此,脾切除术可以作为一种选择。

肾脓肿可能与反复肾盂肾炎有关,特别是在鹿角形肾结石导致的尿路梗阻的情况下。感染源控制方面,可能需要经皮肾造瘘来引流无法从远端排出的被感染的尿液,如果造瘘后疾病仍反复发作,则需要进行肾切除术。

腹腔和盆腔内脓肿

腹腔和盆腔内脓肿可由其他感染引起,包括穿孔性阑尾炎、憩室炎或消化道穿孔术后合并感染。大网膜可以在感染部位周围形成粘连,将其与腹膜腔的剩余部分隔离,导致脓肿形成。增强CT扫描可见腹腔内液体积聚伴边缘强化。对于免疫功能正常的患者,小的脓肿(≈2 cm)可仅使用抗生素治疗。但由于抗生素无法穿透脓肿深部,因此较大的脓肿则需要引流。感染源控制包括经皮穿刺引流,这需要与介入放射科医生沟通,因为周围结构可能会妨碍安全引流。此外,还可通过手术行腹腔镜下冲洗和放置引流管,对感染源进行更好的控制,但由于发炎的肠道很脆弱,存在肠道损伤的风险。小肠常会成为深部脓肿的壁,此情况下,为了清除感染源,常需要肠切除。

结论

尽管早期使用广谱抗生素仍然是治疗腹腔内感染的主要方法,但感染源控制和早期识别游离性穿孔和播散性感染引起的腹膜炎等并发症非常关键。增强CT扫描是大多数腹腔内感染的首选影像学检查方法。老年患者、糖尿病患者、使用类固醇激素的患者或免疫功能低下的患者可能对腹膜炎的反应迟钝,因此必须高度警惕并发症。

推荐阅读

Ahmed M: Acute cholangitis—an update, World J Gastrointest Pathophysiol 9(1):1–7, 2018.

Broad JB, Wu Z, Ng J, et al: Diverticular disease management in primary care: how do estimates from community-dispensed antibiotics inform provision of care? PloS One 14(7):e0219818, 2019.

Eid AI, Mueller P, Thabet A, Castillo CF, Fagenholz P: A step-up approach to infected abdominal fluid collections: not just for pancreatitis, Surg Infect (Larchmt) 21(1):54–61, 2020.

Kumar A, Roberts D, Wood KE, et al: Duration of hypotension before initiation of effective antimicrobial therapy is the critical determinant of survival in human septic shock, Crit Care Med 34(6):1589–1596, 2006.

Kumar V, Fischer M: Expert opinion on fecal microbiota transplantation for the treatment of clostridioides difficile infection and beyond, Expert Opin Biol Ther 20(1):73–81, 2020.

Maconi G, Barbara G, Bosetti C, Cuomo R, Annibale B: Treatment of diverticular disease of the colon and prevention of acute diverticulitis: a systematic review, Dis Colon Rectum 54(10):1326–1338, 2011.

Martinez ML, Ferrer R, Torrents E, et al: Impact of source control in patients with severe sepsis and septic shock, Crit Care Med 45(1):11–19, 2017.

Mazuski JE, Tessier JM, May AK, et al: The surgical infection society revised Guidelines on the management of intra-abdominal infection, Surg Infect (Larchmt) 18(1):1–76, 2017.

McDonald LC, Gerding DN, Johnson S, et al: Clinical practice guidelines for clostridium difficile infection in adults and children: 2017 update by the Infectious Diseases Society of America (IDSA) and society for Healthcare Epidemiology of America (SHEA), Clin Infect Dis 66(7):987–994, 2018.

Mourad MM, Evans R, Kalidindi V, Navaratnam R, Dvorkin L, Bramhall SR: Prophylactic antibiotics in acute pancreatitis: endless debate, Ann R Coll Surg Engl 99(2):107–112, 2017.

Podda M, Cillara N, Di Saverio S, et al: Antibiotics-first strategy for uncomplicated acute appendicitis in adults is associated with increased rates of peritonitis at surgery. A systematic review with meta-analysis of randomized controlled trials comparing appendectomy and non-operative management with antibiotics, Surgeon 15(5):303–314, 2017.

Riccio LM, Popovsky KA, Hranjec T, et al: Association of excessive duration of antibiotic therapy for intra-abdominal infection with subsequent extra-abdominal infection and death: a study of 2,552 consecutive infections, Surg Infect (Larchmt) 15(4):417–424, 2014.

Sawyer RG, Claridge JA, Nathens AB, et al: Trial of short-course antimicrobial therapy for intraabdominal infection, N Engl J Med 372(21):1996–2005, 2015.

Schlottmann F, Gaber C, Strassle PD, Patti MG, Charles AG: Cholecystectomy vs. Cholecystostomy for the management of acute cholecystitis in elderly patients, J Gastrointest Surg 23(3):503–509, 2019.

Riccio LM, Popovsky KA, Hranjec T, et al: Association of excessive duration of antibiotic therapy for intra-abdominal infection with subsequent extra-abdominal infection and death: a study of 2,552 consecutive infections, Surg Infect (Larchmt) 15(4):417–424, 2014.

Sawyer RG, Claridge JA, Nathens AB, et al: Trial of short-course antimicrobial therapy for intraabdominal infection, N Engl J Med 372(21):1996–2005, 2015.

Schlottmann F, Gaber C, Strassle PD, Patti MG, Charles AG: Cholecystectomy vs. Cholecystostomy for the management of acute cholecystitis in elderly patients, J Gastrointest Surg 23(3):503–509, 2019.

Infectious Diarrhea

Awewura Kwara

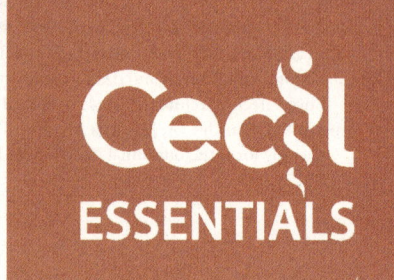

DEFINITION AND EPIDEMIOLOGY

Diarrhea is defined as the passage of three or more unformed stools or more than 250 g of unformed stools per day. Based on duration, diarrhea can be classified as *acute* (less than 14 days), *persistent* (14 to 29 days), or *chronic* (30 or more days). *Infectious diarrhea* is diarrhea that has an infectious etiology and is often associated with symptoms and signs of enteric involvement, such as nausea, vomiting, abdominal cramps, passage of bloody stool (dysentery), or systemic symptoms. Organisms responsible for infectious diarrhea include bacteria, viruses, and parasites.

In the United States (US), acute diarrhea is common, with an estimated annual burden of 179 million outpatient visits, nearly 500,000 hospitalizations, and more than 5000 deaths. The Foodborne Diseases Active Surveillance Network (FoodNet) maintained by the Centers for Disease Control and Prevention (CDC) provides data on pathogen-specific burden of diarrheal diseases in the United States by monitoring cases of laboratory-diagnosed infections caused by eight enteric pathogens transmitted through food in 10 US sites. During 2018, FoodNet identified 25,606 infections, 5893 hospitalizations, and 120 deaths. *Campylobacter*, *Salmonella*, and Shiga toxin–producing *Escherichia coli* (STEC) were the most common identified infections.

PATHOLOGY

Diarrhea is an alteration of movement of ions and water that leads to an increase in water content, volume, or frequency of stools. Under normal conditions, up to 9 L of fluid is passed through the adult gastrointestinal tract daily. Almost 98% of this fluid is absorbed, and only 100 to 200 mL is excreted in stools. Enteric pathogens or microbial toxins that are ingested can overcome host defenses and alter this balance toward a net secretion, leading to diarrhea. A large number of microorganisms are normally ingested with every meal. Host defense mechanisms against enteric pathogens include low gastric pH, rapid transit of bacteria through the proximal small intestine, cellular immune responses, and antibody production. In addition, large numbers of normal bacterial flora inhabit the intestines and prevent colonization by enteric pathogens.

Alteration of the normal defense mechanisms can put individuals at risk for infectious diarrhea. Individuals with gastric resection or achlorhydric states have increased frequency of infection due to *Salmonella*, *Giardia lamblia*, and helminths, whereas some organisms, such as *Shigella* or rotavirus, survive the extreme acidity of the gastric environment. Some viral, bacterial, and parasitic infections are more common in patients with impaired cellular or humoral immunity. More than 99% of the normal colonic flora is made up of anaerobic bacteria; they produce fatty acids and cause acidic pH, which is important for resistance to colonization. Alteration of the bacterial flora due to broad-spectrum antibiotic therapy predisposes some individuals to the development of *Clostridioides difficile* infection (CDI).

The virulence factors employed by enteric pathogens include inoculum size, adherence factors, toxin production, and invasion. Organisms such as *Shigella*, enterohemorrhagic *Escherichia coli* (EHEC), *G. lamblia*, and *Entamoeba histolytica* need as few as 10 to 100 organisms to produce infection, whereas *Vibrio cholerae* needs 10^5 to 10^8 organisms to cause disease. Infectious diarrhea can be classified as noninflammatory or inflammatory based on pathogenesis. Noninflammatory diarrhea is caused by pathogens that adhere to the mucosa of small intestine, disrupting the absorptive and/or secretory processes without causing inflammation or destruction. Pathogens that cause noninflammatory diarrhea include viruses, enterotoxin-producing organisms, *G. lamblia*, and *Cryptosporidium parvum*. Inflammatory diarrhea is cause by pathogens that target the distal ileum or the colon and cause acute inflammatory reaction by secreting cytotoxins or invading the intestinal epithelium. Cytotoxin-producing bacteria include enteroaggregative *E. coli* (EAEC), EHEC, and *C. difficile* and invasive organisms include *Salmonella*, *Shigella*, and *Campylobacter*.

Enterotoxin-Induced Secretory Diarrhea

Ingested enterotoxin-producing bacteria colonize the small bowel, and then produce enterotoxin, which binds to the mucosa and causes watery diarrhea through hypersecretion of isotonic fluid that overwhelms the absorptive capacity of the colon. *V. cholerae* produces the cholera toxin, a heterodimeric protein composed of a single toxic active A subunit (CTA) and a B subunit pentamer (CTB), which is responsible for binding of the toxin to the intestinal mucosa. The bound toxin through a series of processes activates adenylate cyclase to produce cyclic adenosine monophosphate (cAMP), which causes increased chloride secretion and decreased sodium absorption, leading to hypersecretion of fluid. Enterotoxigenic *E. coli* (ETEC) produces both a heat-labile enterotoxin that acts by the same mechanism as the cholera toxin and a heat-stable enterotoxin that causes secretory diarrhea through activation of guanylate cyclase to produce cyclic guanosine monophosphate (cGMP).

Cytotoxin-Induced Diarrhea

In contrast to enterotoxins, cytotoxins elaborated by enteric pathogens destroy mucosal epithelial cells, causing acute inflammatory reaction and bloody diarrhea (dysentery). *Shigella dysenteriae* produces the Shiga toxin, which causes dysenteric diarrhea in patients with shigellosis. Other toxin-producing bacteria include *Vibrio parahaemolyticus*, *C. difficile*, and STEC.

感染性腹泻

田地 译　王芳 肖江 张福杰 审校　张福杰 通审

定义和流行病学

腹泻是指每天排3次或3次以上不成形的粪便，或250 g以上不成形的粪便。根据腹泻持续的时间，可将其分为急性腹泻（少于14天）、持续性腹泻（14～29天）和慢性腹泻（30天或以上）。感染性腹泻是指由各种病原体感染而引起的腹泻，通常伴有肠道受累的症状和体征，如恶心、呕吐、腹部绞痛、排血便（痢疾）或全身症状。引起感染性腹泻的病原体包括细菌、病毒和寄生虫。

在美国，急性腹泻是很常见的，估计每年门诊量可达1.79亿人次，住院人数近50万人次，死亡人数超过5000人。由美国疾病控制与预防中心（CDC）建立的食源性疾病主动监测网络（FoodNet）在美国10个地点通过监测8种实验室确诊的经食物传播的肠道病原体感染病例，提供美国腹泻疾病的病原体特异性负担数据。2018年，FoodNet共监测到感染患者25 606例、住院患者5893例以及死亡患者120例。弯曲菌属、沙门菌属和产志贺毒素大肠埃希菌（STEC）是最常见的感染病原体。

病理学

腹泻是指离子和水分的运动发生改变，导致粪便的含水量、体积或排便次数增加。正常情况下，成人每天通过胃肠道的液体高达9 L，其中近98%的液体被吸收，只有100～200 ml液体随粪便排出体外。肠道病原体或微生物毒素可以克服宿主的防御能力，改变这种平衡，使肠道过多分泌液体，从而导致腹泻。人们通常每餐都会摄入大量微生物，针对肠道病原体，宿主防御机制包括胃内低pH、使细菌快速通过近端小肠以及产生细胞免疫反应和抗体。此外，大量正常菌群栖息在肠道中，也可以防止肠道病原体的定植。

正常防御机制的改变会使人面临感染性腹泻的风险。胃切除术或无胃液状态的患者感染沙门菌属、蓝氏贾第鞭毛虫和蠕虫的概率会增加，而志贺菌或轮状病毒等一些微生物则能在极酸的胃环境中存活下来。一些病毒、细菌和寄生虫感染在细胞或体液免疫受损的患者中更为常见。结肠中正常菌群的99%以上由厌氧菌组成；厌氧菌可产生脂肪酸并导致酸性pH，这对抵抗定植很重要。使用广谱抗生素可导致肠道菌群的改变，使一部分患者更易患上艰难梭菌感染（CDI）。

肠道病原体的致病因素包括病原体数量、黏附因子、产生的毒素和侵袭力。志贺菌、肠出血性大肠埃希菌（EHEC）、蓝氏贾第鞭毛虫和溶组织内阿米巴等只需要10～100个病原体就能产生感染，而霍乱弧菌则需要10^5～10^8个菌体才能致病。根据发病机制，感染性腹泻可分为非炎症性腹泻和炎症性腹泻。非炎症性腹泻是由于病原体附着在小肠黏膜上，破坏了小肠的吸收和（或）分泌过程，但不会引起炎症或破坏。引起非炎症性腹泻的病原体包括病毒、产肠毒素的病原体、蓝氏贾第鞭毛虫和隐孢子虫。引起炎症性腹泻的病原体以回肠远端或结肠为目标，通过分泌细胞毒素或侵入肠上皮细胞引起急性炎症反应。产生细胞毒素的细菌包括肠聚集性大肠埃希菌（EAEC）、EHEC和艰难梭菌，侵入性细菌包括沙门菌属、志贺菌和弯曲杆菌。

肠毒素诱导的分泌性腹泻

摄入的产肠毒素的细菌在小肠内定植后产生肠毒素，这种毒素与肠黏膜结合可引起等渗液体过度分泌，超过结肠的吸收能力，从而引起水样腹泻。霍乱弧菌产生的霍乱毒素是一种异源二聚体蛋白，由一个具有毒性的活性A亚基（CTA）和一个B亚基五聚体（CTB）组成，后者负责将毒素与肠黏膜结合。结合后的毒素通过一系列过程激活腺苷酸环化酶，产生环磷酸腺苷（cAMP），导致氯化物分泌增加和钠吸收减少，从而导致液体分泌过多。肠产毒性大肠埃希菌（ETEC）会产生一种作用机制与霍乱毒素相同的不耐热的肠毒素和一种可通过激活鸟苷酸环化酶产生环磷酸鸟苷（cGMP）而引起分泌性腹泻的热稳定性肠毒素。

细胞毒素诱导的腹泻

与肠毒素不同，肠道病原体产生的细胞毒素会破坏肠黏膜上皮细胞，引起急性炎症反应和血性腹泻（痢疾）。痢疾志贺菌可产生志贺毒素，导致感染者出现痢疾样腹泻。其他产生毒素的细菌包括副溶血弧菌、艰难梭菌和STEC。

TABLE 11.1 Epidemiologic and Clinical Characteristics of Common Enteric Pathogens

Organism	Epidemiologic Features	Common Clinical Features
Campylobacter jejuni	Consumption of undercooked poultry, travel to tropical and semitropical regions	Acute watery diarrhea, fever, abdominal pain, fecal evidence of inflammation (positive fecal leukocytes or lactoferrin)
Vibrio cholerae	Inadequately cooked seafood, travel to endemic regions	Acute dehydrating watery diarrhea; fever is usually absent
Clostridioides difficile	Antibiotic use, recent hospitalization, elderly patients with coexisting conditions	Diarrhea with fever, fecal evidence of inflammation, marked leukocytosis
Enterotoxigenic Escherichia coli	Travel to tropical and semitropical regions	Watery diarrhea, abdominal cramps, nausea and vomiting; leukocytes absent in stools
Nontyphoidal Salmonella	Food-borne outbreaks, exposure to animals	Acute watery diarrhea, fever, abdominal pain, evidence of inflammation
Shigella	Person-to-person transmission, daycare center contact	Severe diarrhea with fever, abdominal pain, bloody diarrhea, fecal evidence of inflammation
Shiga toxin–producing E. coli	Food-borne outbreaks, undercooked hamburgers, raw seed sprouts, water and wading pool exposure	Abdominal pain, bloody stools, absence of fever, fecal evidence of inflammation
Noncholeraic Vibrio	Ingestion of shellfish and undercooked seafood	Watery diarrhea, abdominal cramps, nausea; fever and vomiting are less frequent
Yersinia enterocolitica	Contaminated food or water, inadequately cooked meats, unpasteurized milk	Acute watery diarrhea, fever, abdominal pain, bloody diarrhea
Norovirus	Winter outbreaks in congregate settings, outbreaks on cruise ships	Watery diarrhea, nausea, vomiting, abdominal pain
Cyclospora	Food-borne outbreaks, travel to tropical and subtropical regions (especially Nepal)	Persistent noninflammatory diarrhea
Cryptosporidium	Waterborne outbreaks, travel to tropical and subtropical regions	Persistent noninflammatory diarrhea
Entamoeba histolytica	Travel to tropical regions, recent immigration from endemic regions	Bloody diarrhea, extraintestinal involvement (liver abscess)
Giardia lamblia	Waterborne outbreaks, travel to mountainous areas of North America, Russia	Abdominal pain, persistent watery diarrhea, flatulence, steatorrhea, nausea and vomiting

Invasive Diarrhea

Some bacteria cause dysentery through direct invasion and destruction of intestinal mucosa. *Shigella* and enteroinvasive *E. coli* (EIEC) invade and multiply in epithelial cells and spread to adjacent cells. Diarrhea is often accompanied by fever, abdominal cramps, and small amounts of bloody mucoid stools. Other bacteria, such as *Salmonella typhi* and *Yersinia enterocolitica*, penetrate the mucosa before disseminating into the bloodstream to cause a systemic illness.

Bacterial Food Poisoning

Bacterial food poisoning is caused by ingestion of preformed toxins in food that results in a toxic illness. The toxins may include cytotoxins, enterotoxins, and neurotoxins. Pathogens that cause bacterial food poisoning include *Staphylococcus aureus*, *Clostridioides perfringens*, and *Bacillus cereus*. These organisms grow in food and produce toxins that are ingested directly in the food. Symptoms occur soon after food ingestion, with incubation periods of 1 to 16 hours. The illness is rarely associated with fever, and symptoms usually resolve within 12 to 24 hours after onset.

The staphylococcal and *B. cereus* toxins act on the nervous system to cause vomiting. *S. aureus* causes vomiting and diarrhea within 2 to 7 hours after ingestion of improperly cooked or stored food containing its heat-stable enterotoxin. *C. perfringens* produces secretory and cytotoxin-induced watery diarrhea within 8 to 14 hours after ingestion of contaminated vegetables, meat, or poultry. *B. cereus* often contaminates fried rice, vegetables, or sprouts; it produces one of two toxins that cause disease resembling that of *S. aureus* or *C. perfringens* infection within 1 to 6 hours after ingestion.

SPECIFIC PATHOGENS

The epidemiologic and clinical features of common enteric pathogens and the recommended methods for diagnosis and treatment are summarized in Tables 11.1 and 11.2.

Shigella

Diarrhea due to *Shigella* spp (shigellosis) occurs after ingestion of fecally contaminated food or water. The main strains include *S. dysenteriae*, *S. flexneri*, *S. boydii*, and *S. sonnei*. Ingestion of as few as 10 to 100 microorganisms can lead to infection because the bacteria are relatively resistant to gastric acid. Person-to-person transmission is common, and the attack rate is highest among infants and young children in child-care centers. The incubation period is 6 to 72 hours. Illness may initially manifest as noninflammatory watery diarrhea caused by enterotoxin production or multiplication of bacteria in the small intestines. Invasion of the colonic epithelium and mucosa often manifests as dysentery. Complications of *S. dysenteriae* type 1 shigellosis include hemolytic-uremic syndrome (HUS). Reactive arthritis is associated with *S. flexneri* infection.

Salmonella

Salmonella enterica serovars typhi and paratyphi cause enteric fever whereas nontyphoidal *Salmonella* spp cause diarrhea. Nontyphoidal salmonellosis results from ingestion of contaminated meat, dairy, or poultry products or from direct contact with animals such as birds, pet turtles, snakes, and other reptiles. An oral inoculum of 10^5 to 10^8 organisms is needed but smaller inocula can cause disease in patients

表 11.1 常见肠道病原体的流行病学和临床特点

病原体	流行病学特点	常见的临床特征
空肠弯曲菌	食用未煮熟的家禽、前往热带和亚热带地区旅行	急性水样腹泻、发热、腹痛、粪便有炎症表现（粪便白细胞或乳铁蛋白呈阳性）
霍乱弧菌	食用未充分煮熟的海鲜、前往流行地区旅行	急性脱水型水样腹泻；通常无发热表现
艰难梭菌	使用抗生素、近期住院、有并发症的老年患者	腹泻伴发热、粪便有炎症表现、白细胞明显增多
肠产毒性大肠埃希菌	前往热带和亚热带地区旅游	水样腹泻、腹部绞痛、恶心和呕吐；粪便中无白细胞
非伤寒沙门菌	经食物传播、接触动物	急性水样腹泻、发热、腹痛、炎症表现
志贺菌	人际传播、接触日托中心	严重腹泻伴有发热、腹痛、血样便、粪便中有炎症表现
产志贺毒素大肠埃希菌	经食物传播，食用未煮熟的汉堡、生的种子芽，接触水和涉水池	腹痛、血便、不发热、粪便中有炎症表现
非霍乱弧菌	食用贝类和未完全煮熟的海产品	水样腹泻、腹部绞痛、恶心；发热和呕吐较少发生
小肠结肠炎耶尔森菌	摄入受污染的食物或水、未煮熟的肉类、未消毒的牛奶	急性水样腹泻、发热、腹痛、血样便
诺如病毒	多见于冬季聚集性场所、游轮	水样腹泻、恶心、呕吐、腹痛
环孢子虫	经食物传播、前往热带和亚热带地区（尤其是尼泊尔）旅行	持续非炎症性腹泻
隐孢子虫	经水源传播、前往热带和亚热带地区旅行	持续非炎症性腹泻
溶组织内阿米巴	前往热带地区，近期曾在流行地区生活	血性腹泻、肠外受累（肝脓肿）
蓝氏贾第鞭毛虫	经水源传播、前往北美山区、俄罗斯	腹痛、持续水样腹泻、腹胀、脂肪泻、恶心和呕吐

侵袭性腹泻

有些细菌可通过直接侵入和破坏肠黏膜引起痢疾。志贺菌和肠侵袭性大肠埃希菌（EIEC）会侵入肠上皮细胞并在其中繁殖，然后扩散到邻近的细胞。腹泻通常伴有发热、腹痛和少量黏液血便。其他细菌，如伤寒沙门菌和小肠结肠炎耶尔森菌，会先侵入黏膜，然后扩散到血液中，引起全身性疾病。

细菌性食物中毒

细菌性食物中毒是由于摄入食物中的毒素而导致中毒性疾病。毒素可能包括细胞毒素、肠毒素和神经毒素。引起细菌性食物中毒的病原体包括金黄色葡萄球菌、产气荚膜梭菌和蜡样芽孢杆菌。这些病原体在食物中生长，并产生毒素，患者可直接从食物中摄入。进食后很快出现症状，潜伏期为 1～16 h，很少出现发热，通常在发病后 12～24 h 症状缓解。

葡萄球菌和蜡样芽孢杆菌毒素能作用于神经系统导致呕吐。金黄色葡萄球菌感染引起的呕吐和腹泻在进食烹饪或储存不当的含有其热稳定性肠毒素的食物后 2～7 h 出现。产气荚膜梭菌引起的分泌性、细胞毒素诱导的水样泻在进食受污染的蔬菜、肉类或家禽后 8～14 h 出现。蜡样芽孢杆菌经常污染炒饭、蔬菜或芽菜；它会产生两种毒素中的一种，在进食 1～6 h 引起类似于金黄色葡萄球菌或产气荚膜梭菌感染所致的疾病表现。

特异性病原体

表 11.1 和表 11.2 总结了常见肠道病原体的流行病学和临床特点以及推荐的诊断和治疗方法。

志贺菌

志贺菌引起的腹泻（志贺菌病）发生于进食被粪便污染的食物或水之后。主要菌株包括痢疾志贺菌、福氏志贺菌、鲍氏志贺菌和宋氏志贺菌。由于志贺菌对胃酸有较强的抵抗力，因此只要摄入 10～100 个细菌就可导致感染。人际传播很常见，幼托中心的婴幼儿发病率最高。潜伏期为 6～72 h，疾病早期可表现为非炎症性水样腹泻，由肠毒素或细菌在小肠繁殖引起。结肠上皮和黏膜受侵袭后通常表现为痢疾。痢疾志贺菌 1 型志贺菌病引起的并发症包括溶血性尿毒综合征（HUS）。反应性关节炎与福氏志贺菌感染有关。

沙门菌属

伤寒沙门菌和副伤寒沙门菌会引起肠热症，而非伤寒沙门菌则会引起腹泻。非伤寒沙门菌病是由于进食受污染的肉类、奶制品或家禽产品，或直接接触鸟类、宠物龟、蛇和其他爬行动物等引起。发病需要摄入 10^5～10^8 个细菌，但少量细菌也会导致胃酸受损或免疫力低下的患者发病。细菌侵入回肠远端引起腹泻，

TABLE 11.2 Diagnosis and Recommended Antimicrobial Treatment for Diarrhea With Specific Pathogens in Adults

Organism	Diagnosis	Recommendations
Campylobacter jejuni	Routine stool culture	Azithromycin 500 mg PO daily for 3 days. Alternative ciprofloxacin 500 mg PO bid for 3 days
Vibrio cholerae O1	Stool culture in special salt-containing media (TCBS), test isolate for O1 serotype	Doxycycline 300 mg or azithromycin 1000 mg PO single dose, or tetracycline 500 mg PO qid or TMP-SMZ 160/800 mg PO bid or ceftriaxone 1–2 g IV/IM q24h for 3 days
Clostridioides difficile	Stool test for C. difficile toxin A or B by EIA, or PCR for the B toxin gene	Stop implicated antibiotic. Vancomycin 125 mg PO qid or fidaxomicin 200 mg PO bid for 10 days. For fulminant CDI, vancomycin 500 mg four times daily orally or by NGT is recommended.
Enterotoxigenic Escherichia coli	Stool culture for E. coli, with assay for enterotoxin	Azithromycin 1000 mg PO single dose or 500 mg PO daily for 3 days or ciprofloxacin 500 mg PO bid for 3 days
Nontyphoidal Salmonella	Routine stool culture	Antimicrobials not recommended except for groups at risk of invasive disease. Ciprofloxacin 500 mg bid for 5 to 7 days or ceftriaxone 100 mg/kg/day in one or two divided doses for 5 to 7 days, or longer if endovascular infection or relapsing
Shigella	Routine stool culture	Ciprofloxacin 500 mg bid for 3 days or ceftriaxone 1–2 g IV/IM for 3 days or azithromycin 500 mg PO daily for 3 days
Shiga toxin–producing E. coli	Stool culture with sorbitol-MacConkey agar, followed by serotyping for O157, then H7, with EIA for Shiga toxins	Antibiotics and antimotility drugs should be avoided
Noncholeraic Vibrio	Stool culture in special salt-containing media (TCBS)	Ceftriaxone 1–2 g IV/IM q24h plus doxycycline 100 mg PO bid for 3 days
Yersinia enterocolitica	Stool culture on MacConkey media incubated at 25° to 28° C	Antibiotics usually not required. For severe infection or bacteremia, treat with TMP-SMZ or fluoroquinolone or doxycycline plus aminoglycoside
Cyclospora	Stool trichrome or acid-fast stain for parasites	TMP-SMZ 160/800 mg bid for 7–10 days
Cryptosporidium	Stool trichrome or acid-fast stain for parasites, EIA for Cryptosporidium species	Self-limited in immunocompetent persons. If severe or if patient is immunocompromised, nitazoxanide 500 mg PO bid for 3 to 14 days
Isospora	Stool trichrome or acid-fast stain for parasites	TMP-SMZ 160/800 mg PO bid for 7–10 days
Entamoeba histolytica	Stool examination for ova and parasites, EIA for E. histolytica	Metronidazole 750 mg tid for 5–10 days, plus iodoquinol 650 mg tid for 20 days or paromomycin 500 mg tid for 7 days
Giardia	Stool examination for ova and parasites, EIA for Giardia species	Single dose tinidazole 2 g or nitazoxanide 500 mg bid for 3 days. Metronidazole 250 to 750 mg tid for 5 to 10 days

EIA, Enzyme immunoassay; *PCR*, polymerase chain reaction; *PO*, per oral; *bid*, twice a day; *qid*, four times a day; *TCBS*, thiosulfate-citrate-bile salts-sucrose agar; *tid*, three times a day; *TMP-SMZ*, trimethoprim-sulfamethoxazole.

with impaired gastric acidity or compromised immunity. The organisms invade the distal ileum and cause diarrhea with fever, nausea, or vomiting. Diarrhea usually resolves in 2 to 3 days. Complications include bacteremia and metastatic seeding of atherosclerotic plaques and prostheses. Antibiotic treatment does not shorten the duration of diarrhea and may prolong intestinal carriage in stools. Antibiotics are indicated only for cases of severe disease or extraintestinal involvement.

Campylobacter

Disease caused by *Campylobacter jejuni* usually results from ingestion of undercooked poultry or direct contact with animals. The infective dose is 10^4 to 10^6 organisms, with an incubation period of 1 to 5 days. Acute watery, noninflammatory diarrhea is the most common presentation. Less frequently, acute inflammatory enterocolitis with systemic symptoms may occur. Prodromal symptoms such as fever, myalgia, headache, and malaise may precede diarrhea. Complications include postinfectious irritable bowel syndrome, reactive arthritis, especially associated with the human leukocyte antigen B27 (HLA-B27), and Guillain-Barré syndrome, which can occur 2 to 3 weeks after diarrhea has resolved. Antibiotic therapy shortens the carriage state.

Vibrio

V. cholerae can be divided by the O-antigen of lipopolysaccharide into more than 150 strains. The toxigenic strains *V. cholerae* O1 and O139 produce cholera toxin and are associated with clinical illness. The infectious oral inoculum is about 10^5 to 10^8 organisms, with an incubation period of 6 hours to 5 days. Classic cholera starts with vomiting, abdominal pain, and diarrhea. Diarrhea progresses to voluminous watery stools that have been described as "rice water" because they are clear with flecks of mucus. Massive diarrhea can lead to dehydration and shock within a few hours. The illness may be fulminant, with death occurring 3 to 4 hours after onset. Fever and bacteremia are rare. In endemic areas, the diagnosis is usually made on clinical grounds. Toxigenic *V. cholerae* non-O1, non-O139 produces cholera toxin and has caused sporadic cases of diarrhea or small outbreaks in some parts of the United States through consumption of contaminated seafood or water. *V. parahaemolyticus* has also been reported to cause acute gastroenteritis from consumption of contaminated seafood. The characteristics of noncholeraic *Vibrio* species are covered in Tables 11.1 and 11.2.

Listeria

Listeria monocytogenes is an uncommon cause of diarrhea in the United States. The two major clinical syndromes of *Listeria* infection are

表 11.2 成人特异性病原体腹泻的诊断和推荐的抗感染治疗

病原体	诊断	推荐治疗
空肠弯曲菌	常规粪便培养	阿奇霉素每日 500 mg PO，连续 3 天。环丙沙星 500 mg PO bid，连续 3 天
霍乱弧菌 O1 群	在特殊含盐培养基（TCBS）中进行粪便培养，检测分离出的 O1 血清型	多西环素 300 mg 或阿奇霉素 1000 mg 单次 PO，或四环素 500 mg PO qid，或 TMP-SMZ 160/800 mg PO bid，或头孢曲松 1～2 g 每 24 h IV/IM，持续 3 天
艰难梭菌	粪便通过 EIA 对艰难梭菌毒素 A 或 B 进行检测，或通过 PCR 对 B 型毒素基因进行检测	停用相关抗生素。万古霉素 125 mg PO qid，或非达霉素 200 mg PO bid，连续 10 天。对于暴发性艰难梭菌感染，建议万古霉素 500 mg qid PO 或通过 NGT 服用
肠产毒性大肠埃希菌	粪便培养大肠埃希菌，检测肠毒素	阿奇霉素 1000 mg 单次 PO 或 500 mg 每日 PO，连续 3 天，或环丙沙星 500 mg PO bid，连续 3 天
非伤寒沙门菌	常规粪便培养	不建议使用抗菌药物，有侵袭性疾病风险的人群除外。环丙沙星 500 mg bid，5～7 天；或头孢曲松每日 100 mg/kg，或分为每日两次，使用 5～7 天；如果是血管内感染或复发，则需更长时间
志贺菌	常规粪便培养	环丙沙星 500 mg bid，连续 3 天；或头孢曲松 1～2 g IV/IM，连续 3 天；或阿奇霉素 500 mg PO，连续 3 天
产志贺毒素大肠埃希菌	用山梨醇-麦康凯琼脂进行粪便培养，然后先后检测 O157 和 H7 血清分型，并进行志贺毒素 EIA 检测	应避免使用抗生素和肠动力抑制药物
非霍乱弧菌	在特殊含盐培养基（TCBS）中行粪便培养	头孢曲松 1～2 g 每 24 h IV/IM 联合多西环素 100 mg PO bid，持续 3 天
小肠结肠炎耶尔森菌	在 25～28℃麦康凯培养基上进行粪便培养	通常无须使用抗生素。对于严重感染或菌血症，可使用 TMP-SMZ 或氟喹诺酮类药物或多西环素联合氨基糖苷类药物治疗
环孢子虫	粪便三色染色法或抗酸染色检测寄生虫	TMP-SMZ 160/800 mg bid，7～10 天
隐孢子虫	粪便三色染色法或抗酸染色检测寄生虫，EIA 检测隐孢子虫	免疫功能正常者可自行缓解。如果病情严重或患者免疫力低下，可服用硝唑尼特 500 mg PO bid，连续 3～14 天
等孢球虫属	粪便三色染色法或抗酸染色检测寄生虫	TMP-SMZ 160/800 mg bid，7～10 天
溶组织内阿米巴	粪便卵和寄生虫检查，EIA 检测溶组织内阿米巴	甲硝唑 750 mg tid，连续 5～10 天联合双碘亏喹啉 650 mg tid，连续 20 天，或巴龙霉素 500 mg tid，连续 7 天
蓝氏贾第鞭毛虫	粪便检测虫卵和寄生虫，EIA 检测贾第虫	单次替硝唑 2 g 或硝唑尼特 500 mg bid，连续 3 天。甲硝唑 250～750 mg tid，连续 5～10 天

EIA，酶免疫分析；PCR，聚合酶链反应；PO，口服；bid，每日 2 次；qid，每日 4 次；TCBS，硫代硫酸盐-柠檬酸盐-胆盐-蔗糖琼脂；tid，每日 3 次；TMP-SMZ，甲氧苄啶-磺胺甲噁唑。

伴有发热、恶心或呕吐，腹泻通常在 2～3 天缓解。并发症包括菌血症以及动脉粥样硬化斑块和假体的转移性播散。抗生素治疗不会缩短腹泻的持续时间，还可能延长细菌在粪便中的携带时间。抗生素仅适用于病情严重或肠道外受累的患者。

弯曲杆菌

空肠弯曲菌引起的疾病通常是由于进食未煮熟的家禽或直接接触动物所致。感染剂量为 10^4～10^6 个病菌，潜伏期为 1～5 天。最常见的症状是急性非炎症性水样腹泻，较少见伴有全身症状的急性炎症性小肠结肠炎。腹泻前可能会出现发热、肌痛、头痛和乏力等前驱症状。并发症包括感染后肠易激综合征、反应性关节炎，尤其与人类白细胞抗原 B27（HLA-B27）有关，以及吉兰-巴雷综合征，后者可在腹泻缓解后 2～3 周发生。抗生素治疗可缩短带菌状态。

霍乱弧菌

霍乱弧菌可根据其脂多糖 O 抗原分为 150 多个菌株。产毒素的菌株 O1 和 O139 可产生霍乱毒素，与临床疾病相关。霍乱弧菌的感染剂量为 10^5～10^8 个病菌，潜伏期为 6 h～5 天。典型的霍乱起病时主要表现为呕吐、腹痛和腹泻。腹泻发展为大量水样便，由于粪便清澈并带有黏液，呈"米泔水"样。大量腹泻可在几小时内导致脱水和休克。疾病可能呈暴发性，发病后 3～4 h 死亡。本病发热和菌血症很少见。在霍乱流行地区，通常根据患者的临床症状可做出诊断。非 O1、非 O139 产毒素霍乱弧菌也可产生霍乱毒素，在美国一些地区因进食受污染的海鲜或水而引起散发腹泻病例或小规模疫情。据报道，因食用受污染的海产品副溶血弧菌也可引起急性肠胃炎。非霍乱弧菌的特征见表 11.1 和表 11.2。

李斯特菌

在美国，单核细胞增生李斯特菌引起的腹泻并不常见。李斯特菌感染后可引起胃肠炎和李斯特菌病两种临床综合征。疫情暴发可能是由于摄入了受污染的即食食品，如未经巴氏消毒的牛奶、奶酪、肉类、蔬菜和未经清洗的生鲜农产品。胃肠炎通常是轻微的、

gastroenteritis and listeriosis. Outbreaks may be due to ingestion of contaminated ready-to-eat foods such as unpasteurized milk, cheeses, meats, vegetables, and unwashed raw produce. Gastroenteritis is usually mild, noninvasive, and generally self-limiting. Symptoms including diarrhea, fever, chills, headache, joint pains, and myalgia that may occur 9 to 32 (median, 20) hours after ingestion of contaminated food. The diagnosis of gastroenteritis is often missed, as stool is not routinely cultured. In febrile gastroenteritis where traditional pathogens are not isolated using standard media, culture of stools with selective media for *L. monocytogenes* may demonstrate the organism. If diagnosed in a susceptible host, Listeria gastroenteritis may be treated with amoxicillin 500 mg orally three times a day or TMP/SMX 160/800 mg for 7 days.

Listeriosis is a more severe invasive illness, which may manifest as bacteremia, central nervous system disease, or sepsis in pregnant women with fetal loss. Risk factors for listeriosis include extremes of age, pregnancy, and immunocompromised state. In 2019, the FoodNet reported 134 laboratory-diagnosed cases of listeriosis in the United States, of which 131 (98%) were hospitalized and 21 (16%) died. The overall incidence was 0.3 per 100,000 population.

Diarrhea-Causing *Escherichia coli*

There are several types of diarrheagenic *E. coli*, each with a different pathogenesis leading to diarrhea. These include ETEC, STEC, enteropathogenic (EPEC), EIEC, EAEC, and diffusely adherent *E. coli*. ETEC is the most common cause of traveler's diarrhea. EPEC has been associated with epidemic diarrhea in neonates.

EHEC is acquired by eating contaminated food or water. The oral inoculum is 10 to 100 organisms, with an incubation period of 3 to 4 days. Most disease in the United States is caused by *E. coli* O157:H7. Infection with EHEC, including *E. coli* O157:H7 and other STEC serotypes can cause hemorrhagic colitis. It is classically associated with bloody diarrhea, abdominal pain, and fecal leukocytes. Systemic complications include HUS in children and thrombotic thrombocytopenia purpura in adults. Antibiotic therapy may increase the risk of HUS.

Clostridioides difficile

C. difficile infection is the main cause of nosocomial diarrhea among adults in the United States. The main risk factor for CDI is antibiotic use. Advanced age and severe underlying disease contribute to susceptibility. Virtually all antibiotics have been implicated in the development of CDI, but the most common agents are clindamycin, cephalosporins, fluoroquinolones, ampicillin, and amoxicillin. Infection is transmitted by spores, which occur in the environment and are resistant to alcohol-based handwashing solutions. The spores of toxigenic *C. difficile* are ingested, survive gastric acidity, geminate, and colonize the lower intestinal tract, where they elaborate two exotoxins, toxin A (an enterotoxin) and toxin B (a cytotoxin). The toxins disrupt cell and tight junctions, leading to fluid leakage. The cellular toxicity results in neutrophilic colitis and formation of a pseudomembrane in some cases.

The hypervirulent strain referred to as the North American pulsed-field gel electrophoresis type 1 (NAP1/027) strain is associated with a severe course, higher mortality, and increased risk of relapse. Bacterial factors implicated in outbreaks of CDI caused by the NAP1/027 strain include increased production of toxins A and B, fluoroquinolone resistance, and production of a binary toxin. Patients often have abdominal pain and watery diarrhea but may also have bloody stools. Markers of severe or fulminant CDI include pseudomembranous colitis, acute renal failure, marked leukocytosis, hypotension, and toxic megacolon. The indigenous intestinal microbiota is important for colonization resistance and for recovery from antibiotic-associated CDI.

Yersinia enterocolitica

Y. enterocolitica is a zoonosis caused by ingestion of contaminated food or water or undercooked meats. Oral inoculation requires 10^9 organisms for infection, with an incubation period of 3 to 7 days. The illness may mimic acute appendicitis and may be complicated by ileal perforation, mesenteric adenitis, or terminal ileitis. Postinfectious reactive arthritis may occur.

Viral Causes of Diarrhea

Viruses cause diarrhea by adhering to the intestinal mucosa and disrupting the absorptive and secretory processes without causing inflammation. They may invade intestinal villous epithelial cells and cause sloughing of villi. Rotavirus is a common cause of severe diarrhea in children younger than 5 years of age. The incidence of rotavirus disease has fallen in many countries following the introduction of the rotavirus vaccine. Rotavirus still results in greater than 200,000 deaths annually, mostly in low-income countries. Norovirus is highly contagious and is a very common cause of food-borne gastroenteritis in adults and children in the United States. It has been the cause of epidemic diarrhea on cruise ships. Other viruses that cause diarrhea are adenoviruses, sapoviruses, and astroviruses. The incubation period is usually longer than 14 hours, and vomiting may be a prominent feature of diarrheal disease caused by viral agents.

Protozoan Causes of Diarrhea

Important parasitic causes of diarrhea include *G. lamblia*, *C. parvum*, and *E. histolytica*. Contaminated water sources tend to be the cause of outbreaks. *G. lamblia* trophozoites adhere to the epithelium of the upper small intestine and damage the mucosal brush border without invasion. Ingestion of a few organisms can lead to disease. *C. parvum*, *Isospora belli*, and *Cyclospora cayetanensis* occasionally cause self-limited diarrhea in immunocompetent individuals but may cause severe disease in patients with advanced acquired immunodeficiency syndrome (AIDS). *E. histolytica* causes a syndrome ranging from mild diarrhea to fulminant amebic colitis and extraintestinal amebic abscesses.

Traveler's Diarrhea

Traveler's diarrhea affects 10% to 40% of travelers from industrialized countries who visit tropical and semitropical developing countries. The causative agent is identified in about 85% of cases, and 90% of those identified are bacterial pathogens, most often ETEC or EAEC. Less common bacterial causes include EIEC, diffusely adherent *E. coli*, *Shigella* spp, *Salmonella* spp, *Campylobacter* spp, *Aeromonas*, *V. cholerae*, noncholeraic *Vibrio*, and *Plesiomonas*. The viral etiologies include rotavirus and norovirus. Protozoal causes are rare. Travelers to high-risk areas should be counseled to wash hands, avoid uncooked food, and drink bottled water. Patients with traveler's diarrhea should be treated empirically with antibiotics without stool examination.

CLINICAL PRESENTATION

The epidemiologic and clinical characteristics are important to identify the potential etiologic agent and to guide management (see Table 11.1). The initial evaluation should consider the severity of illness, signs of dehydration, and intestinal inflammation indicated by the fever, abdominal pain, blood in stools (dysentery), or tenesmus. Important epidemiologic clues in the history include age, travel history, ingestion of undercooked or raw food and meat, antibiotic use, sexual activity, daycare attendance, and outbreaks involving others with similar exposure (see Table 11.1). Fever (temperature 38.5° C or 101.3° F or higher) is associated with invasive pathogens that cause

非侵入性的，而且一般是自限性的。症状包括腹泻、发热、畏寒、头痛、关节痛和肌痛，可在摄入受污染食物 9～32 h（中位数为 20 h）后出现。由于没有常规对粪便进行培养，因此胃肠炎常常被漏诊。在发热、胃肠炎的患者中，如果使用标准培养基无法分离出传统病原体，用选择性的单核细胞增生李斯特菌培养基对粪便进行培养可能会有帮助。如果易感宿主确诊为李斯特菌胃肠炎，可口服阿莫西林 500 mg 每日 3 次，或口服 TMP-SMZ 160/800 mg，连续 7 天。

李斯特菌病是一种较严重的侵袭性疾病，可表现为菌血症、中枢神经系统感染或孕妇感染中毒症，导致胎儿死亡。李斯特菌病的危险因素包括极端年龄、怀孕和免疫力低下。2019 年，美国 FoodNet 报告了 134 例实验室确诊的李斯特菌病，其中 131 例（98%）住院治疗，21 例（16%）死亡。总发病率为每 10 万人中 0.3 例。

引起腹泻的大肠埃希菌

致泻性大肠埃希菌有多种类型，每种致泻性大肠埃希菌都有不同的致病机制。其中包括 ETEC、STEC、肠致病性大肠埃希菌（EPEC）、EIEC、EAEC 和弥漫黏附性大肠埃希菌。ETEC 是导致旅行者腹泻的最常见原因。EPEC 与新生儿流行性腹泻有关。

EHEC 感染主要是通过进食受污染的食物或水。感染剂量为 10～100 个病菌，潜伏期为 3～4 天。在美国，大多数疾病是由大肠埃希菌 O157：H7 引起的。感染 EHEC（包括大肠埃希菌 O157：H7 和其他 STEC 血清型）可引起出血性结肠炎。出血性结肠炎通常伴有血性腹泻、腹痛和粪便白细胞。全身并发症包括儿童的 HUS 和成人血栓性血小板减少性紫癜。抗生素治疗可能会增加发生 HUS 的风险。

艰难梭菌

艰难梭菌感染是造成美国成年人院内腹泻的主要原因。CDI 的主要危险因素是抗生素的使用，高龄和患有严重基础疾病的患者易感。几乎所有抗生素的使用都与 CDI 的发生有关，但最常见的药物是克林霉素、头孢菌素类、氟喹诺酮类、氨苄西林和阿莫西林。感染主要通过芽孢进行传播，芽孢存在于环境中，对含酒精的洗手液有抗药性。艰难梭菌芽孢摄入后可在胃酸中存活，并在下消化道定植，产生两种外毒素：毒素 A（肠毒素）和毒素 B（细胞毒素）。毒素破坏细胞和细胞间的紧密连接，导致液体渗出。在一些患者中，细胞毒性可导致嗜中性粒细胞结肠炎并形成伪膜。

被称为北美脉冲场凝胶电泳 1 型（NAP1/027）的高毒力菌株与严重的病程、较高的死亡率和复发风险增加有关。由 NAP1/027 菌株引起的 CDI 暴发与细菌因素有关，包括毒素 A 和毒素 B 的产生增加、氟喹诺酮类药物耐药性以及二元毒素的产生。患者通常会出现腹痛和水样腹泻，但也可能出现血便。严重或暴发性 CDI 的标志包括伪膜性结肠炎、急性肾衰竭、白细胞明显增多、低血压和中毒性巨结肠。肠道正常菌群对于抗定植和抗生素相关 CDI 恢复都是非常重要的。

小肠结肠炎耶尔森菌

小肠结肠炎耶尔森菌是一种人畜共患病，由进食受污染的食物、水或未煮熟的肉类引起。摄入 10^9 个菌体才能导致感染，潜伏期为 3～7 天。该病可表现为急性阑尾炎，并可能并发回肠穿孔、肠系膜腺炎或末端回肠炎，还可能会出现感染后反应性关节炎。

病毒性病因导致的腹泻

病毒通过在肠黏膜上附着干扰吸收和分泌过程而导致腹泻，但不会引起炎症。它们可能侵入肠绒毛上皮细胞，导致绒毛脱落。轮状病毒感染是引起 5 岁以下儿童严重腹泻的常见原因。许多国家在引入轮状病毒疫苗后，轮状病毒病的发病率有所下降。但轮状病毒每年仍会导致 20 多万人死亡，主要发生在低收入国家。诺如病毒具有高度传染性，是美国成人和儿童食源性胃肠炎的常见病因，它也是游轮上流行性腹泻的病因。可引起腹泻的其他病毒还有腺病毒、沙波病毒和星状病毒。潜伏期一般超过 14 h，呕吐可能是病毒性腹泻的一个显著特点。

原生动物病因导致的腹泻

导致腹泻的重要寄生虫包括蓝氏贾第鞭毛虫、隐孢子虫和溶组织内阿米巴。水源污染往往是疫情暴发的原因。蓝氏贾第鞭毛虫滋养体可附着在小肠上皮细胞上，不用侵入而损害黏膜刷状缘，摄入少量病原体可导致发病。隐孢子虫、等孢子球虫和环孢子虫偶尔会引起免疫力低下患者出现自限性腹泻，但可能会导致晚期获得性免疫缺陷综合征（AIDS）患者出现严重疾病。溶组织内阿米巴会引起的疾病可从轻度腹泻到暴发性阿米巴结肠炎和肠外阿米巴脓肿的综合征。

旅行者腹泻

10%～40% 来自工业化国家的旅行者在前往热带和亚热带发展中国家旅游后患上腹泻。约 85% 的患者可有确定的致病菌，其中 90% 的致病菌为细菌，最常见的病原体是 ETEC 或 EAEC，较少见的细菌病原体包括 EIEC、弥漫黏附性大肠埃希菌、志贺菌、沙门菌、弯曲杆菌、气单胞菌、霍乱弧菌、非霍乱弧菌和邻单胞菌。病毒性病因包括轮状病毒和诺如病毒，原生动物病原很少见。前往高风险地区的旅行者应注意洗手，避免食用未煮熟的食物，并饮用瓶装水。旅行者腹泻患者应在未进行粪便检查的情况下经验性使用抗生素进行治疗。

临床表现

流行病学和临床特点对于确定潜在病原体和指导治疗非常重要（表 11.1）。初步评估应考虑疾病的严重程度、脱水表现，以及肠道炎症的表现，如发热、腹痛、便血（痢疾）或里急后重感。病史中重要的流行病学线索包括年龄、旅行经历、进食未煮熟或生的食

intestinal inflammation. The examination should determine the severity of dehydration and need for rehydration as well as the likely cause. Signs of dehydration or hypovolemia include lax skin turgor and tenting, dry mucus membranes, decreased urination, tachycardia, and hypotension.

DIAGNOSIS AND DIFFERENTIAL DIAGNOSIS

The approach to diagnosis and management of infectious diarrhea is shown in Fig. 11.1. Most cases of diarrheal illnesses are self-limiting with almost half resolving within 1 day. Therefore, microbiologic investigation is usually not necessary for patients who are seen within 24 hours of the onset of illness unless certain conditions are present.

The indications for stool culture include severe diarrhea (six or more stools per day), diarrhea lasting longer than 1 week, fever, dysentery, hospitalization, inflammatory diarrhea, and multiple cases in a suspected outbreak. Routine stool culture will identify *Shigella*, *Salmonella*, *Campylobacter*, and *Aeromonas*. Polymerase chain reaction (PCR)–based diagnostic tests are now available and include a multiplex approach that allows several bacterial, viral, and parasitic enteropathogens to be detected in a single test simultaneously. The Luminex xTAG Gastrointestinal Pathogens Panel tests for 14 viruses, bacteria, and parasites and the FilmArray Gastrointestinal panel (Biofire Diagnostics) tests for 22 viruses, bacteria, and parasites. These methods are faster and have higher sensitivity than culture-based methods but they do not distinguish pathogenic and nonpathogenic organisms. If the patient has bloody diarrhea or HUS, stool culture for *E. coli* O157:H7 and tests for Shiga-like toxin (or the genes that encode them) should be performed. If there is a history of recent antibiotic use, hospitalization, or age greater than 65 years with coexisting conditions, immunosuppression, or neutropenia, stool samples should be tested for *C. difficile* toxin. Available tests for *C. difficile* toxin include enzyme immunoassay (EIA), nucleic acid amplification test (NAAT) and glutamate dehydrogenase (GDH plus toxin) test. No single test is suitable as a stand-alone test and often a multistep algorithm testing is used. Consider protozoa, and check stools for ova and parasites (e.g., trophozoites) and/or for *Giardia* antigen test if diarrhea duration is greater than 7 days. If a patient has AIDS, stools should be checked for *Cryptosporidium*, *Microsporidium*, and *Mycobacterium avium* complex.

TREATMENT

Initial therapy should include fluid and electrolyte repletion with or without antimicrobial therapy. Oral rehydration is often adequate unless the patient is comatose or severely dehydrated. Nutritional support with continued feeding improves outcomes in children.

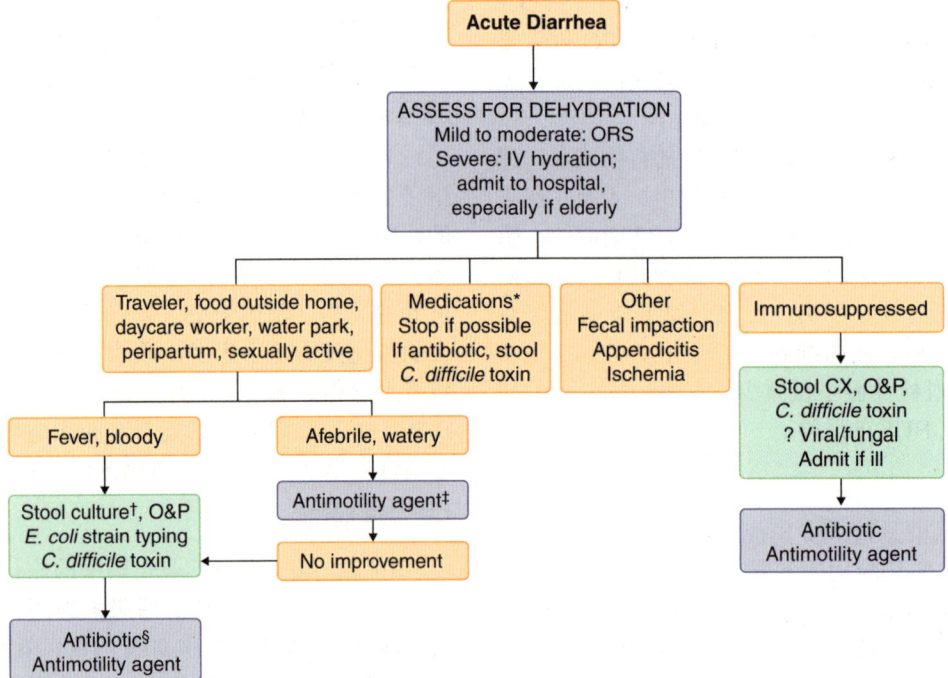

Fig. 11.1 Approach to the diagnosis and management of acute infectious diarrhea. *More than 700 medications cause diarrhea, including furosemide, caffeine, protease inhibitors, thyroid preparations, metformin, mycophenolate mofetil, sirolimus, cholinergic drugs, colchicine, theophylline, selective serotonin reuptake inhibitors, proton pump inhibitors, histamine-2 blockers, 5-ASA derivatives, angiotensin-converting enzyme inhibitors, bisacodyl, senna, aloe, anthraquinones, and magnesium- or phosphorus-containing medications. †Specifically request culture for *Yersinia*, *Plesiomonas*, enterohemorrhagic *Escherichia coli* serotype O157:H7, and *Aeromonas* if suspected. ‡If high suspicion for *Clostridioides difficile* or invasive bacterial infection, wait for stool culture and toxin studies before starting. Racecadotril has antisecretory effects without paralyzing intestinal motility and can be used if available. §Not recommended for patients with bloody diarrhea due to *E. coli* O157:H7. *CX*, Culture; *IV therapy*, intravenous rehydration; *O&P*, ova and parasites; *ORS*, oral rehydration solution. (From Goldman L, Schaefer AI: *Goldman-Cecil Medicine*, 25th ed. Philadelphia, Elsevier, 2016, Fig. 140-1.)

物和肉、抗生素的使用、性行为、参加日托以及涉及其他有类似暴露患者的疫情（表11.1）。发热（体温38.5℃或101.3℉或更高）与引起肠道炎症的侵入性病原体有关。检查应确定脱水的严重程度、补液的必要性以及可能的病因。脱水或血容量不足的体征包括皮肤张力松弛、黏膜干燥、排尿减少、心动过速和低血压。

诊断及鉴别诊断

感染性腹泻的诊断和处理方法如图11.1所示。大多数腹泻都是自限性的，近一半的患者可在1天内痊愈。因此，对于发病后24 h内就诊的患者，除非存在某些特殊情况，否则通常无须进行微生物学检查。

行粪便培养的指征包括严重腹泻（每天6次或更多）、腹泻持续时间超过1周、发热、痢疾、住院、炎症性腹泻以及疑似疫情中有多个病例的情况。常规粪便培养可确定志贺菌、沙门菌、弯曲杆菌和气单胞菌。基于聚合酶链反应（PCR）的诊断检测现已上市，可在一次检测中同时测出多种细菌、病毒和肠致病性寄生虫。Luminex xTAG胃肠道病原体检测试剂盒可检测14种病毒、细菌和寄生虫，FilmArray 胃肠道检测试剂盒（Biofire Diagnostics）可检测22种病毒、细菌和寄生虫。这些方法比培养法更快、敏感性更高，但不能区分病原体是致病还是非致病。如果患者出现血性腹泻或HUS，则应进行大肠埃希菌O157∶H7粪便培养和志贺样毒素（或其编码基因）检测。如果近期有抗生素使用史、住院史，或年龄超过65岁有基础疾病、免疫抑制或中性粒细胞减少症，则应对粪便样本进行艰难梭菌毒素检测。现有的艰难梭菌毒素检测方法包括酶免疫分析（EIA）、核酸扩增试验（NAAT）和谷氨酸脱氢酶（GDH 加毒素）检测。没有任何一种检测适合作为独立的检测，通常需要采用多流程检测。如果腹泻持续时间超过7天，应考虑原虫，并需要检查粪便中的虫卵和寄生虫（如滋养体）和（或）贾第鞭毛虫抗原检测。如果患者患有AIDS，则应检查粪便中是否含有隐孢子虫、小孢子虫和鸟分枝杆菌复合群。

治疗

初始治疗应包括补充液体和电解质，同时或不同时进行抗菌治疗。除非患者昏迷或严重脱水，通常口服补液即可。持续喂养营养支持可改善儿童的预后。

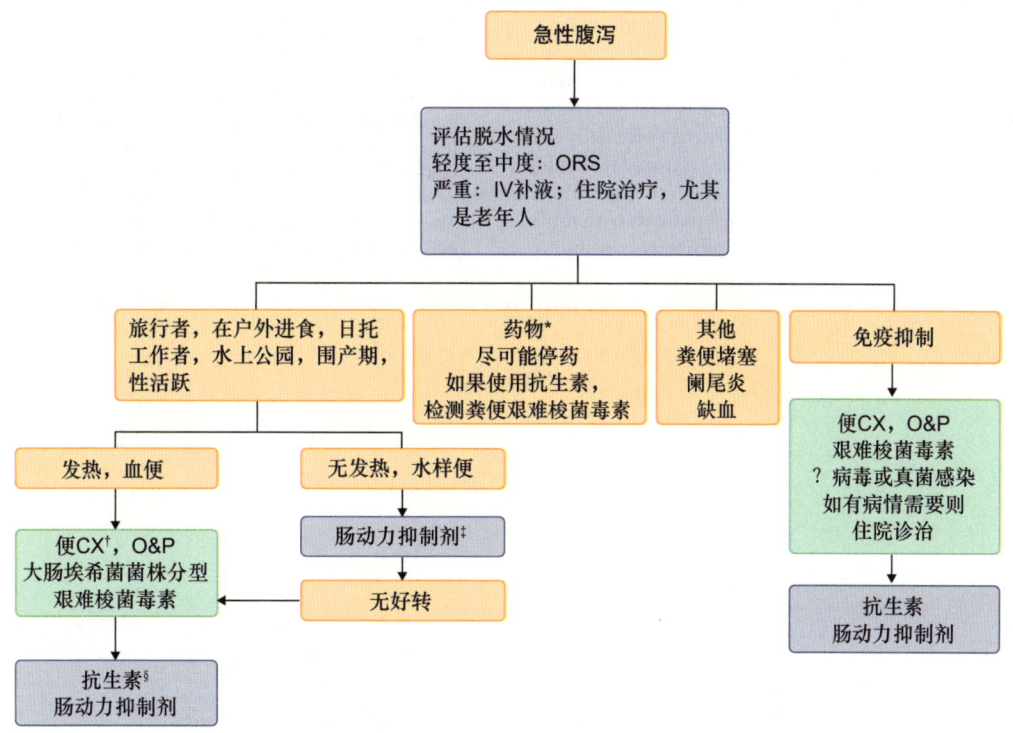

图11.1 急性感染性腹泻的诊断和处理方法。* 超过700种药物会导致腹泻，包括呋塞米、咖啡因、蛋白酶抑制剂、甲状腺制剂、二甲双胍、霉酚酸酯、西罗莫司、胆碱能药物、秋水仙碱、茶碱、选择性血清素再吸收抑制剂、质子泵抑制剂、组胺-2阻滞剂、5-ASA 衍生物、血管紧张素转换酶抑制剂、比沙可啶、番泻叶、芦荟、蒽醌类药物以及含镁或磷的药物。† 如果怀疑有耶尔森菌、邻单胞菌、肠出血性大肠埃希菌血清型 O157∶H7 和气单胞菌，应特别要求进行培养。‡ 如果高度怀疑有艰难梭菌或侵袭性细菌感染，应等待粪便培养和毒素检测后再开始用药。脑啡肽酶抑制剂具有抗分泌作用，但不会麻痹肠道蠕动，如有条件可使用。§ 不推荐用于大肠埃希菌 O157∶H7 引起的血性腹泻患者。CX，培养；IV，静脉注射；O&P，虫卵和寄生虫；ORS，口服补液盐（引自 Goldman L, Schaefer AI：Goldman-Cecil Medicine, 25th ed. Philadelphia, Elsevier, 2016, Fig. 140-1.）

Oral Fluid Therapy

In most patients with diarrhea, fluid repletion can be achieved with oral rehydration therapy using isotonic fluids containing glucose and electrolytes. An effective solution can be prepared by the addition of 2 tablespoons of sugar, one fourth of a teaspoon of salt (NaCl), and one-fourth of a teaspoon of baking soda ($NaHCO_3$) to 1 L of boiled drinking water. In the United States, fluids such as Pedialyte or Rehydrolyte solutions are recommended. Fluid should be administered in large quantities until there is clinical evidence that fluid balance is restored and then as maintenance therapy. Oral rehydration therapy can be life-saving for patients in developing countries with severe diarrhea.

Intravenous Fluid Therapy

Massive fluid loss due to diarrhea should be rapidly replaced by the administration of intravenous fluids. Lactated Ringer's solution is the fluid of choice because the composition is similar to electrolyte loss during diarrhea. The rate of fluid administration and maintenance should be guided by clinical signs including vital signs, appearance of the mucosa, neck veins, and skin turgor.

Antimicrobial Therapy

Most cases of infectious diarrhea do not require antimicrobial therapy. However, antibiotics may decrease the volume of diarrhea (e.g., in cholera) or the duration and severity of the illness. Antibiotics are effective in the treatment of shigellosis, traveler's diarrhea, and *Campylobacter* infection. In uncomplicated salmonellosis, antibiotics may prolong the shedding of *Salmonella*. The choice and dose of antimicrobials for specific pathogens are described in Table 11.2. For traveler's diarrhea in adults, empiric therapy with azithromycin 500 mg daily, or ciprofloxacin 500 mg twice a day, or trimethoprim-sulfamethoxazole (TMP-SMZ) 160/800 mg twice a day, for 3 days is adequate. For antibiotic-associated *C. difficile* colitis, broad-spectrum antibiotics should be discontinued, if possible. Preferred therapy for an initial episode of CDI is oral vancomycin 125 mg four times a day or fidaxomicin 200 mg twice daily for 10 days. If those antibiotics are not available, metronidazole 500 mg three times daily for 10 days is an alternative therapy. Fecal microbiota transplantation may be indicated for patients with multiple recurrences of CDI who have failed appropriate antibiotic treatments. Antibiotics must be avoided in patients with STEC O157 or other STEC that produce Shiga toxin.

Symptomatic Therapy

Antidiarrheal agents such as loperamide and bismuth subsalicylate can be used in some instances for symptomatic relief. Loperamide inhibits intestinal peristalsis and has some antisecretory properties. When used with or without antibiotics in cases of traveler's diarrhea, it may reduce the duration of diarrhea by about 1 day. Antimotility agents should be avoided in patients with bloody or suspected inflammatory diarrhea. The use of these agents has been implicated in prolonging the duration of fever in shigellosis, development of toxic megacolon in CDI, and development of HUS in children with STEC infection.

PROGNOSIS

The prognosis is generally good but is variable depending on the etiology and the severity of illness. Most patients recover completely within 3 to 5 days. However, serious complications, including death, can be seen in individuals who become severely dehydrated, infants, elderly patients, and those with underlying medical conditions or immunosuppression. Untreated severe dehydration may lead to shock, renal failure, and death. Postinfectious reactive polyarthritis can complicate cases due to *Yersinia*, *Campylobacter*, and *Shigella*, and Guillain-Barré syndrome may occur after diarrhea caused by *Campylobacter*.

SUGGESTED READINGS

DuPont HL: Acute infectious diarrhea in immunocompetent adults, N Engl J Med 370:1532–1540, 2014.

DuPont HL: Persistent diarrhea: a clinical review, J Am Med Assoc 315:2712–2723, 2016.

McDonald LC, Gerding DN, Johnson S, et al: Clinical practice guidelines for clostridium difficile infection in adults and children: 2017 update by Infectious Diseases Society of America (IDSA) and Society for Healthcare Epidemiology of America (SHEA). Clin Infect Dis 66:987-994.

Shane AL, Mody RK, Crump JA, et al: 2017 infectious Diseases Society of America clinical practice guidelines for diagnosis and management of infectious diarrhea, Clin Infect Dis 65:e45–e79, 2017.

口服液体疗法

对于大多数腹泻患者来说，可以使用含有葡萄糖和电解质的等渗液体进行口服补液治疗。在 1 L 煮沸的饮用水中加入 2 汤匙糖、1/4 茶匙盐（NaCl）和 1/4 茶匙小苏打（$NaHCO_3$）即可配制出有效的补充液。在美国，建议使用电解质水或 Rehydrolyte 溶液等液体。应大量补液直至有临床证据表明体液平衡得到恢复，然后继续维持治疗。口服补液疗法可挽救发展中国家严重腹泻患者的生命。

静脉输液治疗

腹泻导致的大量体液流失应通过静脉输液迅速补充。乳酸林格液是首选液体，因为其成分与腹泻时流失的电解质相似。输液和维持输液的速度应根据临床体征来确定，包括生命体征、黏膜外观、颈部静脉和皮肤张力的情况。

抗菌治疗

大多数感染性腹泻不需要抗菌治疗。不过，抗生素可减少腹泻量（如霍乱）或缩短病程并减轻病情。抗生素对治疗志贺菌病、旅行者腹泻和弯曲杆菌感染有效。在非复杂的沙门菌病中，抗生素可能会延长沙门菌的转阴时间。表 11.2 列出了针对特定病原体的抗菌药物的选择和剂量。对于成人旅行者腹泻，经验性疗法包括：阿奇霉素每天 500 mg 或环丙沙星 500 mg 每日 2 次或甲氧苄啶-磺胺甲噁唑（TMP-SMZ）160/800 mg 每日 2 次，连续 3 天即可。对于抗生素相关的艰难梭菌结肠炎，应尽可能停用广谱抗生素。CDI 初发患者的首选疗法是口服万古霉素 125 mg 每日 4 次，或非达霉素 200 mg 每日 2 次，连续 10 天。如果没有这些抗生素，也可以选择甲硝唑 500 mg 每日 3 次，持续 10 天。肠道菌群移植可能适用于多次复发以及经适当抗生素治疗无效的 CDI 患者。对于 STEC O157 或其他产生志贺毒素的 STEC 患者，应避免使用抗生素。

对症治疗

在某些情况下，可使用洛哌丁胺和次水杨酸铋等止泻剂来缓解症状。洛哌丁胺可抑制肠道蠕动，并具有一定的止泻作用。在旅行者腹泻的患者中，联用或不联用抗生素，可将腹泻持续时间缩短 1 天左右。血性腹泻或疑似炎症性腹泻患者应避免使用肠动力抑制剂。使用这些药物可能会延长志贺菌病的发热时间、导致 CDI 中毒性巨结肠症的发生以及 STEC 感染的儿童发生 HUS。

预后

预后一般良好，但因病因和病情严重程度而异。大多数患者可在 3～5 天内完全康复。然而，严重脱水者、婴儿、老年患者以及患有基础疾病或使用免疫抑制的患者可能会出现严重并发症以及死亡。未经治疗的严重脱水可能会导致休克、肾衰竭和死亡。耶尔森菌、弯曲杆菌和志贺菌感染的患者可并发感染后反应性多关节炎，弯曲杆菌感染引起腹泻后可出现吉兰-巴雷综合征。

推荐阅读

DuPont HL: Acute infectious diarrhea in immunocompetent adults, N Engl J Med 370:1532–1540, 2014.

DuPont HL: Persistent diarrhea: a clinical review, J Am Med Assoc 315:2712–2723, 2016.

McDonald LC, Gerding DN, Johnson S, et al: Clinical practice guidelines for clostridium difficile infection in adults and children: 2017 update by Infectious Diseases Society of America (IDSA) and Society for Healthcare Epidemiology of America (SHEA). Clin Infect Dis 66:987-994.

Shane AL, Mody RK, Crump JA, et al: 2017 infectious Diseases Society of America clinical practice guidelines for diagnosis and management of infectious diarrhea, Clin Infect Dis 65:e45–e79, 2017.

Infections Involving Bone and Joints

Jerome Larkin

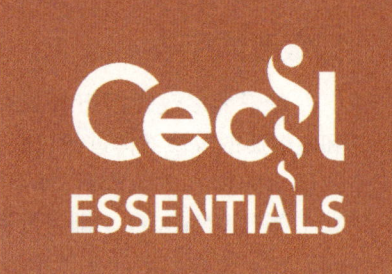

DEFINITION

Osteomyelitis refers to infection of any component of the bony skeleton, whereas *septic arthritis* refers to that of native or prosthetic joints. Tendons, ligaments, and bursae can also become infected, especially if they involve prosthetic or bio-grafted material. Osteomyelitis and septic arthritis can occur by seeding during bacteremia, due to extension from a contiguous focus of infection in an adjacent tissue or structure, as a consequence of vascular insufficiency or as a complication of trauma. In the case of hematogenous infection, the bacteremia itself may be relatively transient and of little clinical consequence. Hematogenous osteomyelitis is common in children but accounts for only 20% of osteomyelitis in adults. The vertebrae and pelvis are the most commonly involved sites of hematogenous osteomyelitis in adults. Peripheral vascular disease leading to tissue hypoxia and related to diabetes, hypertension, hyperlipidemia, and smoking is the biggest risk factor for the development of osteomyelitis in adults older than 50. There is often preceding soft tissue infection or destruction as a result of vascular insufficiency and neuropathy. It is most common in the lower extremities, particularly in the feet, and often occurs in diabetics. Trauma, especially when it involves open fracture with its attendant disruption of the bony architecture and vascular supply, is a second major risk factor for the development of osteomyelitis and septic arthritis. This is particularly true when an open fracture, as may be experienced in a fall or motor vehicle accident, is heavily contaminated with soil or other environmental materials. Such fractures often require internal fixation (i.e., the placement of rods, screws, and other metal devices to stabilize the bone). The presence of such internal fixation provides a nidus for bacteria and other microorganisms including fungi to elude the immune system and incubate. Chronic osteomyelitis is a possible complication of such injuries and is often a result of multiple or unusual organisms. It may occur despite aggressive débridement and prophylactic antibiotic treatment at the time of injury and can arise months or even years afterwards. Individuals who experience prolonged periods of immobility such as those suffering from paraplegia are also at risk for osteomyelitis. Infection typically involves the pelvis, sacrum, and lower spine corresponding to areas of unrelieved pressure as a result of the immobility.

Osteomyelitis may be conceptualized as acute or chronic. The former is typically hematogenous, associated with signs of inflammation in the overlying soft tissue and with an onset over the course of days to a week. Radiographs are usually normal at presentation. Chronic osteomyelitis is more indolent with onset over the course of months, is more likely to exhibit bony destruction on plain radiograph at the time of presentation, and is often associated with a draining sinus tract. Sequestra (areas of dead bone) and involucra (new bone formed around sequestra) may also be seen. Whereas acute osteomyelitis may require a 6-week course of antibiotics alone to effect cure, chronic osteomyelitis more typically requires surgical intervention and a prolonged (3 or more months) course of antibiotic therapy.

PATHOPHYSIOLOGY

Aspects of the vascular supply of the bone as well as properties of the most common pathogen, *Staphylococcus aureus*, may combine to lead to infection. Although bone is generally resistant to infection, the vasculature of the metaphysis contains capillary loops composed of a single layer of discontinuous endothelial cells, which may allow bacteria to enter the extracellular matrix. These capillary beds lack functionally active phagocytes. *S. aureus* can elaborate proteins expressed on its surface that promote adherence to tissues of the extracellular matrix. When engulfed by osteoblasts, *S. aureus* can survive for prolonged periods of time in an almost spore-like state leading to potential recurrences of infection. Finally, many bacteria can elaborate biofilms that allow them to elude clearance by the immune system. Prosthetic material such as in joint replacements and other grafts can serve as a platform for the formation of such biofilms.

In the case of septic arthritis there is usually some underlying abnormality in the joint, but this abnormality may be as mundane as osteoarthritis. It is hypothesized that relatively trivial injury, which may in fact go unnoticed or unremembered by the patient, leads to minor bleeding into the joint, which in turn provides a hospitable environment for bacteria to incubate.

CLINICAL PRESENTATION AND DIAGNOSIS

Patients with osteomyelitis will often present with pain at the site of infection. The overlying soft tissue may have signs of inflammation or tissue destruction, the latter often seen in diabetics with soft tissue ulceration. Historically, the diagnosis of osteomyelitis relied on the presence of lucency on plain radiograph of the affected area. Diagnosis could be confirmed histologically by bone biopsy with culture to identify the pathogenic organism. Currently, diagnosis is typically made by MRI with gadolinium, which demonstrates marrow edema with or without bony destruction. Alternatively, diagnosis may be made by three-phase bone scan or CT. These may be especially helpful in patients with renal insufficiency who cannot undergo gadolinium-enhanced studies due to the risk of nephrogenic systemic fibrosis. An elevated C-reactive protein (CRP) or erythrocyte sedimentation rate (ESR) supports the diagnosis. Microbiologic diagnosis is made either by positive blood cultures or bone biopsy and culture. Culture of cutaneous ulcers is typically not helpful because results of such studies usually demonstrate multiple colonizing organisms and do not correlate with organisms isolated on bone culture. An exception is the isolation of *S. aureus* or *Salmonella* from a draining fistula or on occasion *Pseudomonas* from an ulcer. In the former case, the bacterium can then

累及骨和关节的感染

鲁炳怀 杨雯婷 译 黄磊 宁永忠 审校 曹彬 通审

定义

骨髓炎是指骨骼各部分的感染，而化脓性关节炎是指天然关节或人工关节的感染。感染也可累及肌腱、韧带和滑囊，特别是在假体或生物移植材料部位。骨髓炎和化脓性关节炎可以是菌血症播散、邻近组织或结构感染病灶蔓延、血管功能不全或创伤后并发症。血源感染时，因菌血症相对短暂，其本身对临床结局影响较小。血源性骨髓炎在儿童中很常见，但在成人骨髓炎中仅占20%。成人血源性骨髓炎最常累及的部位是椎骨和骨盆。外周血管疾病可导致组织缺氧，与糖尿病、高血压、高脂血症和吸烟有关，是50岁以上成年人发生骨髓炎的最重要的危险因素。由于血管功能不全和神经病变引起的骨髓炎，通常会先出现软组织感染或破坏。最常见于下肢，尤其是足部，常见于糖尿病患者。创伤，尤其是导致骨结构破坏和血供受损的开放性骨折，是引起骨髓炎和化脓性关节炎的第二大危险因素。坠落或交通事故引起的开放性骨折，并受到土壤或环境中其他物质的严重污染时更易发生。这类骨折通常需要内固定（即放置棒状内置物、螺钉和其他金属装置以稳定骨骼）。内固定的存在为细菌和包括真菌在内的其他微生物提供了逃避免疫系统清除和繁殖的微环境。慢性骨髓炎可能是这种损伤的并发症，通常由多种微生物或少见微生物引起。即使受伤时进行了积极的清创术和预防性抗生素治疗，仍可能在数月甚至数年后出现慢性骨髓炎。长时间不能活动的人，如截瘫患者，也有患骨髓炎的风险。感染好发于因不活动而压力无法缓解的部位，如骨盆、骶骨和下脊柱。

骨髓炎可分为急性和慢性。前者通常是血源性的，伴有上覆软组织的炎症症状，病程数天至一周。就诊时X线片通常表现正常。慢性骨髓炎发病较为迟缓，可数月内起病，就诊时X线片常表现为骨破坏，多伴有窦道。也可见死骨（死骨区域）和包壳（在死骨周围形成的新骨）。急性骨髓炎可能需要6周抗生素疗程治愈，而慢性骨髓炎则需要手术干预和更长疗程的抗生素治疗（3个月或更长时间）。

病理生理学

骨的血供特点和骨感染中最常见的病原体金黄色葡萄球菌的特性，相互促进而导致骨感染。虽然骨通常具有抵御感染的能力，但干骺端的血管系统含有由单层不连续的内皮细胞组成的毛细血管祥，使细菌可进入细胞外基质。这些毛细血管床缺乏功能活跃的吞噬细胞。金黄色葡萄球菌可以表达促进其在细胞外基质黏附的蛋白。金黄色葡萄球菌被成骨细胞吞噬，以"类孢子"的状态长期存活，导致潜在感染的复发。许多细菌也可以生成生物膜，逃避免疫系统的清除。假体材料，如人工关节和其他植入物，可以作为生物膜形成的附着物。

化脓性关节炎中，关节常存在某些潜在的异常情况，但这种异常可能像骨关节炎中一样常见。据推测，患者忽视或忘记的相对轻微的损伤，导致的关节微出血，可为细菌繁殖提供适宜环境。

临床表现和诊断

骨髓炎患者通常表现为感染部位疼痛。上覆软组织可能有炎症或组织破坏的症状，后者常见于有软组织溃疡的糖尿病患者。既往的骨髓炎诊断，依赖于受累部位的X线片是否有透亮区。通过骨活检结合培养鉴定病原微生物的组织学方法确诊。目前，骨髓炎诊断通常有赖于注射钆剂的增强MRI检查，表现为骨髓水肿伴或不伴骨破坏。其他的方法包括三相骨扫描或CT，这些方法更适用于肾功能不全的患者，这类患者存在肾源性系统性纤维化的风险，不能进行钆剂增强MRI检查。C反应蛋白（CRP）或红细胞沉降率（ESR）升高也有助于诊断。微生物学诊断依赖血培养或骨活检与培养的阳性结果。皮肤溃疡的培养价值有限，因为相关研究显示该培养所得到的通常是多种定植微生物，与骨培养中分离的微生物无关。然而，例外的情况是从引流瘘管中分离出金黄色葡萄球菌或沙门菌，或偶

be presumed to be the pathogen; in the latter, a decision would then need to be made to include coverage for this organism in an empiric antibiotic regimen. If cultures of bone obtained by noninvasive techniques under radiographic guidance are negative, either the procedure should be repeated or an open biopsy with culture performed.

Septic arthritis of native joints typically will present with the cardinal features of inflammation (i.e., erythema, swelling, warmth, and pain) when involving joints of the extremities. Fever may often be present and septic arthritis is more likely to present with an associated bacteremia. Septic arthritis of the spine, pelvis, and hip may require imaging, usually MRI, because these may be difficult to assess by examination alone. Persistent back, pelvic or hip pain that is otherwise unexplained should prompt radiographic evaluation even in the absence of fever. Diagnosis ultimately relies on joint aspiration with débridement. Such procedures should occur prior to the administration of antibiotics. Fluid should be sent for cell count with differential, crystal analysis, Gram stain, anaerobic culture, and fungal and acid-fast stains and cultures. Positive stains and/or cultures are taken as evidence of infection in most cases in which an appropriate clinical syndrome is also present. White blood cell (WBC) counts higher than 50,000 cells/mL are suggestive of infection. In cases that are difficult to diagnose or instances where antibiotics have been given prior to aspiration, it may be appropriate to have cultures held for up to 14 days. Specialized culture techniques for fastidious organisms such as anaerobes and nutritionally deficient streptococci may be required. Ultimately, tagged WBC scans may help to clarify the presence or absence of septic arthritis in difficult cases. Evolving molecular technologies such as PCR, especially microarray assays that detect multiple pathogens, and 16-S ribosomal sequencing may offer alternative and more rapid and precise diagnosis in the future.

Prosthetic joint infections (PJI) are defined by their timing following implantation: acute (less than 3 months), delayed (3 to 12 months) or late (12 months). Early PJI presents similarly to native joint infections. Delayed and late infections are more indolent, presenting with pain, decreased function, and evidence of loosening of the prosthesis on plain films. More overt signs of inflammation or systemic infection may be subtle or absent altogether. Diagnosis relies on the presence of either a draining sinus tract that communicates with the prosthesis or two or more periprosthetic cultures harboring the same organism. Minor criteria have been proposed with three or more of the following used to diagnose PJI: elevated CRP or ESR, synovial fluid WBC greater than 3000, elevated synovial polymorphonuclear cells (PMNs), a single positive culture or greater than five PMNs per high-power field on examination of periprosthetic tissue. A point scoring system as advanced by Parvizi and colleagues may increase the sensitivity of the use of minor criteria or be used as a tool in more diagnostically obscure cases.

Most cases of osteomyelitis and septic arthritis are due to *Staphylococcus*, *Streptococcus*, and aerobic gram-negative bacilli, although virtually any pathogenic microorganism can cause such infections in the appropriate circumstance. Infecting staphylococci include both *S. aureus* and coagulase-negative staphylococci. Coagulase-negative staphylococci are often implicated in prosthetic joint infections or infections associated with orthopedic hardware. *Streptococcus* spp causing bone and joint infections include groups A, B, C, G and F as well as *Abiotrophia* and *Gemella* (formerly termed nutritionally deficient streptococci). Gram-negative organisms account for as much as 30% of hematogenous infections. Gram-negative infections are seen more commonly in the elderly as a result of urinary tract infections with associated bacteremia. Isolated species include *Escherichia coli*, *Haemophilus influenza*, and *H. parainfluenza*. Infections with *Serratia marcescens* and *Pseudomonas* are associated with exposure to water and are usually nosocomial or related to intravenous drug use. Fungi such as *Candida*, *Aspergillus*, and *Zygomycetes* may cause bone and joint infections, particularly in immune-compromised patients, diabetics or those who have suffered trauma. *Nocardia* and other acid-fast organisms may be seen following trauma or in association with prosthetic joints and may require several attempts at débridement before being isolated. *Cutibacterium acnes* is often isolated from shoulder infections, especially those involving prosthetic joints. The variety of potential pathogens underscores the need to obtain appropriate specimens for culture prior to the administration of antibiotics.

Infection with *Borrelia burgdorferi*, the causative agent of Lyme disease, can lead to a multifocal or monoarticular septic arthritis. Fluid analysis is consistent with bacterial septic arthritis but is negative for typical organisms on culture. Associated findings of erythema migrans, diffuse myalgias and arthralgias, cranial nerve palsies, fever, and aseptic meningitis may also be present. Polymerase chain reaction of joint fluid has a reported sensitivity of between 30% and 75%. Diagnosis relies on serology and associated findings in patients who reside in endemic areas. Later-stage disease may present with a less inflammatory-appearing effusion, often without any other symptoms. Treatment is with either doxycycline or ceftriaxone depending on the stage of disease.

Neisseria gonorrhea may cause a solitary or multifocal septic arthritis. It is usually seen in sexually active younger adults. Culture of the joint fluid may be negative but testing of specimens from the pharynx, urethra or rectum are usually positive by nucleic acid amplification. The treatment of choice is ceftriaxone.

DIFFERENTIAL DIAGNOSIS

The differential diagnosis of both osteomyelitis and septic arthritis includes other noninfectious inflammatory disorders such as gout, pseudogout, rheumatoid arthritis, inflammatory bowel disease, and other inflammatory and autoimmune disorders. Occasionally, neoplasms such as sarcomas or metastatic lesions may present similarly to osteomyelitis. Several viruses such as rubella, parvovirus B19, Chikungunya and hepatitis B can cause arthritis. Chronic recurrent multifocal osteomyelitis is a noninfectious inflammatory lesion of bone thought to be autoimmune in nature and characterized by findings on MRI similar to osteomyelitis. It is culture-negative and unresponsive to antibiotics. It is a diagnosis of exclusion often made only after several attempts at diagnosing and treating presumed bacterial osteomyelitis. Although typically seen in children, with peak incidence between 7 and 12 years of age, it can also occur in adults.

TREATMENT

Treatment of osteomyelitis involves débridement of appropriate infected and/or necrotic tissue as well as the administration of antibiotics. It is critically important to remove all necrotic or devitalized tissue, which may serve as a nidus of chronic or recurrent infection if not removed. In this regard, it is often necessary to remove any fixating hardware, plastic devices, bone grafts or other donor tissue if infection has been present for greater than one month or is recurrent. Cadaveric donor tissue infections often are caused by atypical organisms such as *Clostridioides* spp. Historically, sequestra developed in the site of chronically infected bone. These are produced by the action of the immune system and histologically are characterized by granulomatous tissue that serves to isolate the infection. While effective in containing infection, they also represented a risk for recurrence as well as an area of bone weakening. When present, they should be surgically excised. Infection that occurs in the immediate postoperative period (i.e., within 1 month after placement of hardware and grafts)

尔从溃疡中分离出假单胞菌。前者可推定细菌为病原体；后者则需要决策应用经验性抗生素治疗覆盖该菌。如果在放射学指导下通过无创技术获得的骨组织培养为阴性，则应重复该过程或进行开放活检并进行培养。

累及四肢关节时，天然关节的化脓性关节炎通常会表现为典型炎症特征（即红、肿、热、痛）。通常可出现发热。化脓性关节炎更可能伴有相关的菌血症。由于很难单独通过体格检查进行评估，脊柱、骨盆和髋关节的化脓性关节炎需要影像学检查，多采用MRI。对于无法解释的持续性背部、骨盆或髋关节疼痛，即使没有发热，也应及时进行影像学检查。最终的诊断依赖于关节穿刺联合清创。此类手术应在使用抗生素之前进行。穿刺液应该进行细胞计数与分类、晶体分析、革兰氏染色、厌氧培养、真菌染色与抗酸染色和培养。在大多数情况下，阳性染色和（或）培养结果联合相应的临床症状可作为感染的证据。白细胞（WBC）计数高于 50 000/ml 提示感染。在难以诊断的病例中，或在穿刺前使用过抗生素时，可以考虑延长培养到 14 天。对厌氧菌和营养缺乏性链球菌等苛养微生物需采用特殊的培养技术。在化脓性关节炎诊断困难的病例中，WBC 标记扫描是最终的诊断方法。随着分子技术的发展，如 PCR 和 16S rRNA 测序，特别是检测多种病原体的芯片检测，在未来可能提供可供选择的、更快速和精确的诊断。

假体关节感染（PJI）根据关节植入术后时间分为：急性 PJI（少于 3 个月），迟发性 PJI（3～12 个月）或慢性 PJI（12 个月）。早期 PJI 表现与天然关节感染相似。迟发性和慢性 PJI 更缓慢，表现为疼痛、功能减退，X 线片显示假体松动。更明显的炎症或全身性感染征象可能很轻微或缺如。诊断依赖于与假体相通的窦道或两个或更多假体周围培养物有相同的微生物。PJI 诊断的次要标准至少包括下述三个标准：CRP 或 ESR 升高，滑液 WBC 大于 3000（译者注：原文 3000 后无单位，*Harrison's Infectious Diseases* 提到"关节滑液中 WBC 为 25 000～250 000/μl，中性粒细胞 90%，是急性细菌性关节感染的特征"）；滑膜多形核细胞（PMNs）升高，单个阳性培养或假体周围组织显微镜检每个高倍视野大于 5 个 PMN。Parvizi 和同事提出的评分系统可能会增加使用上述标准的敏感性，可用于不明病例的诊断。

事实上，虽然任何病原微生物都可在适宜条件下引起骨髓炎和化脓性关节炎，但大多是由葡萄球菌、链球菌和需氧革兰氏阴性杆菌引起的。导致感染的葡萄球菌包括金黄色葡萄球菌和凝固酶阴性葡萄球菌。凝固酶阴性葡萄球菌常与假体关节感染或骨科器械相关的感染有关。引起骨、关节感染的链球菌包括 A、B、C、G 和 F 组，以及乏养菌属和孪生球菌属（以前称为营养缺陷链球菌）。革兰氏阴性菌占血流感染 30% 以上，常见于老年人，是尿路感染合并菌血症的结果。分离的菌种包括大肠埃希菌、流感嗜血杆菌和副流感嗜血杆菌。黏质沙雷菌和假单胞菌感染与水源暴露有关，多为院内感染，或静脉用药所致。念珠菌、曲霉菌和接合菌等真菌可引起骨和关节感染，特别是免疫功能低下的患者、糖尿病患者或创伤患者。诺卡菌和其他抗酸杆菌可见于创伤后或与假体关节感染，可能需要多次清创采样后才可分离。痤疮丙酸杆菌常从肩部感染中分离出来，特别是假体关节感染。潜在病原体的多样性凸显了使用抗生素之前获取适宜标本进行培养的必要性。

莱姆病由伯氏疏螺旋体感染引起，可导致多灶性或单关节化脓性关节炎。穿刺液分析与细菌性化脓性关节炎一致，但典型病原体的培养呈阴性。可伴有移行性红斑、弥漫性肌痛和关节痛、脑神经麻痹、发热和无菌性脑膜炎。关节液 PCR 检测的敏感性为 30%～75%。诊断赖于血清学结果以及患者是否居住于流行地区。疾病晚期炎性渗出常较少，往往不伴其他症状。根据疾病的分期，使用多西环素或头孢曲松治疗。

淋病奈瑟球菌可引起单发性或多灶性化脓性关节炎。通常见于性活跃的年轻人。关节液培养可能呈阴性，但咽、尿路或直肠标本经核酸扩增检测通常呈阳性。治疗选用头孢曲松。

鉴别诊断

骨髓炎和化脓性关节炎的鉴别诊断包括其他非感染性炎症性疾病，如痛风、假性痛风、类风湿关节炎、炎症性肠病和其他炎症性和自身免疫性疾病。有时肿瘤表现与骨髓炎相似，如肉瘤或转移灶。风疹、细小病毒 B19、基孔肯亚病毒和乙型肝炎等几种病毒也可引起关节炎。慢性复发性多灶性骨髓炎是一种非感染性骨炎性病变，被认为是自身免疫性疾病，MRI 检查的特征与骨髓炎相似。培养阴性，抗生素无效。该病是一种排除性诊断，通常在多次尝试诊断和治疗疑似细菌性骨髓炎后才会考虑。常见于儿童，发病高峰为 7～12 岁，亦可见于成人。

治疗

骨髓炎的治疗包括适当的感染和（或）坏死组织的清除，以及抗生素的使用。切除所有坏死组织或无活性物至关重要，如果不彻底清除，这些组织可能成为慢性或复发性感染的病灶。若感染已超过 1 个月或复发，通常要移除所有固定装置、塑料装置、骨移植物或其他供体组织。尸体供体组织感染通常是由产气荚膜梭菌属等非典型微生物所致。既往来看，慢性骨感染的病变部位会出现死骨。它是在免疫系统的作用下产生的，组织学上以肉芽肿组织为特征，起到隔离感染的作用。虽然能有效地控制感染，但也有复发的风险，也会导致骨质脆弱。出现此类情况时，应手术切除。术后即刻发生的感染（即放置固定物和植入物后 1 个月内）和只涉及软组织的感染，可以清创，即

and that appears to only involve the soft tissue may be treated with débridement and antibiotics alone with a reasonable chance of success. Occasionally, infected hardware must be left in place in order to stabilize the bone while a fracture is healing. In this instance, it may be necessary to continue antibiotic treatment until hardware removal can be accomplished. Infected spine hardware that must remain in place may require prolonged antibiotic treatment, at times indefinitely. The addition of rifampin for staphylococcal infections with retained hardware to which the infecting organism is susceptible improves overall cure rates.

Septic arthritis requires serial débridement of the joint until active purulence has resolved. This is indicated by decreasing cell count and sterilization of joint fluid cultures. Prosthetic joint infection typically requires removal of the infected prosthesis with placement of an antibiotic spacer for 4 to 6 weeks while antibiotics are administered. This is followed by placement of a new prosthesis once all signs and symptoms of infection have resolved. Selected infections with coagulase-negative staphylococci and *Streptococcus* infections may be treated with débridement, joint retention, and a 6-week or longer course of antibiotics. Consideration should then be given to chronic suppressive antibiotic therapy, assuming an appropriate agent is available.

Antibiotic treatment should be with agents active against the infecting organism if culture and susceptibility data are available. β-Lactams are the preferred agent in most cases. Therapy with quinolones for Enterobacteriaceae and in combination with rifampin for staphylococci may be considered. These drugs have the advantage of high oral bioavailability that approaches or equals tissue levels when given intravenously. Care should be taken regarding drug interactions with rifampin and the risk of *Clostridioides difficile* colitis and Achilles tendon rupture with quinolones. Recent literature also indicates a small increased risk of aortic aneurysm or dissection with this class of antibiotics. In the face of negative cultures, empiric therapy with an agent active against typical pathogens, including methicillin-resistant *S. aureus*, is reasonable. Vancomycin remains the standard agent for empiric therapy. Prior administration of antibiotics may lead to negative cultures even in cases of unequivocal infection. In this situation, empiric therapy should be based on the activity of the agents previously administered, as well as on potential pathogens based on exposure history. In all cases, the clinical response to infection should be monitored and should inform subsequent decision making regarding the need for additional débridement or changes in antibiotic therapy. Monitoring inflammatory markers such as CRP or ESR is helpful in determining the adequacy of response to treatment. If elevated at the start of treatment they should fall to normal or near normal by the time treatment is finished. Signs and symptoms of inflammation at the site of infection should have also resolved at the cessation of treatment.

There are few randomized, controlled trials comparing different durations of antimicrobial therapy. Acute osteomyelitis should be treated for 4 to 6 weeks. Continuing treatment in a patient who is improved but who has failed to resolve elevated inflammatory markers or local signs of inflammation is reasonable. Such patients should be closely monitored and evaluated for the need for additional débridement or other measures aimed at diagnosis and source control. Chronic osteomyelitis may require 12 or more weeks of therapy, and treatment is usually individualized based on the clinical situation. Patients on therapy should also be monitored weekly for toxicity to antibiotics. Assessment of renal and hepatic function, complete blood count, and drug levels are typically followed depending on the specific agent used. In the case of aminoglycosides, renal function and peak and trough levels should be followed twice weekly. Long-acting glycopeptides such as dalbavancin and oritavancin are promising alternatives to daily antibiotic dosing.

A recent open-label study of the treatment of osteomyelitis that included over 1000 randomized patients demonstrated a lack of inferiority of oral therapy when compared with intravenous therapy. Costs were reduced and patient satisfaction was higher in the orally treated group. The incidence of serious side effects and adverse reactions was similar between the two groups. Oral therapy was largely with quinolones. The study encompassed a heterogenous population so, although promising, application of the findings to particular patients should be done thoughtfully. Adjunctive therapies such as bone grafting, revascularization procedures, and the placement of muscle flaps to cover and protect exposed bone may be utilized in the appropriate clinical situation.

Native joint septic arthritis may be treated with a 4-week course of antibiotics; prosthetic joint infections are typically treated for 6 or more weeks. Monitoring for toxicity and response to treatment is similar to that for osteomyelitis.

PROGNOSIS

The prognosis for osteomyelitis and septic arthritis is excellent, assuming adequate diagnosis, débridement, and antimicrobial therapy. The most common complication is residual pain and/or decreased function of the affected bone or joint. These are relatively rare and relatively minor. An exception involves prosthetic joint infections, in which 25% to 50% of patients experience some loss of function as a result of the infection. Recurrence rates for chronic osteomyelitis, especially in diabetics, may be as high as 30%. In more complex cases such as open contaminated fractures or infected hardware that requires retention, complications include nonunion, prosthesis failure, and chronic osteomyelitis. Infections that cannot be controlled may lead to the need for amputation and its attendant loss of function and mobility. Occasionally, bone or joint infections can lead to dissemination to other joints or the bloodstream. Such cases usually involve infection with *S. aureus* and fortunately remain the exception.

SUGGESTED READINGS

American Academy of Orthopedic Surgeons: Diagnosis and prevention of periprosthetic joint infections clinical practice guidelines. March, 2019.

Lew DP, Waldvogel FA: Osteomyelitis, Lancet 364:369–379, 2004.

Li HK, Rombach I, Zambellas R, et al: Oral versus intravenous antibiotics for bone and joint infection, N Engl J Med 380:425, 2019.

Parvizi J, Tan TL, Goswami K, et al: The 2018 definition of periprosthetic hip and knee infection: an evidence-based and validated criteria, J Arthroplasty 33:1309, 2018.

Rappo U, Puttagunta S, Shevchenko V, et al: Dalbavancin for the treatment of osteomyelitis in adult patients: a randomized clinical trial of efficacy and safety, Open Forum Infect Dis 6:331, 2018.

Shuford JA, Steckelberg JM: Role of oral antimicrobial therapy in the management of osteomyelitis, Curr Opin Infect Dis 16:515–519, 2003.

Spielberg B, Lipsky BA: Systemic antibiotic therapy for chronic osteomyelitis in adults, Clin Infect Dis 54:393, 2012.

Stengel D, Bauwens K, Sehouli J, et al: Systematic review and meta-analysis of antibiotic therapy for bone and joint infections. Lancet Infect Dis 201 1: 175-188.

Tande AJ, Steckelberg JM, Osmon DR, Berbari EF: Osteomyelitis. In Bennett JE, Dolin R, Blaser MJ, editors: Principles and practice of infectious diseases, 9th ed, Philadelphia, 2020, Elsevier.

Tice AD, Hoaglund PA, Shoultz DA: Outcomes of osteomyelitis among patients treated with outpatient parenteral antimicrobial therapy, Am J Med 114:723–728, 2003.

Waldvogel FA, Medoff G, Swartz MN: Osteomyelitis: a review of clinical features, therapeutic consideration and unusual aspects, N Eng J Med 282:316–322, 1970.

Wunsch S, Krause R, Valentin T, et al: Multicenter clinical experience of real life dalbavancin use in gram-positive infection, Int J Infect Dis 81:210, 2019.

使单独使用抗菌药物也有成功的机会。有时，在骨折愈合期间，感染的固定物必须留在原处，以便在骨折愈合时稳定骨骼。在这种情况下，需继续进行抗菌药物治疗，直到可以完成移除固定物。而感染的脊柱固定物则必须留在原位，需长时间抗菌药物治疗，疗程不定。对于保留了感染固定物的葡萄球菌感染，加用利福平可提高总体治愈率。

化脓性关节炎需要多次关节清创，直到活动性化脓被控制。细胞计数减少和关节液培养物无微生物生长可提示感染得到控制。假体关节感染通常需要移除受感染的假体，并放置抗生素垫片4～6周，同时给予抗生素治疗。一旦所有的感染体征和症状消失，需要重新植入新的假体。对凝血酶阴性葡萄球菌和链球菌感染可采用清创、关节保留和6周或更长时间的抗生素治疗。如果有合适的药物可用，则应考虑慢性抑制性抗菌药物治疗。

如果有培养和药敏数据，抗菌药物应使用对感染微生物敏感药物。在大多数情况下，β-内酰胺类抗生素作为首选。喹诺酮类药物可用于治疗肠杆菌科细菌，喹诺酮药物联合利福平可用于治疗葡萄球菌。这两种药物具有口服生物利用度高的优点，接近或等于静脉给药时的组织水平。应注意药物与利福平间相互作用，以及喹诺酮类药物引起艰难梭菌性结肠炎和跟腱断裂的风险。最近的文献也表明，使用这类抗生素可小幅增加主动脉瘤或夹层的风险。若培养未见生长，经验性抗菌治疗可选用一种对典型病原体（包括耐甲氧西林金黄色葡萄球菌）有活性的药物。万古霉素仍然是经验性治疗的标准药物。即使在明确感染的情况下，前期使用抗生素也可能导致培养阴性。此种情况下，经验性治疗的选择应基于前期所用药物的活性，以及基于暴露史的潜在病原体。所有病例均应监测对抗感染的临床反应，并为后续决策提供信息，以确定是否需要进行额外的清创或更改抗生素治疗。监测CRP或ESR等炎症标志物有助于确定对治疗的反应是否充分。如果在治疗开始时升高，到治疗结束时应降至正常或接近正常。感染部位的炎症体征和症状也应在治疗停止时消失。

目前比较抗菌药物不同疗程的随机对照试验较少。急性骨髓炎应治疗4～6周。对于病情有所改善但炎症标志物升高或局部炎症症状未能消除的患者，应继续治疗。此类患者需密切监测，并评估是否需要额外的治疗或采取其他措施进一步确定诊断和控制感染源。慢性骨髓炎可能需要12周或更长时间的治疗，治疗通常根据临床情况进行个体化。接受治疗的患者还应每周监测抗生素的毒性。根据所使用的具体药物，评估肾功能和肝功能、全血细胞计数和药物水平。对于氨基糖苷类药物，应每周两次检测肾功能和药物峰谷水平。达巴凡星和奥利万星等长效糖肽类药物有望替代需每日使用的抗生素。

最近一项包括1000多名随机患者的骨髓炎治疗开放标签研究表明，与静脉注射治疗相比，口服治疗没有劣势。口服治疗组降低了治疗成本，患者满意度更高。两组严重副作用和不良反应的发生率相似。口服治疗以喹诺酮类药物为主。尽管该研究涵盖的人群有异质性，但将研究结果应用于特定患者时应深思熟虑。在适当的临床情况下，可以使用诸如骨移植、血运重建术和放置肌肉瓣以覆盖和保护暴露的骨等辅助疗法。

天然关节化脓性关节炎可以用4周疗程的抗菌药物治疗，假体关节感染一般治疗6周或更长时间。监测毒性和治疗反应与骨髓炎类似。

预后

在合理的诊断、清创和抗菌治疗前提下，骨髓炎和化脓性关节炎的预后良好。最常见的并发症是受影响骨或关节的残余疼痛和（或）功能减退，但相对少见且轻微。假体关节感染是一个例外，其25%～50%的患者因感染而导致部分功能丧失。慢性骨髓炎的复发率，尤其是糖尿病患者，可能高达30%。一些更复杂的病例，如开放性污染骨折或需要保留感染固定物者，并发症包括骨不连、假体植入失败和慢性骨髓炎。无法控制的感染可导致截肢以及随之而来的功能和活动能力丧失。偶尔，骨或关节感染可播散至其他关节或血液。这类病例常见于金黄色葡萄球菌感染，但是，此类情况罕见。

推荐阅读

American Academy of Orthopedic Surgeons: Diagnosis and prevention of periprosthetic joint infections clinical practice guidelines. March, 2019.
Lew DP, Waldvogel FA: Osteomyelitis, Lancet 364:369–379, 2004.
Li HK, Rombach I, Zambellas R, et al: Oral versus intravenous antibiotics for bone and joint infection, N Engl J Med 380:425, 2019.
Parvizi J, Tan TL, Goswami K, et al: The 2018 definition of periprosthetic hip and knee infection: an evidence-based and validated criteria, J Arthroplasty 33:1309, 2018.
Rappo U, Puttagunta S, Shevchenko V, et al: Dalbavancin for the treatment of osteomyelitis in adult patients: a randomized clinical trial of efficacy and safety, Open Forum Infect Dis 6:331, 2018.
Shuford JA, Steckelberg JM: Role of oral antimicrobial therapy in the management of osteomyelitis, Curr Opin Infect Dis 16:515–519, 2003.
Spielberg B, Lipsky BA: Systemic antibiotic therapy for chronic osteomyelitis in adults, Clin Infect Dis 54:393, 2012.
Stengel D, Bauwens K, Sehouli J, et al: Systematic review and meta-analysis of antibiotic therapy for bone and joint infections. Lancet Infect Dis 201 1: 175-188.
Tande AJ, Steckelberg JM, Osmon DR, Berbari EF: Osteomyelitis. In Bennett JE, Dolin R, Blaser MJ, editors: Principles and practice of infectious diseases, 9th ed, Philadelphia, 2020, Elsevier.
Tice AD, Hoaglund PA, Shoultz DA: Outcomes of osteomyelitis among patients treated with outpatient parenteral antimicrobial therapy, Am J Med 114:723–728, 2003.
Waldvogel FA, Medoff G, Swartz MN: Osteomyelitis: a review of clinical features, therapeutic consideration and unusual aspects, N Eng J Med 282:316–322, 1970.
Wunsch S, Krause R, Valentin T, et al: Multicenter clinical experience of real life dalbavancin use in gram-positive infection, Int J Infect Dis 81:210, 2019.

13

Urinary Tract Infections

Abdullah Chahin, Steven M. Opal

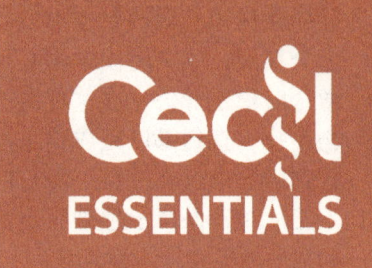

DEFINITION AND DIAGNOSIS

The term *urinary tract infection* (UTI) refers to significant bacteriuria in a patient with symptoms or signs attributable to the urinary tract and no alternative diagnosis. UTI includes asymptomatic bacteriuria, urethritis, cystitis, pyelonephritis, catheter-associated UTI, prostatitis, and urosepsis. This chapter focuses primarily on the two major forms of UTI, cystitis and pyelonephritis.

A practical classification divides these infections into uncomplicated and complicated UTI. Uncomplicated UTIs are episodes of cystitis and mild pyelonephritis occurring in healthy, premenopausal, sexually active, nonpregnant women with no history suggestive of abnormalities in the urinary tract. All other episodes of UTI are deemed to be potentially complicated and deserving of further evaluation.

The term *asymptomatic bacteriuria* refers to isolation of bacteria in an appropriately collected urine specimen from an individual who describes no symptoms for urinary tract infection. In women, asymptomatic bacteriuria is defined as two consecutive voided midstream urine specimens with isolation of the same bacterial strain at levels of at least 10^5 colony-forming units (CFU) per milliliter from patients without genitourinary symptoms. In men, a single clean-catch, midstream voided urine specimen with one bacterial species at a concentration greater than 10^5 CFU/mL defines asymptomatic bacteriuria. The diagnosis of asymptomatic bacteriuria is also established in both women and men from a single catheterized urine specimen (not an indwelling catheter) with one bacterial species isolated at concentrations greater than 10^2 CFU/mL. Although infants and toddlers infrequently have asymptomatic bacteriuria, the incidence increases with age, owing to the incomplete bladder emptying from various obstructive urologic conditions that develop with advanced age, reaching up to 15% or greater in women and men age 65 to 80 years and as high as 50% after age 80. Asymptomatic bacteriuria is therefore commonly encountered in clinical practice, and it frequently poses a challenge in determining the exact source of infection in elderly patients presenting with sepsis. Asymptomatic bacteriuria is a common cause for unnecessary use of antibiotics and the array of complications that can result from antibiotic misuse, ranging from mild adverse reactions to devastating complications such as antibiotic-associated *Clostridioides difficile* infections.

The presence of asymptomatic bacteriuria therefore should not be considered as equivalent to UTI except in neutropenic patients and individuals with anatomic or functional defects in the urinary tract. Asymptomatic bacteriuria in pregnancy has been an indication for treatment. However, the most recent Systematic Review for the US Preventive Services Task Force in September of 2019 showed that screening and treatment for asymptomatic bacteriuria during pregnancy was associated with reduced rates of pyelonephritis and low birth weights, but the available evidence was not current, with only one study conducted in the past 30 years. It is difficult to define asymptomatic bacteriuria in the patient who has undergone renal transplantation, and bacteriuria in such patients often indicates the need to treat for UTI.

To increase the sensitivity of urinalysis and culture, *significant bacteriuria* is defined as greater than 10^2 CFU/mL of urine in a woman with symptoms of uncomplicated cystitis and pyuria (≥ 5 white blood cells per milliliter of urine per high-power field). Among women with symptoms of uncomplicated pyelonephritis and men with UTI, significant bacteriuria is defined as greater than 10^4 CFU/mL plus pyuria. In patients with complicated UTI, a concentration of 10^5 CFU/mL or higher is required for the definition of significant bacteriuria independently of pyuria.

In order for these definitions to be valid, the urine must remain in the bladder for at least 2 hours, and after urine collection the sample should be incubated immediately. If urine is not incubated immediately, it can be refrigerated for up to 8 hours before proper incubation.

Although the presence of bacteriuria is vital for the establishment of the diagnosis of UTI, clinical symptomatology is the hallmark of UTI. The presence of dysuria, increased frequency of urination, suprapubic tenderness, and hematuria associated with bacteriuria or pyuria on urinalysis is unequivocally consistent with the diagnosis of cystitis. Back or flank pain, nausea, vomiting, and the presence of fever or rigors suggest infection of the upper urinary tract, although it is not easy to distinguish cystitis from pyelonephritis on clinical grounds alone. The diagnosis of UTI gets more difficult when patients cannot ascribe symptoms to the urinary tract (e.g., patients with paraplegia or neurogenic bladder, confused elderly or sedated patients) or when they have atypical symptoms, such as changes in mental status, agitation, or hypotension. Sometimes patients have urinary symptoms without bacteriuria (the pyuria-dysuria or "urethral syndrome" commonly caused by *Chlamydia trachomatis* or other difficult-to-culture genitourinary pathogens).

With the widespread utilization of indwelling catheters, *catheter-associated urinary tract infection* (CAUTI) remains a challenge in health care and one of the most common nosocomial infections. Essentially, CAUTI has similar symptoms to a typical UTI but requires the presence of an indwelling urinary catheter for the term to apply. The standard Centers for Disease Control and Prevention (CDC) National Healthcare Safety Network (NHSN) CAUTI definition is complex and subjective. Moreover, it can be difficult to diagnose in patients who are already hospitalized due to the resemblance of the potential signs and symptoms of CAUTI with many other acute disorders that were part of the original reason for hospitalization.

LABORATORY FINDINGS

Young, sexually active women with typical symptoms of UTI have a high pretest probability for UTI. Therefore, no laboratory test is indicated. In this population, pretreatment urine analysis and culture are

13 尿路感染

葛瑛 译　鲁炳怀 刘智博 审校　曹彬 通审

定义与诊断

尿路感染（UTI）一词是指患者尿中存在显著菌尿并出现与尿路相关的症状或体征，而没有其他诊断可以解释。UTI 包括无症状菌尿、尿道炎、膀胱炎、肾盂肾炎、导管相关 UTI、前列腺炎和尿源性感染中毒症。本章主要关注 UTI 的两种主要形式，膀胱炎和肾盂肾炎。

一个实用的分类方法将 UTI 分为非复杂性 UTI 和复杂性 UTI。非复杂性尿路感染是发生在健康、绝经前、性活跃、未怀孕且无尿路异常病史的女性的膀胱炎和轻度肾盂肾炎。所有其他的尿路感染病例被认为是潜在的复杂性尿路感染，需要进一步评估。

无症状菌尿是指在一个没有尿路感染症状的个体中，从合格采集的尿液标本中分离出细菌。在女性患者中，无症状菌尿定义为两个连续的中段尿标本中，分离出相同的细菌菌株，且每毫升至少有 10^5 个菌落形成单位（CFU），并且患者没有生殖泌尿系统症状。在男性患者中，无症状菌尿定义为单一的清洁中段尿标本中，某一细菌种类的浓度超过 10^5 CFU/ml。无症状菌尿的诊断也可以通过女性和男性的单一导尿标本（不是留置导尿管）分离出某一细菌种类，浓度超过 10^2 CFU/ml 来确立。虽然婴儿和幼儿很少有无症状菌尿，但由于随年龄增长出现的各种梗阻性泌尿系统疾病导致膀胱排空不完全，其发生率随年龄增加。在 65～80 岁的女性和男性患者中，无症状菌尿的发生率可达 15% 或更高，80 岁以上的人群中甚至可高达 50%。因此，无症状菌尿在临床很常见，尤其在老年感染中毒症患者中，常常成为确定感染来源的挑战。无症状菌尿是滥用抗菌药物的常见原因，而不合理应用抗菌药物导致的系列的并发症，从轻微的不良反应，到严重灾难性并发症，如与抗生素相关的艰难梭菌感染，均可见。

因此，无症状菌尿的存在不应被视为等同于尿路感染，除非是中性粒细胞减少症患者或有尿路解剖或功能缺陷的个体。妊娠期的无症状菌尿曾被认为需要治疗。然而，2019 年 9 月美国预防服务工作组进行的最新系统评价显示，妊娠期筛查和治疗无症状菌尿可以降低肾盂肾炎发生率和低出生体重患儿的风险，但现有证据不够充分，因为过去 30 年中只有一项相关研究。对于接受肾移植的患者来说，定义无症状菌尿较为困难，这类患者的菌尿通常意味着需要开展 UTI 治疗。

为提高尿液分析和培养的敏感性，对于女性非复杂性膀胱炎患者出现尿路症状和脓尿（高倍视野下尿液白细胞≥5 个）时，显性菌尿定义为尿液中细菌浓度大于 10^2 CFU/ml。对于伴有临床症状的非复杂性肾盂肾炎的女性和男性患者，显性菌尿定义为大于 10^4 CFU/ml 加脓尿。对于复杂性尿路感染患者，不考虑脓尿，显性菌尿的定义需要尿液中细菌浓度达到 10^5 CFU/ml 或更高。

为了使这些定义有效，尿液必须在膀胱中停留至少 2 h，采集尿液后应立即进行培养。如果尿液不能立即培养，可以在冰箱中冷藏最多 8 h，然后进行适当的培养。

虽然菌尿的存在对于确立尿路感染的诊断至关重要，但临床症状是尿路感染的标志。尿液分析显示菌尿或脓尿，伴有排尿困难、尿频、耻骨上区压痛和血尿，这与膀胱炎的诊断一致。如出现背痛或腰痛、恶心、呕吐以及发热或寒战常提示上尿路感染，尽管仅凭临床表现难以区分膀胱炎和肾盂肾炎。当患者无法将症状归因于尿路（例如，患有截瘫或神经源性膀胱的患者、精神错乱的老年人或镇静剂作用下的患者），或者当他们出现非典型症状，如精神状态改变、烦躁或低血压时，诊断尿路感染变得更加困难。有时患者会出现尿路症状但没有菌尿（由沙眼衣原体或其他难以培养的泌尿生殖系统病原体常引起的脓尿-排尿困难综合征或"尿道综合征"）。

随着留置导尿管的广泛应用，导管相关尿路感染（CAUTI）仍然是医疗领域的一个挑战，也是最常见的院内感染之一。基本上，CAUTI 的症状与典型的尿路感染相似，但需要有留置导尿管才能适用该术语。美国疾病控制与预防中心（CDC）国家医疗安全网（NHSN）对 CAUTI 的标准定义复杂且主观。此外，由于 CAUTI 的潜在症状和体征与许多其他导致住院的急性疾病相似，因此在已经住院的患者中诊断 CAUTI 可能会比较困难。

实验室结果

年轻的性活跃女性如果有典型的尿路感染症状，她们患尿路感染的预测概率很高。因此，在这类人群中无须进行实验室检测。仅在诊断不明确或怀疑耐药病原体感染时才需进行治疗前的尿液分析和培养。在所有疑似复杂性尿路感染的病例中，均需进行尿液分

indicated only if the diagnosis is not straightforward or if an antibiotic-resistant organism is suspected. Urinalysis and culture are indicated in all cases of suspected complicated UTI. The presence of white blood cell casts in urinalysis indicates pyelonephritis, and this finding suggests a complicated UTI with possible obstructive lesions within the kidney or collecting system (e.g., papillary necrosis). Blood cultures are mandatory for patients with suspected pyelonephritis. *Staphylococcus aureus* bacteriuria should prompt work-up for *S. aureus* bacteremia and for renal abscesses in non-catheter-related UTIs, particularly in those who are hospitalized and have laboratory evidence of infection. *S. aureus* UTI may also occur without hematogenous seeding in cases of indwelling catheters, with frequent instrumentation, or in the presence of hardware in the genitourinary tract. Candida is a commonly isolated organism on urine cultures (candiduria). Yeasts can be detected in contaminated samples during collection, in patients who have bladder or indwelling catheter colonization, and rarely in patients who have upper urinary tract infection that developed either from retrograde spread from the bladder or hematogenous spread from a distant source. The presence of pyuria and quantitative cultures of urine in cases of candiduria have proved to be of little use in separating infection from colonization. Therefore, clinical symptoms are of great importance, because diagnosing UTI with *Candida* might necessitate an extensive work-up to assess for invasive fungal infections (Candidemia or perinephric abscesses). Imaging studies are indicated if kidney stones, malignancy, obstructive uropathy, and urologic malformations are suspected.

EPIDEMIOLOGY

At the extremes of age, men are more prone to UTI than women. In young boys, urethral malformation is commonly the cause, and in older men, UTI is usually caused by bladder neck obstruction secondary to prostatic hypertrophy. Homosexual men are at increased risk for acquiring UTIs. Teenage girls and sexually active women have more UTIs than their male counterparts. A higher than expected incidence of UTI among young girls might suggest sexual abuse. Sexually active women have the highest rate of UTI. Postmenopausal women have increased prevalence of UTI due to estrogen deficiency and age-related pelvic relaxation with poor bladder emptying.

The most common etiologic agent in patients with uncomplicated UTI is *Escherichia coli* (90% of cases), followed by *Staphylococcus saprophyticus*. Other agents include *Klebsiella* spp, *Enterococcus faecalis*, *Enterococcus faecium*, *Proteus* spp, *Providencia stuartii*, and *Morganella morganii*. In patients with complicated UTI, *E. coli* is still the most frequent uropathogen, but at a lower rate than in uncomplicated UTI. Other causative organisms are *Pseudomonas aeruginosa*, *Acinetobacter baumannii*, *Enterobacter* spp, *Serratia marcescens*, *Stenotrophomonas maltophilia*, *Enterococcus* spp, and *Candida* spp.

Anaerobic agents are infrequent causes of UTI; when present, they represent fistulae between the digestive tract and the urinary tract. *Staphylococcus aureus* UTI most often represents bacteremia with bacteriuria resulting from clearance of bloodstream bacteria by the kidney. Whereas 1% of individuals with a UTI get pyelonephritis, 20% to 40% of pregnant women with a UTI develop pyelonephritis, and 30% of patients with pyelonephritis have bacteremia. In diabetic and transplanted patients with UTI, the incidence of bacteremia is higher.

PATHOGENESIS

There are at least three routes by which bacteria can enter the bladder or kidney: ascending, hematogenous, and lymphatic. Lymphatic spread is the least common route. The hematogenous route is important for gram-positive organisms such as *S. aureus* or *Candida* spp but unimportant for gram-negative bacilli. The ascending route is the most important for enteric bacteria, and this mechanism is supported by higher frequency of UTI in women, given the shorter length of the female urethra, and in individuals with an indwelling Foley catheter.

Before reaching the urinary bladder or kidney, the microorganism must colonize the external part of the urinary tract. Probably the most important aspect in the establishment of UTI is the interaction between host factors (e.g., secretor phenotype, P1 blood group, uroplakin I and II) and bacterial virulence factors (the adhesins, P fimbriae, and type I fimbriae [pili]). The urinary bladder is normally covered by a glycosaminoglycan surface that prevents binding of bacteria that transiently enter the bladder. P-fimbriated uropathogenic *E. coli* bind to alpha 1-4 linked, galactose-galactose disaccharide moieties found on uroepithelial cells, and these gal-gal glycolipids are also expressed on the P1 blood group. People with P1 blood group are overrepresented among individuals with either recurrent UTI or pyelonephritis. Also, people who lack P1 blood group are less prone to complicated UTI.

Studies have shown that P-fimbriated *E. coli* is present in 60% to 100% of isolates from patients with UTI. Ascending UTI infection can be inhibited experimentally by epithelial cell surface receptor analogues. Type I fimbriae bind to glycoprotein uroplakin I and II. *E. coli* expressing type I fimbriae are responsible for most cases of cystitis.

Once *E. coli* is attached to uroepithelial cells, both mechanical and biochemical factors facilitate the development of full-blown UTI. The local trauma and mechanical massage of the urethra during sexual intercourse help deliver bacteria into the bladder and, if vesicoureteral reflux or another ureteral anatomic defect is present, into the kidney. Urinary catheter placement also helps to propel bacteria into the bladder, and all patients with a long-term indwelling catheter in place will eventually develop asymptomatic UTI. All uropathogenic organisms have the ability to multiply in the urine.

From the standpoint of the host, other factors associated with the development of UTI are a new sex partner (within 1 year), use of diaphragms and spermicides, family history of UTI in a first-degree relative, and lower expression of CXCR1, an interleukin 8 receptor. Pathogenic factors associated with the development of UTI are flagellae, diverse adhesins, siderophores, toxins, polysaccharide coating, and the ability to cause a deleterious inflammatory response.

Patient behaviors that are not associated with UTI include precoital or postcoital voiding patterns, daily beverage consumption, frequency of urination, delayed voiding habits, wiping patterns, tampon use, douching, use of hot tubs, and type of underwear.

TREATMENT

The goal of treatment in uncomplicated UTI is to decrease symptoms and prevent complications. Treatment should be guided by two important principles: the prevalence of resistant genitourinary pathogens in the community and collateral damage to ecologic microbiota (i.e., the risk of propagation of resistant organisms). First-line agents for uncomplicated UTI are nitrofurantoin, trimethoprim-sulfamethoxazole (TMP-SMX), and fosfomycin trometamol; alternative agents are the fluoroquinolones (except moxifloxacin) and the β-lactams (Table 13.1).

Treatment of complicated UTI should be based on culture results and the other comorbidities that are present. Recurrent UTI in sexually active women can be prevented with postcoital TMP-SMX 40/200 mg single dose (if the patient has more than two UTIs per year related to coitus) or with daily, every other day, or weekly antibiotic. If the patient has a UTI unrelated to coitus or there are fewer than two UTIs per year related to coitus, the prevention of the UTI recurrence can be achieved with patient-initiated therapy. Daily topical application of intravaginal estriol can be helpful in postmenopausal women. After completion of the treatment, urine culture is indicated for pregnant women and on an individualized basis for other patients with complicated UTI.

析和培养。在尿液分析中发现白细胞管型提示肾盂肾炎，这一发现表明可能存在复杂性尿路感染，可能伴有肾脏或尿集合系统中的阻塞性病变（如肾乳头坏死）。对于疑似肾盂肾炎的患者，必须进行血液培养。对于非导管相关的尿路感染，特别是住院且有感染实验室证据的患者，发现金黄色葡萄球菌菌尿应当进行金黄色葡萄球菌菌血症和肾脓肿的检查。在导管相关感染的病例中，即使没有血源性播散，也可能发生金黄色葡萄球菌尿路感染，特别是在频繁的器械操作或泌尿生殖道存在植入物的情况下。在尿液培养中，念珠菌是常见的分离菌（念珠菌尿）。在收集过程中被污染的标本、膀胱或导尿管留置的住院患者，以及罕见的由膀胱逆行传播或远处来源血源性传播而发展的上尿路感染患者中都可以检测到酵母菌。在念珠菌尿的病例中，脓尿和尿液定量培养在区分感染和定植方面的作用有限。因此，临床症状非常重要，因为诊断念珠菌尿路感染可能需要进行广泛检查以评估侵袭性真菌感染（如念珠菌血症或肾周脓肿）。如果怀疑有肾结石、恶性肿瘤、梗阻性尿路病变和泌尿系统畸形，则需要进行影像学检查。

流行病学

在年龄段两端的患者（老人及幼儿），男性比女性更容易患尿路感染（UTI）。对于男性幼童，尿道畸形是常见原因，而对于老年男性患者，UTI 通常是由前列腺肥大引起的膀胱颈部梗阻所致。男性同性恋患 UTI 的风险增加。少女和性活跃的女性比同龄男性更容易患 UTI。年轻女孩如出现高于预期的 UTI 发病率可能暗示性虐待。性活跃的女性 UTI 的发病率最高。绝经后的女性由于雌激素缺乏和年龄相关的骨盆松弛导致的膀胱排空不良，UTI 的患病率增加。

在患有非复杂性尿路感染的患者中，最常见的病原体是大肠埃希菌（占 90% 的病例），其次是腐生葡萄球菌。其他病原体包括克雷伯菌属、粪肠球菌、尿肠球菌、变形杆菌属、斯氏普鲁威登菌和摩氏摩根菌。在复杂性尿路感染的患者中，大肠埃希菌仍然是最常见的引起尿路感染的病原体，但比非复杂性 UTI 中的发生率要低。其他致病微生物包括铜绿假单胞菌、鲍曼不动杆菌、肠杆菌属、黏质沙雷菌、嗜麦芽窄食单胞菌、肠球菌属和念珠菌属。

厌氧菌引起尿路感染的情况较少见；一旦出现，通常提示消化道和泌尿道之间存在瘘管。金黄色葡萄球菌尿路感染通常提示菌血症，其菌尿是由于肾清除血流中的细菌所致。虽然 1% 的 UTI 患者会患上肾盂肾炎，但在妊娠的 UTI 患者中，20%～40% 会发展为肾盂肾炎，且 30% 的肾盂肾炎患者有菌血症。在糖尿病患者和移植患者的 UTI 病例中，菌血症的发生率更高。

发病机制

细菌进入膀胱或肾至少有 3 种途径：上行、血源性和淋巴播散。淋巴播散最少见。血源性播散对革兰氏阳性菌非常重要，如金黄色葡萄球菌或念珠菌，但对革兰氏阴性杆菌并不重要。上行途径对于肠道细菌来说最重要，这种机制由于女性尿道较短，以及留置导尿管的个体中 UTI 的频率更高而得到支持。

在到达膀胱或肾之前，微生物必须先在尿路的外部定植。可能在 UTI 的发生过程中最重要的方面是宿主因素（例如，分泌型表型、P1 血型、尿路上皮素 I 和 II）与细菌毒力因素（黏附素、P 菌毛和 I 型菌毛）之间的相互作用。膀胱表面通常覆盖有糖胺聚糖层，防止细菌在短暂进入膀胱时附着。具有 P 菌毛的致病性大肠埃希菌与尿路上皮细胞上发现的 α1-4 连接的半乳糖-半乳糖二糖基结合，这些半乳糖-半乳糖糖脂也在 P1 血型中表达。P1 血型的人在反复发作的 UTI 或肾盂肾炎患者中比例更高。而且，缺乏 P1 血型的人不易患复杂性 UTI。

研究表明，在 UTI 患者的分离株中，具有 P 菌毛的大肠埃希菌的比例为 60%～100%。实验表明，通过上皮细胞表面受体的类似物可以抑制上行性 UTI 感染。I 型菌毛与糖蛋白尿路上皮素 I 和 II 结合。表达 I 型菌毛的大肠埃希菌是大多数膀胱炎病例的病因。

一旦大肠埃希菌附着在尿路上皮细胞上，机械和生化因素都会促进全面 UTI 的发展。性交过程中尿路的局部损伤和机械摩擦有助于将细菌送入膀胱，如果存在膀胱输尿管反流或其他输尿管解剖缺陷，则细菌还会进入肾。尿道导管的放置也有助于将细菌推进膀胱，所有长期留置导管的患者最终都会发展成无症状的 UTI。所有泌尿系统致病菌都有能力在尿液中繁殖。

从宿主的角度来看，与 UTI 发展相关的其他因素包括在一年内有新性伴侣、使用子宫帽和杀精剂、一级亲属中有 UTI 家族史以及低表达 CXCR1（一种白介素 8 受体）。与 UTI 发展相关的致病因素包括鞭毛、多种黏附素、铁载体、毒素、多糖涂层，以及引起有害炎症反应的能力。

与 UTI 无关的患者行为包括性交前或性交后的排尿模式、每日饮料摄入、排尿频率、延迟排尿习惯、擦拭方式、使用卫生棉条、阴道冲洗、使用热水浴缸以及内衣类型。

治疗

治疗非复杂性 UTI 的目标是减轻症状并预防并发症。治疗应遵循两个重要原则：社区内泌尿生殖道病原体耐药率和对微生物菌群的附带损害（即耐药病原微生物增殖的风险）。非复杂性 UTI 的一线药物是呋喃妥因、甲氧苄啶-磺胺甲噁唑（TMP-SMX）和磷霉素氨丁三醇；替代药物是氟喹诺酮类（莫西沙星除外）和 β-内酰胺类（表 13.1）

复杂性 UTI 的治疗应基于培养结果和存在的其他合并症。对于性活跃女性的复发性 UTI，可以通过性交后服用单剂量 40/200 mg TMP-SMX（如果患者每年因性交引起的 UTI 超过 2 次），或每天、隔天或每周服用抗生素来预防。如果患者的 UTI 与性交无关或每年因性交引起的 UTI 少于 2 次，则可以通过患者自发治疗来预防

❖ For a deeper discussion on this topic, please see Chapter 268, "Approach to the Patient with Urinary Tract Infection," in *Goldman-Cecil Medicine*, 26th Edition.

COMPLICATIONS

Unrecognized and untreated UTIs can quickly develop grave complications. Recurrent infections, structural damage of the urinary tract and scar tissue formation, loss of renal function, increased risk of delivering low-birthweight or premature infants in pregnant women, and septic shock could all develop in untreated UTI cases. Serious complications include renal abscesses which usually present with fever, back and abdominal pain and may include urinary tract symptoms. Abscesses are usually due to ascending urinary tract infection often with an obstructive process. *E. coli* or other enteric aerobic rods are typical organisms. Renal abscess can also be due to hematogenous spread of *S. aureus*. Prolonged antibiotic therapy directed at the offending organism is usually curative. Perinephric abscess results from rupture of an intrarenal abscess into the perinephric space between the renal capsule and Gerota's fascia. Treatment is drainage and antibiotics. Some other serious complications of urinary tract infections are listed in Table 13.2.

TABLE 13.1 Therapy for Uncomplicated Urinary Tract Infections

Antimicrobial Agent	CYSTITIS			PYELONEPHRITIS		
	Useful Therapeutically	Dose and Duration	Comments	Useful Therapeutically	Dose and Duration	Comments
Nitrofurantoin monohydrate macrocrystals	[a]Yes, first line	100 mg bid for 5 days	Cheap, well tolerated SE: N, H Low impact on microbiome	No	NA	Reduced renal tissue penetration
Trimethoprim-sulfamethoxazole	[a]Yes, first line	160/800 mg bid for 3 days	If resistance is known to be <20% SE: rash, urticaria, N, V	Yes	160/800 mg bid for 14 days	[a]If organism susceptibility is known [c]If not, give an initial LA IV agent
Fosfomycin trometamol	[a]Yes, first line	3 g single-dose sachet	May be less efficient SE: N, D, H	No	NA	Active against MRSA ESBL, VRE
Fluoroquinolones (ciprofloxacin levofloxacin)	[b]Yes, second line	3-day regimen 250 mg bid 250 mg qd	High collateral damage SE: N, V, D, H, tendinitis	[a]Yes, first line	Dose varies; 7–14 days	If resistance is known to be <10%
β-Lactams	[c]Yes, second line	Dose varies by agent; 5–7 days	Less effective, increased side effects SE: N, V, D, rash, urticaria	[c]Yes Use cautiously Less efficient	Dose varies; 10–14 day regimen	[c]Give an initial LA IV agent

Data from Gupta K, Hooton TM, Naber KG, et al: International clinical practice guidelines for the treatment of acute uncomplicated cystitis and pyelonephritis in women: a 2010 update by the Infectious Diseases Society of America and the European Society for Microbiology and Infectious Diseases—executive summary, Clin Infect Dis 52:561-564, 2011.

D, Diarrhea; *ESBL*, extended-spectrum β-lactamase; *H*, headache; *IV*, intravenous; *LA*, long acting; *MSRA*, methicillin-resistant *Staphylococcus aureus*; *N*, nausea; *NA*, not applicable; *SE*, side effects; *V*, vomiting; *VRE*, vancomycin-resistant enterococci.
[a]AI level of evidence from current guidelines.
[b]AIII level of evidence from current guidelines.
[c]BI level of evidence from current guidelines.

TABLE 13.2 Complications of Urinary Tract Infections

Complications	Pathophysiology	Diagnostic Methods/Likely Pathogens	Treatment
Cortico-medullary abscess	Focal abscesses can occur with ascending, generalized pyelonephritis, often occur with anatomic abnormalities of the GU tract	CT scanning is the study of choice. Ultrasound findings are less specific. Likely pathogens are gram-negative bacilli.	Antibiotics alone for lesions <3 cm. Drainage and antibiotics for larger lesions.
Cortical abscess (Renal carbuncle)	Focal abscess within the kidney parenchyma from hematogenous blood stream infection	Ultrasound or CT scanning. *Staphylococcus aureus*, enteric gram-negative bacteria.	Treat source of bacteremia, large lesions need drainage
Septic shock	Urinary tract infections are a common source of gram-negative bacteremia sepsis and septic shock	Blood cultures, imaging studies for possible urinary obstruction/enteric gram-negative bacteria	Urgent antibiotic therapy, urinary drainage if needed, IV fluids and vasopressors
Perinephric abscess	Insidious purulent collection between the kidney capsule and Gerota fascia; secondary to urinary tract obstruction and/or hematogenous spread	CT scan or renal ultrasonography. Fifty percent have accompanying pleural effusion or lung pathology. Gram-negative bacterial pathogens.	Percutaneous drainage and antibiotics. Septation of the perinephric space makes drainage more difficult.

Continued

UTI复发。在绝经后的女性，每日局部应用阴道内雌三醇可能会有所帮助。治疗完成后，对于孕妇应进行尿培养，对于其他复杂性UTI患者则应根据个体情况进行尿培养。复杂尿感染的治疗应以培养结果为依据。

◆ 有关此专题的深入讨论，请参阅 Goldman-Cecil Medicine 第26版第268章"尿路感染患者的处理方法"。

并发症

未被发现和未治疗的尿路感染会迅速发展成严重并发症。未经治疗的UTI病例可能会发展成复发性感染、尿路结构损伤和瘢痕组织形成、肾功能丧失、孕妇低出生体重儿或早产婴儿的风险增加，以及感染中毒性休克。严重并发症包括肾脓肿，通常表现为发热、背部和腹部疼痛，可能还包括尿路症状。脓肿通常是由于上行性尿路感染，通常伴有梗阻的过程。大肠埃希菌或其他肠道需氧杆菌是典型病原体。肾脓肿也可能是由金黄色葡萄球菌的血源性播散引起。针对致病菌的长期抗菌治疗通常可以治愈。肾周脓肿是由于肾内脓肿破裂进入肾包膜和Gerota筋膜之间的肾周间隙。治疗方法是引流和抗菌药物治疗。其他一些尿路感染的严重并发症列在表13.2中。

表13.1 非复杂性尿路感染的治疗

抗微生物药	膀胱炎				肾盂肾炎		
	是否对治疗有帮助	剂量和疗程	评价		是否对治疗有帮助	剂量和疗程	评价
硝基呋喃妥因单水合物微晶体	[a]是，一线药物	100 mg bid 连续5天	便宜，耐受性好 SE：N，H 对正常菌群影响小		否	NA	肾组织穿透性低
甲氧苄啶-磺胺甲噁唑	[a]是，一线药物	160/800 mg bid 连续3天	若已知耐药率 < 20% 可用 SE：皮疹，荨麻疹，N，V		是	160/800 mg bid 连用14天	[a] 如果药敏结果已知 [c] 如果药敏结果未知，给予初始 LA IV 制剂
磷霉素氨丁三醇	[a]是，一线药物	3 g 单剂服用	可能效果不佳 SE：N，D，H		否	NA	对 MRSA ESBL，VRE 有活性
氟喹诺酮类（环丙沙星、左氧氟沙星）	[b]是，二线药物	3天疗法 250 mg bid 250 mg qd	附加伤害大 SE：N，V，D，H，跟腱炎		[a]是，一线药物	剂量不定；7～14天	如果已知耐药率 < 10%
β-内酰胺类	[c]是，二线药物	根据不同药物确定剂量；5～7天	效果差，副作用多 SE：N，V，D，皮疹，荨麻疹		[c]是 慎用，效果差	剂量不定；10～14天	[c] 初始给予 LA IV 制剂

数据引自 Gupta K, Hooton TM, Naber KG, et al: International clinical practice guidelines for the treatment of acute uncomplicated cystitis and pyelonephritis in women: a 2010 update by the Infectious Diseases Society of America and the European Society for Microbiology and Infectious Diseases—executive summary, Clin Infect Dis 52: 561-564, 2011.
D，腹泻；ESBL，超广谱β-内酰胺酶；H，头痛；IV，静脉注射；LA，长效；MRSA，耐甲氧西林金黄色葡萄球菌；N，恶心；NA，不适用；SE，副作用；V，呕吐；VRE，耐万古霉素肠球菌。
[a] 当前指南中 A I 证据水平。
[b] 当前指南中 A III 证据水平。
[c] 当前指南中 B I 证据水平。

表13.2 尿路感染并发症

并发症	病理生理学	诊断方法/可能的病原体	治疗
皮质-髓质脓肿	局部脓肿可发生在上行的、广泛的肾盂肾炎中，通常伴有泌尿系统的解剖异常	CT扫描是首选检查方法，超声检查特异性低，可能的病原体为革兰氏阴性杆菌	小于3 cm的病灶仅需抗菌药物治疗，较大的病灶需要引流和抗菌药物治疗
肾皮质脓肿（肾痈）	局部脓肿发生在肾实质内，由血源性感染引起	超声或CT扫描，病原体为金黄色葡萄球菌和肠道革兰氏阴性菌	通过抗菌药物治疗菌血症来源，大病灶需要引流
感染中毒性休克	尿路感染是革兰氏阴性菌血症、感染中毒症和感染中毒性休克的常见来源	血培养和影像学检查可发现尿路梗阻和肠道革兰氏阴性菌	紧急抗生素治疗，必要时进行尿路引流，静脉输液和血管升压药
肾周脓肿	隐匿性化脓性积聚位于肾包膜和Gerota筋膜之间；由尿路梗阻和（或）血源性播散引起	CT扫描或肾超声检查，50%伴有胸腔积液或肺部病变，革兰氏阴性菌病原体	经皮肾穿刺引流和抗菌药物治疗，肾周间隙的隔膜化使引流更加困难

TABLE 13.2 Complications of Urinary Tract Infections—cont'd

Complications	Pathophysiology	Diagnostic Methods/Likely Pathogens	Treatment
Emphysematous pyelonephritis	Rapid onset, severe infection of the kidney with accumulation of gas in the tissues. Seen in uncontrolled diabetes and impaired host immunity.	Detection of air surrounding the kidney by chest radiography or CT scan. *E. coli* accounts for most cases.	Intravenous antibiotics and drainage; urgent nephrectomy often needed
Papillary necrosis	Necrosis of the renal medullary pyramids and papillae secondary to vascular impairment. Can occur with infectious and noninfectious processes.	CT scanning or intravenous urography (IVU). Associated with a variety of enteric gram-negative and gram-positive bacteria.	Treat the underlying cause and ameliorate the ischemia with hydration and alkalization
Xanthogranulomatis pyelonephritis	Chronic, insidious, and destructive disease of the kidney marked by a granulomatous inflammatory response with lipid-laden macrophages	Rare chronic, infectious, inflammatory disease of the kidney seen in diabetes, lipid storage diseases, obstructive uropathy. *Proteus* sp is the most common bacterial pathogen.	Treat underlying cause, mass effects from kidney can form fistula tracts and be confused for neoplastic disease

SUGGESTED READINGS

Gupta K, Hooton TM, Naber KG, et al: International clinical practice guidelines for the treatment of acute uncomplicated cystitis and pyelonephritis in women: a 2010 update by the Infectious Diseases Society of America and the European Society for Microbiology and Infectious Diseases—executive summary, Clin Infect Dis 52:561–564, 2011.

Gupta K, Trautner B: In the clinic: urinary tract infection [review], Ann Intern Med 156:ITC3-1–ITC3-15, quiz ITC-13–ITC-16, 2012.

Henderson JT, Webber EM, Bean SI: Screening for asymptomatic bacteriuria in adults: updated evidence report and systematic review for the US preventive Services Task Force, J Am Med Assoc 322(12):1195–1205, 2019. https://doi.org/10.1001/jama.2019.10060.

Hooton TM: Clinical practice: uncomplicated urinary tract infection [review], N Engl J Med 366:1028–1037, 2012.

Hooton TM, Bradley SF, Cardenas DD, et al: Diagnosis, prevention, and treatment of catheter-associated urinary tract infection in adults: 2009 International clinical practice guidelines from the infectious Diseases society of America, Clin Infect Dis 50:625–663, 2010.

Nicolle LE, Bradley S, Colgan R, et al: Infectious Diseases Society of America guidelines for the diagnosis and treatment of asymptomatic bacteriuria in adults, Clin Infect Dis 40:643–654, 2005.

表 13.2　尿路感染并发症（续表）

并发症	病理生理学	诊断方法 / 可能的病原体	治疗
气性肾盂肾炎	快速起病，严重的肾感染，组织中气体积聚，见于未控制的糖尿病患者和免疫力低下宿主	胸部 X 线检查或 CT 可见空气征，大肠埃希菌为大多数病例的病原体	静脉注射抗生素和引流；通常需要紧急肾切除术
肾乳头坏死	肾髓质锥体和乳头坏死，继发于血管受损，可发生在感染性和非感染性过程	CT 扫描或静脉尿路造影（IVU），与多种肠道革兰氏阴性和革兰氏阳性菌有关	治疗根本原因，通过补液和碱化改善缺血
黄色肉芽肿性肾盂肾炎	肾的慢性、隐匿性和破坏性疾病，以肉芽肿性炎症反应和含脂质的巨噬细胞为特征	罕见的慢性、感染性、炎症性肾病，见于糖尿病、脂质贮积疾病和梗阻性尿路病变。变形杆菌是最常见的细菌病原体	治疗根本原因，肾的占位效应可能形成瘘管，并容易与肿瘤性疾病混淆

推荐阅读

Gupta K, Hooton TM, Naber KG, et al: International clinical practice guidelines for the treatment of acute uncomplicated cystitis and pyelonephritis in women: a 2010 update by the Infectious Diseases Society of America and the European Society for Microbiology and Infectious Diseases—executive summary, Clin Infect Dis 52:561–564, 2011.

Gupta K, Trautner B: In the clinic: urinary tract infection [review], Ann Intern Med 156:ITC3-1–ITC3-15, quiz ITC-13–ITC-16, 2012.

Henderson JT, Webber EM, Bean SI: Screening for asymptomatic bacteriuria in adults: updated evidence report and systematic review for the US preventive Services Task Force, J Am Med Assoc 322(12):1195–1205, 2019. https://doi.org/10.1001/jama.2019.10060.

Hooton TM: Clinical practice: uncomplicated urinary tract infection [review], N Engl J Med 366:1028–1037, 2012.

Hooton TM, Bradley SF, Cardenas DD, et al: Diagnosis, prevention, and treatment of catheter-associated urinary tract infection in adults: 2009 International clinical practice guidelines from the infectious Diseases society of America, Clin Infect Dis 50:625–663, 2010.

Nicolle LE, Bradley S, Colgan R, et al: Infectious Diseases Society of America guidelines for the diagnosis and treatment of asymptomatic bacteriuria in adults, Clin Infect Dis 40:643–654, 2005.

14

Health Care-Associated Infections

Paul G. Jacob, Thomas R. Talbot

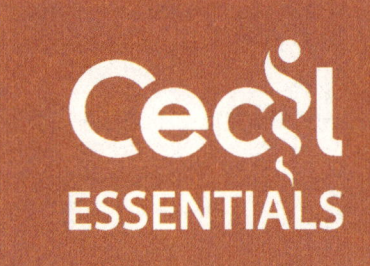

INTRODUCTION

A health care–associated infection (HAI) is an infection that did not exist or was not incubating at the time of admission to the health care facility. These infections can occur in all types of health care settings, including acute care units, long-term care facilities, rehabilitation facilities, outpatient dialysis clinics, and outpatient surgical centers. Surgical site infections (SSI), central line–associated bloodstream infections (CLABSI), and catheter-associated urinary tract infections (CAUTI) are common examples.

HAIs cause a substantial degree of morbidity and mortality. A 2018 study of 199 hospitals found a prevalence rate of 3.2% among a population of 12,299 patients in 2015. Extrapolating from this data, researchers concluded there were approximately 687,200 HAIs in US acute care hospitals in 2015. The Centers for Disease Control and Prevention (CDC) estimates that on any given day, approximately 1 in 31 hospitalized patients has an HAI. Beyond the extensive morbidity and mortality they cause, HAIs are costly, with costs ranging from $896 per catheter-associated urinary tract infection to $45,814 per central line–associated bloodstream infection. These costs are likely to be underestimated because of incomplete estimation of the outpatient costs of parenteral antibiotics, skilled nursing care, physical rehabilitation, and lost work days.

As of January 2011, the Centers for Medicare and Medicaid Services (CMS) required public reporting of certain facility-specific HAI outcomes as part of value-based purchasing. As of August 2019, the following acute care–related HAIs are required for reporting by CDC's National Healthcare Safety Network (NHSN): catheter-associated urinary tract infections and central line–associated bloodstream infections in all adult, pediatric, and neonatal intensive care units (ICU) and from all patient care locations meeting the NHSN definition for adult and pediatric medical, surgical or combined medical/surgical wards, colon and abdominal hysterectomy SSIs, hospital-onset *Clostridioides difficile* infections (CDIs), and hospital-onset methicillin-resistant *Staphylococcus aureus* (MRSA) bacteremias. The importance of preventing HAIs has never been more apparent.

The major types of HAIs include the infections reported to CMS, hospital-acquired pneumonia (HAP) or ventilator-associated pneumonia (VAP), health care–associated respiratory viral infections (e.g., influenza and respiratory syncytial virus acquired within a health care facility) and other multidrug-resistant organisms (MDROs). MDROs are pathogens with resistance to various important antibiotics (e.g., MRSA, vancomycin-resistant *Enterococcus* (VRE), antibiotic-resistant gram-negative bacilli). This chapter reviews the major classes of HAIs, with a focus on prevention, diagnosis, and treatment.

HEALTH CARE EPIDEMIOLOGY AND INFECTION PREVENTION

In the age of increasing MDROs, shortage of new antibiotics, and public reporting of HAIs, the importance of efforts to prevent HAIs is growing. The fields of health care epidemiology and infection prevention focus on the practices of tracking HAIs in a systematic fashion (i.e., surveillance) to implement evidence-based HAI prevention practices.

Although HAIs were once thought to be the cost of being critically ill and receiving care in a hospital, several key events have occurred during the past 20 years that have shifted that perception. In 2006, Pronovost and colleagues implemented a "simple and inexpensive intervention" in 103 ICUs in the state of Michigan while participating in the Michigan Health and Hospital Association Keystone ICU project. This landmark study showed a reduction in the median rate of CLABSIs from 2.7 per 1000 catheter days to zero. These results shifted the discussion from merely controlling HAIs to preventing them. Other major events have included the recognition and effectiveness of using bundles of evidence-based practices to reduce HAIs; the recognition of the HAI burden in nonacute, non-ICU settings (including ambulatory clinics, long-term care facilities, and other venues where healthcare is delivered); and the importance of quality improvement science in reducing HAIs.

The prevention of HAIs has become increasingly possible, and various types of prevention interventions can reduce the HAI burden dramatically. In 2010, Wenzel and Edmund described these interventions as horizontal and vertical strategies (Table 14.1). Horizontal infection prevention strategies are broad practices (e.g., hand hygiene, isolation precautions) aimed at preventing many or all types of HAIs, regardless of the specific pathogen, procedure, or device. Vertical HAI prevention strategies are directed at specific types of HAIs or target a specific organism. Vertical strategies include using procedural checklists or standardized bundles and MRSA decolonization.

CATHETER-ASSOCIATED URINARY TRACT INFECTIONS

CAUTIs were the third most common device-related infection according to a survey performed in 2018. In comparison to data in 2011, the percentage of patients with an HAI due to CAUTI in 2015 declined from 23.6% to 18.7%. The additional cost of a CAUTI, according to a 2013 meta-analysis, has been estimated at approximately $896 (range: $603 to $1189) per episode.

CAUTI complications include cystitis, pyelonephritis, and in up to 4%, bacteremia. Although urinary catheter–associated bacteremias are rare, they are an underappreciated cause of health care–associated bacteremias and have been estimated to cost an additional $3744 per episode. Though surveillance of CAUTI has long been emphasized in the ICU, efforts have increasingly focused on understanding its impact in non-ICU settings. A 2013 study of 506 CAUTIs among 15 hospitals revealed 72% occurred in non-ICU settings.

Most health care–associated urinary tract infections are catheter associated. A catheterized patient's daily risk of developing bacteriuria

医疗照护相关感染

康梅 译 葛瑛 崔晓敬 审校 曹彬 通审

引言

医疗照护相关感染（HAI）是指患者在入院时不存在也不处于潜伏期，而是在医疗照护机构获得的感染。HAI 可能发生在各种类型的医疗机构，包括急症护理病房、长期护理机构、康复机构、血液透析门诊和门诊手术中心。最常见的感染类型为手术部位感染（SSI）、中心静脉导管相关感染（CLABSI）和导管相关尿路感染（CAUTI）等。

HAI 具有极高的发病率和死亡率。2018 年对 199 家医院进行的一项研究发现，2015 年 12 299 名患者中，HAI 的流行率为 3.2%。根据该数据研究人员推断，2015 年美国提供急症照护的医院约有 687 200 例 HAI。据美国疾病控制与预防中心（CDC）估计，单日每 31 名住院患者中就约有 1 人罹患 HAI。除了导致大量发病和死亡外，HAI 导致的医疗花费也极高，从每例次导管相关尿路感染诊治费用 896 美元到每例次中心静脉导管相关感染诊治费用 45 814 美元不等。由于对静脉用抗生素、专业护理、物理康复和工作日损失等门诊费用的估算尚不完全，这些成本很可能被低估。

自 2011 年 1 月起，美国联邦医保和医助服务总局（CMS）要求公开报告某些医疗机构特定的 HAI 结果，作为基于价值的医保采购的一部分。截至 2019 年 8 月，美国 CDC 负责的美国国家医疗安全网（NHSN）要求报告以下急性照护相关的 HAI：所有成人、儿科和新生儿重症监护病房（ICU）以及所有符合 NHSN 定义的成人和儿科医疗护理机构，手术病房或内外科联合病房的 CAUTI 和 CLABSI、结肠和腹部子宫切除术后 SSI、在医院发生的艰难梭菌感染（CDI）以及耐甲氧西林金黄色葡萄球菌（MRSA）菌血症等。由此可见预防 HAI 具有前所未有的重要性。

HAI 的主要类型包括以上须向 CMS 报告的感染、医院获得性肺炎（HAP）或呼吸机相关肺炎（VAP）、医疗照护相关呼吸道病毒感染（如在医疗机构内感染的流感和呼吸道合胞病毒）以及其他多重耐药菌（MDRO）。MDRO 是指对多种重要抗菌药物具有耐药性的病原体［如 MRSA、耐万古霉素肠球菌（VRE）、多重耐药革兰氏阴性杆菌］。本章回顾了主要类别的 HAI，聚焦其预防、诊断和治疗。

医疗照护流行病学和感染预防

在 MDRO 增加、新抗菌药物短缺和公开报告 HAI 的时代，预防 HAI 的重要性与日俱增。医疗照护流行病学和感染预防领域的工作重点是系统跟踪 HAI（即监测），以实施循证为基础的 HAI 预防措施。

虽然 HAI 曾经被认为是危重患者在医院接受治疗的代价，但在过去 20 年中发生的几件关键事情转变了这个观念。2006 年，在密歇根州卫生健康与医院协会的 Keystone ICU 项目中 Pronovost 等在密歇根州 103 个重症监护病房实施了一项"简单而廉价的干预措施"，这项里程碑式研究将 CLABSI 的中位数从每 1000 个导管日 2.7 例降至 0。这样的研究结果也将过去仅讨论如何控制 HAI 转变到了如何预防 HAI。其他重要事件还包括认识到采用集束化循证实践能有效减少 HAI；对非急诊、非 ICU（包括门诊、长期护理机构和其他提供医疗服务的场所）中 HAI 的负担；以及通过科学的质量改进减少 HAIs 的重要性等。

由此可见，预防 HAI 变得越来越可能，各种类型的预防干预措施可以显著减轻 HAI 负担。2010 年，Wenzel 和 Edmund 将这些干预措施描述为横向和纵向策略（表 14.1）。横向预防策略是指预防多种或所有类型 HAI 的通用做法（如手卫生、预防隔离措施），与具体病原体、程序或设备无关。纵向 HAI 预防策略针对特定类型的 HAI 或特定的病原体。纵向策略包括使用程序检查清单或标准集束化措施以及 MRSA 去定植。

导管相关尿路感染

根据 2018 年进行的一项调查，CAUTI 是第三大最常见的设备相关感染。与 2011 年的数据相比，2015 年因 CAUTI 导致 HAI 的患者比例从 23.6% 降至 18.7%。根据 2013 年的一项荟萃分析，CAUTI 的额外费用估计约为每例次 896 美元（范围：603～1189 美元）。

CAUTI 包括膀胱炎、肾盂肾炎，且可并发菌血症（可达 4%）。虽然导管相关菌血症很少见，但它们是医疗照护相关菌血症被低估的原因之一，据估计，每例次发生会产生 3744 美元的额外费用。尽管 CAUTI 的监测长期以来在 ICU 备受重视，但人们也越发关注其在非 ICU

is about 3% to 10%. Indwelling urinary catheters disrupt several mechanisms of the natural defense against infection, including urine flow, length of the urethra, and micturition to prevent attachment of potential pathogens to the uroepithelium. Tamm-Horsfall proteins, the most abundant soluble proteins in the urine, play a significant role by binding uropathogenic bacteria, facilitating wash out, and lowering the threshold for activating local innate immunity. These soluble proteins are prevented from entering the lower urinary tract by the catheters.

An indwelling catheter allows colonization, attachment, and biofilm formation by certain microorganisms. Most of the organisms causing CAUTIs arrive by ascending the urethra from the meatus and perineum. The most common uropathogens identified in CAUTIs are *Escherichia coli*, *Candida* spp, *Klebsiella* spp, *Pseudomonas aeruginosa*, and *Enterococcus* spp (Fig. 14.1).

Common symptoms of a urinary tract infection (e.g., dysuria, urinary frequency) may not be useful in diagnosing a patient with an indwelling catheter. However, the most common clinical manifestations of a CAUTI are fever (≥38° C) and bacteriuria. Other signs and symptoms of a CAUTI can include rigors, altered mental status, pelvic or suprapubic pain, costovertebral angle tenderness, and acute onset of hematuria without another underlying cause. One of these signs or symptoms plus a positive urine culture with a known uropathogen (>10^5 colony-forming units) strongly suggests a CAUTI. Pyuria (>5 leukocytes/mL of urine) is not always a reliable indicator for infection in patients with indwelling catheters; pyuria and asymptomatic bacteriuria are not necessarily indications for treatment. Risk factors for CAUTI acquisition include duration of catheterization, underlying fatal illness, age older than 50 years, having a nonsurgical underlying illness, and nonadherence to proper catheter care.

The most effective method of preventing CAUTIs is to avoid placing urinary catheters unless absolutely necessary and to restrict catheter use to institutionally accepted indications. Proper insertion and care of urinary catheters are paramount (see Table 14.1). Maintenance of unobstructed flow with the collection bag below the bladder, use of a closed catheter system (even when sampling urine), and discontinuation of the catheter as soon as appropriate are key elements for preventing a CAUTI. Nurse-directed discontinuation protocols in which frontline personnel have defined parameters for removing catheters without requiring a provider's order are increasingly used to eliminate unnecessary catheters. The routine use of antimicrobial-coated catheters is not recommended except when infection rates remain elevated despite proper adherence to all other prevention strategies.

Treatment of asymptomatic bacteriuria usually is not recommended, with exception of pregnant women and patients who will undergo urologic procedures. Treatment of CAUTI is based on current Infectious Disease Society of America (IDSA) guidelines, and the choice of antimicrobial regimen should be based on the local antibiogram and identified syndrome (e.g., pyelonephritis). Before treatment, urine culture and sensitivity results are used to evaluate a resistant organism and tailor an empirical antimicrobial regimen. To ensure accurate diagnosis of urinary tract infections, many hospitals have adopted algorithms that will only allow for cultures if there is pyuria demonstrated on urinalysis (also known as reflexive culture).

Most clinicians prefer to replace or discontinue the catheter after a urinary tract infection is diagnosed. Guidelines recommend replacement if it has been in place for more than 2 weeks. There is good evidence based on review by expert committees that duration of treatment can be 7 days if symptoms quickly resolve or 10 to 14 days if resolution is delayed. In nonpregnant women younger than 65 years of age, a 3-day course of antibiotic therapy can be considered after the urinary catheter has been removed.

HOSPITAL-ACQUIRED AND VENTILATOR-ASSOCIATED PNEUMONIA

Pneumonia remains one of the most common HAIs, following *C. difficile* infection. Both HAP and VAP are included in the surveillance of HAIs. As of the most recent American Thoracic Society and IDSA guidelines in 2016, the term "health care–associated pneumonia (HCAP)" has been retired due to overlap with HAP and VAP. Other definitions are given in Table 14.2.

The incidence of HAP or VAP is difficult to determine due to the various definitions that have been used for surveillance and the subjective nature of these diagnoses. Some studies have estimated that the incidence of VAP ranges from 2 to 16 cases per 1000 ventilator days. VAP is associated with an increased length of hospital stay (10 days in one study), costs (approximately $40,000), and mortality (attributable mortality rate of 13%, highest among surgical patients).

Risk factors for VAP include conditions that lead to increased aspiration or impairment of host defenses and bacterial colonization of the respiratory and upper gastrointestinal tracts. In a ventilated patient, the body's natural mechanical defense mechanisms (e.g., ciliated epithelium, mucus, cough) are interrupted, leading to colonization of the lower airways by potentially pathogenic organisms. The most significant source of these organisms tends to be the patient's own oropharynx and upper gastric contents.

The most commonly implicated respiratory pathogens are *S. aureus* and *P. aeruginosa*, followed by several Enterobacteriaceae species and *Acinetobacter baumannii* (see Fig. 14.1). Colonization with MDROs correlates with an increasing duration of hospitalization. Guidelines argue that late (>4 days after admission) compared with early HAP may be the most useful factor when determining empirical antimicrobial therapy. Although bacteria play the largest role in HAP, fungi and viruses also must be considered in immunosuppressed patients.

One definition of HAP or VAP includes clinical, radiographic, and microbiologic criteria. Signs and symptoms indicating an infection include fever (≥38° C), peripheral leukocytosis, purulent sputum, and worsening respiratory status. A tracheal aspirate for Gram stain and culture provides the last piece of diagnostic information. When several of these signs and symptoms exist in the absence of a pulmonary infiltrate, alternative diagnoses should be considered, including ventilator-associated tracheobronchitis.

The greatest risk factor for the prediction of MDRO-related pneumonia is prior intravenous antibiotic therapy, whether for HAP or VAP (see Table 14.2). Longer duration of hospitalization increases the risk for acquisition of multidrug resistant pathogens, though the concept of early- and late-onset pneumonia has been challenged by more recent studies. Prior intravenous antibiotic therapy within the last 90 days is an independent risk factor for both MRSA and MDR *Pseudomonas aeruginosa*. Additional risk factors in VAP include septic shock, acute respiratory distress syndrome (ARDS), 5 or more days prior to occurrence, and prior receipt of acute renal replacement therapy.

INFECTIONS ASSOCIATED WITH VASCULAR CATHETERS

The NHSN collects data on CLABSIs, and public reporting is required for CLABSIs in ICUs and certain non-ICU inpatient units. In 2011, the incidence of CLABSIs ranged from 0 to 3.7 cases per 1000 catheter days. In 2015, CLABSIs made up a smaller percentage of HAIs (16.9%) than in 2011 (18.8%). Although CLABSIs have the lowest prevalence

环境中的影响。2013年对15家医院的506例CAUTI进行的一项研究显示，72%的CAUTI发生在非ICU病房。

大多数与医疗照护相关的尿路感染都与导管有关。患者每导管日发生菌尿的风险为3%~10%。留置导管破坏了机体多种抗感染自然防御机制，这些可防止潜在病原体附着在尿路上皮细胞的防御机制包括尿流、尿道长度和排尿。T-H蛋白是尿液中含量最高的可溶性蛋白，可通过结合尿路致病菌并促进其排泄以及尽早激活局部先天免疫发挥重要作用。导管可阻止这些可溶性蛋白质进入下尿路。

留置导管可导致特定微生物定植、附着和形成生物膜。导致CAUTI的绝大多数微生物都是从尿道口和会阴部进入尿路的。CAUTI最常见的尿路病原菌是大肠埃希菌、念珠菌属、克雷伯菌属、铜绿假单胞菌和肠球菌属（图14.1）。

普通尿路感染的常见症状（如排尿困难、尿频）可能对留置导管患者的诊断没有帮助。CAUTI最常见的临床表现是发热（≥38℃）和菌尿。CAUTI的其他体征和症状还包括寒战、精神状态改变、骨盆或耻骨上疼痛、肋脊角压痛以及不明原因的急性血尿。具有其中一项症状或体征并且有已知尿路病原体的尿培养阳性（>10^5 CFU/ml），则强烈提示为CAUTI。对留置导管患者而言，脓尿（白细胞>5/ml）并非总是尿路感染的可靠诊断指标；脓尿和无症状菌尿也不一定是治疗指征。发生CAUTI的危险因素包括导尿时间长短、潜在的致命疾病、年龄超过50岁、患有非外科基础疾病以及未坚持正确的导管护理。

预防CAUTI的最有效方法是，除非绝对必要，尽量避免安置导管，并将安置导管严格限制在机构认可的适应证范围内。导管的正确安置和护理至关重要（表14.1）。保持集尿袋在膀胱下方的畅通、使用封闭的导管系统（即便在采样尿液时）以及在合适时机尽快停用导管是预防CAUTI的关键因素。护士主导的拔管方案提及一旦满足拔管指标，一线人员无须医嘱即可进行拔管操作，该方案正越来越多地用于移除不必要的导管。不建议常规使用抗菌药物涂层导管，除非在适当遵守所有其他预防策略的情况下感染率仍然上升。

通常不建议治疗无症状性菌尿，孕妇和即将接受泌尿外科手术的患者除外。导管相关尿路感染（CAUTI）的治疗依据当前美国感染病学会（IDSA）的指南，抗菌方案的选择应基于当地的抗菌药物体外药敏谱和确定的综合征（如肾盂肾炎等）。在治疗前，应进行尿培养和药敏试验来评估抗药菌物并调整经验性抗菌治疗方案。为确保尿路感染的诊断准确性，许多医院采用了诊断流程，即仅在尿常规显示脓尿时才进行尿培养。

大多数临床医生诊断尿路感染后，倾向于更换或移除导管。指南推荐，如果导管已安置超过2周，应进行更换。基于专家委员会的抗菌治疗共识指出，有充分的证据支持如果症状迅速缓解，抗菌疗程可持续7天；如果缓解延迟，则疗程可延长至10~14天。对于65岁以下的非孕妇，在移除导管后，可以考虑为期3天的抗菌治疗。

医院获得性肺炎和呼吸机相关肺炎

肺炎是除艰难梭菌感染以外最常见的HAI之一。医院获得性肺炎和呼吸机相关肺炎（VAP）均被纳入HAI监测范围。根据2016年美国胸科学会和IDSA的最新指南，"医疗照护相关肺炎（HCAP）"这一术语因与HAP和VAP重叠而不再使用。其他定义见表14.2。

由于监测的定义各不相同以及诊断的主观性，HAP或VAP的发病率难以确定。有研究估计，VAP的发病率为每1000个呼吸机日2~16例。VAP与住院时间（一项研究显示为10天）、费用（约4万美元）和死亡率（归因死亡率为13%，手术患者死亡率最高）的增加有关。

导致VAP的危险因素包括误吸发生率增高或宿主防御功能受损以及呼吸道和上消化道的细菌定植。对插管患者，机体的天然机械防御机制（如纤毛上皮、黏液、咳嗽）失效，导致潜在病原体在下呼吸道定植。这些病原体的最主要来源往往是患者自身的口咽部和上消化道内容物。

最常见的呼吸道病原体是金黄色葡萄球菌和铜绿假单胞菌，其次是几种肠杆菌和鲍曼不动杆菌（图14.1）。MDRO的定植与住院时长有关。指南认为，晚发（入院后>4天）与早发HAP是指导经验性抗菌治疗选择最有用的因素。虽然导致HAP的病原体中细菌最常见，但免疫抑制患者也必须考虑真菌和病毒。

HAP或VAP的定义包括临床、影像学和微生物学标准。感染相关体征和症状包括发热（≥38℃）、外周血白细胞增多、脓性痰和呼吸状况恶化。气道抽吸物行革兰氏染色和培养可提供最终的诊断信息。如仅有上述症状和体征，但没有肺部浸润，则应考虑其他诊断，包括呼吸机相关气管支气管炎。

无论是HAP还是VAP（表14.2），之前的抗菌药物暴露均是MDRO相关肺炎的最大危险因素。住院时间越长，感染多重耐药菌的风险就越大，不过早发和晚发肺炎的概念已受到最新研究的质疑。过去90天内曾接受过静脉用抗菌药物治疗是MRSA和MDR铜绿假单胞菌肺炎的独立危险因素。VAP的其他危险因素包括感染中毒性休克、急性呼吸窘迫综合征（ARDS）、已发病5天或以上以及曾接受急性肾替代治疗。

血管导管相关感染

NHSN收集有关CLABSI的数据，并要求ICU和某些非ICU住院病房公开报告CLABSI。2011年，每1000个导管日中CLABSI的发生从0例到3.7例不等。2015年，CLABSI占HAI的比例（16.9%）低于2011年（18.8%）。虽然CLABSI在HAI中发病率最低，但

TABLE 14.1 Strategies for Preventing Health Care–Associated Infections

Horizontal Strategies (to Prevent All or Many Types of HAIs)
1. Standard precautions
   - Hand hygiene
   - Use of appropriate PPE
   - Respiratory hygiene and cough etiquette
   - Appropriate environmental cleaning and waste disposal
2. Chlorhexidine bathing in all ICU patients and in non-ICU acute inpatients with central lines[a]
3. Isolation precautions appropriate for pathogen
4. Steps to prevent needlestick injuries
5. Education of health care workers on IC/IP protocols

Vertical Strategies (Specific to HAI Type)

CAUTI
Urinary catheter placed only for appropriate indications:
  Urinary retention or obstruction
  Need for accurate UOP measurement in critical illness
  Incontinence and perineal or sacral wounds
  Comfort care use for terminal illness
Consider alternatives:
  Condom catheters
  Intermittent catheterization
Proper insertion and maintenance:
  Maintain aseptic technique
  Properly secure catheter to patient
  Maintain closed drainage system
  Maintain unobstructed flow
Urinary catheter premeditated stop order or RN-initiated discontinuation policy
Anti-infective catheters if infection rates remain high
Reflexive culture testing algorithms to reduce false diagnosis of urinary tract infection

VAP
Use noninvasive ventilation when able
On intubation:
  Semirecumbent position (30–45 degrees) unless contraindicated
  Hypopharyngeal suctioning
  Avoid gastric overdistention
  Use cuffed ET tube
  Oral care, tooth brushing
  Keep ventilatory circuit closed unless changing for soiling or malfunctioning
  Daily targeted sedation management
  Spontaneous breathing trial if screening finds applicable
Use weaning protocols to minimize duration of ventilation

CLABSI
Use checklist for device insertion:
  Bundle supplies
  All present use at least face mask, then proceduralist uses sterile gown and gloves, mask, and head cap
  Avoid femoral line placement if possible
  Skin antisepsis with alcohol and >0.5% chlorhexidine
  Use of chlorhexidine-impregnated dressing or sponge at insertion site
  Empower personnel to stop nonemergent insertion if improper technique is followed
Maintenance:
  Access as infrequently as feasible
  Scrub the access hub or port with antiseptic
  Daily bathing with chlorhexidine and intranasal antiseptic with mupirocin or povidone-iodine
Daily audits for assessment of device need and potential discontinuation
Interventions to reduce blood culture contamination that may be falsely assessed as true bacteremia

SSI
Preoperative strategies:
  Nonirritative hair removal with clippers on the day of surgery (not razors)
  Eradicate remote infection
  Decolonization of *Staphylococcus aureus*
  CHG bathing
  Smoking cessation
  Glucose control, hemoglobin A_{1c} <7% if possible
  Avoid immunosuppressive medication in perioperative period
  Identify and address malnutrition
Intraoperative strategies:
  In OR: proper ventilation, minimize traffic, proper attire, and surgical scrub
  Proper skin preparation (chlorhexidine plus alcohol or povidone plus alcohol) and draping
  Antimicrobial prophylaxis; proper timing, dosing, and intraoperative redosing
  Maintain normothermia
  Glucose control
  Tissue oxygenation, preoperative and postoperative supplementation

CDI
Prevention of acquisition:
  Antimicrobial stewardship
Prevention of transmission:
  Contact precautions (e.g., empiric placement for those suspected of CDI before confirmation of diagnosis)
  Hand hygiene with soap and water before leaving the patient's room
  Continue contact precautions
  Appropriate environmental cleaning with bleach-containing agents

CAUTI, Catheter-associated urinary tract infection; *CDI*, *Clostridioides difficile* infection; *CHG*, chlorhexidine gluconate; *CLABSI*, central line–associated bloodstream infection; *ET*, endotracheal; *HAI*, health care–associated infection; *IC/IP*, infection control or prevention; *ICU*, intensive care unit; *OR*, operating room; *PPE*, personal protective equipment; *RN*, registered nurse; *SSI*, surgical site infection; *UOP*, urine output; *VAP*, ventilator-associated pneumonia.

[a]Current data are not strong for prevention of CAUTI, VAP, and CDI by this method.

表 14.1 预防医疗照护相关感染的策略

横向策略（预防所有或多种类型的 HAI）

1. 标准预防措施
   - 手卫生
   - 使用适当的 PPE
   - 呼吸道卫生和咳嗽礼仪
   - 适当的环境清洁和废物处理
2. 所有 ICU 患者和中心静脉置管的非 ICU 急性住院患者行氯己定沐浴 [a]
3. 针对不同病原体的隔离预防措施
4. 预防针刺伤的步骤
5. 对医护人员进行 IC/IP 规范教育

纵向策略（针对 HAI 类型）

CAUTI

安置导管适应证：
  尿潴留或梗阻
  需要精确测量危重患者 UOP
  尿失禁和会阴或骶骨伤口
  临终关怀
可考虑得替代方案：
  避孕套导管
  间歇性导尿
正确安置和维护：
  无菌操作
  正确固定
  保持导尿系统封闭
  保持导管畅通
预设拔管规则或 RN 主导的拔管规则
如果感染率居高不下，可使用抗菌涂层导管
采用导向性培养程序以减少尿路感染误诊

VAP

尽可能使用无创呼吸
插管时：
  半卧位（30°～45°），除非有禁忌证
  声门下抽吸
  避免胃过度潴留
  使用带套囊的 ET 管
  口腔护理、刷牙
  保持呼吸回路密闭，除非因脏污或故障需更换
  每天进行有针对性的镇静管理
  一旦条件合适，则进行自主呼吸试验
采用间断方案，尽量缩短机械通气时间

CLABSI

按清单核对插管操作：
  集束化措施
  所有现场人员至少使用面罩，操作员着无菌服、戴手套、口罩和帽子
  尽可能避免股动脉置管
  用酒精和 > 0.5% 氯己定行皮肤消毒
  在插入部位使用浸过氯己定的敷料或海绵
  如出现违反原则的不当操作，授权工作人员可终止非紧急插管
导管维护：
  尽量减少接触频次
  用消毒剂擦洗连接器或端口
  每日氯己定沐浴以及用含莫匹罗星或聚维酮碘的抗菌剂行鼻内冲洗
每日评估持续血管内通路的必要性，以便撤去非必需的导管
采取措施减少可能被误诊为菌血症的血培养污染

SSI

术前策略：
  手术当日使用剪刀无刺激性去除毛发（不能用剃刀）
  根除手术远端部位感染
  金黄色葡萄球菌去定植
  CHG 沐浴
  戒烟
  控制血糖，尽可能控制糖化血红蛋白 $A_{1c} < 7\%$
  围术期避免使用免疫抑制药物
  确定并解决营养不良问题
术中策略：
  OR 内：适当通风，尽量减少人流，穿戴整齐，外科手消毒
  适当的皮肤准备（氯己定加酒精或聚维酮碘加酒精）和手术铺巾
  预防性抗菌药物应用；适当的时间、剂量和术中再用药
  保持体温正常
  控制血糖
  组织供氧、术前和术后支持

CDI

预防感染：
  抗菌药物管理
预防传播：
  接触隔离（如在确诊前对疑似 CDI 患者进行经验性隔离）
  离开隔离病房前用肥皂和水洗手
  继续采取接触隔离措施
采用含漂白剂成分的消毒剂进行适当环境消毒

CAUTI，导管相关尿路感染；CDI，艰难梭菌感染；CHG，葡萄糖酸氯己定；CLABSI，中心静脉导管相关感染；ET，气管内；HAI，医疗照护相关感染；IC/IP，感染控制 / 预防；ICU，重症监护病房；OR，手术室；PPE，个人防护设备；RN，注册护士；SSI，手术部位感染；UOP，尿量；VAP，呼吸机相关肺炎。
[a] 目前的数据还不足以证明该方法能有效预防 CAUTI、VAP 和 CDI。

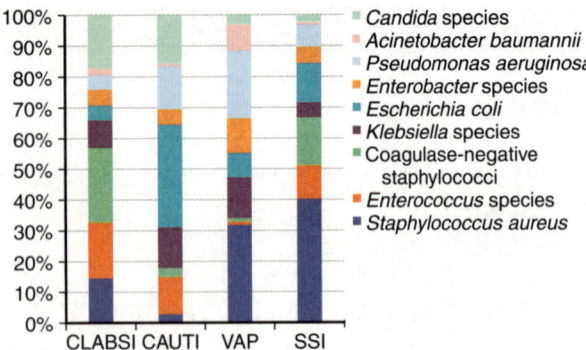

Fig. 14.1 Causative pathogens by specific type of health care–associated infection as reported to the Centers for Disease Control and Prevention National Healthcare Safety Network. *CAUTI*, Catheter-associated urinary tract infections; *CLABSI*, central line–associated bloodstream infections; *SSI*, surgical site infections; *VAP*, ventilator-associated pneumonia. (Modified from Sievert DM, Ricks P, Edwards JR, et al: Antimicrobial-resistant pathogens associated with healthcare-associated infection: summary of data reported to the National Healthcare Safety Network at the Centers for Disease Control and Prevention, 2009-2010, Infect Control Hosp Epidemiol 34:1-14, 2013.)

TABLE 14.2	Definitions of Types of Health Care–Associated Pneumonia
Pneumonia Type	**Definition**
Hospital-acquired pneumonia (HAP)	Pneumonia that occurs at least 48 hours after admission and that was not incubating at the time of admission
Ventilator-associated pneumonia (VAP)	Pneumonia that arises 48–72 hours after endotracheal intubation

Data from American Thoracic Society, Infectious Diseases Society of America: Guidelines for the management of adults with hospital-acquired, ventilator-associated, and healthcare-associated pneumonia, Am J Respir Crit Care Med 171:388-416, 2005.

among HAIs, the cost per episode and morbidity rate remain high. The estimated additional cost of an infection related to an intravenous catheter has been estimated at $45,814 (95% confidence interval [CI]): $30,919 to $65,245) per episode. The attributable increase in length of stay has been between 6.5 and 22 days, and the attributable mortality rate is about 10% among hospitalized patients.

The most common pathogens that cause primary CLABSIs are flora arising at the percutaneous insertion site or from contamination of the catheter hub. Hematogenous seeding from a gastrointestinal or other endovascular source occurs but is less likely. The most common pathogens that cause CLABSIs are coagulase-negative staphylococci, *Candida* species, *S. aureus*, and *Enterococcus* spp (see Fig. 14.1). The rising proportion of infections caused by *Enterococcus* and *Candida* spp since the 2006 to 2007 period suggests that skin colonization is being adequately addressed by the adoption of evidence-based prevention strategies and that an increasing fraction of CLABSIs are caused by secondary hematogenous seeding. Patients who are more severely ill, are neutropenic, have burns, or are on total parenteral nutrition are also at increased risk for candidemia. Other types of catheter-related infections include phlebitis, exit site infection, and pocket infection, tunnel infection, and septic thrombophlebitis.

Many CLABSIs are preventable through the use of evidence-based prevention practices for line insertion and maintenance. Strategies include appropriate decolonization of the skin before insertion with chlorhexidine plus alcohol, use of maximal sterile barriers (i.e., proceduralist wears sterile gloves and gown, cap, and mask, and a large barrier drape is placed over the patient), hand hygiene, and sterile technique (see Table 14.1). Appropriate maintenance of the central line mandates scrubbing the hub with an antiseptic and discontinuing the catheter as soon as it is not needed. Additional strategies with evidence for prevention of CLABSIs in the ICU include daily chlorhexidine bathing and nasal decolonization with mupirocin or povidone-iodine.

For a patient with a fever or systemic symptoms who has a central venous catheter, a bloodstream infection should be suspected. The diagnostic evaluation should begin with paired peripheral and catheter blood samples for culture before initiation of antimicrobial therapy. In a suspected case of bloodstream infection, the exudate at the exit site should be cultured.

The type of device (e.g., peripheral vs. central, short term vs. long term), associated infectious complications, and the implicated organism all play a role in treatment. For CLABSIs associated with short-term, nontunneled catheters and no complicating factors (e.g., suppurative thrombophlebitis, endocarditis, intravascular hardware), it may be appropriate to treat for 7 to 14 days after removal of the catheter. However, for long-term catheters, salvage may be attempted with systemic plus antibiotic lock therapy (as indicated by only a moderate amount of evidence from well-designed clinical trials or cohort or case series). Salvage of catheters associated with *S. aureus* bacteremia and fungemia have largely been unsuccessful, and it is not recommended. In the setting of an endovascular complication, removal of the catheter is strongly recommended, and systemic antibiotic therapy should be prolonged (i.e., 4 to 6 weeks). In many cases, septic thrombophlebitis may require surgical attention. Tunnel and pocket infections may also require débridement, but after the catheter is removed, 7 to 14 days of antimicrobial therapy should be sufficient.

SURGICAL SITE INFECTIONS

Standard definitions of SSIs classify them as superficial incisional, deep incisional (involving fascia or muscle), and organ space depending on the depth of tissue involvement. Most SSIs occur within 30 days of the operation, but some may develop later, especially in the setting of implanted foreign bodies (e.g., arthroplasty). The 2015 HAI Prevalence study from the CDC estimated an annual national burden of over 110,800 SSIs among hospitalized adult patients, a figure that does not include those patients with an SSI that did not require hospitalization. A patient who develops an SSI while hospitalized has a greater than 60% risk of being admitted to the intensive care unit, is 15 times more likely to be readmitted to the hospital within 30 days after discharge, and incurs an attributable extra hospital course of 6.5 days, leading to a direct cost of an additional $3000 per infection.

Endogenous seeding from the patient's skin flora is the most common avenue of infection. *S. aureus* and coagulase-negative *Staphylococcus* cause more than 40% of SSIs. In clean-contaminated operations, including open abdominal surgeries, gram-negative bacilli are predominant. An SSI should be suspected when postoperative patients have wound-associated purulent drainage, pain, tenderness, swelling, or redness. Positive culture growth from an aseptically obtained specimen is most convincing.

Many practices are used to prevent SSIs (see Table 14.1). One of the earliest and most effective strategies has been active surveillance and subsequent reporting of infection rates to the surgeons and staff. Much of the reduction in rates was attributed to the Hawthorne effect (i.e., active monitoring changes the behaviors of those being monitored). Other important interventions designed to reduce SSIs include

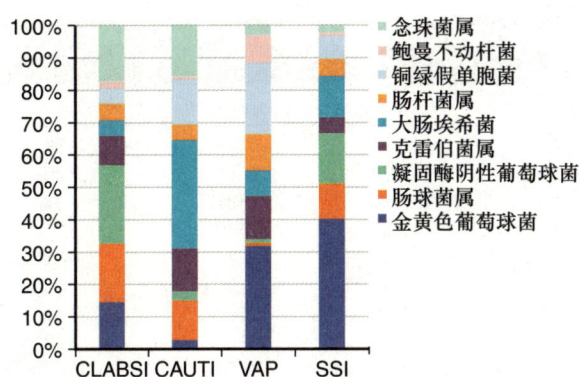

图 14.1 美国疾病控制与预防中心国家医疗安全网报告医疗照护相关感染的致病菌。CAUTI，导管相关尿路感染；CLABSI，中心静脉导管相关感染；SSI，手术部位感染；VAP，呼吸机相关肺炎（改编自 Sievert DM, Ricks P, Edwards JR, et al: Antimicrobial-resistant pathogens associated with healthcare-associated infection: summary of data reported to the National Healthcare Safety Network at the Centers for Disease Control and Prevention, 2009-2010, Infect Control Hosp Epidemiol 34: 1-14, 2013.）

表 14.2 医疗照护相关肺炎类型的定义	
肺炎类型	定义
医院获得性肺炎（HAP）	住院 48 h 后新发的肺炎，不包括入院时处于病原感染潜伏期
呼吸机相关肺炎（VAP）	气管插管 48～72 h 后发生的肺炎

数据引自 American Thoracic Society, Infectious Diseases Society of America: Guidelines for the management of adults with hospital-acquired, ventilator-associated, and healthcare-associated pneumonia, Am J Respir Crit Care Med 171: 388-416, 2005.

其单次发病的医疗负担和发病率仍然很高。据估计，与静脉导管相关的感染所造成的额外花费为每例 45 814 美元［95% 置信区间（CI）：30 919～65 245 美元］。相应住院时间增加 6.5～22 天，归因死亡率约为 10%。

导致原发性 CLABSI 的最常见病原体是导管插入部位的皮肤菌群或导管接口污染菌。胃肠道或其他血管内来源的血源性播散也会发生，但可能性较小。导致 CLABSI 的最常见病原菌是凝固酶阴性葡萄球菌、念珠菌属、金黄色葡萄球菌和肠球菌属（图 14.1）。2006—2007 年期间，由肠球菌和念珠菌属引起感染的比例不断上升，这提示采用基于循证的预防策略已充分解决了皮肤定植问题，进而出现越来越多的由血源播散引起的继发性 CLABSI。病情危重、中性粒细胞缺乏、烧伤或全肠外营养的患者发生念珠菌血症的风险也会增加。其他类型的导管相关感染包括静脉炎、出口部位感染、储袋感染、隧道感染和感染中毒性血栓性静脉炎。

很多 CLABSI 可通过在置管和维护过程中采用循证预防措施防止其发生。这些策略包括在置管前用氯己定和酒精对皮肤进行适当的去定植处理、遵守最大无菌屏障要求（即，专业置管人员戴无菌手套、穿隔离衣、戴工作帽和外科口罩，并将大型防护隔离罩覆盖在患者身上）、手卫生和无菌技术（见表 14.1）。中心静脉导管的适当维护要求使用消毒剂擦洗导管端口，并在不需要时立即停止使用导管。有证据表明可预防 ICU CLABSI 的其他策略包括每日氯己定沐浴和使用莫匹罗星或聚维酮碘进行鼻腔去定植。

中央静脉导管置管的患者一旦出现发热或全身感染症状，应怀疑是血流感染。在启动抗菌治疗前，应首先采集配套的外周血和导管血样本进行培养用以诊断评估。在疑似血流感染的病例中，应对置管部位的渗出物进行培养。

导管类型（如外周与中央、短期与长期）、相关感染并发症和所涉及病原体都会对治疗产生影响。如果没有并发症危险因素（如化脓性血栓性静脉炎、心内膜炎、血管内植入物），短期非隧道导管引起的 CLABSI，在拔除导管后治疗 7～14 天即可。对于长期导管，可尝试采用全身抗菌药物加抗生素封管疗法来抢救治疗（来自设计良好的临床试验、队列研究或病例研究的中等质量证据）。对于导管相关的金黄色葡萄球菌菌血症和真菌血症，这种抢救治疗基本无效，因此不建议采用该方法。一旦出现血管内并发症，强烈建议拔除导管，并延长全身抗菌疗程（即 4～6 周）。在许多情况下，血栓性静脉炎可能需要手术治疗。隧道感染和储袋感染可能需要清创术，但拔除导管后，7～14 天的抗菌疗程即可。

手术部位感染

手术部位感染（SSI）的标准定义将其分为浅部切口感染、深部切口感染（涉及筋膜或肌肉）和器官腔隙感染，具体取决于组织受累的深度。绝大多数 SSI 发生在术后 30 天内，但也有一些可能迟发，尤其是存在植入物的情况下（如关节成形术）。据 2015 年美国 CDC 的 HAI 流行率研究估计，全美每年住院成人患者中发生的 SSI 超过 110 800 例，还不包括不需要住院治疗的 SSI 患者。一旦患者住院期间发生 SSI，有超过 60% 的风险必须转 ICU 抢救，同时出院后 30 天内再入院的可能性是其他患者的 15 倍，住院时间也会增加 6.5 天，导致每例次感染的直接费用会额外增加 3000 美元。

最常见的感染途径是患者皮肤菌群的内源性移位。金黄色葡萄球菌和凝固酶阴性葡萄球菌导致 40% 以上的 SSI。在清洁-污染手术（包括开腹）中，革兰氏阴性杆菌占主导地位。当术后患者出现伤口相关的脓性分泌物、疼痛、触痛、肿胀或发红时，应怀疑是 SSI。无菌操作采集的标本培养阳性最有说服力。

预防 SSI 的方法很多（表 14.1）。最早也是最有效的策略之一是主动监测并且向外科医生和员工报告感染率。感染率的降低在很大程度上归因于霍桑效应（即主动监控会改变被监控者的行为）。旨在减少 SSI 的其他重要干预措施包括抗菌药物预防（如在正确的

TABLE 14.3 Pathogenic Isolates Resistant to Selected Antimicrobial Agents According to the NHSN, 2014

Organism	Antimicrobial	CLABSI	CAUTI	VAP[a]	SSI
Staphylococcus aureus	Oxacillin, methicillin, cefoxitin	50.7%	52.0%	42.4%	42.6%
Enterococcus faecium	Vancomycin	82.2%	85.1%	n/a	58.4%
Klebsiella pneumoniae	Ceftriaxone, ceftazidime, cefotaxime, or cefepime	24.1%	22.5%	21.0%	11.3%
	Carbapenems	10.9%	9.5%	10.1%	3.3%
Escherichia coli	Ceftriaxone, ceftazidime, cefotaxime, or cefepime	22.2%	16.1%	16.7%	15.3%
	Fluoroquinolones	49.3%	34.8%	30.8%	30.9%
Enterobacter spp	Ceftriaxone, ceftazidime, cefotaxime, or cefepime	36.1%	40.5%	26.9%	27.5%
	Carbapenems	6.6%	6.5%	3.2%	3.4%
Pseudomonas aeruginosa	Fluoroquinolones	30.2%	32.6%	31.9%	11.5%
	Piperacillin-tazobactam	18.4%	15.5%	19.4%	7.4%
	Cefepime, or ceftazidime	24.2%	22.5%	25.7%	9.9%
	Carbapenems	25.8%	23.9%	28.4%	7.7%
Acinetobacter baumannii	Carbapenems	46.6%	64.0%	55.5%	33.3%

Modified from Weiner LM, Webb AK, Limbago B, et al. Antimicrobial-resistant pathogens associated with healthcare-associated infections: summary of data reported to the National Healthcare Safety Network at the Centers for Disease Control and Prevention, 2011-2014. Infect Control Hosp Epidemiol. 2016;37(11):1288-1301.

CAUTI, Catheter-associated urinary tract infection; *CLABSI*, central line–associated bloodstream infection; *NHSN*, National Healthcare Safety Network; *SSI*, surgical site infection; *VAP*, ventilator-associated pneumonia.
[a]2012.

antimicrobial prophylaxis (i.e., the right drug at the right dose and right time), appropriate skin antisepsis, and maintenance of glucose control (see Table 14.1).

Management of SSIs often involves opening of the incision, evacuation of infected tissue, and allowing the wound to heal by second intention. The decision for initiating antibiotics is made on an individual basis and depends on the appearance of the wound, systemic signs of infection, depth of the infection, host's immune system, and type of surgery. Culture and Gram stain results help to dictate antibiotic coverage. For SSIs from a clean operation, empirical therapy covering *S. aureus* and *Streptococcus* species is recommended. For procedures involving the perineum, intestinal tract, or urogenital tract, broader coverage is needed to address gram-negative and anaerobic pathogens. When the SSI occurs within 48 hours of the index operation, *Streptococcus pyogenes* and *Clostridioides* spp are often implicated.

CLOSTRIDIOIDES DIFFICILE INFECTION

CDI is defined as diarrhea or toxic megacolon with detection of the *C. difficile* organism or toxin A or B, or both, in the stool or evidence of pseudomembranous colitis detected endoscopically, surgically, or histopathologically. This colonic infection is often accompanied by fever and leukocytosis.

C. difficile is the most common pathogen responsible for HAIs, approximating 12.1% of all HAIs. The incidence and severity of CDIs had been steadily increasing until more recently. Most reports have implicated the emerging BI/NAP1/027 strain, antibiotic overuse, and the aging population of hospitalized patients, who are disproportionately affected by CDI. Virtually every antibiotic has been associated with increasing the risk of CDI. Intensive efforts to combat CDI have also focused on several avenues: accurate diagnosis, reducing vectors for transmission, and judicious use of antimicrobials. Diagnosis of CDI must correctly identify infection versus colonization. The strategy of diagnostic stewardship aims to employ proper testing algorithms to ensure only patients exhibiting clear signs and symptoms receive diagnostic evaluation. Transmission prevention has focused on efforts to reduce the environmental burden of pathogens through environmental cleaning and hand hygiene as well as through the use of transmission-based precautions (e.g., contact precautions).

The continued rise of CDI, increasing resistance to antimicrobials by many different pathogens, and lack of antimicrobials with novel mechanisms of action underscore the importance of antimicrobial stewardship. Antimicrobial stewardship is a strategy that emphasizes optimal selection, dose, and duration of antimicrobial therapy, producing the best clinical outcome while decreasing the risk of subsequent complications.

The consequences of poor stewardship include the emergence of resistance, CDI, and excessive drug expenditures. Antimicrobials have different probabilities of invoking resistance or CDI. Strategies implemented by antimicrobial stewardship programs include provider education and guidelines, de-escalation or tailoring of empirical therapy when possible, use of more appropriate empirical treatments, and front-end restriction of certain antibiotics.

For a deeper discussion of these topics, please see Chapter 267, "Approach to the Patient with Suspected Enteric Infection," and Chapter 280, "Clostridial Infections," in *Goldman-Cecil Medicine*, 26th Edition.

MULTIDRUG-RESISTANT PATHOGENS

MDROs are organisms that are resistant to more than one class of antimicrobial agents, although the names of some (e.g., MRSA, VRE) imply resistance to only one drug. According to NHSN data reported from the 2011 to 2014 period, high rates of resistance persist for a multitude of common bacterial pathogens (Table 14.3).

Infections caused by MDROs lead to increased length of hospitalization, health care costs, and mortality rates for patients compared with those who are infected by antimicrobial-susceptible organisms. Kollef and colleagues found that patients who received inadequate antimicrobial therapy for their HAIs had an infection-related mortality rate 2.37 times that of those in the ICU who received adequate coverage. The principal reason for inadequate coverage was multidrug resistance.

The predominant gram-positive MDRO pathogens are MRSA and VRE. Methicillin resistance in *S. aureus* is caused by the production of an alternative penicillin-binding protein (PBP2A) that has a low affinity

表14.3 病原菌对常见抗菌药物的耐药性（数据来自NHSN 2014）

病原菌	抗菌药物	CLABSI	CAUTI	VAP[a]	SSI
金黄色葡萄球菌	苯唑西林，甲氧西林，头孢西丁	50.7%	52.0%	42.4%	42.6%
屎肠球菌	万古霉素	82.2%	85.1%	n/a	58.4%
肺炎克雷伯菌	头孢曲松，头孢他啶，头孢噻肟或头孢吡肟	24.1%	22.5%	21.0%	11.3%
	碳青霉烯类	10.9%	9.5%	10.1%	3.3%
大肠埃希菌	头孢曲松，头孢他啶，头孢噻肟或头孢吡肟	22.2%	16.1%	16.7%	15.3%
	氟喹诺酮类	49.3%	34.8%	30.8%	30.9%
肠杆菌属	头孢曲松，头孢他啶，头孢噻肟或头孢吡肟	36.1%	40.5%	26.9%	27.5%
	碳青霉烯类	6.6%	6.5%	3.2%	3.4%
铜绿假单胞菌	氟喹诺酮类	30.2%	32.6%	31.9%	11.5%
	哌拉西林-他唑巴坦	18.4%	15.5%	19.4%	7.4%
	头孢吡肟或头孢他啶	24.2%	22.5%	25.7%	9.9%
	碳青霉烯类	25.8%	23.9%	28.4%	7.7%
鲍曼不动杆菌	碳青霉烯类	46.6%	64.0%	55.5%	33.3%

改编自 Weiner LM，Webb AK，Limbago B，et al. Antimicrobial-resistant pathogens associated with healthcare-associated infections: summary of data reported to the National Healthcare Safety Network at the Centers for Disease Control and Prevention，2011-2014. Infect Control Hosp Epidemiol. 2016；37（11）：1288-1301.

CAUTI，导管相关尿路感染；CLABSI，中心静脉导管相关感染；NHSN，国家医疗安全网；SSI，手术部位感染；VAP，呼吸机相关肺炎。
[a] 2012。

时间、正确剂量使用正确的药物）、适当的皮肤消毒以及控制血糖（表14.1）。

SSI的处理通常包括开放切口、感染组织清创并通过二次干预促进伤口愈合。是否使用抗生素要根据个体情况而定，取决于伤口外观、全身感染症状、感染深度、宿主免疫系统和手术类型。培养和革兰氏染色结果有助于确定抗菌药物的覆盖范围。对于清洁手术引起的SSI，建议采用可覆盖金黄色葡萄球菌和链球菌的经验治疗方案。对于涉及会阴部、肠道或泌尿生殖道的手术，需要使用覆盖更广泛的抗菌药物来应对革兰氏阴性菌和厌氧菌感染。当SSI发生在手术后48 h内时，化脓性链球菌和梭状芽孢杆菌往往与之有关。

艰难梭菌感染

CDI是指临床表现为腹泻或中毒性巨结肠，或经内镜、手术或病理证实为假膜性结肠炎，同时粪便中艰难梭菌和毒素（A、B）阳性或其中一项阳性。这种结肠感染通常伴有发热和白细胞增多。

艰难梭菌是导致HAI的最常见病原体，约占所有HAIs的12.1%。近年来，艰难梭菌感染的发病率和严重程度一直在稳步上升。大多数报告都认为，新出现的BI/NAP1/027毒株、抗菌药物的过度使用以及住院患者的老龄化对CDI的发病率影响极大。几乎所有抗菌药物都能增加CDI风险。CDI的防控也聚焦在准确诊断、减少传播媒介和合理使用抗菌药物等几方面。诊断CDI必须正确识别感染与定植。诊断管理策略旨在确保只对有明确体征和症状的患者采用适当的检测程序进行诊断评估。预防传播的重点是通过环境清洁和手卫生以及使用基于预防传播的措施（如接触隔离）来减少病原体的环境负荷。

CDI发病率持续上升、很多不同病原菌对抗菌药物耐药性的不断增加，以及具有新作用机制的抗菌药物的缺乏，都凸显了抗菌药物管理的重要性。抗菌药物管理是一种强调优化药物选择、剂量和疗程的策略，可在降低后续并发症风险的同时获得最佳临床疗效。

抗菌药物管理不善的后果包括诱发耐药、CDI和过高的药物支出。不同抗菌药物诱导产生耐药或引发CDI的概率各不相同。抗菌药物管理计划实施的策略包括对医务人员提供教育和指南、在可能的情况下降阶梯或调整经验治疗方案、采用更合适的经验治疗以及某些特殊级抗生素的限制性使用。

有关此专题的深入讨论，请参阅 Goldman-Cecil Medicine 第26版第267章"疑似肠道感染患者的处理方法"和第280章"梭菌感染"。

多重耐药菌

多重耐药菌（MDRO）是指对一类以上抗菌药物产生耐药的微生物，尽管有些病原菌（如MRSA、VRE）的名称意味着只对一种药物产生耐药性。根据NHSN报告的2011—2014年期间的数据，多种常见病原菌的耐药率居高不下（表14.3）。

与敏感菌感染相比，MDRO引起的感染会导致患者住院时间延长、医疗费用增加、死亡率升高。Kollef及其同事发现，抗菌治疗覆盖面不足的HAI患者的感染相关死亡率是接受广覆盖治疗的ICU患者的2.37倍。覆盖面不足的主要原因是病原菌表现为多重耐药。

革兰氏阳性菌中主要的MDRO是MRSA和VRE。金黄色葡萄球菌对甲氧西林耐药是因为产生了一种对β-内酰胺类抗生素的亲和力较低的替代青霉素结合蛋白（PBP2A），这种蛋白在β-内酰胺类抗生素含量充

for β-lactam antibiotics and forms stable peptidoglycan products in the presence of adequate levels of the β-lactam. MRSA infections tend to have worse outcomes compared with methicillin-susceptible *S. aureus* (MSSA), but the typical health care–acquired strains are not necessarily more virulent. However, community-acquired MRSA, the most prevalent of which is the USA-300 strain, tends to be more virulent, and many of these isolates produce the Panton-Valentine leukocidin toxin, which is associated with greater leucocyte destruction and tissue necrosis. The largest reservoirs of MRSA are patients with the greatest contact with the health care system, and most carriers are asymptomatic.

Vancomycin resistance in *S. aureus* is another concern. Vancomycin intermediate-resistant strains, vancomycin heteroresistant strains, and vancomycin-resistant strains have been detected. The intermediate resistance or decreased susceptibility to vancomycin is thought to result from cell wall and biomatrix thickening, making the drug target more difficult to reach. Complete vancomycin resistance occurs by acquisition of the *vanA* gene from VRE. VRE, unlike many MRSA strains, is almost entirely a health care–associated phenomenon. Clusters of *vanA* or *vanB* genes are carried on mobile genetic elements that are readily transmitted between strains. These genes encode peptidoglycan precursors that have a low affinity for vancomycin.

Gram-negative MDROs have a greater tendency to form resistance to multiple antimicrobials, and new antimicrobials to target these pathogens are not available. The Enterobacteriaceae are gram-negative bacteria that usually reside in the gastrointestinal tract, are glucose fermenters, and account for about 29% of HAIs. These organisms tend to be the most common pathogens in SSIs associated with abdominal operations. The non–glucose fermenting organisms, including *P. aeruginosa*, *Acinetobacter baumannii*, and *Stenotrophomonas maltophilia*, account for about 9% of HAIs.

Multidrug-resistant gram-negative bacteria are making their way into the limelight largely due to the emergence of isolates that are resistant to most or all available antimicrobials (e.g., MDROs that exhibit β-lactamases, extended-spectrum β-lactamases (ESBL), carbapenem and fluoroquinolone resistance). The emergence of carbapenem-resistant Enterobacteriaceae (CRE) has become particularly concerning. The predominant carbapenem-resistance mechanisms are the loss of OprD, an outer membrane protein, *Klebsiella pneumoniae* carbapenemases (KPCs), and the metalo-β-lactamases (MBLs), which hydrolyze carbapenems. The New Delhi metalo-β-lactamase 1 (NDM1) is one of the first MBLs to cause outbreaks in the United States. The carbapenemases and MBLs are easily transmissible and tend to be associated with other genes encoding mechanisms of resistance to other antimicrobial classes. Fluoroquinolone resistance can occur by efflux pumps or mutations in genes encoding the drug targets DNA gyrase and topoisomerase IV. Emerging resistance among fungi (e.g., *Candida* spp) is an additional concern. In particular, *Candida auris* has led to outbreaks in ICUs and often harbors high rates of resistance to first- and second-line antifungal agents as well as some routine disinfectants.

Limiting the spread of MDROs in the health care setting should be a comprehensive and system-wide program at any institution. Infection prevention programs should include optimized surveillance practices to identify emerging MDROs and appropriate intervention strategies. The mainstay of these programs includes use of evidence-based prevention practices and antimicrobial stewardship programs. Prevention also necessitates increased communication between hospitals and public health institutions to limit the spread of MDROs, conduct proper surveillance, and implement infection control actions.

SUGGESTED READINGS

Ban KA, Minei JP, Laronga C, et al: American College of Surgeons and Surgical Infection Society: Surgical Site Infection Guidelines, 2016 update, J Am Coll Surg 224(1):59–74, 2017.

Hooton TM, Bradley SF, Cardenas DD, et al: Diagnosis, prevention, and treatment of catheter-associated urinary tract infection in adults: 2009 International Clinical Practice Guidelines from the Infectious Diseases Society of America, Clin Infect Dis 50:625–663, 2010.

Kalil AC, Metersky ML, Klompas M, et al: Management of adults with hospital-acquired and ventilator-associated pneumonia: 2016 Clinical Practice Guidelines by the Infectious Diseases Society of America and the American Thoracic Society, Clin Infect Dis 63(5):e61–e111, 2016.

Kollef MH, Hamilton CW, Ernst FR: Economic impact of ventilator-associated pneumonia in a large matched cohort, Infect Control Hosp Epidemiol 33:250–256, 2012.

Magill SS, O'Leary E, Janelle SJ, et al: Changes in prevalence of health care-associated infections in U.S. Hospitals, N Engl J Med 379(18):1732–1744, 2018.

O'Grady NP, Alexander M, Burns LA, et al: Guidelines for the prevention of intravascular catheter-related infections, Clin Infect Dis 52(9):e162–e193, 2011.

Pronovost P, Needham D, Berenholtz S, et al: An intervention to decrease catheter-related bloodstream infections in the ICU, N Engl J Med 355:2725–2732, 2006.

Scott RD II: The direct medical costs of healthcare-associated infections in U.S. hospitals and the benefits of prevention. Available at: http://www.cdc.gov/hai/pdfs/hai/scott_costpaper.pdf. Accessed November 1, 2014.

Stevens DL, Bisno AL, Chambers HF, et al: Practice guidelines for the diagnosis and management of skin and soft tissue infections: 2014 update by the Infectious Diseases Society of America, Clin Infect Dis 59(2):e10–52, 2014.

Wenzel RP, Edmond MB: Infection control: the case for horizontal rather than vertical interventional programs, Int J Infect Dis 14(Suppl 4):S3–S5, 2010.

足的情况下会形成稳定的肽聚糖产物。与甲氧西林敏感的金黄色葡萄球菌（MSSA）相比，MRSA感染的后果往往更严重，但典型的医疗照护感染菌株并不一定具有更强的毒性。不过，社区获得性MRSA（其中最常见的是USA-300）往往毒性更强，其中许多分离株会产生PVL毒素（杀白细胞毒素），该毒素会导致更严重的白细胞破坏和组织坏死。与医疗系统接触最多的患者是MRSA的最大储存库，大多数携带者都没有症状。

金黄色葡萄球菌对万古霉素耐药是另一个令人担忧的问题。目前已发现万古霉素中等耐药株、万古霉素异质耐药株和万古霉素耐药株。对万古霉素中等耐药或敏感性降低被认为是由于细胞壁和生物基质增厚，使药物更难到达作用靶点所致。对万古霉素完全耐药是通过获得VRE的 vanA 基因产生的。与许多MRSA菌株不同，VRE几乎完全是与医疗照护感染相关。易于在菌株间传播的移动遗传元件上携带有 vanA 或 vanB 基因簇。这些基因编码的肽聚糖前体对万古霉素的亲和力较低。

革兰氏阴性MDRO更容易对多种抗菌药物产生耐药性，目前缺乏针对这些病原菌的新型抗菌药物。肠杆菌科细菌是一大群通常栖息于胃肠道，能发酵葡萄糖的革兰氏阴性杆菌，约占HAI病原菌的29%。这些细菌往往是腹部手术相关SSI中最常见的病原体。非发酵菌，包括铜绿假单胞菌、鲍曼不动杆菌和嗜麦芽窄食单胞菌，约占HAI病原菌的9%。

由于出现了对大多数或所有可用抗菌药物均耐药的菌株，多重耐药的革兰氏阴性菌正成为人们关注的焦点［如产β-内酰胺酶、超广谱β-内酰胺酶（ESBL）、对碳青霉烯类和氟喹诺酮类耐药的MDRO］。耐碳青霉烯类肠杆菌科细菌（CRE）的出现尤其令人担忧。主要的碳青霉烯类耐药机制是外膜蛋白OprD缺失、产可水解碳青霉烯类的肺炎克雷伯菌碳青霉烯酶（KPC）和金属β-内酰胺酶（MBL）。新德里金属β-内酰胺酶1（NDM-1）是最早在美国引起流行暴发的MBL之一。碳青霉烯酶和MBL极容易传播，而且往往与编码对其他抗菌药物耐药的基因相关联。氟喹诺酮类药物耐药机制是药物外排泵或药物靶位DNA回旋酶和拓扑异构酶Ⅳ的编码基因发生突变。真菌（如念珠菌属）新出现的耐药性是另一个令人担忧的问题。尤其是耳念珠菌已导致ICU暴发案例，而且通常对一线和二线抗真菌药物以及一些常规消毒剂具有很高的耐药性。

在任何医疗照护机构，限制MDRO在医疗环境中的传播都应该是一项全面的系统工程。感染防控计划应包括优化的监控措施，用以识别新出现的MDRO并采取适当的干预策略。这些计划的主要内容包括使用循证防控实践和抗菌药物管理计划。防控工作还需要加强医院与公共卫生机构之间的沟通，以限制MDRO的传播、进行适当的监控并实施感染控制措施。

推荐阅读

Ban KA, Minei JP, Laronga C, et al: American College of Surgeons and Surgical Infection Society: Surgical Site Infection Guidelines, 2016 update, J Am Coll Surg 224(1):59–74, 2017.

Hooton TM, Bradley SF, Cardenas DD, et al: Diagnosis, prevention, and treatment of catheter-associated urinary tract infection in adults: 2009 International Clinical Practice Guidelines from the Infectious Diseases Society of America, Clin Infect Dis 50:625–663, 2010.

Kalil AC, Metersky ML, Klompas M, et al: Management of adults with hospital-acquired and ventilator-associated pneumonia: 2016 Clinical Practice Guidelines by the Infectious Diseases Society of America and the American Thoracic Society, Clin Infect Dis 63(5):e61–e111, 2016.

Kollef MH, Hamilton CW, Ernst FR: Economic impact of ventilator-associated pneumonia in a large matched cohort, Infect Control Hosp Epidemiol 33:250–256, 2012.

Magill SS, O'Leary E, Janelle SJ, et al: Changes in prevalence of health care-associated infections in U.S. Hospitals, N Engl J Med 379(18):1732–1744, 2018.

O'Grady NP, Alexander M, Burns LA, et al: Guidelines for the prevention of intravascular catheter-related infections, Clin Infect Dis 52(9):e162–e193, 2011.

Pronovost P, Needham D, Berenholtz S, et al: An intervention to decrease catheter-related bloodstream infections in the ICU, N Engl J Med 355:2725–2732, 2006.

Scott RD II: The direct medical costs of healthcare-associated infections in U.S. hospitals and the benefits of prevention. Available at: http://www.cdc.gov/hai/pdfs/hai/scott_costpaper.pdf. Accessed November 1, 2014.

Stevens DL, Bisno AL, Chambers HF, et al: Practice guidelines for the diagnosis and management of skin and soft tissue infections: 2014 update by the Infectious Diseases Society of America, Clin Infect Dis 59(2):e10–52, 2014.

Wenzel RP, Edmond MB: Infection control: the case for horizontal rather than vertical interventional programs, Int J Infect Dis 14(Suppl 4):S3–S5, 2010.

15

Sexually Transmitted Infections

Philip A. Chan, Susan Cu-Uvin

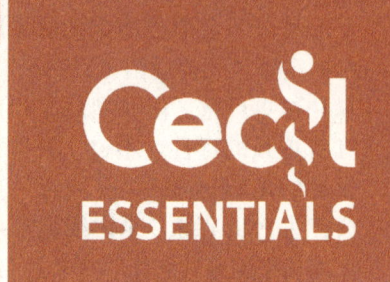

INTRODUCTION

Sexually transmitted infections (STIs) encompass a wide variety of organisms that have been causing human disease for thousands of years. Recognition of STIs can be challenging due to the heterogeneous nature and multiple symptoms of a single disease. Diagnosis and management of STIs is further complicated by underlying social bias and hesitancy by medical providers and patients to discuss issues related to sexuality and disease transmission.

The diagnosis of STIs should be based on a detailed history with special attention to sexual orientation and behaviors, a physical examination, and laboratory confirmation when appropriate. Professional and respectful attitudes by medical providers are essential to obtaining an accurate clinical history pertinent to STIs. Patients often deny risky behavior because of embarrassment or social stigma. Patients may also underestimate risky behaviors, and the diagnosis of STIs should therefore be based on a combination of history, epidemiology, clinical examination, and diagnostic testing.

A detailed sexual history should be obtained from all individuals with a suspected STI. They should be informed that the information is necessary to appropriately diagnose and manage STIs. The history should include sexual preferences for male or female partners; gender identity; the number of main, casual, and one-time partners; the use of condoms, drugs, and alcohol; and use of preexposure prophylaxis (PrEP) for human immunodeficiency virus (HIV) prevention as well as last HIV/STI testing. The history of partners should be elicited, including current symptoms and diagnosed STIs. If possible, counseling and education should be incorporated during the encounter. Prevention topics include abstinence, routine testing, disclosure of STIs to partners, behavior modification (i.e., avoiding risky sexual activities), condom use, prophylactic treatment for STI exposures, and PrEP.

Because of the diverse nature of STIs, it is useful to categorize the infections into a few major groups. There is overlap between different categories, and clinical judgment must be used to accurately diagnose STIs. For example, STIs that typically manifest with an ulcer may occasionally manifest with urethritis. Importantly, many STIs are asymptomatic or have symptoms that go unnoticed. When an individual has one STI, other STIs should be considered. The main categories of STIs are urethritis and cervicitis, genital ulcer disease, and genital warts. Symptomatic individuals with an STI usually fit into one of these categories.

URETHRITIS AND CERVICITIS

Urethritis and cervicitis are characterized by dysuria, burning, and urethral discharge. The discharge may range from barely noticeable to watery or frank pus. Urethritis has been categorized as gonococcal (i.e., caused by *Neisseria gonorrhoeae* and visible on Gram stain) or nongonococcal (i.e., commonly caused by *Chlamydia trachomatis*). Nongonococcal urethritis can be caused by other organisms, many of which are rarely tested for. Urethritis has historically been classified as gonococcal or nongonococcal because *N. gonorrhoeae* can easily be visualized on Gram stain. Most patients with symptomatic urethritis should be treated empirically with antibiotics directed against gonorrheal and chlamydial organisms without waiting for test results.

Chlamydia

Definition and Epidemiology

Chlamydia is the most prevalent bacterial STI in the United States and the world. The infection is caused by the bacterium *C. trachomatis*, which causes 30% to 40% of nongonococcal urethritis and cervicitis cases. In the United States, approximately 1.8 million cases were reported to the Centers for Disease Control and Prevention (CDC) in 2018, with an estimated number of infections that is more than twice the number of reported cases.

Age is a factor. Chlamydia has a 5% to 10% prevalence among adolescents and young adults. Other risk factors include having multiple sex partners, having condomless sex, or living in a lower socioeconomic area. In men, chlamydia is uncommonly associated with complications. In women, untreated chlamydia is associated with potentially severe complications, including pelvic inflammatory disease (PID), ectopic pregnancy, and infertility.

The CDC and USPTF recommends all sexually active women age 24 years or younger and other at-risk women be screened for chlamydia. Screening should also be considered for individuals who have a history of chlamydia or other STIs, have new or multiple sex partners, or exchange sex for drugs or money. All pregnant women should be screened. Men who have sex with men (MSM) should be screened at least annually and more frequently if there are ongoing risk factors such as multiple partners. The rationale for screening men is to prevent symptomatic epididymitis, proctitis, and urethritis. Importantly, MSM should also be screened at sites of exposure, which may include oropharyngeal and rectal screening for men that perform oral sex or have receptive anal sex, respectively. Screening MSM only for urogenital infection will miss up to 80% of chlamydia and gonorrhea infections. The presence of a rectal STI is a notable risk factor for HIV infection.

Pathology

C. trachomatis is an obligate intracellular, gram-negative bacterium that is evolutionary distinct from other bacteria. Several serovars of *C. trachomatis* are associated with human disease. They include serovars A-C (i.e., trachoma or ocular disease), D-K (i.e., anogenital disease), and L1-L3 (i.e., lymphogranuloma venereum [LGV]). *C. trachomatis* exists as an extracellular elementary body before attachment to susceptible epithelial cells and subsequent endocytosis. On entering the cell, the elementary form of *C. trachomatis* reorganizes into a reticulate

性传播感染

李军　刘明娟　译　郑和义　张福杰　张文宏　阮巧玲　审校　张福杰　通审

介绍

性传播感染（STI）涵盖了数千年来导致人类疾病的多种病原体。由于性传播感染的异质性和单一疾病的症状多样性，识别性传播感染具有挑战性。由于潜在的社会偏见以及医患之间讨论性和疾病传播相关问题时的犹豫，性传播感染的诊断和治疗变得更加复杂。

性传播感染的诊断应基于详细的病史，尤其需要关注性取向和性行为、体格检查以及必要时的实验室确认。医护人员的专业素养和尊重态度对于获取准确的性传播感染病史至关重要。患者常因担心尴尬或社会污名化而否认高危性行为。患者也可能会低估高危性行为，因此性传播感染的诊断应结合病史、流行病学、临床检查和诊断测试几个方面综合考虑。

对所有怀疑性传播感染的患者，应详细询问性行为史，并告知患者这些信息对于准确诊断和治疗性传播感染是必要的。采集的病史应包括以下信息：性取向；性别认同；主要、临时和一次性伴侣的数量；避孕套、毒品和酒精的使用情况；为预防人类免疫缺陷病毒（HIV）而使用暴露前预防（PrEP）的情况以及最近一次HIV/STI检测的情况。还应启发患者提供性伴侣的病史，包括当前症状和已确诊的性传播感染。如果可能，应在接诊过程中进行咨询和教育。预防性传播感染的话题包括洁身自好、常规检测、向性伴侣告知性传播感染、性行为修正（如避免高危性行为）、避孕套的使用、性传播感染暴露后的预防性治疗和暴露前预防。

由于性传播感染的多样性，有必要将这类感染分为几个主要类别。不同类别之间存在重叠，需要结合临床评估来准确诊断性传播感染。例如，通常表现为溃疡的性传播感染可能偶尔表现为尿道炎。重要的是，许多性传播感染是无症状的，或症状不明显。当一个人患有一种性传播感染时，也应当考虑其是否患有其他性传播感染。性传播感染的主要类别包括尿道炎和宫颈炎、生殖器溃疡性疾病和生殖器疣。有症状的性传播感染患者通常属于其中一类。

尿道炎和宫颈炎

尿道炎和宫颈炎的特征是排尿困难、烧灼感和尿道分泌物。分泌物从几乎察觉不到至稀薄水样或明显的脓样不等。尿道炎可分为淋球菌性尿道炎（由淋病奈瑟球菌引起，在革兰氏染色中可见）和非淋菌性尿道炎（通常由沙眼衣原体引起）。非淋菌性尿道炎也可由其他病原体引起，其中许多病原体很少进行检测。因为淋球菌在革兰氏染色中容易被观察到，尿道炎历来被分类为淋菌性或非淋菌性。对于大多数有症状的尿道炎患者，应在等待检测结果前，经验性使用针对淋球菌和衣原体的抗生素治疗。

衣原体

定义和流行病学

衣原体感染是美国及全球最常见的细菌性性传播感染。该感染由沙眼衣原体引起，导致30%～40%的非淋菌性尿道炎和宫颈炎病例。在美国，2018年美国疾病控制与预防中心（CDC）报告的患者是180万例，实际感染数量预计为报告病例数的两倍以上。

年龄是一个危险因素。沙眼衣原体在青少年和年轻人中的患病率为5%～10%。其他危险因素包括：多个性伴侣、无安全套性行为或生活在社会经济水平较低的地区。在男性中，沙眼衣原体很少导致相关并发症。但在女性中，未经治疗的沙眼衣原体感染可能导致潜在的严重并发症，包括盆腔炎（PID）、异位妊娠和不孕症。

美国CDC和美国预防医学工作组（UsPTF）建议对所有24岁及以下的性活跃女性和其他高风险女性进行沙眼衣原体筛查。对既往沙眼衣原体或其他性传播感染者、有新性伴侣或多个性伴侣，或以性服务换取毒品、金钱的个体也应考虑进行筛查。所有孕妇应进行筛查。男男性行为者（MSM）应至少每年筛查一次，如果存在多个性伴侣等持续的高风险因素，则应更频繁地进行筛查。筛查男性的目的是预防症状性附睾炎、直肠炎和尿道炎。重要的是，对于男男性行为者，还应对暴露部位进行筛查，可能包括对进行口交或接受肛交的男性分别进行口咽部和直肠筛查。如果仅对男男性行为者进行泌尿生殖系统感染筛查，对沙眼衣原体和淋病感染的漏诊将高达80%。存在直肠性传播感染是HIV感染的显著危险因素。

病理学

沙眼衣原体是一种专性细胞内寄生的革兰氏阴性菌，在进化上与其他细菌有显著不同。沙眼衣原体的某些血清型与人类疾病相关，包括血清型A-C（如沙眼或眼部疾病）、D-K（如肛门生殖器疾病）和L1-L3（如性病性淋巴肉芽肿，LGV）。沙眼衣原体以原体形式进入细胞，在空泡内重组为功能活跃的网状体，进而导

body within vacuoles that is functionally active, leading to growth and replication of the organism.

Clinical Presentation

Chlamydia may manifest with signs and symptoms ranging from none (most common) to life-threatening PID in women. When individuals have symptoms, the most common is urethritis in men and cervicitis in women. The incubation period varies but is usually 7 to 14 days after exposure.

Among men, 40% to more than 90% of chlamydia cases may be asymptomatic. Urethritis usually manifests as dysuria or discharge. *C. trachomatis* and *N. gonorrhoeae* infections are common causes of epididymitis in younger men. The infection typically manifests with unilateral testicular pain, swelling, and tenderness. *C. trachomatis* infection may also cause prostatitis and proctitis; the latter is typically found in MSM. The symptoms of proctitis in MSM should raise the possibility of LGV. The rates of transmission from infected men to women are as high as 65%.

In women and men, more than 85% of infections are asymptomatic. When symptomatic, *C. trachomatis* infection in women can be difficult to diagnose due to the nonspecific nature of symptoms. The classic manifestation is cervicitis, which can cause discharge, bleeding, pelvic pain, cervical friability, and ulcers. Complications of chlamydia include chronic pelvic pain, infertility, ectopic pregnancy, and PID. The lifetime prevalence of PID due to *C. trachomatis* infection depends on the population studied but is approximately 4%. PID usually manifests as abdominal or pelvic pain, cervical motion tenderness, and uterine or adnexal tenderness. Infection may also cause perihepatitis (i.e., Fitz-Hugh–Curtis syndrome), which is inflammation of the liver capsule. It occurs in 5% to 15% of PID cases. Chlamydia is the leading cause of preventable infertility worldwide.

Chlamydia may cause conjunctivitis and ocular trachomatis, the most common cause of preventable blindness worldwide. The disease also may manifest with pharyngitis and LGV. Classically a disease endemic in Africa, Southeast Asia, and the Caribbean, LGV has been identified in the United States and Europe, particularly among MSM with symptoms of proctitis. Typically, LGV manifests with genital ulceration and inguinal lymphadenopathy. Recognition of LGV is important given the longer duration of treatment.

Diagnosis and Differential Diagnosis

C. trachomatis cannot be routinely cultured on growth media, which has made diagnosis difficult. The introduction of nucleic acid amplification testing (NAAT) was a major advance and is now the standard diagnostic test. NAAT encompasses several laboratory methods including polymerase chain reaction (PCR), transcription-mediated amplification, and strand displacement amplification. The reported sensitivity of NAAT is 80% to 90%, with a specificity of 99%. The test may be performed on urine and vaginal or urethral (men) endocervical swab specimens. NAAT may also be performed on rectal and pharyngeal swab specimens.

Individuals who test positive and are treated for chlamydia should not be retested for at least 3 weeks after treatment. NAAT may remain positive during this time due to remnant material that does not signify persistent infection. Repeat testing to demonstrate cure should be performed for pregnant women or those with a concern about persistent infection. Individuals are usually retested at 3 months and then periodically depending on risk behaviors. Having had an STI places individuals at risk for becoming infected again. For individuals with multiple partners, including MSM, general STI testing that includes chlamydia is recommended every 3 to 6 months.

Treatment

Standard treatment regimens for urethritis or cervicitis due to chlamydia are azithromycin (1 g taken once orally) or doxycycline (100 mg twice daily for 7 days). These two medications are effective and cure more than 95% of infections. Azithromycin should be used in situations where adherence is a concern given the simplicity of dosing, which facilitates adherence. However, doxycycline may be more effective in achieving cure. Azithromycin can also be used in pregnancy. Other drugs that are effective in treating chlamydia include quinolones and penicillin. Sulfonamides (e.g., Bactrim) and cephalosporins should not be used. Doxycycline, ofloxacin, and levofloxacin are contraindicated in pregnant women.

Epididymitis due to chlamydia should be treated with doxycycline (100 mg taken orally twice per day for 10 days). Treatment for LGV proctitis depends on the severity of symptoms and should include doxycycline (100 mg orally twice each day for up to 3 weeks). In women, PID should be treated with ceftriaxone (250 mg given once intramuscularly) to cover gonorrhea and doxycycline (100 mg taken orally twice each day for 14 days) for chlamydia. Women who have concerning symptoms should be hospitalized and started on intravenous antibiotics, including cefoxitin (2 g given intravenously every 6 hours) or cefotetan (2 g given intravenously every 12 hours) and doxycycline (100 mg taken orally every 12 hours) (if not pregnant). Alternative treatment regimens include clindamycin (900 mg given intravenously every 8 hours) and gentamicin (2-mg/kg loading dose followed by 1.5 mg/kg every 8 hours). The duration depends on clinical improvement but is usually 2 weeks.

Prognosis

The natural history of untreated *C. trachomatis* infection varies. Individuals may remain asymptomatic for long periods, and the infection may resolve spontaneously or progress to symptoms and complications. Approximately 20% of individuals diagnosed with chlamydia but without symptoms may clear the infection before returning for treatment. Infection does not translate to protective immunity, and reinfection is common (10% to 20%). Therefore treatment of sex partners is important. In many areas, expedited partner therapy is allowed, and medical providers may prescribe treatment for sex partners without seeing them.

Gonorrhea
Definition and Epidemiology

Gonorrhea is caused by the bacterium *N. gonorrhoeae* and is the second most common reportable STI in the United States behind chlamydia. Similar to chlamydia, gonorrhea is a significant cause of urethritis in men and cervicitis in women and has the same complications. In the United States, the rate of gonorrhea declined in 2009 to a nadir of 98.1 cases per 100,000 people. Much of this was attributed to screening and treatment programs. Since 2009, however, cases of gonorrhea have increased each year to 104.2 cases per 100,000, with almost 600,000 cases reported in 2018.

Most individuals diagnosed with gonorrhea are adolescents or young adults. Cases among males are now more common than among females. MSM have also emerged as an important at-risk group. Risk factors for infection include younger age, multiple sexual partners, race or ethnicity, low socioeconomic status, and previous STIs. African Americans and Hispanic/Latinos have significantly higher rates of gonorrhea than white individuals in the United States.

Pathology

N. gonorrhoeae is a gram-negative bacterium with an outer membrane, peptidoglycan cell wall, and cytoplasmic membrane. Several

致该病原体的生长和复制。

临床表现

衣原体感染的临床症状与体征从最为常见的无症状到危及生命的女性盆腔炎不等。当感染者出现症状时，最常见的是男性尿道炎和女性宫颈炎。潜伏期长短不一，但通常为接触后的7～14天。

在男性中，40%～90%以上的衣原体感染可能是无症状的。尿道炎通常表现为排尿困难或分泌物。沙眼衣原体和淋病奈瑟球菌感染是年轻男性患附睾炎的常见病因。感染通常表现为单侧睾丸疼痛、肿胀和触痛。沙眼衣原体感染还可能导致前列腺炎和直肠炎；后者通常见于男男性行为者。在男男性行为者中，直肠炎症状的出现应考虑到性病性淋巴肉芽肿的可能。男性感染者传染给女性的概率高达65%。

在女性中，超过85%是无症状感染。当出现症状时，女性的沙眼衣原体感染由于症状缺乏特异性而有时难以诊断。典型的表现是宫颈炎，这种炎症可能引起分泌物增多、出血、盆腔疼痛、宫颈脆弱和溃疡。衣原体感染的并发症包括慢性盆腔疼痛、不孕、异位妊娠和盆腔炎。沙眼衣原体感染导致终生盆腔炎的患病率因研究人群不同而异，但大约为4%。盆腔炎通常表现为腹痛或盆腔痛、宫颈举痛以及子宫或附件区压痛。感染还可能导致肝周炎（即Fitz-Hugh-Curtis综合征），即肝包膜的炎症，在盆腔炎病例中发生率为5%～15%。衣原体感染是全球可预防性不孕的主要原因。

衣原体可引起结膜炎和沙眼，是全球可预防失明的最常见原因。衣原体感染还可能表现为咽炎和性病性淋巴肉芽肿。性病性淋巴肉芽肿传统上为非洲、东南亚和加勒比地区的地方性疾病，但在美国和欧洲也发现了性病性淋巴肉芽肿，尤其是在有直肠炎症状的男男性行为者中。通常，性病性淋巴肉芽肿表现为生殖器溃疡和腹股沟淋巴结肿大。由于治疗时间较长，识别性病性淋巴肉芽肿非常重要。

诊断和鉴别诊断

沙眼衣原体无法在培养基上进行常规培养，因此诊断困难。核酸扩增试验（NAAT）的引入是一项重大进展，目前已成为标准诊断检测方法。核酸扩增试验包括多种实验室方法，如聚合酶链反应（PCR）、转录介导扩增和链置换扩增。据报道，核酸扩增试验的敏感性为80%～90%，特异性为99%。该检测可以对尿液、阴道或尿道（男性）通过宫颈拭子取材的样本进行检测，也可对直肠拭子和咽拭子取材的标本进行检测。

检测结果阳性并接受抗衣原体治疗的患者在治疗后至少3周内不应接受复检。核酸扩增试验在此期间可能因为体内残留物质而仍显示阳性，但并不代表持续感染。对孕妇或担心持续感染的患者，应进行重复检测以确认治愈。通常在3个月时进行复检，然后根据高危行为情况定期复检。曾有性传播感染史的患者再次感染风险较高。对有多个性伴侣（包括男男性行为者）的个体，建议每3～6个月进行一次包括衣原体在内的常规性传播感染检测。

治疗

衣原体感染引起的尿道炎或宫颈炎的标准治疗方案是阿奇霉素（1 g，单次口服）或多西环素（100 mg，每日两次口服，连续7天）。这两种药物很有效，可治愈95%以上的衣原体感染。在依从性存在问题的情况下应使用阿奇霉素，因为其简单的给药方式有助于提高患者依从性。但多西环素可能在治愈方面更有效。妊娠时阿奇霉素也可服用。其他有效治疗衣原体的药物包括喹诺酮类和青霉素。不应使用磺胺类药物（如甲氧苄啶-磺胺甲噁唑）和头孢菌素。多西环素、氧氟沙星和左氧氟沙星在孕妇中禁用。

衣原体引起的附睾炎应使用多西环素（100 mg，口服，每日2次，连续10天）。以直肠炎为表现的性病性淋巴肉芽肿的治疗应视症状的严重程度而定，应包括多西环素（100 mg，口服，每日2次，最多连续3周）。女性盆腔炎应使用头孢曲松（250 mg，单次肌内注射）覆盖淋病，使用多西环素（100 mg，口服，每日两次，连续14天）覆盖衣原体。症状严重的女性应住院并开始静脉输注抗生素，包括头孢西丁（2 g，每6 h一次，静脉输注）或头孢替坦（2 g，每12 h一次，静脉输注），若未怀孕，加用多西环素（100 mg，口服，每12 h一次）。替代治疗方案包括克林霉素（900 mg，每8 h一次，静脉输注）和庆大霉素（初始剂量2 mg/kg，之后每8 h 1.5 mg/kg），治疗时间取决于临床改善情况，但通常为2周。

预后

未经治疗的沙眼衣原体感染的自然病程各不相同。患者可能长时间无症状，感染可能自发消退或进展为临床症状和并发症。被诊断为无症状衣原体感染者中，大约20%患者在接受治疗前能自行清除感染。感染并不意味着获得保护性免疫，重复感染很常见（10%～20%）。因此，治疗性伴侣很重要。许多地区允许对患者的性伴侣进行快速治疗，医护人员可以在未见到患者性伴侣的情况下为其开具治疗。

淋病

定义和流行病学

淋病由淋病奈瑟球菌引起，是美国报道的第二常见性传播感染，发病率仅次于衣原体。与衣原体类似，淋病是男性尿道炎和女性宫颈炎的重要原因，并具有相同的并发症。在美国，2009年淋病的发病率降至最低点，为98.1/10万，很大程度上得益于筛查和治疗项目的开展。然而，自2009年以来，淋病病例逐年增加，到2018年，发病率上升至104.2/10万人，报告病例接近60万例。

大多数诊断为淋病的个体是青少年或年轻人。目前男性病例比女性病例更为常见。男男性行为者也已成为重要的高危群体。感染的危险因素包括：年轻、多个性伴侣、种族或民族、社会经济地位低和既往性传播感染史。美国非裔和西班牙裔/拉美裔的淋病发病率显著高于白人。

病理学

淋病奈瑟球菌是一种革兰氏阴性菌，具有外膜、肽

components contribute to the virulence of the organism. Attachment to columnar epithelial cells is facilitated by pili, which extend from the cell surface and allow entry into the host cell by endocytosis. Organisms without pili are thought to be noninfectious. Gonococci are able to replicate within host epithelial cells and phagocytes. After mucosal infection, immune activation of neutrophils produces significant inflammation and exudate as pus.

Clinical Presentation

Gonorrhea is transmitted during sex with an infected partner. The risk of infection ranges from 20% to 50% per single act of sexual intercourse and increases with multiple acts. The incubation period is 2 to 7 days. When symptomatic, individuals with gonorrhea tend to have more purulent discharge than individuals with nongonococcal urethritis. In men, urethritis is the most common symptom at clinical presentation. Ten percent of men may be asymptomatic. Other manifestations of gonorrhea include epididymitis, proctitis, and pharyngitis. Rare but severe complications include abscesses and urethral strictures.

Between 50% and 80% of women with gonorrhea are asymptomatic. Typical symptoms include those of cervicitis, such as pelvic or adnexal pain, discharge, dysuria, and abnormal bleeding. As in men, gonorrhea can cause proctitis and pharyngitis in women. Most of these infections are asymptomatic. The most common complication of gonorrhea is PID. It may result in severe infection, chronic pelvic pain, and infertility. Infection during pregnancy may lead to complications such as premature labor, rupture of membranes, and spontaneous abortions.

Gonorrhea infection may also be associated with perihepatitis (Fitz-Hugh–Curtis syndrome). In less than 3% of individuals, disseminated gonococcal infection can lead to a classic triad of tenosynovitis (i.e., affecting multiple tendons), dermatitis (i.e., painless, few transient pustular lesions), and polyarthralgias (i.e., nonpurulent forms). Alternatively, individuals with disseminated infection may have purulent arthritis alone. Clinical presentation usually includes fever and other nonspecific systemic symptoms.

Diagnosis and Differential Diagnosis

N. gonorrhoeae is a gram-negative diplococcic that can be visualized easily on Gram stain of purulent material. However, the most common method of diagnosis is NAAT, which has more than 98% sensitivity. NAAT testing can be performed on urethral, cervical, oropharyngeal, and rectal specimens. The major disadvantage of NAAT is the inability to evaluate antibiotic susceptibilities. *N. gonorrhoeae* can also be cultured from swab specimens from the rectum, urethra, pharynx, or cervix. Samples often contain many different microorganisms. Selective media such as modified Thayer-Martin media (with vancomycin, colistin, nystatin, and trimethoprim) is used to inhibit growth of indigenous flora. The sensitivity of cultures varies from 65% to 95%. When drug resistance is a concern, cultures should be sent for sensitivity testing.

Treatment

Antibiotic resistance of *N. gonorrhoeae* continues to be a worldwide problem. In the last decade, treatment of gonorrhea has been complicated by an increase in higher minimum inhibitory concentrations (MICs) for commonly used antibiotics, including first-line cephalosporins. The resistance patterns of gonorrhea vary by region.

To address the concern of antibiotic resistance, uncomplicated urogenital gonorrhea should be treated with dual therapy; one agent should be ceftriaxone (250 mg given once intramuscularly) and the other azithromycin (1 g taken once orally). This regimen is 99% effective in curing gonorrhea. Azithromycin can also treat concurrent chlamydia. Alternatively, doxycycline (100 mg taken orally twice each day for 7 days) may be given instead of azithromycin. High resistance rates (10% to 20%) limit the use of tetracyclines. Cefixime (400 mg taken once orally) should be reserved only if ceftriaxone is unavailable and given with azithromycin (1 g taken once orally). Cefixime may be less effective in the treatment of pharyngeal gonorrhea. In patients allergic to ceftriaxone, dual treatment with single doses of gentamicin (240 mg intramuscular once) and azithromycin (2 g taken orally once) may be used cautiously. Gastrointestinal side effects are common with the higher dose of azithromycin.

Other antibiotics with activity against gonorrhea include spectinomycin. Antibiotics that should not be used to treat gonorrhea due to resistance include penicillins and fluoroquinolones. Disseminated or complicated gonococcal infections should be treated with intravenous ceftriaxone and doxycycline or azithromycin. The duration of these regimens depends on the clinical course and response to therapy.

Prognosis

Gonorrhea is curable with proper antibiotic therapy. Untreated disease often resolves over several weeks, but prompt treatment halts transmission and prevents complications.

Vaginitis
Definition and Epidemiology

The term *vaginitis* refers to disorders of the vagina characterized by inflammation or irritation of the vulva and an abnormal vaginal discharge. Although a separate entity from urethritis, there is significant overlap of symptoms and the organisms that cause vaginitis and urethritis. The three main types of infectious vaginitis are *Candida* vulvovaginitis, bacterial vaginosis, and trichomoniasis. The latter two are strongly associated with sexual transmission.

Trichomoniasis is the most common nonviral STI worldwide. In the United States, 3.1% of women between the ages of 14 and 49 years are infected with *Trichomonas vaginalis*. Screening is recommended for trichomoniasis in women who are at high risk for other STIs as determined by commonly accepted measures (i.e., having new or multiple partners). Screening for bacterial vaginosis in pregnant women is a controversial topic.

Pathology

Candida albicans and *Candida glabrata* are the most common organisms responsible for *Candida* vulvovaginitis. These species may colonize asymptomatic women but their presence does not necessarily mean infection. Symptomatic cases are caused by an overgrowth of the species and penetration of the superficial vaginal epithelial cells. Overgrowth can result from increased estrogen levels or suppression of other vaginal flora by antibiotics.

Trichomoniasis is caused by the protozoan *T. vaginalis*, which infects the squamous epithelium in the urogenital tract. *T. vaginalis* is not normally present in the vagina and has an incubation period of a few days.

Bacterial vaginosis is caused by a variety of organisms flourishing in the vaginal ecosystem in conjunction with a reduction of normally occurring lactobacilli. The bacterium *Gardnerella vaginalis* is especially prominent in cases of bacterial vaginosis and is thought to infect the vaginal epithelium, creating a biofilm to which other bacteria may adhere. *G. vaginalis* is also the organism thought to play the most likely role in sexual transmission of bacterial vaginosis.

聚糖细胞壁和细胞质膜。多个组成成分共同决定了这种微生物的毒力。从细胞表面伸出的菌毛协助细菌黏附于柱状上皮细胞，使细菌通过内吞作用进入宿主细胞。没有菌毛的细菌被认为是不具备传染性的。淋病奈瑟球菌能够在宿主上皮细胞和吞噬细胞内复制。黏膜感染后，中性粒细胞的免疫激活产生显著的炎症和脓液。

临床表现

淋病是通过与感染者性伴侣的性接触传播的。单次性交感染风险为20%～50%，并随着性交次数的增加而上升。潜伏期为2～7天。当出现症状时，淋病患者的脓性分泌物通常比非淋菌性尿道炎患者更多。对男性患者而言，尿道炎是临床表现中最为常见的症状。约10%的男性可能无症状。淋病的其他表现包括附睾炎、直肠炎和咽炎。罕见但严重的并发症包括脓肿和尿道狭窄。

在女性中，50%～80%淋病无症状。典型症状包括宫颈炎，如盆腔或附件区疼痛、分泌物、排尿困难和异常出血。与男性类似，淋病在女性中也可以引起直肠炎和咽炎，这些感染大多无症状。淋病最常见的并发症是盆腔炎，可导致严重感染、慢性盆腔疼痛和不孕症。妊娠期间的感染可能导致早产、胎膜早破和自然流产等并发症。

淋病感染还可能与肝周炎（Fitz-Hugh-Curtis综合征）相关。在不到3%的病例中，播散性淋病感染可以导致经典的三联征：腱鞘炎（影响多条肌腱）、皮炎（无痛、散在的暂时性脓疱性皮损）和多关节痛（非化脓性），或者，播散性感染的患者可能仅表现为化脓性关节炎。临床表现通常包括发热和其他非特异性全身症状。

诊断和鉴别诊断

淋病奈瑟球菌是一种革兰氏阴性双球菌，在脓液的革兰氏染色中易于观察到。然而，最常见的诊断方法是核酸扩增试验，其敏感性超过98%。核酸扩增试验可以对尿道、宫颈、口咽和直肠的标本进行化验。核酸扩增试验的主要缺点是无法评估抗生素敏感性。淋病奈瑟球菌也可以从直肠、尿道、咽喉或宫颈的拭子样本中培养出来。这些样本通常含有许多不同的微生物。使用改良的Thayer-Martin培养基（含有万古霉素、多黏菌素、制霉菌素和甲氧苄啶）作为选择性培养基，可用于抑制定植菌群的生长。培养的敏感性为65%～95%。当我们关注耐药性时，应将培养物送检以进行药物敏感性测试。

治疗

淋病奈瑟球菌的抗生素耐药性仍然是全球性问题。在过去十年中，由于包括一线头孢菌素在内的常用抗生素最低抑菌浓度（MIC）的上升，淋病的治疗变得更加困难。淋病的耐药谱因地区而异。

为应对抗生素耐药性问题，无并发症的泌尿生殖道淋病应采用二联治疗方案，其中一种药物应为头孢曲松（250 mg，单次肌内注射），另一种药物为阿奇霉素（1 g，单次口服）。这方案对淋病的治愈有效率为99%。阿奇霉素还能同时治疗合并的衣原体感染。或者，可以使用多西环素（100 mg，口服，每日2次，持续7天）代替阿奇霉素。高达10%～20%的耐药率限制了四环素类药物的应用。仅在无法获得头孢曲松的情况下，才应使用头孢克肟（400 mg，单次口服），并与阿奇霉素（1 g，单次口服）联合应用。头孢克肟治疗咽部淋病的效果可能较差。对头孢曲松过敏的患者，可以谨慎选用庆大霉素（240 mg，单次肌内注射）和阿奇霉素（2 g，单次口服）的二联治疗。较高剂量的阿奇霉素常见副作用是胃肠道不良反应。

其他对淋病有效的抗生素包括大观霉素。由于耐药性，不应使用青霉素和氟喹诺酮类药物治疗淋病。播散性或复杂性淋病感染应使用静脉输注头孢曲松和多西环素或阿奇霉素进行治疗。治疗方案的持续时间取决于临床病程和对治疗的反应。

预后

使用合适的抗生素治疗，淋病是可以治愈的。未经治疗的情况下通常在几周内自愈，但及时治疗可以阻止传播并预防并发症。

阴道炎

定义与流行病学

阴道炎一词指的是以外阴炎症或刺激和异常阴道分泌物为特征的阴道疾病。虽然阴道炎与尿道炎是两种不同的疾病，但阴道炎和尿道炎的症状和致病菌有很大的重叠。三种主要的感染性阴道炎类型是念珠菌性外阴阴道炎、细菌性阴道病和滴虫病。后两种与性传播密切相关。

滴虫病是全球最常见的非病毒性性传播感染。在美国，14～49岁女性中，3.1%感染了阴道毛滴虫。建议对被公认的确定有其他性传播感染高危因素（如有新性伴侣或多个性伴侣）的女性进行滴虫病筛查。是否对孕妇进行细菌性阴道病筛查有争议。

病理学

白念珠菌和光滑念珠菌是引起念珠菌性外阴阴道炎的最常见病原体。这些菌种可能在无症状的女性中定植，但菌种的存在并不一定意味着感染。有症状患者是这些菌种的过度生长和侵入浅表阴道上皮细胞引起的。念珠菌的过度生长可能是雌激素水平升高或抗生素抑制其他阴道菌群所致。

滴虫病由原生动物阴道毛滴虫感染引起，滴虫会感染泌尿生殖道的鳞状上皮。阴道中通常不会存在毛滴虫，其潜伏期为几天。

伴随着正常存在的乳酸杆菌的减少，多种在阴道生态系统中繁殖的微生物引起细菌性阴道病。在细菌性阴道病病例中，阴道加德纳菌非常重要，被认为能感染阴道上皮细胞，并形成供其他细菌附着的生物膜。阴道加德纳菌也被认为在细菌性阴道病的性传播中最有可能发挥作用。

Clinical Presentation

Symptoms of vaginitis may include pruritus (i.e., primary feature of *Candida* vulvovaginitis); a change in the volume, color, or odor of discharge; burning; irritation; erythema; dyspareunia; spotting; and dysuria. In the case of trichomoniasis and bacterial vaginosis, infection is often asymptomatic but can be associated with sex. Symptomatic trichomoniasis in women most commonly includes a purulent vaginal discharge, erythema, and irritation of the vulva. An abnormal odor is also often associated with infection.

Bacterial vaginosis manifests with milder symptoms of irritation and erythema and is rarely associated with dysuria or dyspareunia. Patients with bacterial vaginosis most commonly have a notably fishy odor in the vaginal discharge, which may also be abnormally colored or textured.

Diagnosis and Differential Diagnosis

Laboratory testing and microscopy are needed for a diagnosis of vaginitis. Examination of vaginal pH can be a helpful differentiating tool. *Candida* vulvovaginitis typically does not cause a change in vaginal pH, whereas bacterial vaginosis and trichomoniasis do increase the pH up to 6. The identification of *Candida* organisms on a wet mount or culture of discharge from women with characteristic clinical symptoms indicates *Candida* vulvovaginitis.

The diagnosis of trichomoniasis may be based on laboratory testing (NAAT), motile trichomonads on a wet mount, or positive culture results. NAAT testing for vaginitis is also available that evaluates for *Candida*, trichomoniasis, and bacterial vaginosis. Amsel criteria or Nugent criteria may be used to diagnose bacterial vaginosis when Gram stain or microscopy is not available.

Treatment

Vaginitis is curable with proper antibiotic therapy. Trichomoniasis is treated with metronidazole (500 mg orally twice each day for 7 days or 2 g taken orally once) or tinidazole. Pregnant women can be treated with 2 g of metronidazole in a single dose at any stage of pregnancy. The safety of tinidazole has not been fully established.

Treatment of all recent sexual partners is recommended because trichomoniasis is almost exclusively transmitted by sexual contact. The same twice-daily regimen of 500 mg of oral metronidazole is the primary treatment for bacterial vaginosis; however, the single 2-g oral dose is *not* recommended for treatment of bacterial vaginosis. Treatment of *Candida* vulvovaginitis with a single 150-mg dose of fluconazole is highly effective. Use of a topical agent depends on whether the case is considered complicated or uncomplicated. Only topical azole therapies, applied for 7 days, are recommended for use by pregnant women.

Prognosis

Bacterial vaginosis is treatable with various antibiotics, but the primary concern is failure of normal *Lactobacillus* flora to reestablish colonization in the vagina. This leads to repeated infections and necessitates prolonged treatment. Oral and vaginal administration of *Lactobacillus* bacteria is sometimes recommended. Bacterial vaginosis increases risk of infection with HIV, herpes simplex virus type 2 (HSV-2), and *N. gonorrhoeae*, making treatment critical for the management of other STIs.

Other Causes of Nongonococcal Urethritis

There are several other known causes of urethritis and cervicitis and likely more that are unknown. Significant causes may include *Mycoplasma genitalium*, HSV-1/2, *Treponema pallidum*, adenovirus, and *Ureaplasma urealyticum*. *U. urealyticum* can be part of the normal flora, and its role in urethritis has not been validated.

The most common of these organisms is *M. genitalium*. It is a bacterium that lacks a cell wall, cannot be Gram stained, and is very difficult to grow in culture. The organism accounts for 15% to 25% of men with nongonococcal urethritis in the United States and is thought to be a cause of cervicitis and PID in women. NAAT testing of urine, urethral, vaginal, and cervical specimens for *M. genitalium* is available and is the recommended diagnostic test. Testing for *M. genitalium* should be considered for individuals with persistent urethritis or cervicitis. Treatment of *M. genitalium* is complicated by concerns of emerging resistance across the world. Empirical treatment of symptomatic individuals includes azithromycin (1 g taken orally once or a 500-mg dose followed by 250 mg daily for 4 days; a longer duration of azithromycin may be more effective). Moxifloxacin (400 mg daily for 7 to 14 days) is also effective and should be used if individuals have persistent symptoms.

GENITAL ULCER DISEASE

Genital ulcers are a major manifestation of several STIs. Genital ulcers are best classified as painful (e.g., HSV, chancroid) or nonpainful (e.g., syphilis). LGV due to *Chlamydia* also manifests with ulcerations. Ulcers may be classified as single (e.g., syphilis, chancroid) or multiple or grouped (e.g., HSV-1/2). All of these STIs manifest with diverse signs and symptoms, and clinical examination alone may be inadequate for accurate diagnosis (Table 15.1).

Syphilis
Definition and Epidemiology

Syphilis is caused by the spirochete *T. pallidum*, which can result in a wide spectrum of clinical disease. At the beginning of the 20th century, it was thought that an astounding 10% of the general population in the United States had syphilis. The CDC began reporting rates of syphilis in 1941. The rates peaked in the early 1940s at almost 600,000 cases and subsequently reached a nadir in 2000 with a rate of 2.1 cases per 100,000 people in the general population. However, since that time, the number of reported syphilis cases has been increasing. The major at-risk group is MSM, but the disease is observed in people across all ages, genders, sexual orientations, socioeconomic status, and racial and ethnic classes.

The resurgence of a generalized syphilis epidemic among MSM with HIV infection has had important consequences. Clinicians at STI clinics and those treating individuals with HIV need to be aware of guidelines for the diagnosis and treatment of syphilis in this population. Furthermore, clinicians need to be aware of less common presentations of syphilis and have a high degree of suspicion. Given the increasing number of MSM living with HIV, it is not uncommon to see coinfection in this population. All MSM, regardless of HIV status, should be considered for syphilis screening on an annual basis and more frequently if they have other risk factors.

Pathology

T. pallidum organisms are thinly coiled bacteria that move in a corkscrew motion. *T. pallidum* cannot be easily cultured, hindering diagnosis and study of the organism. *T. pallidum* infects and penetrates mucosal membranes, resulting in the classic chancre lesion. The organism then infects local lymph nodes and disseminates systemically. The median incubation period is approximately 3 weeks. In more than 60% of infected individuals, syphilis does not progress to tertiary stages. Immune host factors are thought to contribute to the development of tertiary syphilis.

Clinical Presentation

Primary syphilis classically involves the genitals, although lesions may also be observed in the rectum or oropharynx. The estimated risk of

临床表现

阴道炎的症状可能包括瘙痒（念珠菌性外阴阴道炎的主要特征），分泌物的量、颜色或气味改变，灼热感，刺激感，红斑，性交痛，点状出血以及排尿困难。滴虫性阴道炎和细菌性阴道病的感染通常没有症状，但可能与性传播相关。女性滴虫病最常见的症状是脓性阴道分泌物、外阴红斑和刺激感。异常气味也常与感染相关。

细菌性阴道病表现为较轻微的刺激和红斑症状，很少伴有排尿困难或性交疼痛。细菌性阴道病患者的阴道分泌物通常有明显的鱼腥味，颜色或质地也可能异常。

诊断和鉴别诊断

阴道炎的诊断需要实验室检测和显微镜观察。阴道 pH 的检测可以作为一种有用的鉴别方法。念珠菌性外阴阴道炎通常不会引起阴道 pH 的变化，而细菌性阴道病和滴虫病则会使 pH 升高到 6。对于具有典型临床症状的女性，在分泌物湿片镜检或培养物中观察到念珠菌，则表明存在念珠菌性外阴阴道炎。

滴虫病的诊断可以通过实验室检测（核酸扩增试验）、湿片镜检下观察到的活动性毛滴虫或阳性的培养结果来确定。针对阴道炎的核酸扩增试验也可以评估念珠菌、滴虫病和细菌性阴道病。当无法进行革兰氏染色或显微镜检查时，可以使用 Amsel 标准或 Nugent 标准来诊断细菌性阴道病。

治疗

经过适当的抗生素治疗阴道炎可治愈。滴虫病的治疗包括甲硝唑（500 mg，口服，每日 2 次，连续 7 天；或 2 g 单次口服）或替硝唑。孕妇可以在妊娠期任何阶段接受单次的 2 g 甲硝唑治疗。替硝唑的安全性尚未完全确定。

建议对患者近期的所有性伴侣进行治疗，因为滴虫病几乎完全通过性接触传播。对细菌性阴道病的首选治疗也是每日 2 次口服 500 mg 的甲硝唑，但不推荐单次口服 2 g 剂量来治疗细菌性阴道病。使用单次 150 mg 剂量的氟康唑治疗念珠菌性外阴阴道炎非常有效。外用药物的使用取决于是否为复杂性病例。对于孕妇，仅推荐局部外用唑类治疗，连续 7 天。

预后

细菌性阴道病可用各种抗生素进行治疗，但主要问题是正常乳酸杆菌菌群无法重新在阴道内定植以重建阴道微生态，导致反复感染并需要长期治疗。有时会推荐口服和阴道给予乳酸杆菌。细菌性阴道病会增加 HIV、单纯疱疹病毒 2 型（HSV-2）以及淋病奈瑟球菌感染的风险，因此治疗细菌性阴道病对防治其他性传播感染很重要。

其他非淋菌性尿道炎的原因

尿道炎和宫颈炎还有其他几种已知的病因，可能还有更多未知的病因。重要的病因可能包括生殖支原体、单纯疱疹病毒 1/2 型、梅毒螺旋体、腺病毒和解脲支原体。解脲支原体可以是正常菌群的一部分，它在尿道炎中的作用尚未得到证实。

这些微生物中最常见的是生殖支原体。它是一种没有细胞壁、无法进行革兰氏染色，且很难在培养中生长的细菌。在美国，这种病原体引起了 15%～25% 的男性非淋菌性尿道炎，也被认为能够导致女性宫颈炎和盆腔炎。可使用尿液、尿道、阴道和宫颈样本进行生殖支原体核酸扩增试验，是推荐的诊断检测。对于顽固性尿道炎或宫颈炎患者，应考虑进行生殖支原体检测。生殖支原体的治疗因全球范围内出现的耐药问题而变得复杂。对有症状的个体的经验治疗包括阿奇霉素（1 g，单次口服；或首次 500 mg 口服，以后每日 250 mg，连续 4 天；更长的阿奇霉素疗程可能更为有效）。莫西沙星（每日 400 mg，连续 7～14 天）也是一种有效的治疗方案，应在患者有持续症状时使用。

生殖器溃疡性疾病

生殖器溃疡是多种性传播疾病的主要表现形式。生殖器溃疡最好应分类为疼痛性（如单纯疱疹病毒感染，软下疳）或无痛性（如梅毒）。由衣原体感染导致的性病性淋巴肉芽肿也表现为溃疡。溃疡可以分为单发（如梅毒、软下疳）或多发或成簇（如单纯疱疹 1/2 型）。所有这些性传播感染都表现出多样化的症状和体征，仅凭临床检查可能不足以进行准确诊断（表 15.1）。

梅毒

定义和流行病学

梅毒是由梅毒螺旋体引起的疾病，可以导致多种临床表现。20 世纪初，人们认为美国普通人群中约有 10% 患有梅毒。美国 CDC 自 1941 年开始报告梅毒发病率。梅毒发病率在 20 世纪 40 年代初达到顶峰，几乎有 60 万病例，随后在 2000 年降至最低点，当时普通人群的发病率为每 10 万人中有 2.1 例。然而，从那时起，梅毒报告病例数开始增加。主要的高危人群是男男性行为者，但该疾病在各个年龄、性别、性取向、社会经济地位以及种族和族裔群体中均有发现。

在男男性行为者中，梅毒在 HIV 感染者中的再度广泛流行产生了重要影响。性病门诊的临床医生以及治疗 HIV 感染的医生需要了解针对该人群的梅毒诊断和治疗指南。此外，临床医生需要对梅毒的非典型表现保持高度警惕。鉴于越来越多的男男性行为者携带 HIV，在这类人群中 HIV 与梅毒合并感染常见。所有男男性行为者，无论有无 HIV 感染，都应每年进行一次梅毒筛查，如果有其他危险因素，应更频繁地进行筛查。

病理学

梅毒螺旋体是一种细长的螺旋状细菌，以螺旋运动的方式移动。梅毒螺旋体难以培养，阻碍了我们对这种微生物的诊断和研究。梅毒螺旋体感染并进入黏膜，导致典型的硬下疳病变。随后，病原体感染局部淋巴结并扩散全身。感染中位潜伏期约为 3 周。超过 60% 的感染者，梅毒并不会进展到晚期。宿主的免疫因素被认为在晚期梅毒的发展中起到了一定作用。

TABLE 15.1 Differential Diagnosis of Genital Ulcer Disease

Disease	Primary Lesion	Adenopathy	Systemic Features	Diagnosis and Treatment
Genital herpes (HSV-1/2)				
Primary	Incubation 2-7 days; multiple, painful vesicles on erythematous base; lasts 7-14 days	Tender, soft, and usually bilateral	Fever, malaise	Viral cultures, DFA, antibody testing, Tzanck smear
Recurrent	Grouped, painful vesicles on erythematous base; lasts 3-10 days	None	None	Tx: acyclovir, famciclovir, or valacyclovir for 7-10 days (shorter for recurrent cases)
Primary syphilis (*Treponema pallidum*)	Incubation 10-90 days (average, 21) Chancre: painless papule that ulcerates with firm, raised border and smooth base; usually single; may be genital or almost anywhere; heals in 3-6 weeks without treatment	1 week after chancre appears; bilateral or unilateral; firm, discrete, no overlying skin changes, painless, nonsuppurative	During later stages	Nontreponemal tests (RPR, VDRL), treponemal tests (FTA-ABS), darkfield microscopy; cannot be cultured Tx: see Table 15.3
Chancroid (*Haemophilus ducreyi*)	Incubation 3-5 days; vesicle or papule to pustule to ulcer; soft, not indurated; very painful	1 week after primary in 50%; painful, unilateral in two thirds; suppurative	None	Gram stain and culture. Tx: azithromycin, ceftriaxone, ciprofloxacin
Lymphogranuloma venereum (*Chlamydia trachomatis* serovars L1, L2, L3)	Incubation 5-21 days; self-limited, painless papule, vesicle, or ulcer; lasts 2-3 days; found in only 10-40%	5-21 days after primary; one third bilateral, tender, matted iliac or femoral groove sign; multiple abscesses; coalescent, caseating, suppurative; thick yellow pus; sinus tracts; fistulas; strictures; genital ulcerations	Fever, arthritis, pericarditis, proctitis, meningoencephalitis, keratoconjunctivitis, preauricular adenopathy, erythema nodosum	NAAT for *Chlamydia*. Samples can be sent to the CDC to evaluate for LGV specific serotypes. Tx: incision and drainage, doxycycline
Granuloma inguinale (donovanosis)	Incubation 9-50 days; at least one painless papule that gradually ulcerates; ulcers are large (1-4 cm), irregular, nontender, with thickened; rolled margins and beefy red tissue at base; older portions of ulcer show depigmented scarring, white areas; advancing edge contains new papules	No true adenopathy; in one fifth of patients, subcutaneous spread through lymphatics leads to indurated swelling or abscesses of groin (pseudobuboes)	Metastatic infection of bones, joints, liver	Wright or Giemsa staining with short, plump, bipolar staining pattern, Donovan bodies in macrophage vacuoles Tx: doxycycline
Condyloma acuminatum (genital warts)	Characteristic large, soft, fleshy, cauliflower-like excrescences around vulva, glans, urethral orifice, anus, perineum	None	None	Clinical diagnosis, biopsy if necessary Tx: topical podophyllin, surgery, others

DFA, Direct fluorescent antibody test; *FTA-ABS*, fluorescent treponemal antibody absorption test; *HSV*, herpes simplex virus; *NAAT*, nucleic acid amplification test; *RPR*, rapid plasma reagin; *Tx*, treatment; *VDRL*, venereal disease research laboratory.

transmission from an individual with primary syphilis to an uninfected individual is 30% per sexual act. Syphilis may also be transmitted to others sites (i.e., rectum, oropharynx) through exposure with any contact of a primary lesion. Inoculation of the organism by surgeons through needlesticks has been well documented and typically does not result in a chancre at the site of infection (i.e., syphilis d'emblee).

The four classic stages of syphilis are primary, secondary, latent, and tertiary. Staging is best thought of as a continuum rather than discrete stages of infection. The states can manifest individually, but individuals often have symptoms consistent with primary and secondary symptoms. The primary and secondary stages of syphilis are extremely infectious, and cases of transmission during the tertiary stage have been reported.

It can be very difficult to diagnose primary syphilis based solely on the physical examination. The primary chancre is generally described as a painless, clean-based, indurated ulcer. The borders are firm and raised. However, the presentation of a primary chancre may vary and any dermatologic manifestation in the right clinical setting (i.e., sexually active MSM) should be tested for syphilis. The chancre is teeming with spirochetes and should be considered extremely infectious. It is rare for a primary chancre to be absent, but it may go unnoticed. The chancre spontaneously heals without treatment over several weeks.

表 15.1 生殖器溃疡性疾病的鉴别诊断

疾病	原发皮损	淋巴结肿大	全身特征	诊断和治疗
生殖器疱疹 (HSV-1/2)				
原发	潜伏期 2~7 天；红斑基础上多发水疱伴疼痛；持续 7~14 天	触痛，柔软，通常为双侧	发热、周身不适	病毒培养、DFA、抗体检测、Tzanck 涂片
复发	红斑基础上成簇的痛性水疱；持续 3~10 天	无	无	Tx：阿昔洛韦、泛昔洛韦或伐昔洛韦 7~10 日（复发病例治疗时间较短）
一期梅毒（梅毒螺旋体）	潜伏期 10~90 天（平均 21 天）；硬下疳：无痛性丘疹溃疡，边缘坚硬隆起，基底光滑；通常单发；可能出现在生殖器或几乎任何部位；未治疗可在 3~6 周内自愈	在硬下疳出现 1 周后；双侧或单侧；坚硬，不连续，没有表面皮肤变化，无痛，非化脓性	疾病后期	非梅毒螺旋体试验（RPR, VDRL），梅毒螺旋体试验（FTA-ABS），暗视野显微镜检查；无法培养 Tx：见表 15.3
软下疳（杜克雷嗜血杆菌）	潜伏期 3~5 天；从水疱或丘疹到脓疱再到溃疡；质地柔软，无硬化；非常疼痛	50% 的患者在原发感染 1 周后出现；疼痛，2/3 为单侧；化脓性	无	革兰氏染色和培养 Tx：阿奇霉素、头孢曲松、环丙沙星
性病性淋巴肉芽肿（沙眼衣原体 L1、L2、L3 血清型）	潜伏期 5~21 天；自限性，无痛丘疹、水疱或溃疡；持续 2~3 天；仅 10%~40% 的患者有此表现	原发感染后 5~21 天出现；1/3 为双侧，触痛，粘连的髂窝或腹股沟体征；多发脓肿；融合性、干酪样化脓性；黄色稠脓；窦道瘘管、狭窄；生殖器溃疡	发热、关节炎、心包炎、直肠炎、脑膜脑炎、角膜结膜炎、耳前淋巴结肿大、结节性红斑	衣原体 NAAT，样本可送至 CDC 评估特定血清型。 Tx：切开引流，多西环素
腹股沟肉芽肿（杜诺凡病）	潜伏期 9~50 天；至少一个无痛的丘疹逐渐形成溃疡，溃疡大（1~4 cm），不规则，无触痛，边缘厚，呈卷边状，基底呈牛肉红色组织；溃疡陈旧部分呈色素减退性疤痕、白色区域；进展边缘有新丘疹	无真正淋巴结肿大；1/5 患者通过淋巴管的皮下扩散导致腹股沟肿胀或脓肿（假性淋巴结肿大）	骨、关节、肝转移感染	瑞氏染色和吉姆萨染色显示病原体为短小，丰满的双极染色模式，在巨噬细胞空泡中有杜诺凡小体。 Tx：多西环素
尖锐湿疣（生殖器疣）	特征性大而柔软的肉色菜花状赘生物；出现在外阴、龟头、尿道口、肛门、会阴周围	无	无	临床诊断，必要时活检 Tx：局部涂抹鬼臼毒素、手术等

DFA，直接免疫荧光试验；FTA-ABS，荧光螺旋体抗体吸收试验；HSV，单纯疱疹病毒；NAAT，核酸扩增试验；RPR，快速血浆反应素环状卡片试验；Tx，治疗；VDRL，性病研究实验室。

临床表现

虽然也可能在直肠或口咽部观察到病变，但是经典的一期梅毒通常累及生殖器。据估计，每次性行为中，一期梅毒患者将梅毒传染给未感染个体的风险约为 30%。梅毒也可能通过与原发病灶的任何接触而传染到其他部位（如直肠、口咽）。有详细记载外科医生通过针刺接种感染该病原体，通常不会在感染部位形成硬下疳（即 syphilis d'emblee）。

梅毒的四个经典分期分别是：一期、二期、潜伏和晚期。最好将梅毒分期视为一个连续的感染过程，而不是相互独立的感染阶段。各阶段可以单独出现，但患者经常同时表现出符合一期和二期梅毒的症状。一期和二期梅毒传染性极强，也有在晚期梅毒期间发生传染的病例报道。

仅凭查体很难诊断一期梅毒。一期梅毒硬下疳通常描述为一个无痛、基底干净、质地坚硬的溃疡。其边缘坚实并隆起。然而，硬下疳的表现也可以有所不同。在合适的临床情境下（如针对性活跃的男男性行为者），任何皮肤病变都应当进行梅毒检测。硬下疳中充满螺旋体，传染性极强。一期梅不出现硬下疳的情况非常罕见，但出现的硬下疳可能会被忽视。硬下疳即使未治疗，也可在数周内自愈。

Secondary syphilis usually manifests as a diffuse, maculopapular rash that classically involves the palms and soles. However, a wide range of early skin manifestations exists, including macular, papular, pustular, vesicular, or any combination of these. Vesicular lesions may easily be confused with other STIs, including HSV-1/2. Syphilis may also have late skin manifestations, including nodular, squamous, or gummous appearances.

The rash typically develops a few weeks after the chancre and results from dissemination of the organism. Up to 80% of patients have some cutaneous manifestations of disease. The rash is usually symmetrical and pink, with no pain or burning, and it usually spares the face. It resolves on its own over weeks to months and may be confused with pityriasis rosea, erythema multiforme, drug rashes, tinea, measles, and seborrheic dermatitis. The maculopapular rash of secondary syphilis is considered noninfectious, although lesions in axillary or inguinal folds or other regions exposed to chaffing may erode and become infectious.

Syphilis then enters a latent stage, during which an infected individual has no symptoms but does have positive serologic test results (Table 15.2). Tertiary syphilis may then develop at any point from years to decades after the initial infection.

Approximately 30% to 40% of individuals with untreated syphilis infection develop tertiary disease, which can include neurosyphilis, cardiovascular syphilis, and gummatous disease. Neurosyphilis has classically been thought of as a complication of tertiary syphilis. However, *T. pallidum* may invade and cause symptoms of the central nervous system at the time of initial infection. Early neurosyphilis may be characterized by signs and symptoms of meningitis and milder symptoms, including headache. Other manifestations of neurosyphilis include otosyphilis (i.e., hearing loss) and ocular syphilis, which is classically characterized as posterior uveitis. Late neurosyphilis may manifest with general paresis (i.e., progressive dementia, forgetfulness, psychiatric disease, and personality change), Argyll-Robertson pupils (i.e., no response to light but normal accommodation), and tabes dorsalis (i.e., ataxia and lancinating pains). The most common finding in late neurosyphilis is irregular pupils.

Gummas, a result of immune system activation, may develop in any tissue or organ in the body. Classic cardiovascular symptoms of syphilis include aortitis, which often affects the ascending thoracic aorta causing a tree-bark appearance with dilation and aortic valve regurgitation.

Diagnosis and Differential Diagnosis

The diagnosis of syphilis is limited by the inability of *T. pallidum* to grow on standard laboratory media. Diagnostic testing for syphilis relies on the direct and indirect measurement of antibodies against treponema. Nontreponemal tests such as the rapid plasma reagin (RPR) and venereal disease research laboratory (VDRL) test rely on anticardiolipin antibodies, which usually resemble antibodies against treponema. These tests are usually sensitive but nonspecific, and false-positive results are relatively common, especially in individuals with other autoimmune diseases or who are pregnant. Nontreponemal tests report antibodies in terms of dilutions; a titer of 1:2 is extremely low compared with a titer of 1:1024. This measurement can be used as a general representation of spirochete load in the patient. With treatment, nontreponemal test results may revert to nonreactive. However, some individuals may not have a serologic response (12%) or may have persistent nontreponemal titers ("serofast"; 35% to 44%) despite appropriate treatment.

Treponemal tests such as the fluorescent treponemal antibody absorption (FTA-ABS) test rely on antibodies that directly target the organism and are therefore more specific. Test results may be positive or negative, and a positive result usually remains so for life. The normal testing algorithm employs the sensitive, nontreponemal tests, followed by a more specific treponemal test to confirm the diagnosis. However, the "reverse" algorithm, which employs a treponemal test first followed by a nontreponemal test, is also commonly used. In the case of a discordant result (i.e., a positive treponemal test and a negative nontreponemal test), a third different treponemal test is used (*Treponema pallidum* particle agglutination assay, TP-PA). The inherent limitation of antibody testing results in many cases of unclear diagnoses.

Several mistakes may be made by clinicians in the diagnosis of syphilis. In primary syphilis, the initial nontreponemal test result may be negative up to 30% of the time. A patient with a lesion suspicious for syphilis should undergo repeat testing or empirical treatment regardless of the serologic results. In the event of a recent exposure, a patient should be counseled that a syphilis and HIV antibody test may be negative. A patient who is treated early in the course of disease may never develop an antibody response and may therefore never have a positive test result.

After successful treatment, patients with an initial episode of syphilis should see a 4-fold decrease in nontreponemal titers at approximately 6 to 12 months. Titers may never return to normal and should be followed periodically. For MSM, CDC guidelines suggest yearly STI testing and more frequent testing (3 to 6 months) for patients with multiple partners, anonymous partners, or other risk factors for infection.

TABLE 15.2 Serologic Testing for Syphilis

Features	Nontreponemal	Treponemal
Technique	Antibody to cardiolipin-lecithin (RPR, VDRL)	Antibody to *Treponema pallidum* (FTA-ABS, EIA)
Indications	Screening and assessing response to therapy; should be quantified by diluting serum and reporting in titers	Confirmatory test; usually remains positive for life; may be used as a screening test
Positive for syphilis		
Primary	77%	86%
Secondary	98%	100%
Early latent	95%	99%
Late latent	73%	96%
False positives	1-2% of the population may have a false-positive RPR/VDRL; common in pregnancy, recent immunization, autoimmune diseases, acute infectious illness, HIV, chronic liver disease, prozone reaction (negative result due to high antibody titers)	Borderline positive is common in pregnancy, and test should be repeated

EIA, Enzyme immunoassay; *FTA-ABS*, fluorescent treponemal antibody absorption test; *HIV*, human immunodeficiency virus infection; *RPR*, rapid plasma reagin; *VDRL*, venereal disease research laboratory test.

二期梅毒表现为弥漫性斑丘疹，典型皮损累及掌跖。然而，早期皮损表现形式多样，包括斑疹、丘疹、脓疱、水疱，或这些的任意组合。水疱性皮损容易与其他性传播感染（如 HSV-1/2）混淆。梅毒还可能出现晚期皮肤表现，包括结节性、鳞屑性或树胶肿样病变。

皮疹通常在硬下疳出现几周后发生，是病原体播散的结果。高达 80% 的患者会出现皮肤表现。皮疹通常对称且呈粉红色，没有疼感或灼热感，通常不会累及面部。皮疹会在几周到几个月内自行消退，皮疹容易与玫瑰糠疹、多形红斑、药疹、真菌感染性皮肤病、麻疹和脂溢性皮炎混淆。二期梅毒的斑丘疹认为不具有传染性，尽管腋窝、腹股沟及易受摩擦区域的皮损可能会糜烂而具有传染性。

梅毒随后进入潜伏期，在此期间感染者没有任何症状，但血清学试验结果呈阳性（表 15.2）。晚期梅毒可能在初次感染后数年到数十年的任何时候出现。

未经治疗的梅毒感染者有 30%～40% 进展到晚期梅毒，其中包括神经梅毒、心血管梅毒和树胶肿类疾病。神经梅毒通常被认为是晚期梅毒的并发症。然而，梅毒螺旋体可能在初次感染时即侵袭中枢神经系统并引起症状。早期神经梅毒可能表现为特征性的脑膜炎症状体征，包括头痛在内的轻度症状。神经梅毒的其他表现还包括耳梅毒（听力丧失）和眼梅毒，眼梅毒典型特征为后葡萄膜炎。晚期神经梅毒可能表现为麻痹性痴呆（即进行性痴呆、健忘、精神疾病和人格改变）、阿-罗瞳孔（对光反射消失，调节反射正常）和脊髓痨（共济失调和刺痛）。晚期神经梅毒最常见的表现是瞳孔不规则。

树胶肿是一种机体免疫系统激活的结果，可能出现在身体的任何组织或器官中。梅毒典型心血管症状包括主动脉炎，通常影响胸升主动脉，导致外观呈现树皮样伴主动脉扩张和主动脉瓣反流。

诊断和鉴别诊断

由于梅毒螺旋体无法在标准实验室培养基上生长，梅毒的诊断受到了限制。梅毒的诊断检测依靠对梅毒螺旋体抗体的直接和间接检测。非梅毒螺旋体试验［如快速血浆反应素（RPR）和性病研究实验室（VDRL）试验］依赖于对抗心磷脂抗体的检测，这些抗体通常类似于抗梅毒螺旋体抗体。这类检测通常具有高敏感性但缺乏特异性，假阳性结果较为常见，特别是在患有其他自身免疫性疾病或妊娠的个体中。非梅毒螺旋体试验以稀释倍数形式报告抗体滴度；与 1∶1024 的滴度相比，1∶2 的滴度极低。该测量可以大致反映患者体内螺旋体的载量。治疗后，非梅毒螺旋体试验的结果可能会阴转。然而，即使给予正规治疗，一些患者可能无血清学反应（约 12%）或者非梅毒螺旋体试验的滴度仍可能保持不变（"血清固定"；35%～44%）。

梅毒螺旋体试验［如荧光密螺旋体抗体吸收（FTA-ABS）试验］依靠直接针对病原体的抗体进行检测，因此具有更高的特异性。检测结果可能为阳性或阴性，阳性结果通常会保持终身。常规的检测流程是先采用敏感的非特异性梅毒检测，然后再进行更具特异性的梅毒螺旋体试验以确认诊断。然而，所谓的"反向"流程也常用，即首先进行梅毒螺旋体试验，然后再进行非梅毒螺旋体试验。在结果不一致的情况下（即梅毒螺旋体试验阳性而非梅毒螺旋体试验阴性），会使用第三种不同的梅毒螺旋体试验［如梅毒螺旋体颗粒凝集试验（TP-PA）］。抗体检测的固有局限性导致许多病例诊断不清。

在梅毒诊断中，临床医生容易犯几个错误。在一期梅毒中，最初的非梅毒螺旋体试验结果可能高达 30% 为阴性。因此，无论血清学结果如何，对于有疑似梅毒皮损的患者，都应进行重复检测或经验性治疗。如果患者近期有过性接触，则应告知其梅毒和 HIV 抗体检测结果可能为阴性。在疾病早期接受治疗的患者可能永远不会产生抗体，因此可能永远不会出现阳性检测结果。

成功治疗后，首次感染梅毒的患者在约 6～12 个月内非梅毒螺旋体滴度应下降 4 倍。滴度可能永远不会恢复正常，因此应定期随访。针对男男性行为者，疾病控制与预防中心指南建议每年进行性传播感染检测，对于有多个性伴侣、陌生性伴侣或其他感染危险因素的患者，建议应进行更频繁的检测（3～6 个月）。

表 15.2　梅毒血清学检测

特征	非梅毒螺旋体	梅毒螺旋体
技术	抗心磷脂-卵磷脂抗体（RPR，VDRL）	梅毒螺旋体抗体（FTA-ABS，EIA）
适应情况	用于筛查及评估治疗反应；应通过稀释血清进行滴度定量	确认性测试；通常结果终身持续为阳性；可作为筛查试验
梅毒检测阳性		
一期	77%	86%
二期	98%	100%
早期潜伏	95%	99%
晚期潜伏	73%	96%
假阳性	人群中 1%～2% 可能出现 RPR/VDRL 假阳性；常见于妊娠、近期免疫接种、自身免疫病、急性感染、HIV、慢性肝病和高抗体滴度导致的梅毒检测阴性反应（前带现象）[a]	妊娠时可疑阳性常见，应重复检测

EIA，酶免疫分析；FTA-ABS，荧光螺旋体抗体吸收试验；HIV，人类免疫缺陷病毒；RPR，快速血浆反应素试验；VDRL，梅毒研究实验室。
[a] 译者注：前带现象应为假阴性现象。

Treatment

Despite the classic staging of syphilis as primary, secondary, latent, or tertiary, the disease is best thought of in terms of early infection (<1 year) or late infection (≥1 year) when considering treatment. Early infection consists of primary, secondary, and early latent stages. Late infection consists of late latent and tertiary disease. *T. pallidum* remains sensitive to penicillin. Individuals with early syphilis can be treated with a single intramuscular injection of benzathine penicillin G (Bicillin), which achieves high and prolonged serum concentrations. Individuals with late syphilis or disease of unknown duration should be treated with three weekly injections of intramuscular benzathine penicillin G (Table 15.3). This cures most patients. Importantly, other formulations of penicillin are less effective and should not be used.

Although penicillin remains the drug of choice, doxycycline may also be used in individuals who have severe allergies to penicillin. However, every effort should be made to use penicillin because of the sensitivity of the organism. For pregnant women who are allergic to penicillin, penicillin desensitization should occur in collaboration with a pharmacist and an allergist specialist. As a result of treatment, individuals may experience a febrile reaction (i.e., Jarisch-Herxheimer reaction). Symptoms are caused by killing of the spirochetes and should not be confused with an allergic reaction.

The co-epidemic of syphilis and HIV has led to an increase in individuals with manifestations of neurosyphilis. In cases of syphilis with neurologic symptoms, a lumbar puncture and CSF examination is warranted to rule out neurologic involvement. Any pleocytosis or increase in protein concentration warrants treatment for neurosyphilis. A cerebrospinal fluid (CSF) sample should be sent for VDRL testing, but the test lacks sensitivity (50%), and a negative test result does not rule out neurosyphilis. Usually, HIV-negative individuals with syphilis without neurologic symptoms should not undergo a lumbar puncture. Many HIV-infected individuals with syphilis, however, have asymptomatic neurosyphilis. The clinical implications of this are unclear, but these individuals may fail intramuscular therapy at a high rate. Some experts recommend CSF examination in all HIV-infected individuals with a $CD4^+$ count lower than 350 cells/μL or a nontreponemal titer greater than 1:32. These criteria capture almost everyone with asymptomatic neurosyphilis.

Individuals with neurosyphilis should be treated with intravenous penicillin G for 10 to 14 days. In tertiary disease with manifestations of neurologic disease, treatment with intravenous penicillin halts disease progression but does not reverse existing structural damage. Ocular disease or other similar neurologic manifestations should be treated as neurosyphilis. Nontreponemal titers should be followed to ensure an appropriate response. Repeat treatment may be necessary in a small number of cases.

Prognosis

Although penicillin is the treatment of choice for syphilis, it has not been validated in clinical trials but is based on a long history of clinical use. However, a significant number of individuals with syphilis do not respond with the recommended decline in nontreponemal titer. Individuals who do not respond should be retreated.

For a deeper discussion of these topics, please see Chapter 303, "Syphilis," in *Goldman-Cecil Medicine*, 26th Edition.

Herpes Simplex Virus

Definition and Epidemiology

HSV-1/2 cause a wide variety of clinical disease. HSV-1 is historically the cause of herpes labialis (i.e., cold sores), and HSV-2 is the cause of genital herpes, although there is overlap. After infection occurs, HSV-1/2 enters a latent state and may later reactivate to cause disease in a subset of individuals.

The overall prevalence of HSV-1 and HSV-2 in the population is approximately 60% and 20%, respectively. However, the incidence of HSV-1 infection approaches 90% to 100% among middle-aged adults. Seroprevalence of HSV-2 is associated with a patient's sexual activity, including number of partners and history of other STIs, and with age, gender (women are at higher risk than men), and race or ethnicity. More than 50 million people in the United States are infected with genital HSV-1/2, and most are asymptomatic. CDC guidelines do not recommend routine screening for HSV-1/2 in people without symptoms. There is no evidence that screening for HSV-1/2 reduces its spread or has an impact on the disease. HSV-1/2 is not a reportable disease in the United States.

Pathology

HSV-1 and HSV-2 are two of eight double-stranded DNA human herpesviruses. Others include varicella-zoster virus (VZV), cytomegalovirus (CMV), Epstein-Barr virus (EBV), and human herpesviruses 6, 7, and 8. Infection with one type of HSV does not prevent or increase the chances of infection with other types. After initial infection, HSV-1/2 enters a latent state within neuronal cells of sensory or autonomic peripheral ganglia. Reactivation can occur at any time and is mediated in part by immune factors. HSV-1 most commonly infects the trigeminal ganglia and HSV-2 the sacral nerve root ganglia (S2-S5).

Clinical Presentation

Transmission of HSV-1/2 is through skin-to-skin contact, including sexual contact at mucosal surfaces such as the oropharynx, vagina, rectum, cervix, and conjunctivae. Importantly, transmission may occur in the absence of symptoms.

TABLE 15.3 Syphilis Treatment

Clinical Category	Regimen of Choice	Alternative[a]
Early syphilis (<1 year)	Benzathine penicillin, 2.4 million units IM, given once	Penicillin desensitization Doxycycline, 100 mg PO bid for 14 days Tetracycline, 500 mg PO qid for 14 days Azithromycin 2 g PO qd
Late syphilis (≥1 year) or unknown duration	Benzathine penicillin, 2.4 million units IM, given once each week for 3 wk	Penicillin desensitization Doxycycline, 100 mg PO bid for 28 days Tetracycline, 500 mg PO qid for 28 days
Neurosyphilis	Penicillin G, 4 million units IV q4h or 24 million units by continuous infusion qd for 10-14 days	Penicillin desensitization Ceftriaxone 2 g qd IM or IV for 10-14 days

[a]If patient has a penicillin allergy.

治疗

尽管梅毒传统上分为一期梅毒、二期梅毒、潜伏梅毒和晚期梅毒，但在考虑治疗时，最好还是从早期感染（＜1年）或晚期感染（≥1年）的角度来考虑（译者注：在我国，早期与晚期梅毒的划分以2年为分界。早期梅毒指感染梅毒螺旋体2年内的梅毒感染，包括一期、二期和早期潜伏梅毒。晚期梅毒的病程是指病程超过2年的梅毒感染，包括晚期三期梅毒、晚期潜伏梅毒）。早期感染包括一期梅毒、二期梅毒和早期潜伏梅毒，晚期感染则包括晚期潜伏梅毒和晚期梅毒。梅毒螺旋体对青霉素仍然敏感。早期梅毒患者可以通过单次肌内注射苄星青霉素G进行治疗，这种药物能够在血清中维持高浓度，而且效果持久。晚期梅毒或病程不明的患者应接受每周1次、连续3周的肌内注射苄星青霉素G治疗（表15.3）。这种治疗方案可以治愈大多数患者。需要注意的是，其他形式的青霉素疗效不佳，不推荐使用。

尽管青霉素仍然是首选药物，但对于严重青霉素过敏的患者，也可以使用多西环素进行治疗。然而，鉴于梅毒螺旋体对青霉素的高敏感性，应该尽量使用青霉素。对于青霉素过敏的孕妇，应在药师和变态反应科专家的协作下对患者进行青霉素脱敏治疗。治疗过程中，患者可能会出现发热反应（即吉海反应），是梅毒螺旋体被杀灭而引起的症状，不应与过敏反应混淆。

梅毒和HIV感染的共同流行导致出现神经梅毒表现的患者增多。对于伴有神经系统症状的梅毒病例，需要进行腰椎穿刺和脑脊液检查，以除外神经系统受累。这种情形下，任何脑脊液细胞增多或蛋白含量增加的情况都需要按神经梅毒治疗。应该送检脑脊液样本进行VDRL检测，但该检测的敏感性低，仅为50%，阴性检测结果并不能除外神经梅毒。通常情况下，没有神经系统症状且HIV阴性的梅毒患者不需要接受腰椎穿刺。然而，许多HIV感染的梅毒患者存在无症状神经梅毒，其临床意义尚不明确，但这些患者使用肌内注射治疗失败率较高。一些专家建议对所有CD4+计数低于350/μl或者非梅毒螺旋体抗体滴度大于1∶32的HIV感染者进行脑脊液检查。这些标准几乎涵盖了所有无症状神经梅毒患者。

神经梅毒患者应给予10～14日的青霉素G静脉输注治疗。对于伴有神经系统疾病表现的晚期梅毒患者，静脉输注青霉素可以阻止疾病进展，但不能逆转现有的结构性损害。眼部疾病或其他类似的神经系统表现应当按照神经梅毒进行治疗。应随访非梅毒螺旋体抗体滴度以确保治疗效果。少数病例可能需要重复治疗。

预后

尽管青霉素是梅毒的首选治疗药物，但它的疗效尚未在临床试验中得到验证，而是基于长期的临床使用经验得来。然而，仍有相当一部分梅毒患者未能达到非梅毒螺旋体抗体滴度推荐的下降程度。对于治疗无反应的患者，应进行复治。有关此专题的深入讨论，请参阅 Goldman-Cecil Medicine 第26版第303章"梅毒"。

单纯疱疹病毒

定义和流行病学

HSV-1/2 可引起多种临床疾病。既往认为，HSV-1主要导致唇疱疹（即感冒疮），HSV-2导致生殖器疱疹，尽管两者存在重叠。感染后，HSV-1/2会进入潜伏状态，并可能在部分患者中重新激活导致疾病。

HSV-1 和 HSV-2 在人群中的总体发病率分别约为60%和20%。然而，在中年人中，HSV-1感染的发病率接近90%～100%。HSV-2的血清阳性率与患者的性活动（性伴侣数量和其他性传播感染史）、年龄、性别（女性比男性风险更高）、种族或民族有关。美国有超过5000万人感染了HSV-1/2，大多数无症状。美国CDC指南不建议对无症状者进行常规的HSV-1/2筛查。没有证据表明HSV-1/2筛查可以减少其传播或对疾病产生影响。在美国，HSV-1/2是一种不需要报告的疾病。

病理学

HSV-1 和 HSV-2 是 8 种双链DNA人类疱疹病毒中的两种。其他疱疹病毒包括水痘-带状疱疹病毒（VZV）、巨细胞病毒（CMV）、EB病毒（EBV）以及人类疱疹病毒6、7和8。感染一种HSV并不会预防或增加感染其他疱疹病毒的可能性。初次感染后，HSV-1/2 在感觉或自主神经周围神经节的神经元细胞内进入潜伏状态。病毒可能在任何时候再激活，其中部分

表15.3 梅毒的治疗方案

临床分类	首选方案	替代方案[a]
早期梅毒（＜1年）	苄星青霉素，240万单位，肌内注射，单次给药	青霉素脱敏 多西环素，100 mg，口服，每日2次，连续14日 四环素，500 mg，口服，每日4次，连续14日 阿奇霉素，2 g，口服，日1次
晚期梅毒（≥1年）或未知病程	苄星青霉素，240万单位，肌内注射，每周1次，连续3周	青霉素脱敏 多西环素，100 mg，口服，每日2次，连续28日 四环素，500 mg，口服，每日4次，连续28日
神经梅毒	青霉素G，400万单位，静脉输注，每4 h一次或2400万单位，持续输液，每日1次，连续10～14日	青霉素脱敏 头孢曲松，2 g，肌内注射或静脉输注，每日1次，连续10～14日

[a] 如果该患者存在青霉素过敏。

The stages of HSV-1/2 infection include primary, latent, and recurrent. Primary infection of genital HSV-1/2 may include fever, headache, other systemic symptoms, and the classic local symptoms of painful genital vesicles or ulcers (multiple) and lymphadenopathy. Oral infections of HSV-1 may include gingivostomatitis and pharyngitis. Symptoms may vary from none to serious and require hospitalization. HSV-1/2 then enters a latent state. Reactivation occurs in a subset of individuals with symptoms less severe than those of primary infection. Some individuals have no reactivation, and others have multiple reactivations per year.

Complications of HSV-1/2 infection include meningitis and proctitis. Recurrent episodes of meningitis (i.e., Mollaret meningitis) may be caused by HSV-1/2. Other manifestations of HSV-1/2 include herpetic whitlow (e.g., infection of a finger of a health care worker), herpes gladiatorum (e.g., HSV-1/2 skin infections in athletes such as wrestlers), and ocular disease (e.g., keratitis, acute retinal necrosis). HSV-1/2 infection may rarely be associated with erythema multiforme, hepatitis, and encephalitis.

Diagnosis and Differential Diagnosis

The diagnosis of HSV-1/2 is typically made clinically. If possible, lesions should be tested for HSV-1/2 using viral culture (50% sensitivity), PCR, or direct fluorescent antibody (DFA) testing. Alternatively, serology testing for immunoglobulin M (IgM) and immunoglobulin G (IgG) antibodies is available. This test should be reserved for individuals with suspected primary infection or to document chronic infection, and it should usually not be used for screening purposes.

Treatment

Recommended regimens for primary HSV-1/2 infection include acyclovir (400 mg orally three times per day for 7 to 10 days or 200 mg orally five times per day for 7 to 10 days), famciclovir (250 mg orally three times each day for 7 to 10 days), or valacyclovir (1 g orally twice each day for 7 to 10 days). Treatment can also be used for reactivation disease: acyclovir (400 mg orally three times each day for 5 days, 800 mg orally twice each day for 5 days, or 800 mg orally three times each day for 2 days), famciclovir (125 mg orally twice each day for 5 days or 1000 mg orally twice each day for 1 day or 500 mg once followed by 250 mg twice each day for 2 days), or valacyclovir (500 mg twice each day for 3 days or 1 g orally once each day for 5 days).

Individuals with frequent recurrences may be candidates for suppressive therapy. Severe disease should be treated with intravenous acyclovir (5 to 10 mg/kg intravenously every 8 hours). Duration and transition to oral medication should be based on clinical improvement. Total treatment duration is usually at least 10 days. The safety of systemic acyclovir, valacyclovir, and famciclovir therapy in pregnant women is not established.

Prognosis

Although HSV-1/2 infection cannot be cured, most people are asymptomatic, and suppressive therapy is available. Individuals with HSV-1/2 infection should be educated regarding the disease, including transmission and available treatments. They should be encouraged to discuss their status with sexual partners, including the possibility that transmission may occur in the absence of symptoms. Individuals should abstain from sex during an outbreak.

Chancroid

Chancroid is a rare cause of genital ulceration in the United States. The infection is caused by the gram-negative rod *Haemophilus ducreyi* and is endemic in parts of Africa and the Caribbean. Classic symptoms include a single or multiple painful, nonindurated genital ulcers and inguinal lymphadenopathy. Growth of the organism in cultures requires hemin-containing media, and it may appear as a school of fish on Gram stain. PCR may be available in certain areas.

Testing for HSV-1/2 and syphilis should always be performed. Recommended treatment regimens include azithromycin (1 g orally once), ceftriaxone (250 mg intramuscularly once), or ciprofloxacin (500 mg orally twice each day for 3 days). Ciprofloxacin is contraindicated in pregnant and lactating women.

Granuloma Inguinale

Granuloma inguinale is also known as donovanosis. It is caused by the gram-negative bacterium *Klebsiella granulomatis*. The disease is rare in the United States but endemic in regions of Africa, India, Oceania, and the Caribbean. Clinical manifestations include painless, ulcerative genital lesions with erythema. Classic Donovan bodies may be observed on histopathology.

The recommended treatment regimen is doxycycline (100 mg orally twice each day for at least 3 weeks). Alternative regimens include azithromycin, ciprofloxacin, and sulfamethoxazole-trimethoprim. Azithromycin may be useful for treating granuloma inguinale during pregnancy. Doxycycline and ciprofloxacin are contraindicated in pregnant women.

Other Causes of Genital Ulcers

Other causes of genital ulcers should be considered when the results of routine testing are negative. Noninfectious causes include trauma, Behçet's disease, malignancy, and drug-mediated disease.

OTHER SEXUALLY TRANSMITTED INFECTIONS

Genital Warts

Human papillomavirus (HPV) is responsible for a spectrum of cutaneous and mucosal disease, ranging from genital warts to invasive cancer. HPV has been linked to cervical, anal, and oropharyngeal cancer. There are more than 100 types of HPV. Sexually transmitted HPV infection is responsible for genital warts and anogenital carcinoma. More than 80% of sexually active adults acquire HPV infection in their lifetime. Genital warts tend to be benign and asymptomatic, and 90% are caused by HPV types 6 and 11. The HPV types most often linked to anogenital carcinoma are 16 and 18; HPV-16 is the most common.

Warts are usually described as flat and papular in the genital regions. Diagnosis of genital warts is usually made by clinical examination. If unclear, a biopsy may be performed. Treatment of genital warts may include podofilox (0.5% solution or gel), imiquimod (5% cream), sinecatechins (15% ointment), cryotherapy, podophyllin resin (10% to 25% concentration), trichloroacetic acid (TCA), and surgical excision.

HPV vaccination is available with Gardasil (quadrivalent vaccine) and Cervarix (bivalent vaccine). The main objective of vaccination is to prevent cervical and other cancers. The vaccines are also effective in preventing genital warts. The vaccines are most effective before sexual debut. Guidelines suggest vaccination of males and females between the ages of 11 to 26 years. Vaccines may be administered to individuals as young as 9 years old. HPV vaccination is approved for men and women up to 45 years of age. In several countries including the United States, there has been a decline in anogenital warts in adolescents, young women, older women, heterosexual men, as well as men who have sex with men.

Pubic Lice

Pubic lice (i.e., *Pediculosis pubis*) may spread from the genitalia to other areas of the body. The most common symptom is pruritus. Small macules and localized lymphadenopathy may occur. Diagnosis of this STI is made by light microscopy of the organism.

是由免疫因素介导。HSV-1 最常感染三叉神经节，而 HSV-2 则常感染骶神经根神经节（S2～S5）。

临床表现

HSV-1/2 通过皮肤接触传播，包括口咽、阴道、直肠、子宫颈和结膜等黏膜表面的性接触。需要注意的是，无症状感染者也可以传播。

HSV-1/2 感染分为初发、潜伏和复发感染阶段。HSV-1/2 的初发感染可能包括发热、头痛及其他全身症状和痛性生殖器水疱或多发溃疡和淋巴结肿大等典型局部症状。HSV-1 的口腔感染可引起齿龈口腔炎和咽炎，症状可能从无到严重到需要住院治疗。随后，HSV-1/2 感染会进入潜伏状态。部分患者会复发，其症状通常不如原发感染严重。有些个体不会复发，而有些则可能一年多次复发。

HSV-1/2 感染的并发症包括脑膜炎和直肠炎。复发性脑膜炎（莫拉雷脑膜炎）可能由 HSV-1/2 感染所致。HSV-1/2 的其他表现形式包括疱疹性化脓性指头炎（例如医护人员手指感染）、格斗性疱疹（例如摔跤运动员间的 HSV-1/2 皮肤感染）和眼部疾病（例如角膜炎、急性视网膜坏死）。HSV-1/2 感染极少数情况下可能与多形红斑、肝炎和脑炎有关。

诊断和鉴别诊断

通常根据临床表现诊断 HSV-1/2。如果条件允许，应当使用病毒培养（敏感性为 50%）、聚合酶链反应或直接荧光抗体试验对皮损进行 HSV-1/2 检测。此外，也可进行免疫球蛋白 M（IgM）和免疫球蛋白 G（IgG）抗体的血清学检测，该检测应仅用于检测疑似原发感染或记录慢性感染的个体，通常不适用于筛查。

治疗

针对原发 HSV-1/2 感染，推荐的治疗方案包括阿昔洛韦（400 mg，每日口服 3 次，连续 7～10 日；或 200 mg，每日 5 次口服，连续 7～10 日）、泛昔洛韦（250 mg，每日口服 3 次，连续 7～10 日）或伐昔洛韦（1 g，每日口服 2 次，连续 7～10 日）。治疗也可用于复发感染：阿昔洛韦（400 mg，每日口服 3 次，连续 5 日；或 800 mg，每日口服 2 次，连续 5 日，或 800 mg，每日口服 3 次，连续 2 日）、泛昔洛韦（125 mg，每日口服 2 次，连续 5 日；或 1000 mg，每日口服 2 次，1 日，或首次 500 mg 口服，之后 250 mg，每日 2 次，连续 2 日）或伐昔洛韦（500 mg，每日口服 2 次，连续 3 日；或 1 g，每日口服 1 次，连续 5 日）。

频繁复发的个体可能适合采用抑制疗法。病情严重的患者应使用静脉输注阿昔洛韦治疗（5～10 mg/kg，每 8 h 静脉输注 1 次）。治疗疗程和转为口服药物的时机取决于患者的临床改善情况。总治疗时间通常至少 10 日。妊娠期女性系统应用阿昔洛韦、伐昔洛韦和泛昔洛韦的安全性尚不明确。

预后

虽然 HSV-1/2 感染无法治愈，但大多数人没有症状，而且可以采用抑制疗法。对于 HSV-1/2 感染者，应该进行疾病教育，包括感染的传播途径和可采用的治疗方法。应鼓励患者与性伴侣讨论自己的感染状况，包括在无症状情况下发生传播的可能性。在疾病发作期，患者应避免性行为。

软下疳

在美国，软下疳是生殖器溃疡的一种罕见病因。该感染由革兰氏阴性杆菌杜克雷嗜血杆菌引起，在非洲和加勒比地区流行。典型症状包括单个或多个疼痛性、非硬化性生殖器溃疡和腹股沟淋巴结肿大。该菌株在含血红素的培养基生长，培养出的菌株可能在革兰氏染色中呈"鱼群"状。某些地区可使用聚合酶链反应检测。

对于软下疳患者，一定要进行 HSV-1/2 和梅毒检测。软下疳的推荐治疗方案包括阿奇霉素（1 g，单次口服）、头孢曲松（250 mg，单次肌内注射）或环丙沙星（500 mg，每日口服 2 次，连续 3 日）。妊娠期和哺乳期妇女禁用环丙沙星。

腹股沟肉芽肿

腹股沟肉芽肿也被称为杜诺凡病，由革兰氏阴性肉芽肿克雷伯杆菌引起。该病在美国罕见，但在非洲、印度、大洋洲和加勒比地区流行。临床表现包括无痛性溃疡性生殖器皮损伴有红斑。组织病理学或可观察到典型的杜诺凡小体。

推荐治疗方案是多西环素（100 mg，每日口服 2 次，至少 3 周）。替代方案包括阿奇霉素、环丙沙星和甲氧苄啶-磺胺甲噁唑。阿奇霉素可能有助于治疗妊娠期腹股沟肉芽肿。孕妇禁用多西环素和环丙沙星。

其他原因所致生殖器溃疡

当常规检测结果为阴性时，应考虑其他原因导致的生殖器溃疡。非感染性原因包括创伤、白塞病、恶性肿瘤和药疹。

其他性传播感染

生殖器疣

人乳头瘤病毒（HPV）会导致一系列皮肤黏膜病变，从生殖器疣到侵袭性癌症。HPV 与宫颈癌、肛门癌和口咽癌有关。HPV 有 100 多种类型。性传播的 HPV 感染会导致生殖器疣和肛门生殖器癌。超过 80% 的性活跃成年人在其一生中感染过 HPV。生殖器疣通常是良性无症状的，90% 由 HPV 6 型和 11 型引起。与肛门生殖器癌最相关的 HPV 类型是 16 型和 18 型；其中 HPV-16 型是最常见的。

生殖器部位的疣通常被描述为扁平和丘疹样。通常通过临床检查即可诊断生殖器疣。如果诊断不明确，可进行活检。生殖器疣的治疗方法包括鬼臼毒素

Treatment includes permethrin (1% cream applied to affected areas, rinsed off in 10 minutes) or pyrethrins (similar application). Alternative medications include malathion (0.5% lotion) or ivermectin. Clothing, bed sheets, and other linens should be thoroughly washed.

Scabies

Scabies is caused by the skin mite *Sarcoptes scabiei*. Transmission occurs by skin contact, and among adults, it is usually sexual. Clinical presentation usually includes pruritus and small erythematous papules that are classically present on the wrists, forearms, fingers, and genital areas.

Diagnosis is usually based on clinical presentation and examination of skin scrapings. Recommended treatment regimens include permethrin (5% cream applied from the neck down and washed off after 8 to 14 hours) or ivermectin.

SUGGESTED READINGS

Centers for Disease Control and Prevention: Sexually transmitted diseases surveillance 2012, Atlanta, 2013, U.S. Department of Health and Human Services.

Cook RL, Hutchison SL, Østergaard L, et al: Systematic review: noninvasive testing for *Chlamydia trachomatis* and *Neisseria gonorrhoeae*, Ann Intern Med 142:914–925, 2005.

Geisler WM, Lensing SY, Press CG, et al: Spontaneous resolution of genital *Chlamydia trachomatis* infection in women and protection from reinfection, J Infect Dis 207:1850–1856, 2013.

Jensen JS: *Mycoplasma genitalium*: the aetiological agent of urethritis and other sexually transmitted diseases, J Eur Acad Dermatol Venereol 18:1–11, 2004.

Platt R, Rice PA, McCormack WM: Risk of acquiring gonorrhea and prevalence of abnormal adnexal findings among women recently exposed to gonorrhea, J Am Med Assoc 250:3205–3209, 1983.

Rockwell DH, Yobs AR, Moore Jr MB: The Tuskegee study of untreated syphilis: the 30th year of observation, Arch Intern Med 114:792–798, 1964.

Schroeter AL, Lucas JB, Price EV, et al: Treatment for early syphilis and reactivity of serologic tests, J Am Med Assoc 221:471–476, 1972.

Vall-Mayans M, Caballero E, Sanz B: The emergence of lymphogranuloma venereum in Europe, Lancet 374:356, 2009.

（0.5%溶液或凝胶）、咪喹莫特（5%乳膏）、茶多酚（15%软膏）、冷冻治疗、鬼臼毒素树脂（10%～25%浓度）、三氯乙酸（TCA）和外科切除。

HPV疫苗有Gardasil（四价疫苗）和Cervarix（二价疫苗）[译者注：除了Gardasil和Cervarix，当今市面上还有Gardasil 9（九价疫苗），可预防6、11、16、18、31、33、45、52和58型HPV]。疫苗接种的主要目的是预防宫颈癌和其他癌症。这些疫苗也能有效预防生殖器疣。疫苗在初次性行为前接种最为有效。指南建议11～26岁的男性和女性接种疫苗。疫苗接种最早可以从9岁开始，最晚被批准用于45岁的男性和女性。在包括美国在内的几个国家，青少年、年轻女性、老年女性、异性恋男性以及男男性行为人群肛门生殖器疣的发病率有所下降。

阴虱

阴虱可能从生殖器部位传播到身体其他部位。最常见的症状是瘙痒。可能出现小斑疹和局部淋巴结肿大。这种性传播感染可通过光学显微镜下观察到病原体来确诊。

治疗包括使用扑灭司林（1%乳膏涂抹在患处，10 min后冲洗掉）或除虫菊酯（类似用法）。其他药物选择包括马拉硫磷（0.5%乳液）或伊维菌素。应彻底清洗衣物、床单和其他床上用品。

疥疮

疥疮由皮肤疥螨引起。疥疮通过皮肤接触传播，在成人中通常是通过性传播。临床表现通常包括瘙痒和较小的红斑丘疹，通常出现在手腕、前臂、手指和生殖器部位。

通常根据临床表现和皮肤刮片检查来诊断疥疮。推荐的治疗方案包括使用扑灭司林（5%乳膏，从颈部向下涂抹，8～14 h后洗掉）或伊维菌素。

推荐阅读

Centers for Disease Control and Prevention: Sexually transmitted diseases surveillance 2012, Atlanta, 2013, U.S. Department of Health and Human Services.

Cook RL, Hutchison SL, Østergaard L, et al: Systematic review: noninvasive testing for *Chlamydia trachomatis* and *Neisseria gonorrhoeae*, Ann Intern Med 142:914–925, 2005.

Geisler WM, Lensing SY, Press CG, et al: Spontaneous resolution of genital *Chlamydia trachomatis* infection in women and protection from reinfection, J Infect Dis 207:1850–1856, 2013.

Jensen JS: *Mycoplasma genitalium*: the aetiological agent of urethritis and other sexually transmitted diseases, J Eur Acad Dermatol Venereol 18:1–11, 2004.

Platt R, Rice PA, McCormack WM: Risk of acquiring gonorrhea and prevalence of abnormal adnexal findings among women recently exposed to gonorrhea, J Am Med Assoc 250:3205–3209, 1983.

Rockwell DH, Yobs AR, Moore Jr MB: The Tuskegee study of untreated syphilis: the 30th year of observation, Arch Intern Med 114:792–798, 1964.

Schroeter AL, Lucas JB, Price EV, et al: Treatment for early syphilis and reactivity of serologic tests, J Am Med Assoc 221:471–476, 1972.

Vall-Mayans M, Caballero E, Sanz B: The emergence of lymphogranuloma venereum in Europe, Lancet 374:356, 2009.

16

Human Immunodeficiency Virus Infection

Joseph Metmowlee Garland, Timothy Flanigan, Edward J. Wing

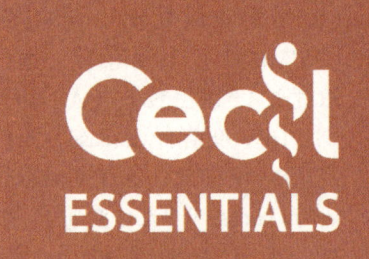

HISTORY

Human immunodeficiency virus (HIV) infection was first diagnosed in 1981 in the United States, when it was recognized as an immunodeficiency syndrome in young gay men and people who inject drugs. Soon after, the disease was recognized in patients with hemophilia, others who had received blood transfusions, previously healthy women, and rarely, health care workers. Patients with the syndrome were susceptible to unusual opportunistic infections such as *Pneumocystis jirovecii* pneumonia and unusual tumors such as Kaposi's sarcoma. Tragically, once patients had clinically identified disease, mortality over several years was very high. Patients developed recurrent infections, progressive tumors such as Kaposi's sarcoma and B cell lymphoma, wasting, and progressive neurologic syndromes including dementia. The immunodeficiency was characterized by weakened cell-mediated immunity marked by low CD4 T cells in the peripheral blood. Subsequently this disease was labeled the acquired immunodeficiency syndrome, or AIDS. In 1983, the causative agent, the human immunodeficiency virus, was identified by Luc Montagnier in France (winner of the Nobel Prize in Medicine) and Robert Gallo in the United States. By 1985, there was a serum test to identify the virus. Transmission in the United States was primarily through sex, particularly anal sex in men who had sex with men (MSM), through sharing needles during injection drug use, and through infusion of blood products.

The effect on a generation of young people was devastating. Initially, the cause was unknown, the modes of transmission uncertain, and the infectivity unclear. There was no treatment available, other than specific therapy for the opportunistic infections and tumors. All classes, races, and ethnic groups were affected. The incidence of the disease rose to greater than 50,000/year, and the number infected in the United States increased to over 1 million. Discrimination against people living with HIV (PLWH) was widespread. The government's response was slow. The early epidemic is poignantly described in Randy Shilts' book *And The Band Played On*. In 1987 the first drug, zidovudine or AZT, was approved for use against HIV and heralded a new era of virus-directed treatment. Unfortunately because of the virus' ability to mutate, resistance developed in most patients after several months of use. Other drugs with other mechanisms were developed over the next decade so that by 1995, with the discovery and approval of protease inhibitors, widespread use of effective combinations of antiretroviral therapy (ART) became available (initially called highly active antiretroviral therapy [HAART] or combination ART [cART]). This transformed HIV from a progressive disease to a manageable chronic condition in those diagnosed and engaged in treatment. Even patients with severe end-stage AIDS could resolve their opportunistic infections and recover CD4 T cell counts.

Once the virus was identified, there was a vigorous search for the geographic and animal origins of the virus. By the late 1980s, AIDS was recognized as a worldwide pandemic. Because early cases had been identified in Africa, particularly West Africa, and because HIV was closely related to endemic simian viruses, early samples from West Africa were sought and tested. The earliest human case was identified retrospectively from serum taken from a sailor in 1959 in Kinshasa, now in the Democratic Republic of Congo. Because the virus mutates at a very fast rate, a retrospective "molecular clock" technique with mathematical modeling was used to project that the origin of HIV occurred in the early 20th century during several cross-species transmission events from chimpanzees, which harbor simian immunodeficiency virus (SIV), to humans, likely in southeast Cameroon. Such transmission occurred presumably in hunters during the killing and butchering of primates for food. Sexual transmission between humans followed, and the disease progressed along rivers and highways in West Africa during a time of social change and development in the early 20th century. Spread throughout the world eventually occurred due to increased international travel and interaction.

Subsequent virologic studies of HIV have demonstrated that HIV-1 can be divided into four groups that include group M (90% to 95% of all infections) and groups N, O, and P that account for much small numbers. Group M is further divided into subgroups or clades labeled A through D, F through N, and J and K. Clade B is the most frequent in the United States and Europe, whereas C and A are found in Africa, where they account for 50% and 12% of all HIV cases, respectively. A separate distinct retrovirus, HIV-2, was identified in 1986. Confined primarily to West Africa, it causes a less severe form of AIDS.

EPIDEMIOLOGY

The course of the HIV epidemic in the United States is shown in Fig. 16.1. Stage 3 (AIDS) classification refers to those with CD4 count less than 200 or with specific opportunistic infections/tumors. As can be seen, the incidence of HIV/AIDS rose until 1993, and the death rate until 1995. Subsequently, both fell dramatically with the widespread use of multidrug effective ART. From 1998 onward, there was a leveling off, with little change in the death rate but a slow decline in number of AIDS diagnoses. Overall there has been a linear increase in the prevalence, that is, in PLWH.

人类免疫缺陷病毒感染

肖江　张福杰　译　代丽丽　郑和义　审校　张福杰　通审

历史

人类免疫缺陷病毒（HIV）感染于 1981 年在美国首次被诊断，当时它被认为是一种免疫缺陷综合征，发病人群是年轻的男同性恋者和注射毒品者。不久之后，在血友病患者、接受过输血者、曾经健康的妇女以及极少数医护人员中也发现了这种疾病。该病的患者易患不寻常的机会性感染，如肺孢子虫肺炎和罕见的肿瘤，如卡波西肉瘤。可悲的是，一旦患者在临床上发现该疾病，几年内的死亡率非常高。患者会出现反复感染、进展性肿瘤（如卡波西肉瘤和 B 细胞淋巴瘤）、消瘦以及进展性神经综合征（如痴呆）。免疫缺陷的特点是细胞免疫减弱，以外周血 $CD4^+$ T 细胞减少为主要标志。随后，这种疾病被称为获得性免疫缺陷综合征，或 AIDS。1983 年，法国的 Luc Montagnie（诺贝尔医学奖得主）和美国的 Robert Gallo 确定了致病物质——人类免疫缺陷病毒。到 1985 年，已经可以通过血清检测方法识别这种病毒。在美国，病毒主要通过性传播，尤其是男男性行为者（MSM）的肛交、注射吸毒时共用针头以及输注血液制品传播。

这对一代年轻人的影响是毁灭性的。起初，该疾病的病因不明，传播方式不确定，传染性也不明确。除了针对机会性感染和肿瘤的特异性治疗外，没有有效的治疗方法。所有阶层、种族和民族都受到了影响。这种疾病的发病率逐渐上升到每年 5 万例以上，美国的感染人数增加指数到 100 万例以上。对 HIV 感染者（PLWH）的歧视十分普遍，然而政府对此反应非常迟缓。Randy Shilts 的 *And The Band Played On* 一书深刻地描写了早期的流行状况。1987 年，第一种药物齐多夫定（AZT）被批准用于对抗 HIV，这预示着一个以病毒为导向的治疗新时代的到来。不幸的是，由于病毒具有变异能力，大多数患者在用药几个月后就产生了抗药性。在接下来的十年中，其他机制的药物也相继问世，到 1995 年，随着蛋白酶抑制剂的发现和获批，有效的抗逆转录病毒治疗（ART）开始得到广泛使用，最初被称为高效抗逆转录病毒治疗（HAART）或联合抗逆转录病毒治疗（cART）。这使 HIV 感染从一种进展性疾病，转变为一种在得到诊治的患者中可控的慢性疾病，甚至严重的 AIDS 晚期患者也可以治疗机会性感染，以及获得 $CD4^+$ T 细胞计数的恢复。

HIV 被发现后，人们开始积极寻找病毒的地理和动物来源。到 20 世纪 80 年代末，AIDS 被认定为一种全球性的流行病。由于早期病例是在非洲，特别是西非发现的，而且 HIV 与当地流行的猿类病毒关系密切，因此人们开始寻找和检测西非的早期样本。最早的人类病例是 1959 年在金沙萨（现属刚果民主共和国）的一名水手身上提取的血清中发现的。由于病毒的变异速度非常快，因此采用了一种通过数学建模的回顾性分子时钟技术，推测 HIV 的起源发生在 20 世纪初，从携带猴免疫缺陷病毒病（SIV）的黑猩猩到人类的几次跨物种传播过程中，很可能发生在喀麦隆东南部。这种传播可能发生于猎人捕杀灵长类动物作为食物的过程中，随后通过性传播继续播散。在 20 世纪初的社会变革和发展时期，这种疾病沿着西非的河流和高速公路传播，随着国际旅行和往来，疾病最终传播到世界各地。

后续的 HIV 病毒学研究表明，HIV-1 毒株可分为四组，其中包括 M 组（占所有感染病例的 90%～95%）、N、O 和 P 组，后者感染人数要少得多。M 组后续被进一步分类为 A 至 D、F 至 N、J 及 K 亚型。其中 B 亚型在美国和欧洲最为常见，而 C 亚型和 A 亚型则常见于非洲，分别占所有 HIV 感染病例的 50% 和 12%。一种独立的逆转录病毒 HIV-2 于 1986 年被发现。它主要分布在西非，引起的 AIDS 程度较轻。

流行病学

HIV 在美国的流行过程如图 16.1 所示。第 3 阶段（艾滋病期）指 $CD4^+$ T 细胞计数低于 200 或患有特殊机会性感染或肿瘤的患者。可以看出，HIV/AIDS 的发病率在 1993 年之前一直在上升，死亡率在 1995 年之前也一直在上升。随后，随着多种有效抗逆转录病毒治疗（ART）的广泛使用，这两种疗法的发病率都急剧下降。从 1998 年起，情况开始趋于平稳，死亡率变化不大，但 HIV 感染确诊人数却在缓慢下降。总体而言，PLWH 呈直线上升趋势。

CHAPTER 16 Human Immunodeficiency Virus Infection

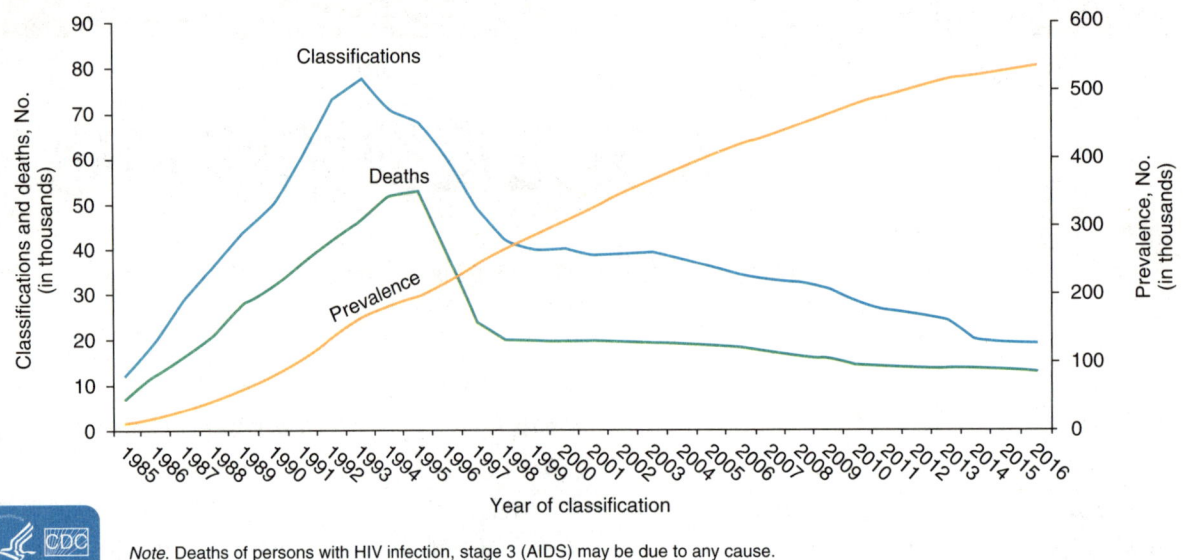

Fig. 16.1 Stage 3 (AIDS) classifications, deaths, and persons living with diagnosed HIV infection ever classified as stage 3 (AIDS) 1985–2016: United States and six dependent areas. (From the Centers for Disease Control and Prevention; National Center for HIV/AIDS, Viral Hepatitis, STD, and TB Prevention Division of HIV/AIDS Prevention. *Trends in HIV Infection Stage 3 [AIDS]*. https://npin.cdc.gov/publication/trends-hiv-infection-stage-3-aids. Accessed January 23, 2019.)

In 2017, there were 38,739 new cases of HIV infection in the United States, a rate that has been unchanged since 2012. In 2017 it was estimated that 1.2 million people were living with HIV in the United States and 86% had been diagnosed. Sixty-three percent of those who had been diagnosed had a suppressed viral load. Geographically, the rates of new HIV diagnoses are highest in the South followed by the Northeast, the West, and finally the Midwest. Those at greatest risk remain MSM, accounting for 66% of all HIV diagnoses in 2017. The risk of acquiring HIV is 22 times higher than in the general population in men who have sex with men. Women are at risk primarily through heterosexual contact (17% of new diagnoses), with African American women being at greatest risk. Minority populations, particularly African American and Hispanic individuals are at greater risk for HIV compared to other races/ethnicities. In 2017 African Americans accounted for 43% of new HIV diagnoses, though they accounted for only 13% of the entire population. Hispanic individuals accounted for 26% of new diagnoses but were only approximately 17% of the total population.

Though still considered a traditional risk factor, injection drug use has fallen markedly as a cause of HIV transmission, largely through the use of syringe exchange programs and other harm reduction practices among people who inject drugs. In 2017, injection drug use accounted for only 9% of new HIV diagnoses in the United States. The risk of acquiring HIV is 22 times higher in those who inject drugs and 21 times higher in sex workers. Unfortunately, in 2018, only 18% of persons at high risk with indications had been prescribed medications for preexposure prophylaxis (PrEP, see later section) for prophylaxis.

Since the 1980s, HIV infection has become a worldwide pandemic and HIV continues to spread throughout all continents. Since the late 1990s, rapid transmission has occurred throughout Africa, India, Southeast Asia, the former Soviet Union, and some parts of Eastern Europe. Today, approximately 70% of PLWH live in Africa; the Americas and South-East Asia account for slightly more than 9% each, and Europe accounts for 6%. Because of latency between HIV infection and the development of AIDS-associated illnesses, the clinically recognized epidemic of AIDS has lagged 6 to 8 years behind the spread of the virus into new populations.

Since the start of the epidemic, according to UNAIDS, 74.9 million people have become infected with HIV and 32 million people have died from HIV. In 2018 it was estimated that 37.9 million people globally were living with HIV and of those, 1.7 million people were younger than 15 years of age. In that year 1.7 million people were newly infected and 770,000 people died from HIV. In 2018, 23.3 million people living with HIV were taking ART. As a result of increasing availability of ART, the number of new infections has been reduced by 40% since 1997 and AIDS-related deaths have been reduced by more than 56% since 2004. With more access to ART worldwide and increasing efforts at availability and adherence, incidence and mortality rates should continue to fall. Tuberculosis remains the leading cause of death among PLWH, accounting for approximately one in three deaths due to HIV. It is estimated that almost half of people infected with HIV and TB are unaware of their coinfection and therefore are not receiving appropriate care.

VIROLOGY

HIV contains two single-stranded copies of the viral RNA genome, together with the virus-encoded enzymes reverse transcriptase, protease, and integrase (Fig. 16.2). Surrounding the structural (p24 and p18) proteins is a lipid bilayer derived from the host cell, through which protrude the transmembrane (gp41) and surface (gp120) envelope glycoproteins. The HIV envelope glycoproteins have a high affinity for the

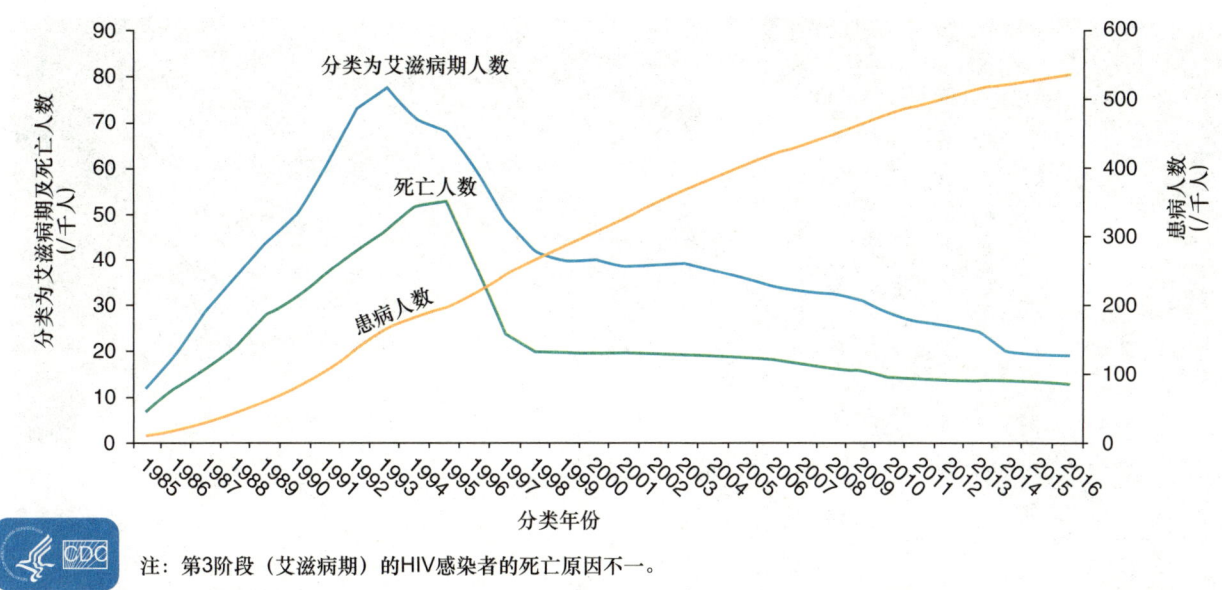

注：第3阶段（艾滋病期）的HIV感染者的死亡原因不一。

图16.1　1985—2016年分类为第3阶段（艾滋病期）人数、死亡人数和曾被归类为第3阶段（艾滋病期）的确诊HIV感染者：美国和六个附属地区统计数据（引自 the Centers for Disease Control and Prevention；National Center for HIV/AIDS, Viral Hepatitis, STD, and TB Prevention Division of HIV/AIDS Prevention. Trends in HIV Infection Stage 3［AIDS］. https://npin.cdc.gov/publication/trends-hivinfection-stage-3-aids. Accessed January 23, 2019.）

2017年美国报告新发HIV感染者38 739人，这一新发比例自2012年以来一直未有变化。据估计，2017年美国有约120万HIV感染者，其中86%已确诊。在确诊者中，63%的患者病毒载量得到抑制。从地域上看，南部地区新诊断出的HIV感染率最高，其次是东北部、西部，最后是中西部。风险最大的仍然是男男性行为者，占2017年所有HIV感染确诊病例的66%。男男性行为者感染HIV的风险是普通人群的22倍。女性主要通过异性性接触面临风险（占新诊断病例的17%），其中非裔美国女性面临的风险最大。与其他种族相比，少数种族，尤其是非裔美国人和西班牙裔美国人感染HIV的风险更大。2017年，非洲裔美国人占新诊断HIV病例的43%，尽管他们在总人口中仅占13%。西班牙裔个体占新诊断病例的26%，但在整个总人口中只约占17%。

尽管注射吸毒仍被视为一种传统的危险因素，但其作为HIV传播因素的比例已明显下降，这主要得益于注射吸毒者实施的注射器交换项目和其他减少伤害的措施。2017年，在美国新确诊的HIV感染者中，注射吸毒者仅占9%。与一般人群相比，注射吸毒者感染HIV的风险高达22倍，性工作者则高达21倍。遗憾的是，2018年，仅有18%有适应证的高危人群使用了暴露前预防药物（PrEP，见后文）用于预防。

自20世纪80年代以来，HIV感染已成为世界性流行病，HIV持续在各大洲间传播。自20世纪90年代末以来，非洲、印度、东南亚、苏联和东欧部分地区出现了快速传播。如今，大约70%的HIV感染者生活在非洲，在美洲和东南亚各约占9%，欧洲占6%。由于HIV感染和AIDS相关疾病的进展之间存在潜伏期，临床上公认的AIDS流行比病毒传播到新的人群滞后6～8年。

据联合国艾滋病规划署（UNAIDS）统计，自AIDS流行以来，已有7490万人感染HIV，3200万人死于HIV。据估计，2018年全球有3790万人感染HIV，其中170万人年龄小于15岁。当年有170万人新发感染，77万人死于HIV感染。2018年，有2330万HIV感染者正在接受抗逆转录病毒治疗（ART）。由于抗逆转录病毒治疗的普及率不断提高，自1997年以来，新发感染人数减少了40%，自2004年以来，与AIDS相关的死亡人数减少了56%以上。随着抗逆转录病毒治疗在全球范围内的普及，以及在药物可及性和依从性方面的不断努力，发病率和死亡率应会继续下降。结核病仍然是HIV感染者的主要死因，约占HIV导致死亡人数的1/3。据估计，几乎有一半的HIV和结核病合并感染者不知道自己同时感染了HIV和结核病，因此没有得到适当的治疗。

病毒学

HIV由两个单链RNA病毒核酸、病毒编码的逆转录酶、蛋白酶和整合酶组成（图16.2）。在结构蛋白（p24和p18）周围有一层来自宿主细胞的脂质双分子层，跨膜（gp41）蛋白和表面（gp120）包膜糖蛋白从脂质双分子层结构中穿入。HIV病毒包膜糖蛋白对辅

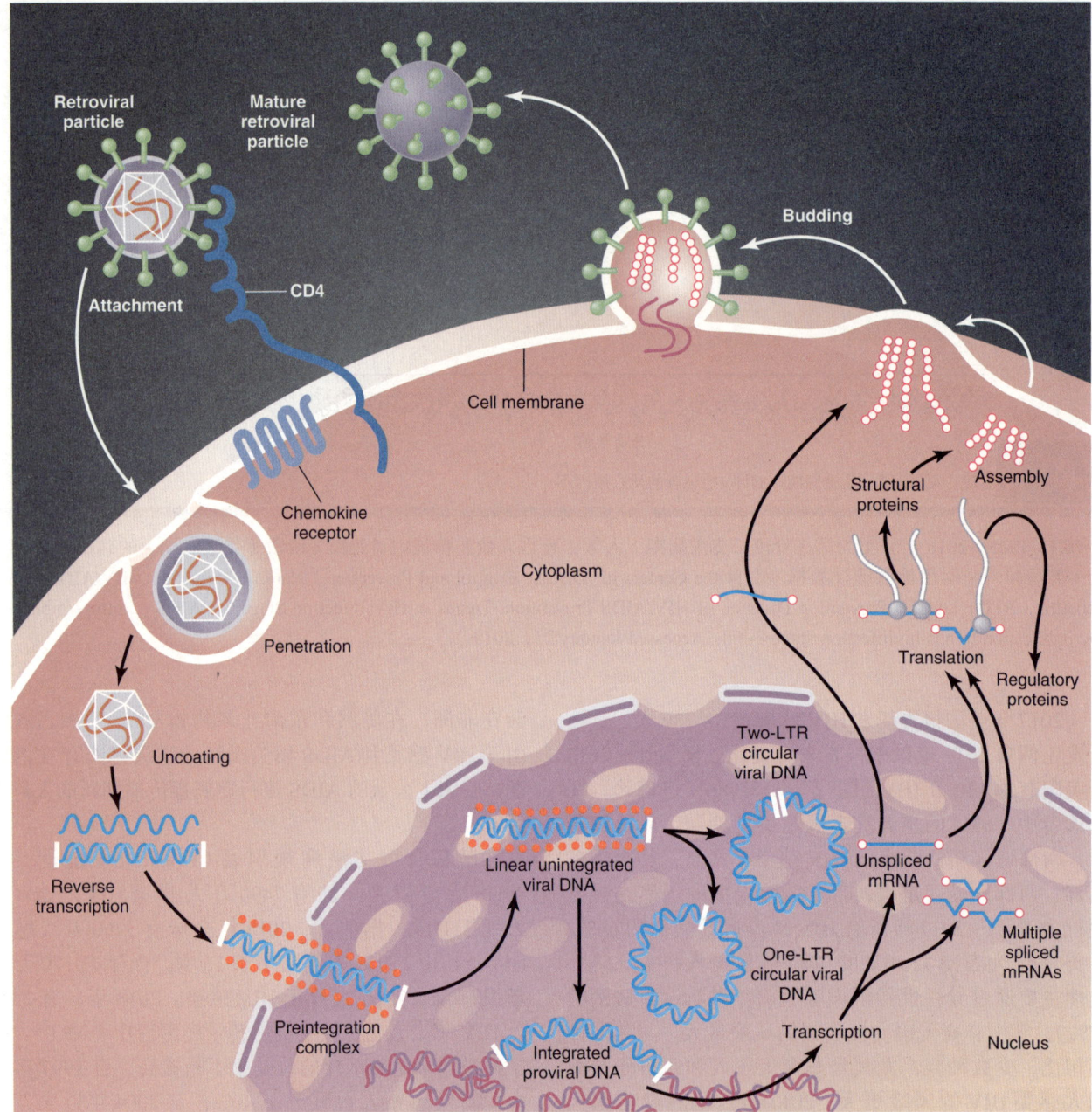

Fig. 16.2 HIV viral replication. Key steps in the pathway targeted by antiretroviral therapy include membrane binding and fusion, reverse transcription, integration of proviral DNA, and protein synthesis. *LTR*, Long terminal repeat; *mRNA*, messenger RNA. (Modified from Furtado MR, Callaway DS, Phair JP, et al: Persistence of HIV-1 transcription in patients receiving potent antiretroviral therapy, N Engl J Med 340:1614–1622, 1999.)

CD4 molecule on the surface of T-helper lymphocytes and other cells of monocyte-macrophage lineage. After HIV binds to the CD4 molecule, the envelope undergoes a conformational change that facilitates binding to another cellular coreceptor; the most important of these are the chemokine receptors CCR5 and CXCR4. This second binding event promotes a major conformational change that causes approximation of the viral and cellular membranes; fusion of these membranes is mediated by insertion of the newly exposed fusion domain of the envelope gp41 into the host cell membrane.

As a result of these processes, the HIV nucleoprotein complex enters the cytoplasm, where the RNA viral genome undergoes reverse transcription by the virally encoded reverse transcriptase. The resulting double-stranded viral DNA enters the nucleus, where proper localization of the viral preintegration complex is mediated by host proteins, and integration of the DNA provirus into the host chromosome is catalyzed by the retroviral integrase. Latently infected resting memory CD4 lymphocytes serve as reservoirs of persistent infection for the life of the patient even with effective ART (see later discussion). However, the bulk of viral replication takes place in activated T cells, which are both more susceptible to HIV infection and more capable of supporting productive HIV replication.

When a CD4+ lymphocyte is activated, expression of HIV messenger RNA (mRNA) is enhanced. Core proteins, viral enzymes, and envelope proteins are encoded by the *gag*, *pol*, and *env* genes of HIV, respectively. More than 100 host proteins, in addition to the viral proteins,

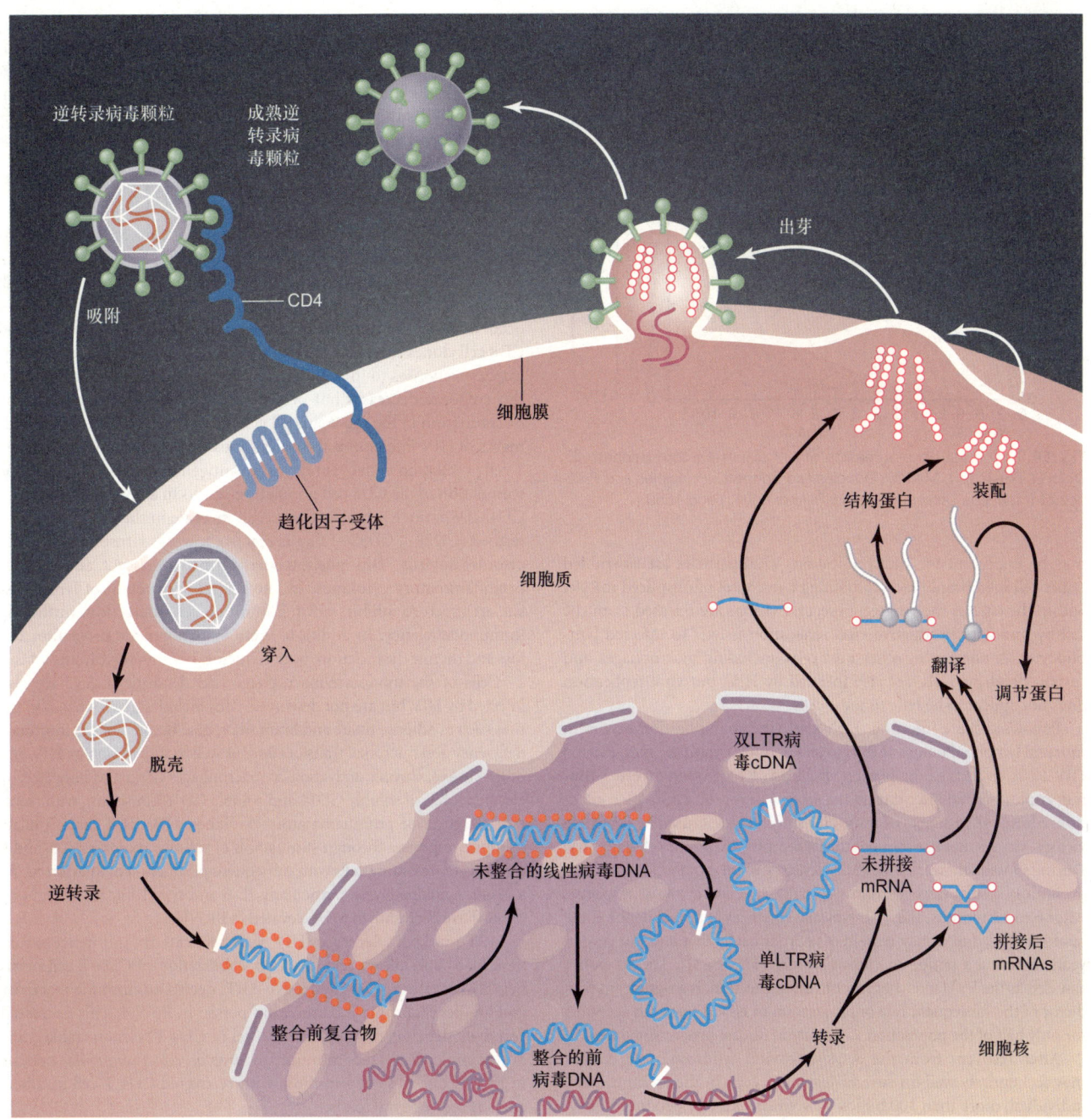

图16.2 HIV病毒复制过程。抗逆转录病毒治疗所针对的途径中的关键步骤包括膜结合和融合、逆转录、前病毒DNA整合和蛋白合成。LTR, 长末端重复序列; mRNA, 信使RNA（改编自 Furtado MR, Callaway DS, Phair JP, et al: Persistence of HIV-1 transcription in patients receiving potent antiretroviral therapy, N Engl J Med 340: 1614-1622, 1999.）

助性T淋巴细胞和单核巨噬细胞谱系的其他细胞表面的CD4分子具有高亲和力。HIV与CD4分子结合后，包膜发生构象变化，从而与另一个细胞核受体结合，其中最重要的是趋化因子受体CCR5和CXCR4。第二次结合会促进包膜构象发生重大变化，使病毒膜和细胞膜近似，包膜gp41新暴露的融合结构域插入宿主细胞膜，介导膜的融合。

在这些过程中，HIV核蛋白复合物进入细胞质，病毒RNA在这里通过病毒编码的逆转录酶进行逆转录。由此产生的双链病毒DNA进入细胞核，病毒整合前复合物在宿主蛋白质的介导下正确定位，前病毒DNA在逆转录病毒整合酶的催化下整合到宿主染色体上。即便使用有效的抗逆转录病毒治疗，潜伏感染的静息记忆$CD4^+$ T细胞也会成为持续感染的病毒储存库（见后文）。然而，大部分病毒复制发生在活化的T淋巴细胞中，这些细胞更容易受到HIV感染，也更能够支持HIV的有效复制。

当$CD4^+$ T细胞被激活时，HIV mRNA的表达增强，*gag*、*pol* 和 *env* 基因进行编码翻译核心蛋白、病毒酶和包膜蛋白。除病毒蛋白外，还有100多种宿主蛋白可能对病毒复制产生重要影响。病毒颗粒在细胞膜上组装，每个颗粒的核心含有两个未拼接的mRNA，病毒颗粒则通过出芽的方式从细胞中释放出来。病毒复制对受

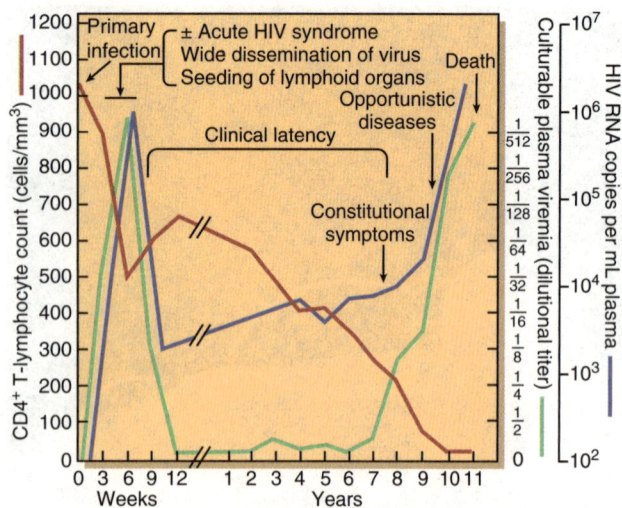

Fig. 16.3 The natural progression of HIV disease. (From Bennett JE, Dolin R, Blaser MJ. Mandell Douglas and Bennett's Principles and Practice of Infectious Diseases, 9th ed. Figure 122.1, page 1659.)

may be important for viral replication. Viral particles are assembled at the cell membrane, each containing two copies of unspliced mRNA within the core as the viral genome, and virions are released from the cell by budding. Productive viral replication is lytic to infected lymphocytes. A number of other host cells, including macrophages and certain dendritic cells, are also infected by HIV, but viral replication does not appear to be lytic to these cells.

Following acute infection, high-level viral multiplication occurs in mucosal lymphoid tissues of the gut and in other lymphatic sites. Plasma HIV RNA levels (i.e., the plasma viral load [PVL]) often exceed 1 million copies per milliliter during the second to fourth weeks after infection. Almost all instances of acute HIV infection are caused by R5 tropic viruses, viruses that use the chemokine receptor CCR5 for cellular entry. During subsequent weeks, the PVL decreases, often rapidly. This decrease in viremia results largely from a partially effective immune response. After 6 to 12 months, the PVL typically stabilizes at a level denoted the viral *set point*, and it may remain at approximately that level for several years, entering a period of clinical latency (Fig. 16.3). The set point, assessed as the PVL at 6 to 12 months after infection, is a significant predictor of the subsequent rate of progression of HIV disease but accounts for only half of the population variability in disease progression rates.

After recovery from the acute retroviral syndrome, the patient may feel entirely well for several years, but even in the asymptomatic individual, more than 100 billion new virions may be produced daily. Rapid production and turnover of circulating $CD4^+$ cells also occurs throughout the course of HIV infection, and a progressive decline in circulating $CD4^+$ cells occurs in most individuals. Cell lysis associated with HIV replication accounts only partially for this progressive loss of CD4 cells. During the years of clinical latency, virions are present in large numbers in the follicular dendritic processes of the germinal centers of the lymph nodes, which undergo both hyperplasia and progressive fibrosis. As HIV disease progresses over several years, the lymphatic tissue atrophies and plasma viremia intensifies. In later-stage HIV disease, a more dramatic CD4 cell decline is observed, following a sharp rise in the PVL (see Fig. 16.3).

The decline in the number of CD4 cells is accompanied by profound functional impairment of the remaining lymphocyte populations. Anergy may develop early in HIV infection and eventually occurs in almost all persons with AIDS. T-helper lymphocyte proliferation in response to antigenic stimuli is dramatically impaired, T cell cytotoxic responses are diminished, and natural killer cell activity against virus-infected cells is greatly impaired. Decrease in function as well as number of CD4 cells is central to the immune dysfunction, and this impairment partly underlies the failure of B-lymphocyte function, as measured by impaired capacity to synthesize antibody in response to new antigens.

IMMUNOLOGY AND INFLAMMATION

Acute HIV infection results in massive destruction of T cells in lymphoid tissue throughout the body, particularly in the intestinal wall, and the decrease can be easily quantified in the peripheral blood. Partial recovery of T cell numbers and partial control of HIV viral load occurs due to the initial immune response in which both CD4 and CD8 cell clones react to HIV antigens (see Fig. 16.3). Robust inflammatory responses to initial infection occur. Within weeks to months, this response decreases but persists above baseline compared to the inflammation in the age-matched general population. One of the hallmarks of HIV infection is the continuous slow destruction of the CD4 T cell population with eventual loss of antigenic reactivity. Continuous stimulation of the CD8 cell population results in a reversal of the usual CD4:CD8 ratio. Eventually there is an increase in the CD8 phenotype termed (CD28−, CD57+) that is reactive towards viruses, particularly cytomegalovirus. This phenotype is termed senescent and secretes proinflammatory cytokines. In late stages, destruction of lymph tissue architecture inhibits normal immune cell interaction, furthering immunodeficiency. In addition, there is hemopoietic progenitor cell loss and thymic dysfunction, both reducing T lymphocyte homeostasis.

Cells of the monocyte/macrophage and dendritic lineage are also infected by HIV but are not destroyed. This includes macrophages in tissues such as adipose tissue and brain microglia. Because of gut immunodeficiency and microbial translocation, as well as stimulation by HIV and other viruses, chronic activation of macrophages occurs, as indicated by elevated levels of soluble CD14 and soluble CD163 in serum, with resultant secretion of proinflammatory cytokines. HIV itself can stimulate immune responses through stimulation of toll-like receptors 7, 8, and 9 on antigen presenting cells with subsequent production of interferons. As a result, cytokine levels, particularly IL-6 and type I interferons among others have been shown to be elevated in PLWH.

ART markedly decreases HIV viral replication (and hence serum viral load) and allows recovery and stabilization of CD4 T cell numbers. However, even with effective ART, decreased immune reactivity and low-level chronic inflammation persist in PLWH. This decreased reactivity depends roughly on the level of CD4 T cells on stable ART. For example, decreased immunity to *Streptococcus pneumoniae* persists in PLWH on ART even in those with recovered CD4 T cell numbers and suppressed viral loads.

Persistent chronic inflammation in people living with HIV, even in those on effective ART, is presumed to be multifactorial in etiology including: (1) low levels of HIV replication; (2) gut immunodeficiency allowing continuous exposure to microbial antigens resulting in macrophage activation; (3) reactivation of herpes viruses, particularly CMV and EBV; and (4) cytokine production by cells including macrophages and senescent CD8 T cells. This low-level inflammation is linked in part to increased risk for chronic diseases including cardiovascular, bone, kidney, and other morbidities associated with aging.

CLINICAL DIAGNOSIS OF HIV

Since 2013, the US Preventive Services Task Force has recommended routine HIV testing in all persons ages 15 to 65, to be offered in primary care settings. Despite this recommendation, almost a quarter of new

免疫学和炎症

急性HIV感染会导致全身淋巴组织（尤其是肠壁）中的T淋巴细胞大量破坏，外周血中的T淋巴细胞减少情况也很容易量化监测。由于最初的免疫反应，$CD4^+$ T细胞和$CD8^+$ T细胞克隆都会对HIV抗原产生反应，因此T淋巴细胞数量会部分恢复，HIV病毒载量也会得到部分控制（图16.3）。初始感染时会出现强烈的炎症反应，而在数周至数月内，这种反应会减弱，但仍高于年龄匹配的普通人群的炎症反应。其中HIV感染的一个标志是$CD4^+$ T细胞的持续缓慢破坏，最终会丧失抗原反应活性。对$CD8^+$ T细胞的持续刺激通常会导致CD4：CD8比例发生逆转。最终，被称为（$CD28^-$、$CD57^+$）的$CD8^+$ T细胞表型会增加，这种表型对病毒，尤其是巨细胞病毒会产生免疫反应。这种表型的细胞被称为衰老型，会分泌促炎细胞因子。在晚期，淋巴管结构的破坏抑制了正常免疫细胞的相互作用，进一步导致免疫缺陷加剧。此外，造血祖细胞丢失和胸腺功能障碍也会降低T淋巴细胞的稳态。

单核细胞、巨噬细胞和树突状细胞也会感染HIV，但不会导致细胞凋亡，这些细胞包括脂肪组织和大脑小胶质细胞等组织中的巨噬细胞。由于肠道免疫缺陷和微生物易位以及HIV和其他病毒的刺激，巨噬细胞发生慢性活化，表现为血清中可溶性CD14和可溶性CD163水平升高，继而分泌促炎细胞因子。HIV本身可通过刺激抗原提呈细胞上的Toll样受体7、8和9以及随后产生的干扰素来刺激免疫反应。因此，细胞因子的水平，尤其是IL-6和I型干扰素的水平会随着时间的推移而升高，其他一些指标在HIV感染者中也显示升高。

抗逆转录病毒治疗可显著降低HIV病毒复制，进而降低血清病毒载量，并使$CD4^+$ T细胞数量得以恢复和稳定。然而，即使抗逆转录病毒治疗有效，HIV感染者的免疫反应性下降和低水平慢性炎症依然存在。这种反应性的降低大致取决于接受稳定抗逆转录病毒治疗时的$CD4^+$ T细胞计数水平。例如，在接受抗逆转录病毒治疗的HIV感染者中，即使$CD4^+$ T细胞计数得到恢复、病毒载量得到抑制，他们对肺炎链球菌的免疫力也会降低。

即使是接受有效抗逆转录病毒治疗的HIV感染者，其体内也会持续存在慢性炎症状态，目前推测是由多种因素造成，包括：①HIV低水平复制；②肠道免疫缺陷导致持续暴露于微生物抗原，从而导致巨噬细胞活化；③疱疹病毒，尤其是CMV和EBV的重新激活；④包括巨噬细胞和衰老$CD8^+$ T细胞在内的细胞产生的细胞因子。这种低水平的炎症反应在一定程度上与慢性疾病风险的增加有关，包括心血管、骨骼、肾及其他与衰老相关的疾病。

HIV感染的临床诊断

自2013年以来，美国预防服务工作组一直建议在初级卫生机构中对所有15～65岁人群进行常规HIV

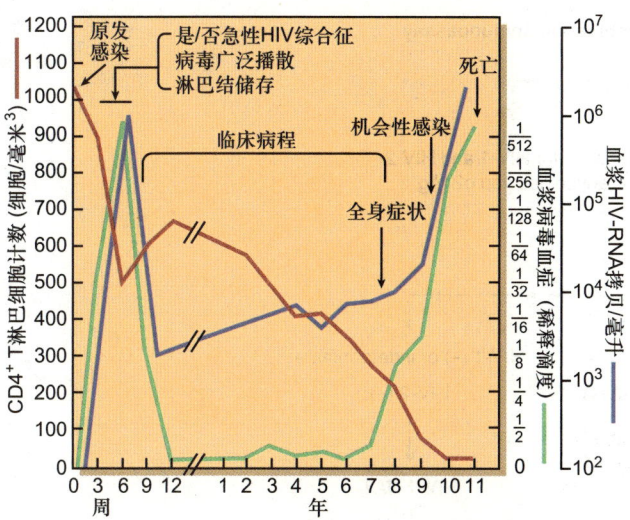

图16.3　HIV疾病的自然病程（引自Bennett JE, Dolin R, Blaser MJ. Mandell Douglas and Bennett's Principles and Practice of Infectious Diseases, 9th ed. Figure 122.1, page 1659.）

感染的淋巴细胞具有杀伤作用。其他一些宿主细胞，包括巨噬细胞和某些树突状细胞，也会被HIV感染，但病毒复制似乎不会对这些细胞产生裂解作用。

发生急性HIV感染后，病毒会在肠道黏膜淋巴组织和其他淋巴部位大量繁殖。血浆HIV-RNA水平［即血浆病毒载量（PVL）］在感染后的第2～4周往往超过每100万拷贝/毫升。几乎所有急性HIV感染都是由利用趋化因子受体CCR5进入细胞的病毒引起。在随后的几周内，病毒载量通常会迅速下降，主要是由于部分有效的免疫反应发挥作用。6～12个月后，病毒载量通常会稳定在固定水平，并可能在近似该水平上维持数年，进入临床潜伏期（图16.3）。病毒感染后6～12个月的病毒载量即为病毒设定值，它是AIDS病情进展速度的重要预测因素，但仅在半数人群中具有预测性。

HIV感染者从急性逆转录病毒综合征好转后，可能在数年内感觉完全康复，但即使是无症状的患者，每天也可能产生超过1000亿个新病毒。在整个HIV感染过程中，外周循环中的$CD4^+$ T细胞也会迅速发生更替，大多数人的循环$CD4^+$ T细胞会逐渐减少。与HIV复制相关的细胞裂解仅是$CD4^+$ T细胞逐渐减少的部分原因。在临床潜伏期，病毒大量存在于淋巴结生发中心的滤泡树突中，这些滤泡树突会发生增生和纤维化。随着HIV感染的进展，淋巴组织萎缩，血浆病毒血症加剧；在HIV感染晚期，$CD4^+$ T细胞的下降更为显著，而病毒载量则急剧上升（图16.3）。

$CD4^+$ T细胞数量的减少伴随着剩余淋巴细胞群功能受损。HIV感染初期可能会出现无反应性，最终几乎所有AIDS患者都会出现这种现象。患者的辅助性T淋巴细胞增殖对抗原刺激的反应明显减弱，T淋巴细胞的细胞毒性反应减弱，自然杀伤细胞对受病毒感染细胞的活性也大大减弱。$CD4^+$ T细胞功能和数量的减少是免疫功能失调的核心，这种损伤也是导致B淋巴细胞功能失调的部分原因，表现为对新抗原合成抗体的能力减弱。

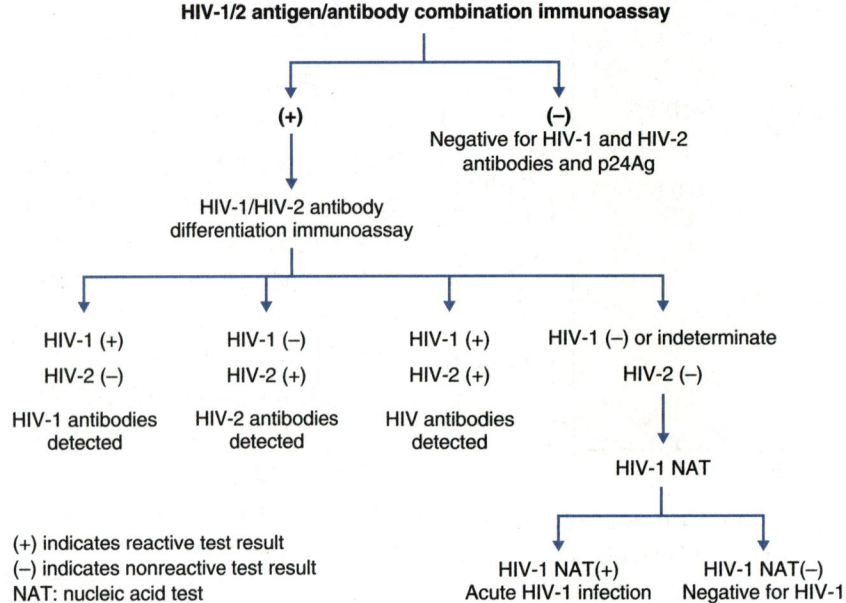

Fig. 16.4 Recommended HIV testing algorithm (CLSI).

HIV diagnoses are made when the patient already has an AIDS diagnosis (CD4 count <200 or AIDS-defining condition), indicating late diagnosis and missed opportunities for earlier testing remain an issue. All pregnant women should be offered HIV testing as well. Standard testing for HIV in the United States is through use of a fourth-generation immunoassay for HIV-1 and HIV-2 antibodies and an HIV early antigen (p24). Confirmation is by an HIV-1 and HIV-2 antibody differentiation immunoassay and nucleic acid testing if these are both negative or indeterminate (Fig. 16.4). The "window period" from disease acquisition to test positivity has greatly reduced as compared with earlier generations of the test; fourth-generation testing is usually positive within 18 to 45 days. Rapid point-of-care testing methods also exist and may play an important role in HIV testing in many clinical and community settings. These rapid tests are lateral-flow (immunochromatographic) or vertical-flow (immunofiltration) assays that detect the presence of HIV-1/2 antibodies and/or HIV p24 antigen and can be performed on oral fluid or a drop of serum ("finger stick") to provide results within 30 minutes. They do require confirmation by serum antibody-based tests. If HIV is diagnosed, it is important to pursue further testing to characterize the stage of disease, including a CD4 count and PVL.

Identification of persons with HIV and linkage to effective care are critical public health priorities. Early identification of infection affects prognosis; patients who have AIDS at diagnosis have a lower predicted life expectancy than those with higher CD4 counts. Further, studies have demonstrated that patients who are diagnosed and treated with effective ART do not transmit virus to others once their serum viral load is undetectable, therefore HIV treatment is also a cornerstone of HIV prevention efforts.

Any discussion of HIV diagnosis raises the important question of disclosure. Respect for patients' right to confidentiality is important to remember at all points of contact with the health care system, particularly given the often-stigmatized nature of HIV infection in society. Communication of a new diagnosis, and any subsequent discussion of treatment, prognosis, transmission, or other aspects of care, must be performed in a confidential setting. Whether and how to disclose to partners or family members is a patient decision, and disclosure should be done by the patient or by the patient with the provider's assistance. State-by-state laws differ on the legality of disclosing patients' HIV status without their consent, but best practices generally discourage this practice because it will damage the patient-provider relationship and increases the risk of losing the patient to care entirely. After establishing a relationship with a patient, providers should also discuss designating a health care proxy (HCP) and gain an understanding of what the HCP knows about the patient's health, so that the patient's wishes around confidentiality can be respected even in the setting of incapacitation.

THE NATURAL PROGRESSION OF HIV DISEASE

Acute Retroviral Syndrome

Up to 50% of PLWH report a mononucleosis-like syndrome (acute retroviral syndrome) occurring 2 to 6 weeks after initial infection. The symptoms may include fever, sore throat, gastrointestinal symptoms, diffuse lymph node enlargement, rash, arthralgias, and headache that usually persist for several days to 3 weeks (Table 16.1). The rash is typically maculopapular and short-lived and usually affects the trunk or face. Ten percent of infected individuals experience an acute, self-limited, aseptic meningitis, which on lumbar puncture can be characterized by cerebrospinal fluid (CSF) pleocytosis with detectable HIV in the CSF; however, this syndrome is often not recognized. Rarely, patients may present with opportunistic infections during this period, most commonly thrush (*Candida* pharyngitis). The acute retroviral syndrome is often sufficiently severe that the patient seeks medical attention, though it is uncommon to require hospitalization. During acute infection, the plasma viral load can be extremely high, often greater than 1 million copies per mL, and the CD4 count will dip lower than where it will eventually settle (see Fig. 16.3). It is critical to maintain a high index of suspicion for acute HIV retroviral syndrome because the very high plasma HIV RNA level during this period confers a high likelihood of HIV transmission to sexual or needle-sharing partners, or from mother to infant (e.g., during breast-feeding).

Natural Clinical Progression of Untreated Disease

Untreated HIV infection usually results in a slow, nonlinear progression to severe immunodeficiency over the course of years. However, the progression of disease varies greatly among individuals. Within

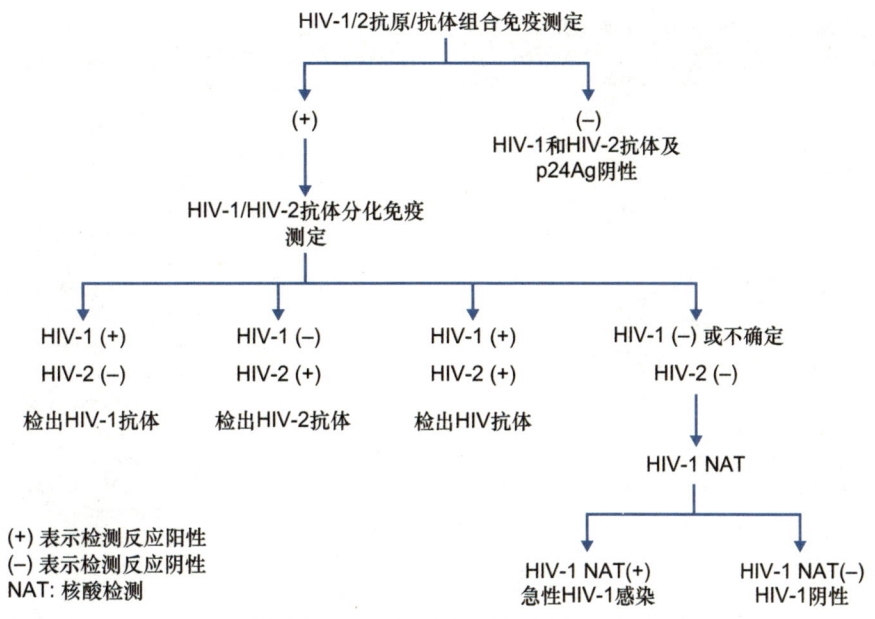

图 16.4　HIV 检测流程推荐（CLSI）

筛查。尽管有这一建议，但近 1/4 的新诊断 HIV 感染者是在进入艾滋病期（CD4$^+$ T 细胞计数小于 200 或出现 AIDS 指征性疾病）后才得到诊断，这表明晚期诊断和错失早期检测机会仍是一个问题。所有孕妇也应接受 HIV 检测。在美国，HIV 的标准检测方法是使用第四代免疫测定法检测 HIV-1、HIV-2 抗体以及 HIV 早期抗原（p24）。如果 HIV-1 和 HIV-2 抗体均为阴性或不确定，则通过 HIV-1 和 HIV-2 抗体分化免疫测定和核酸检测进行确证实验（图 16.4）。与早期的检测方法相比，从感染疾病到检测结果呈阳性的窗口期大幅缩短，第四代检测方法通常在 18～45 天检测结果呈阳性。此外，还有一些快速的即时检测方法应用于临床和社区环境中的 HIV 检测中。这些快速检测方法是通过免疫层析或免疫过滤检测法，从而检测 HIV-1/2 抗体和（或）HIV p24 抗原的存在，并可通过采集口腔唾液或一滴血清（末梢指血）来进行检测，在 30 min 内得出结果，但需要通过血清抗体检测进行确认。如果确诊为 HIV 感染，必须进行进一步检测以确定疾病的阶段，包括 CD4$^+$ T 细胞计数和血清病毒载量。

识别 HIV 感染者并与医疗体系建立联系是公共卫生的首要事项。早期发现感染状态有助于改善预后，与 CD4$^+$ T 细胞计数较高的患者相比，诊断时已进入艾滋病期的患者的预期寿命较短。此外，研究表明，经诊断并接受有效抗逆转录病毒治疗的患者，一旦其血清病毒载量检测不到，就不会将病毒传染给他人。因此，HIV 抗病毒治疗也是 HIV 预防工作的基石。任何有关 HIV 诊断的讨论都会导致信息暴露，因此在医护人员与患者的接触中，尊重隐私是非常重要的方面，特别是考虑到 HIV 感染者在社会上往往会伴随病耻感。

告知 HIV 感染者诊断结果，以及随后讨论治疗、预后、传播或护理的其他方面，都必须在保密的情况下进行。是否及如何告知患者伴侣或家庭成员，均应由患者决定，且应由患者本人或在医护人员的协助下进行。对于不经患者允许即披露 HIV 感染状态，不同地区的法律规定不同，但通常不鼓励，因为这会破坏患者与医护人员之间的关系及可能导致失访。在与患者建立关系后，医护人员还应讨论指定一名患者委托人，明确委托人对患者健康状况的了解程度，以便即使在患者丧失自主能力的情况下，也能尊重患者的保密意愿。

HIV 感染的自然病程

急性逆转录病毒综合征

多达 50% 的 HIV 感染者报告在初次感染后 2～6 周，出现类似单核细胞增多症的综合征，即急性逆转录病毒综合征。症状可能包括发热、咽痛、胃肠道症状、弥漫性淋巴结肿大、皮疹、关节痛和头痛，通常持续数天至 3 周（表 16.1）。皮疹通常为斑丘疹，持续时间短，通常累及躯干或面部。10% 的感染者会出现急性自限性无菌性脑膜炎，腰椎穿刺时可发现脑脊液细胞增多、HIV 检测阳性。但这种综合征往往不容易被发现。极少数患者在此期间会出现机会性感染，最常见的是鹅口疮（念珠菌性咽炎）。急性逆转录病毒综合征通常病情严重，需要立即就医，但往往不需住院治疗。在急性感染期间，血浆病毒载量可能会非常高，通常超过 100 万拷贝/毫升，CD4$^+$ T 细胞计数也会下降，但最终会稳定在较低水平（图 16.3）。面对急性 HIV 逆转录病毒综合征应保持高度警惕，因为在此期间极高的血浆 HIV-RNA 载量极有可能导致 HIV 传播给性接触者或共用针头者，或由母亲传播给婴儿（如母乳喂养）。

未经治疗的 HIV 感染的自然病程

未经治疗的 HIV 感染通常会在数年内缓慢、非线性地发展为严重的免疫缺陷状态。然而，疾病的进展存在

TABLE 16.1	Symptoms and Signs of Acute Retroviral Syndrome in 209 Patients	
Symptom or Sign	No. With Finding	Frequency (%)
Fever	200	96
Adenopathy	154	74
Pharyngitis	146	70
Rash	146	70
Myalgia or arthralgia	112	54
Thrombocytopenia	94	45
Leukopenia	80	38
Diarrhea	67	32
Headache	66	32
Nausea, vomiting	56	27
Elevated aminotransferase levels	38	21
Hepatosplenomegaly	30	14
Thrush	24	12
Neuropathy	13	6
Encephalopathy	12	6

Modified from Niu MT, Stein DS, Schnittman SM. Primary human immunodeficiency virus type 1 infection: review of pathogenesis and early treatment intervention in human and animal retrovirus infections. J Infect Dis 1993;168:1490-1501.

TABLE 16.2	Progressive Complications of HIV Infection by CD4 Count
CD4 Count (cells/mm^3)	Opportunistic Infection or Neoplasm
>500	Herpes zoster
	Tuberculosis
200-500	Oral hairy leukoplakia
	Candida pharyngitis (thrush)
	Kaposi's sarcoma, mucocutaneous
	Bacterial pneumonia, recurrent
	Cervical or anal neoplasia
100-200	*Pneumocystis jirovecii* pneumonia
	Histoplasmosis capsulatum infection, disseminated
	Kaposi's sarcoma, visceral
	Progressive multifocal leukoencephalopathy
	Lymphoma, non-Hodgkin's
<100	*Candida* esophagitis
	Cytomegalovirus retinitis
	Mycobacterium avium-intercellulare
	Toxoplasma gondii encephalitis
	Cryptosporidium parvum enteritis
	Cryptococcus neoformans meningitis
	Herpes simplex virus, chronic, ulcerative
	Cytomegalovirus esophagitis or colitis
	Primary central nervous system lymphoma

10 years after infection, approximately 50% of untreated individuals will develop AIDS, 30% will have milder symptoms, and fewer than 20% will be entirely asymptomatic (see Fig. 16.3). Children and adolescents progress to AIDS at a slower rate than older persons. The rate of progression of immunodeficiency is not influenced by the route of HIV transmission and appears mostly to be inherent to characteristics of the individual rather than the transmitted virus. In the long term, disease does not appear to differ by gender, although typically women with HIV infection tend to experience more rapid disease progression with lower levels of HIV in plasma.

Clinically recognized lymph node enlargement occurs in 35% to 40% of asymptomatic HIV-infected persons but is not significantly associated with either rate of progression of immunodeficiency or with subsequent development of lymphoma. During early HIV infection, thrombocytopenia, probably caused by autoimmune platelet destruction, is common. Most PLWH remain asymptomatic until their CD4 count falls to less than 200 cells/mm^3, a fact that contributes to the late diagnosis of disease.

Patients with moderate immunodeficiency (CD4 counts between 200 and 500 cells/mm^3) exhibit diminished antibody response to protein and polysaccharide antigens, as well as decreased cell-mediated immune function. These functional impairments are manifested clinically by a 3-fold to 4-fold increase in the incidence of bacteremic pneumonias caused by common pulmonary pathogens (especially *Streptococcus pneumoniae* and *Haemophilus influenzae*) and by a marked increase in incidence of active pulmonary tuberculosis in endemic areas (Table 16.2). Mucocutaneous lesions may be the first manifestations of immune dysfunction; these include reactivation of varicella zoster (shingles), recurrent genital herpes simplex virus (HSV) infections, oral or vaginal candidiasis, and oral hairy leukoplakia (see later discussion). Women living with HIV show an increased prevalence of high-grade squamous intraepithelial lesions on Papanicolaou (Pap) smear. Both men and women may show similarly increased rates of dysplasia or neoplasia on anal Pap smear.

With advanced immunodeficiency, indicated by CD4 counts lower than 200 cells/mm^3, patients are at high risk for development of opportunistic diseases, including infections and malignancies (see Table 16.2). Prior to the advent of antiretroviral therapy, time from diagnosis of AIDS to death was on average 1.3 years; death was generally due to opportunistic disease, including *Pneumocystis jirovecii* pneumonia and *Toxoplasma* meningitis, among many others. CD4 counts lower than 50 cells/mm^3 indicate profound immunosuppression and, in the absence of effective ART, are associated with a high mortality rate within the subsequent 12 to 24 months. Cytomegalovirus (CMV) retinitis, which can lead rapidly to blindness, and disseminated *Mycobacterium avium* complex (MAC) infection occur frequently in the absence of therapy at these low CD4 counts. They respond adequately to specific therapy only if it is accompanied by effective control of viral replication.

Opportunistic Infections
Candida Infections

Perhaps one of the earliest indications of HIV disease in many patients is the development of *Candida* disease. Both oropharyngeal and esophageal candidiasis are common in PLWH. Angular cheilosis may also be a manifestation of *Candida* infection. Typically, but not exclusively, caused by *Candida albicans*, oropharyngeal candidiasis may manifest as painless, creamy white, plaque-like lesions on the buccal surface, classically on an erythematous base. Esophageal disease is often symptomatic, usually presenting with odynophagia and/or retrosternal burning pain. In women living with HIV, *Candida* vulvovaginitis usually presents with white adherent vaginal discharge and a burning or itching sensation. *Candida*-associated disease may occur at any CD4 count, but esophageal disease is generally associated with lower CD4 counts. Treatment with oral fluconazole is as effective as or superior to localized topical therapy and is generally better tolerated and therefore preferred. Primary and secondary prophylaxis against *Candida* infection is generally not recommended unless patients have severe or frequent recurrences because therapy for acute disease is rapidly effective, mortality is extremely low, therapy is costly, and potential for development of resistance is of concern.

表 16.1　209 例患者中急性逆转录病毒综合征的常见症状及体征

症状或体征	发现人数	发生率（%）
发热	200	96
腺体疾病	154	74
咽炎	146	70
皮疹	146	70
肌痛或关节痛	112	54
血小板减少	94	45
白细胞减少	80	38
腹泻	67	32
头痛	66	32
恶心呕吐	56	27
转氨酶升高	38	21
肝脾大	30	14
鹅口疮	24	12
神经疾病	13	6
脑病	12	6

改编自 Niu MT, Stein DS, Schnittman SM. Primary human immunodeficiency virus type 1 infection: review of pathogenesis and early treatment intervention in human and animal retrovirus infections. J Infect Dis 1993; 168: 1490-1501.

表 16.2　按 $CD4^+$ T 细胞计数分类的 HIV 感染进展期并发症

$CD4^+$ T 细胞计数（$/mm^3$）	机会性感染或肿瘤
> 500	带状疱疹
	肺结核
200～500	口腔毛状白斑
	念珠菌性咽炎（鹅口疮）
	皮肤黏膜卡波西肉瘤
	复发性细菌性肺炎
	宫颈或肛门肿瘤
100～200	耶氏肺孢子虫肺炎
	播散性荚膜组织胞浆菌感染
	内脏卡波西肉瘤
	进行性多灶性白质脑病
	非霍奇金淋巴瘤
< 100	念珠菌性食管炎
	巨细胞病毒视网膜炎
	鸟-胞内分枝杆菌
	刚地弓形虫脑炎
	隐孢子虫肠炎
	新型隐球菌性脑膜炎
	慢性溃疡性单纯疱疹病毒感染
	巨细胞病毒食管炎或结肠炎
	原发性中枢神经系统淋巴瘤

极大个体差异。在感染 10 年后，未经治疗的人中约有 50% 会发展为获得性免疫缺陷综合征（AIDS），30% 症状较轻，只有不足 20% 完全没有症状（图 16.3）。儿童和青少年的 AIDS 进展速度比老年人慢。免疫缺陷的进展速度不受 HIV 传播途径的影响，而是由个体因素决定。从远期来看，疾病似乎没有性别差异，但 HIV 感染的女性通常在血浆中 HIV 水平较低时反而疾病进展更快。

35%～40% 的无症状 HIV 感染者会出现淋巴结肿大，但该症状与免疫缺陷的进展或淋巴瘤的发病无明显关联。在 HIV 感染早期，血小板减少非常常见，这可能是由自身免疫性血小板破坏引起的。大多数 HIV 感染者在 $CD4^+$ T 细胞计数降至 $200/mm^3$ 以下之前都没有症状，这也是导致疾病诊断较晚的原因之一。

在 $CD4^+$ T 细胞计数为 200～$500/mm^3$ 的中度免疫缺陷患者中观察到，该类患者对蛋白和多糖抗原的抗体反应减弱，且细胞介导的免疫功能也会下降。这些免疫功能障碍状态，在临床上表现为由常见肺部病原体（尤其是肺炎链球菌和流感嗜血杆菌）引起的细菌性肺炎的发病率增加 3～4 倍，以及在流行地区活动性肺结核发病率明显增加（表 16.2）。皮肤黏膜病变可能是免疫功能失调的最初表现，这些病变包括这些包括带状疱疹［水痘-带状疱疹病毒（VZV）的再激活］、生殖器单纯疱疹病毒（HSV）反复感染、口腔或阴道念珠菌病以及口腔毛状白斑（见后文）。HIV 感染妇女在巴氏涂片检查中发现高级别鳞状上皮内病变的概率增加；且在肛门巴氏涂片检查中，男性和女性的非典型增生或肿瘤的发生率增加。

当 $CD4^+$ T 细胞计数低于 $200/mm^3$ 时，即为免疫缺陷晚期，患者出现感染及恶性肿瘤等机会性疾病的风险升高（表 16.2）。在抗逆转录病毒治疗出现之前，从确诊 AIDS 到死亡平均需要 1.3 年时间，死亡原因通常是机会性感染的发生，包括耶氏肺孢子虫肺炎和弓形虫脑膜炎等。$CD4^+$ T 细胞计数低于 $50/mm^3$ 表明严重免疫抑制状态，在缺乏有效抗逆转录病毒治疗的情况下，在随后的 12～24 个月死亡率极高。巨细胞病毒视网膜炎会导致快速失明，巨细胞病毒性视网膜炎和鸟分枝杆菌感染在 $CD4^+$ T 细胞计数过低且缺乏治疗的情况下极易发生。只有在有效控制病毒载量的情况下，这些疾病才会对特异性治疗产生积极反应。

机会性感染

念珠菌感染

许多 HIV 感染患者的最早表现可能为念珠菌感染。口咽和食管念珠菌病在 HIV 感染者中都很常见。口角干裂也可能是念珠菌感染的一种表现。口咽部念珠菌病大部分由白念珠菌引起，但也不完全是由白念珠菌引起的，其通常是在红斑的基础上，可表现为口腔表面无痛、乳白色、斑块状的病变；食管疾病通常表现为吞咽困难或胸骨后灼痛。在 HIV 感染的女性中，念珠菌性外阴阴道炎通常表现为白色黏稠的阴道分泌物和灼热或瘙痒感。念珠菌相关疾病可发生于任何 $CD4^+$ T 细胞计数水平的患者，但食管疾病通常与低 $CD4^+$ T 细胞计数相关。口服氟康唑的治疗效果与局部外用治疗效果相同或更佳，而且一般耐受性更好，通常为首选治疗。除非患者病情严重或经常复发，否则一般不建议对念珠菌感染进行一级和二级预防，因为急性期的治疗很快就能见效、死亡率极低但是治疗费用高，而且预防性治疗有产生耐药性的风险。

TABLE 16.3 Primary Antimicrobial Prophylaxis for Adults Living With HIV and a Low CD4 Count

Opportunistic Infection	Treatment	When to Start	When to Stop
Pneumocystis jirovecii	TMP/SMX 1 DS or SS daily Alt: TMP/SMX 1 DS TIW Alt: Dapsone 100 mg daily or 50 mg BID Alt: Nebulized pentamidine 300 mg monthly Alt: Atovaquone 1500 mg daily	CD4 <200 or CD4% <14%	CD4 >200 for >3 mo (AI) or CD4 between 100-200 if HIV VL is undetectable >3 mo (BII)
Toxoplasma gondii	TMP/SMX 1 DS daily Alt: TMP/SMX 1 DS TIW Alt: TMP/SMX 1 DS daily Alt: Dapsone-pyrimethamine + leucovorin Alt: Atovaquone 1500 mg daily	CD4 <100	CD4 >200 for >3 mo (AI) or CD4 between 100-200 if HIV VL is undetectable >3 mo (BII)
Mycobacterium avium complex	Azithromycin 1200 mg weekly Clarithromycin 500 mg BID Alt: Rifabutin	Not recommended if effective ART initiated immediately. Recommended for those who are not on fully suppressive ART, after ruling out active disseminated MAC disease	CD4 >100 for >3 mo
Mycobacterium tuberculosis	Isoniazid (INH) 300 mg daily × 9 months Alt: Rifapentine + INH 900 mg once weekly for 12 weeks Alt: Rifampin 10 mg/kg/day (600 mg max) × 4 months	Positive screening test for LTBI with no evidence of active TB, and no prior treatment for active TB or LTBI	Stop after completion of recommended LTBI treatment duration
Histoplasmosis	Itraconazole 200 mg daily	CD4 <150 if high-risk environmental or occupational exposure exists	CD4 >150 for >6 mo
Cryptococcosis	Fluconazole	Not recommended in United States	

Pneumocystis Pneumonia

Pneumocystis jirovecii is a ubiquitous yeast in the environment. It is not associated with disease except in the setting of immunocompromise. Before the widespread use of ART and prophylactic medications, *Pneumocystis jirovecii* pneumonia (PJP or PCP; both abbreviations are still used) occurred in 70% of patients with AIDS, and the course of treated PCP was still associated with 20% to 40% mortality. The typical presentation is subacute, with progressive fever, shortness of breath, and weight loss over weeks. Profound desaturation with exertion is a common clinical sign, as is a substernal catch on inspiration. Hypoxemia is the most common laboratory abnormality. A serum LDH greater than 500 is common, and a serum 1,3-β-D-glucan is commonly elevated as well. Both of these can be helpful diagnostically. Definitive diagnosis can be made on sputum sample; induced sputum may be positive, though often bronchoscopic sampling for DFA and/or PCR testing is needed. Radiographic findings are classically described as diffuse, bilateral, symmetrical "ground-glass" interstitial infiltrates emanating from the hila in a "butterfly" pattern. However, it is important to remember that 10% of patients will have a normal radiograph, and 30% will have nonspecific findings. Atypical findings such as nodules, blebs, or cysts, can occur, as can spontaneous pneumothorax. Early initiation of treatment is crucial, and treatment should not be delayed while waiting for diagnostic results in patients with a high index of suspicion. First-line therapy is trimethoprim-sulfamethoxazole 15 to 20 mg/kg/day in divided doses over a 21-day course. Steroids should be added in patients with moderate or severe disease, generally defined as a PO_2 of less than 70 or an Aa gradient of 35 mm Hg or greater. Alternative treatments for mild-to-moderate disease include primaquine with clindamycin, dapsone with trimethoprim, or atovaquone. Alternative treatments for moderate-to-severe disease include primaquine with clindamycin or intravenous pentamidine. Due to the high prevalence of *Pneumocystis*, prophylaxis with trimethoprim-sulfamethoxazole is recommended for all patients with a CD4 count less than 200. Alternatives include dapsone, atovaquone, or inhaled pentamidine. In patients with a CD4 count between 100 and 200, prophylaxis can be discontinued once the serum HIV viral load is undetectable for 3 to 6 months. See Table 16.3 for prophylaxis guidelines.

Cryptococcal Disease

Cryptococcus neoformans is a yeast that generally affects immunocompromised individuals. It enters the body through the lungs, though pulmonary disease is often asymptomatic. Meningitis is the most common clinical presentation of cryptococcal disease, but cutaneous manifestations, classically presenting as umbilicated papules, may be present in 10% of patients. Cryptococcal meningitis occurs in about 1 million cases per year worldwide, with an estimated 600,000 deaths annually. Classic meningeal symptoms occur in only 25% of patients; more commonly, patients present with progressive headache, lethargy progressive to encephalopathy, personality changes, memory loss, coma, and death. A serum cryptococcal antigen test is generally positive, but a lumbar puncture must be performed both for diagnosis and for therapeutic purposes to evaluate CSF pressure (and relieve it, if elevated). CSF studies will generally show an elevated total protein and low glucose, and CSF cryptococcal antigen testing will be positive. India ink staining of the CSF, though uncommon now in the United States, will show encapsulated yeast forms. CSF lymphocyte counts may be elevated or may be normal. A minimal inflammatory response is common; in fact, 55% of patients with AIDS-related cryptococcal meningitis have a CSF lymphocyte count of less than 10 cells/mL. This lack of immunologic response is associated with a poorer prognosis. Treatment is focused on (1) management of CSF pressures through serial lumbar puncture with removal of CSF until pressures return to normal range and (2) antifungal therapy. Therapy is generally divided into three phases: induction, consolidation, and maintenance. Induction therapy is with amphotericin B and flucytosine. Once CSF cultures have cleared and patients have completed at least 2 weeks of therapy, consolidation with high-dose oral fluconazole is continued

表 16.3　低 CD4⁺ T 细胞计数的成人 HIV 感染者的主要抗感染药物预防措施

机会性感染	治疗	启动时机	停药时机
耶氏肺孢子虫	TMP/SMX 1 片或 2 片 qd 替代方案： TMP/SMX 2 片 tiw 氨苯砜 100 mg qd 或 50 mg bid 雾化吸入喷他脒 300 mg 每月一次 阿托伐醌 1500 mg qd	CD4 < 200 或 CD4% < 14%	CD4 > 200 持续 3 个月以上（AⅠ），或 CD4 为 100 ～ 200 且 HIV 病载未检出持续 3 个月以上（BⅡ）
弓形虫	TMP/SMX 2 片 qd 替代方案： TMP/SMX 2 片 tiw 氨苯砜-乙胺嘧啶+亚叶酸 阿托伐醌 1500 mg qd	CD4 < 100	CD4 > 200 持续 3 个月以上（AⅠ），或 CD4 为 100 ～ 200 且 HIV 病载未检出持续 3 个月以上（BⅡ）
鸟分枝杆菌复合群	阿奇霉素 1200 mg qw 克拉霉素 500 mg bid 替代方案： 利福布汀	如果立即开始有效的抗逆转录病毒治疗（ART），则不推荐；对于没有接受完全抑制病毒的 ART 治疗的患者，在排除活动性播散性鸟分枝杆菌复合群（MAC）疾病后，推荐使用	CD4 > 100 持续 3 个月以上
结核分枝杆菌	异烟肼（INH）300 mg qd×9 个月 替代方案： 利福喷丁+异烟肼 900 mg qw×12 周 利福平 10 mg/kg qd（最大 600 mg）×4 个月	对潜伏结核感染（LTBI）的筛查试验呈阳性，但没有活动性结核病（TB）的证据，并且之前没有接受过活动性结核病或潜伏结核感染的治疗	完成疗程后即停止
组织胞浆菌病 隐球菌病	伊曲康唑 200 mg qd 氟康唑	CD4 < 150（高危环境或存在职业暴露） 在美国不建议使用	CD4 > 150 持续 6 个月以上

肺孢子虫肺炎

耶氏肺孢子虫是一种在环境中无处不在的酵母菌，因此仅在免疫功能低下的情况下致病。在广泛使用抗逆转录病毒治疗和预防性药物之前，70% 的 HIV 感染者都会患上耶氏肺孢子虫肺炎（PJP 或 PCP），而且经过治疗的 PCP 病程仍有 20% ～ 40% 的死亡率。典型的表现是亚急性病程，数周内出现进行性发热、呼吸急促和体重减轻，剧烈运动后气短是常见的临床症状之一，还可出现吸气时胸骨内侧的刺痛感。低氧血症是最常见的实验室异常。血清 LDH 常大于 500 U/L，血清 1,3-β-D 葡聚糖通常也会升高，这两点均有助于诊断。明确诊断 PCP 可通过病原学检查如痰液或支气管肺泡灌洗/肺组织活检，取样进行 DFA 或 PCR 检测。胸部 X 线检查通常提示弥漫性、双侧、对称性的"磨玻璃"间质浸润，呈"蝴蝶"状从肺叶向外扩展。然而，10% 的患者可能会有正常的影像学表现，30% 的患者可能呈非特异性的表现，也可出现结节、出血点或囊肿、自发性气胸等非特异性征象。尽早开始治疗至关重要，在高度怀疑患者等待诊断结果期间不应延误治疗。一线治疗为甲氧苄啶-磺胺甲噁唑（TMP/SMZ）15 ～ 20 mg/(kg·d)，分次服用，疗程为 21 天；中度或重度患者（PaO₂ < 70 mmHg 或肺泡-动脉血氧分压差 > 35 mmHg），应加用激素治疗。轻度至中度疾病的替代治疗方法包括：伯氨喹联合克林霉素、氨苯砜联合甲氧苄啶或阿托伐醌；中度至重度疾病的替代治疗方法包括：伯氨喹联合克林霉素或静脉注射喷他脒。由于 PCP 发病率高，建议所有 CD4⁺ T 细胞计数低于 200/mm³ 的患者使用 SMZ-TMP 进行预防。替代药物包括氨苯砜、阿托伐醌或吸入喷他脒。对于 CD4⁺ T 细胞计数为 100 ～ 200/mm³ 的患者，一旦血清 HIV 病毒载量在 3 ～ 6 个月内保持稳定，即可停止预防。预防建议见表 16.3。

隐球菌病

新型隐球菌是一种酵母菌，通常免疫力低下人群容易感染。它通过肺部进入人体，但肺部通常没有症状。脑膜炎是隐球菌病最常见的临床表现，但也有 10% 的患者会出现皮肤症状，通常表现为脐丘疹。全世界每年约有 100 万例隐球菌脑膜炎病例，估计每年有 60 万人死亡。只有 25% 的患者会出现典型的脑膜症状，更常见的症状为进行性头痛、嗜睡并逐渐发展为脑病、性格改变、记忆力减退、昏迷和死亡。血清隐球菌抗原检测通常呈阳性，但为了明确诊断及治疗，必须进行腰椎穿刺，以评估脑脊液压力，必要时需降颅压治疗。脑脊液检查常提示总蛋白升高和葡萄糖降低，脑脊液隐球菌抗原检测呈阳性。脑脊液墨汁染色镜检可发现隐球菌。脑脊液淋巴细胞计数可能升高，也可能正常，55% 的 HIV 相关隐球菌脑膜炎患者的 CSF 淋巴细胞计数低于 10/ml，这种免疫应答的缺乏与较差的预后相关。治疗的重点为：①通过腰椎穿刺控制脑脊液压力，直至压力恢复到正常范围；②抗真菌治疗。治疗一般分为 3 个阶段：诱导、巩固和维持。诱导治疗使用两性霉素 B 和氟尿嘧啶。一旦脑脊液培养病原转阴，且患者完成至少 2 周的治疗，应继续使用大剂量口服氟康唑进行巩固治疗 8 周。维持治疗每天口服氟康唑 200 mg，疗程至少 1 年。

for 8 additional weeks. Maintenance therapy is with oral fluconazole 200 mg daily for a minimum of 1 year.

Toxoplasma Encephalitis

Toxoplasma gondii is an obligate intracellular protozoan that most commonly causes encephalitis in patients with AIDS, though it may also present with retinitis or in skeletal muscle or myocardium. Primary infection occurs from eating undercooked meat containing tissue cysts or ingesting oocysts that have been shed in cat feces and sporulated into the environment. Clinical disease in PLWH is usually due to reactivation. Patients present with a focal encephalitis with headache, confusion, motor weakness, and fever. In the absence of treatment, disease will progress to seizures, stupor, coma, and death. Imaging is usually the means of diagnosis, with contrast-enhanced MRI showing multiple contrast-enhancing lesions in the gray matter of the cortex or basal ganglia, often associated with edema. Because disease is usually due to reactivation of latent disease, patients may have a positive serum anti-toxoplasma IgG. CSF testing for toxoplasma PCR may be positive as well. Treatment is initiated based on high clinical suspicion rather than definitive diagnosis. If repeat imaging in 1 to 3 weeks does not show response to treatment in all visualized lesions, brain biopsy may be necessary. In this scenario, biopsy is important to rule out alternative diagnoses such as CNS lymphoma, progressive multifocal leukoencephalopathy (PML), or tuberculosis, among others. Treatment consists of pyrimethamine and sulfadiazine with leucovorin to reduce hematologic toxicity. Treatment is for a minimum of 6 weeks; then patients should be put on chronic maintenance therapy until the CD4 has been greater than 200 for over 6 months. Primary prophylaxis for *Toxoplasma* with trimethoprim-sulfamethoxazole should be initiated in any patient with a CD4 count less than 100, with atovaquone as an alternative. See Table 16.3 for prophylaxis guidelines.

Mycobacterium Tuberculosis

Tuberculosis is the most common opportunistic infection seen worldwide in people living with HIV disease and in fact is the leading cause of death due to infectious disease worldwide. PLWH may either acquire acute disease through inhaling droplet nuclei or suffer reactivation disease due to impaired cellular immunity. The annual risk of reactivation tuberculosis disease in people living with HIV is estimated to be 3% to 16% per year. Reactivation can occur at any CD4 count but is higher risk the more significant the immunodeficiency. The greatest risk in people living in the United States is birth or residence outside the United States because global rates of tuberculosis are much higher than in the United States itself. Clinical presentations of people living with HIV are generally not different than in people who do not have HIV, but presentations of severe systemic disease and disseminated disease are more common. Clinical manifestations can be protean, but classic symptoms of fever, cachexia, and night sweats remain common. Pulmonary disease is still the most common presentation. Chest radiographs in patients may show features of primary tuberculosis, including hilar adenopathy, lower or middle lobe infiltrates, miliary pattern, or pleural effusions, as well as classic patterns of reactivation with upper lobe disease. Less common presentations include pericarditis, pericardial effusions, meningitis, CNS lesions, and bony disease. Diagnosis is determined in the same manner as in HIV-negative patients, and treatment does not differ, though careful review of medications is important to avoid significant drug/drug interactions that can occur between antiretrovirals and antituberculous medications. See Chapter 7 for more details.

Nontuberculous Mycobacterial Disease

A number of different nontuberculous mycobacteria are associated with advanced HIV disease, though far and away the most common is *Mycobacterium avium* complex (MAC). The incidence of MAC in patients with severe AIDS-associated immunosuppression is 20% to 40% in the absence of effective ART or chemoprophylaxis. Disease tends to occur with a CD4 count less than 50 and a high HIV viral load (usually greater than 100,000). MAC often presents as a disseminated disease with fever, night sweats, weight loss, diarrhea, and abdominal pain. On physical examination, hepatosplenomegaly and lymphadenopathy are common. Laboratory testing is often initially nonspecific, though anemia and an increased alkaline phosphatase are common. Diagnosis is usually made on a compatible clinical syndrome and isolation of MAC on culture or AFB stain on tissue with confirmation on culture. Cultures can be sent from blood, lymph node biopsy, bone marrow, or other tissues or fluids felt to be infected. Treatment is with two or more drugs, usually clarithromycin or azithromycin with ethambutol. Rifabutin may be added as a third agent in some cases. Treatment is for a minimum of 12 months and may then be discontinued when patients are asymptomatic and have a CD4 count greater than 100 for over 6 months. Prophylaxis against MAC is no longer recommended routinely for those who are immediately initiating ART, based on literature demonstrating no added benefit when ART is initiated promptly. Prophylaxis is therefore only recommended in those with a CD4 count less than 50 who are not receiving ART or who are not on fully suppressive ART, and only once active MAC disease has been ruled out based on clinical assessment, including a baseline AFB blood culture. Prophylaxis is generally with azithromycin 1200 mg once weekly.

Progressive Multifocal Leukoencephalopathy

PML is an opportunistic infection of the CNS caused by JC virus, a polyoma virus that causes focal demyelination. JC virus is common throughout the world and demonstrates a seroprevalence of 39% in healthy adults. PML is a disease that occurs with profound immunosuppression in people with HIV (CD4 <50) or in people receiving certain immunomodulatory humanized antibodies (e.g., natalizumab, rituximab). Prior to the advent of ART, PML developed in 3% to 7% of patients with advanced AIDS. PML manifests with focal neurologic deficits, usually of slow and insidious onset, that become progressive. Seizures occur in 20% of patients. Patients do not have headache or fever. Diagnosis is suspected based on MRI findings of distinct nonenhancing white matter lesions in areas of the brain corresponding to clinical deficits. Confirmation of diagnosis is usually through testing of the CSF for JC virus DNA by PCR, which is positive in 70% to 90% of patients. In some patients, however, brain biopsy is required to establish the diagnosis. There are no specific therapies for treating JC virus or PML. Initiation of antiretroviral therapy is the cornerstone of treatment; over 50% of patients will experience remission, though some neurologic deficits often persist.

Cytomegalovirus Disease

Cytomegalovirus (CMV) is a ubiquitous DNA virus. In patients with advanced AIDS and a CD4 count less than 50, it may present with end-organ disease. Before the advent of ART, 30% of patients with advanced AIDS developed CMV retinitis. Retinitis often begins unilaterally but then progresses to bilateral disease. This may be asymptomatic or present with floaters, scotomata, or visual field deficits. Ophthalmologic exam is generally diagnostic, with fluffy, yellow-white retinal lesions with or without intraretinal hemorrhage, and absent or minimal vitreous inflammation. Other manifestations of CMV can occur, including colitis, esophagitis, and CNS disease. CMV pneumonitis is extremely uncommon in patients with HIV. For these other manifestations, diagnosis based on biopsy is still necessary. An elevated CMV viral load in serum may be present but does not confirm disease. Treatment is oral valganciclovir or intravenous ganciclovir.

弓形虫脑炎

弓形虫是一种必须在胞内存活的原生动物，是HIV患者脑炎最常见的致病原因，但也可能导致视网膜炎、骨骼肌或心肌炎。原发性弓形虫感染是由于食用了含有组织包囊的未煮熟的肉类，或摄入了猫粪中脱落并孢子化到环境中的卵囊。HIV感染者的临床起病通常是由再激活引起的。患者表现为局灶性脑炎，伴有头痛、意识模糊、运动无力和发热。在未治疗的情况下，病情会进展到癫痫发作、昏迷和死亡。通常通过影像学检查来诊断，表现为增强磁共振成像显示皮层或基底节灰质中存在多个对比增强病灶，且常伴有水肿。由于疾病通常是由于潜伏期疾病的再激活所致，因此患者的血清抗弓形虫IgG可能呈阳性，脑脊液弓形虫PCR检测也可呈阳性。临床上高度怀疑时就应开始治疗，不应等待至明确诊断后。如果1～3周后重复影像学检查仍未显示病灶对治疗的反应，则可能需要进行脑活检。活检对于排除中枢神经系统淋巴瘤、进行性多灶性白质脑病（PML）或结核病等其他诊断非常重要。治疗包括使用乙胺嘧啶、磺胺嘧啶以及亚叶酸，以减少血液系统毒性。治疗至少持续6周，然后患者应接受慢性维持治疗，直到$CD4^+$ T细胞计数超过$200/mm^3$且持续6个月以上。对于$CD4^+$ T细胞计数小于$100/mm^3$的患者，应开始使用TMP/SMZ对弓形虫进行一级预防，也可使用阿托伐醌作为替代药物。预防建议见表16.3。

结核分枝杆菌

结核病是全球HIV感染者最常见的机会性感染，也是全球传染病致死的主要原因。HIV感染者由于细胞免疫功能低下，可能通过吸入飞沫出现急性感染，也可通过再激活导致感染。据估计，HIV感染者每年再次感染结核病的风险为3%～16%。任何$CD4^+$ T细胞计数的患者都可能发生再激活，但免疫缺陷程度越严重则风险越高。对于美国居民而言，最大的感染风险来自出生或居住在美国境外人群，因为国际结核病的发病率远远高于美国。HIV感染者的临床表现一般与非HIV感染者无异，但严重的全身性疾病和播散性疾病更为常见。临床表现可多种多样，但发热、恶病质和盗汗等典型症状仍然常见。肺部征象仍然是最常见的表现，患者的胸片可显示原发性肺结核的特征，包括肺门腺病、下叶或中叶浸润、粟粒型或胸腔积液，以及典型的上叶疾病再激活的表现。较少见的表现包括心包炎、心包积液、脑膜炎、中枢神经系统病变和骨骼疾病。诊断及治疗方法与HIV阴性患者相同，但必须仔细审查药物成分，以避免抗逆转录病毒药物和抗结核药物之间可能发生的严重药物相互作用。详见第7章。

非结核分枝杆菌病

许多的非结核分枝杆菌感染都与晚期HIV疾病有关，但最常见的是鸟分枝杆菌复合群（MAC）。MAC在缺乏有效抗逆转录病毒治疗或预防的情况下，严重HIV相关免疫抑制患者的发病率为20%～40%。疾病往往发生在$CD4^+$ T细胞计数低于$50/mm^3$或HIV病毒载量较高（通常大于100 000拷贝/毫升）的情况下。MAC通常表现为播散性疾病，伴有发热、盗汗、体重减轻、腹泻和腹痛。体格检查常见肝脾大和淋巴结病变。实验室检查最初往往没有特异性，但贫血和碱性磷酸酶增高很常见。诊断通常是根据相符的临床综合征和病原学培养中的MAC或组织染色以确认。可从血液、淋巴结活检、骨髓或其他受感染的组织或体液中进行培养。治疗使用两种或两种以上药物，通常是克拉霉素或阿奇霉素加乙胺丁醇。在某些情况下，利福布汀可作为第三种药物加入。治疗至少持续12个月，如果患者无症状且$CD4^+$ T细胞计数大于$100/mm^3$且持续6个月以上，则可停止治疗。对于立即开始抗逆转录病毒治疗的患者，不再建议常规使用预防药物，因为有文献表明，立即开始抗逆转录病毒治疗并不会带来额外的益处。因此，仅建$CD4^+$ T细胞计数低于$50/mm^3$且未接受抗逆转录病毒治疗或未完全抑制病载的患者进行预防，并且仅在根据临床评估（包括基线AFB血液培养）排除活动性MAC疾病后进行预防。通常使用阿奇霉素1200 mg进行预防，每周一次。

进行性多灶性白质脑病

PML是由JC病毒引起的中枢神经系统机会性感染，JC病毒是一种多瘤病毒，可导致局灶性脱髓鞘表现。JC病毒在世界各地都很常见，健康成年人的血清阳性反应率为39%。PML是一种在HIV感染者（$CD4^+$ T细胞计数 < $50/mm^3$）或接受某些免疫调节人源化抗体（如那他珠单抗、利妥昔单抗）治疗的患者出现严重免疫抑制时发生的疾病。在抗逆转录病毒治疗出现之前，3%～7%的晚期AIDS患者会出现PML。PML表现为局灶性神经功能障碍，通常起病缓慢而隐匿，并呈进行性发展，20%的患者会出现癫痫发作，通常没有头痛或发热等症状。根据核磁共振成像（MRI）可发现与临床症状相应的脑部区域有明显的非增强性白质病变，即可疑似诊断。确诊通常需要通过PCR检测CSF中的JC病毒DNA检测来确认，70%～90%的患者检测结果呈阳性，但有些患者需要进行脑活检才能确诊。目前还没有治疗JC病毒或PML的特效疗法。开始抗逆转录病毒治疗是治疗的基础，50%以上的患者病情会得到缓解，但一些神经功能障碍通常会持续存在。

巨细胞病毒病

巨细胞病毒（CMV）是一种无处不在的DNA病毒。在$CD4^+$ T细胞计数低于$50/mm^3$的晚期AIDS患者中，CMV可能会导致内脏器官疾病。在抗逆转录病毒治疗出现之前，30%的晚期AIDS患者会出现CMV视网膜炎。视网膜炎通常从单侧开始，然后发展为双侧；可能是无症状的，也可能伴有浮游物、光斑或视野缺损。眼科检查通常可以确诊，视网膜病变呈绒毛状、黄白色，伴有或不伴有视网膜内出血，玻璃体无炎症或炎症反应轻微。CMV感染还可能伴有结肠炎、食管炎和中枢神经系统疾病。CMV肺炎在HIV感染者中极为罕见。对于这些其他表现，仍需根据活组织检查进行诊断。血清中CMV病毒载量升高可能存在，但并不能确诊疾病。治疗方法是口服或静脉注射更昔洛韦。

Varicella-Zoster Disease

Varicella-zoster is a ubiquitous virus known to have infected over 95% of adults in the United States. Reactivation varicella (termed herpes zoster, or "shingles") occurred at a 15-fold higher rate in PLWH prior to the advent of ART, and rates remain elevated in PLWH. Varicella reactivation can occur at any CD4 count, but reactivation is strongly associated with CD4 counts less than 200 and with active HIV viremia. Herpes zoster, or reactivation varicella virus, manifests as a painful vesicular eruption on the skin in a dermatomal distribution; 50% are in thoracic dermatomes, but cranial nerves and cervical nerves are also common, and any nerve distribution can be involved. The probability of a recurrence within 1 year is 10% in PLWH. If the eye is involved, acute retinal necrosis (ARN) or progressive outer retinal necrosis (PORN) can occur; both are associated with high rates of vision loss. In patients with CD4 counts less than 200, disseminated herpes zoster can also occur, including with CNS involvement that may manifest with CNS vasculitis, multifocal leukoencephalitis, ventriculitis, myelitis, optic neuritis, cranial nerve palsies, focal brainstem lesions, or aseptic meningitis. Diagnosis of varicella reactivation can be made based on clinical exam demonstrating classic dermatologic manifestations; VZV PCR of an unroofed vesicle can assist with diagnosis of unclear cases. PCR can also be performed on CSF or vitreous humor to help diagnose disease in those locations. Treatment of uncomplicated herpes zoster is similar to HIV-negative patients with use of oral valacyclovir, famciclovir, or acyclovir for 7 to 10 days. Intravenous acyclovir is recommended for treatment of severe or complicated varicella disease. Ophthalmologic disease should be managed by an experienced ophthalmologist. Current recommendations regarding primary vaccination (in patients with no reported history of childhood illness or vaccination) and to prevent reactivation disease are addressed in Table 16.6.

Other Opportunistic Infections

A number of other infections are considered opportunistic in patients living with HIV disease. These infections include bacterial and parasitic intestinal infections (including *Cryptosporidium*, *Cystoisospora*, and *Microsporidia* spp). Other bacterial infections, such as *Bartonella* spp, syphilis, and bacterial pneumonias, also occur at increased rates in patients living with HIV. Systemic fungal infections, including endemic fungi such as *Coccidioides*, *Histoplasma*, and *Talaromyces* infections, occur regionally. Viral diseases, including hepatitis B, hepatitis C, HSV, and HPV, are associated with worsened disease in PLWH, as is reactivation of varicella virus (herpes zoster).

HIV and Malignancy

Early in the HIV epidemic, rates of certain cancers were noted to be high in PLWH. Kaposi's sarcoma (KS) and non-Hodgkin's B-cell lymphoma were recognized as markers of the disease. Other AIDS-defining tumors, including invasive cervical cancer and primary central nervous system lymphoma, were also detected early. These AIDS-defining tumors were associated with viral coinfections, and the interplay of the immune dysregulation of advanced HIV disease and other viruses with potential for oncogenesis raise the risk of an opportunistic malignancy.

Kaposi's Sarcoma

In the early days of the HIV epidemic, rates of KS, a rare angiogenic cutaneous tumor found previously in elderly men, were present at rates 1000 times that of the general population. In the United States, KS occurred predominantly in young MSM infected with HIV and human herpes virus 8 (HHV-8). In Africa, rates of KS were particularly high in people living with HIV, accounting in some series for as much as 40% of all cancers in men. Ninety-five percent of patients with KS will have skin lesions characterized as violaceous, red macules or nodules with a wide distribution. Thirty percent will also have oral lesions and 40% will have gastrointestinal disease. Pulmonary disease and rarely visceral disease can also occur. Rates of KS have fallen dramatically with the widespread use of ART, although they remain significantly higher than in the non-HIV population. The mainstay of treatment is initiation of ART. Of note, paradoxical worsening of disease after initiation of ART is well described (see section on Immune Reconstitution Inflammatory Syndrome). Radiotherapy and intralesional chemotherapy may be used for skin disease, and chemotherapy, usually with liposomal doxorubicin, is used for widespread disease.

Non-Hodgkin's Lymphoma

The incidence of non-Hodgkin's B-cell lymphoma (NHL) early in the epidemic was 100 times the incidence seen in the general population. This has fallen significantly with the use of ART. Similar to other AIDS-defining malignancies, lymphoma in PLWH is usually associated with a viral coinfection, in this instance, Epstein-Barr virus (EBV). The most common types of lymphoma in patients living with HIV in decreasing order of prevalence include diffuse large B-cell lymphoma, Burkitt's lymphoma, and primary CNS lymphoma. Primary CNS lymphoma complicates advanced HIV infection in 3% to 6% of cases and is almost invariably associated with detectable EBV DNA in the CSF. Lesions may be single or multiple and are often weakly ring enhancing. Irradiation often provides remission, which may be sustained as immune function is restored by effective ART. Treatment for other types of lymphoma in HIV is with standard chemotherapy and radiation regimens.

HPV-Associated Cancers

Cervical and anal cancers appear at increased rates in people living with HIV. This is related to both HPV persistence and the degree of immunodeficiency. It appears that ART decreases the persistence of cervical HPV and the rate of invasive cervical cancer. Screening for cervical cancer with Pap smear and/or high-risk HPV according to guidelines for cervical cancer remains very important for HIV-positive women throughout their lives (see recommendations later). Anal cancer is also increased in both men and women with HIV. At this time, no national recommendations exist for screening for anal cancer, though the Infectious Disease Society of America (IDSA) HIV Primary Care Guidelines do recommend anal Pap smear testing. Treatment for both cervical and anal cancer, if found, is per guidelines, and treatment is not different for people living with HIV disease. Rates for oropharyngeal cancer, related to both smoking and HPV, are also increased in PLWH.

Non-AIDS–Defining Cancers

Non-AIDS–defining cancers (NADC) in PWLH include lung, liver, renal, colorectal, and oropharyngeal cancer, as well as Hodgkin's disease. The incidence of many of these malignancies has historically been increased for PLWH and although they have fallen recently with the use of ART, many persist with higher incidence than in the general population.

- *Lung cancer* is increased 2 to 3 times in PLWH compared with the general population, primarily because of high rates of smoking (42% to 59% of PLWH smoke), though the risk for lung cancer in PLWH is increased even when smoking is controlled for. Non–small cell carcinoma is the most common form of lung cancer in PLWH, as with the general population. Treatment follows guidelines for the general population, but it should be noted that protocols for lung cancer therapy have historically excluded PLWH, and thus data do not exist specifically for this population. The effect of ART on lung cancer risk or prognosis is not clear. Unfortunately,

水痘-带状疱疹感染

水痘-带状疱疹病毒是一种无处不在的病毒，美国95%以上的成年人都曾感染过这种病毒。在抗逆转录病毒治疗出现之前，水痘-带状疱疹病毒再激活在HIV感染者中的发生率比现在高出15倍，而且目前仍然很高。水痘再活化可发生在任何$CD4^+$ T细胞计数水平，但再激活与$CD4^+$ T细胞计数低于$200/mm^3$和活跃的HIV病毒血症密切相关。带状疱疹或水痘病毒再活化，可表现为皮肤上疼痛的水泡状疹子，呈皮节分布，50%发生在胸部皮节，但脑神经和颈神经也很常见，任何神经都可能受累。HIV感染者1年内复发的概率为10%。如果累及眼部，则可能发生急性视网膜坏死（ARN）或进行性外层视网膜坏死（PORN），都可能会导致视力丧失。$CD4^+$ T细胞计数低于$200/mm^3$的患者也可能出现播散性疱疹，可能表现为中枢神经系统血管炎、多灶性白质脑炎、脑室炎、脊髓炎、视神经炎、脑神经麻痹、局灶性脑干病变或无菌性脑膜炎。VZV再激活的诊断，可依据临床检查显示的典型皮肤表现；通过PCR检测未破损的水疱液可以帮助诊断不明确的病例，还可以对脑脊液或玻璃体液进行PCR检测以帮助诊断。轻度的带状疱疹的治疗方法与HIV阴性患者类似，口服伐昔洛韦、泛昔洛韦或阿昔洛韦7~10天；建议严重或复杂的患者，采用静脉注射阿昔洛韦治疗。眼科疾病应由经验丰富的眼科医生处理。表16.6列出了目前关于初次接种（针对无儿童疾病史或接种史的患者）和预防疾病再激活的建议。

其他机会性感染

在HIV感染者中，还有一些其他机会性感染，包括细菌性和寄生虫性肠道感染（包括隐孢子虫、囊孢子虫和小孢子虫）等。其他细菌感染，如巴尔通体、梅毒和细菌性肺炎在HIV感染者中的发病率也有所上升。全身性真菌感染，包括地方性真菌，如球孢子菌、组织胞浆菌和塔拉菌感染，在各地区均有发生。病毒性疾病，包括乙型肝炎、丙型肝炎、单纯疱疹病毒和人乳头瘤病毒，与水痘病毒（带状疱疹）的再激活一样，都与HIV感染者的病情恶化有关。

HIV与恶性肿瘤

在HIV流行的早期，人们注意到HIV感染者中某些癌症的发病率很高。卡波西肉瘤（KS）和非霍奇金淋巴瘤被认为是标志性疾病，其他艾滋病标志性肿瘤还包括浸润性宫颈癌和原发性中枢神经系统淋巴瘤等。这些艾滋病标志性肿瘤与病毒合并感染有关，晚期HIV疾病的免疫调节失调与其他具有肿瘤发生潜能的病毒相互作用，增加了机会性恶性肿瘤的风险。

卡波西肉瘤

在HIV流行的早期，KS作为多发于老年男性的罕见血管性皮肤肿瘤，其发病率是普通人群的1000倍。在美国，KS主要发生在感染HIV和人类疱疹病毒8（HHV-8）的年轻男男性行为者。在非洲，HIV感染者的KS患病率特别高，在某些男性人群中高达40%。95%的KS患者会有的皮肤表现为广泛分布的紫红色斑丘疹或结节，30%的患者还会出现口腔病变，40%的患者会出现胃肠道疾病，肺部疾病和极少数内脏疾病也会发生。随着抗逆转录病毒治疗的广泛使用，KS的发病率已大幅下降，但仍明显高于非HIV感染人群。治疗的重点在于尽早启动抗逆转录病毒治疗。值得警惕的是，抗逆转录病毒治疗启动后可能反而出现疾病恶化的现象（参见"免疫重建炎症综合征"部分）。皮肤病变可采用放疗和鞘内化疗，全身表现通常采用脂质体多柔比星化疗。

非霍奇金淋巴瘤

在HIV流行早期，非霍奇金B细胞淋巴瘤（NHL）在HIV感染者中的发病率是普通人群的100倍；而随着抗逆转录病毒治疗的使用，发病率已大幅下降。与其他艾滋病标志性的恶性肿瘤类似，HIV携带者的淋巴瘤通常与病毒合并感染有关，例如EB病毒（EBV）。HIV感染者最常见的淋巴瘤包括弥漫大B细胞淋巴瘤、伯基特淋巴瘤和原发性中枢神经系统淋巴瘤。原发性中枢神经系统淋巴瘤是晚期HIV疾病的并发症，占3%~6%，几乎无一例外地与脑脊液中可检测到的EBV-DNA相关。病变可为单发或多发，影像学表现通常呈弱环状增强。放射治疗通常可以缓解病情，随着有效的抗逆转录病毒治疗恢复免疫功能，病情可持续达到缓解。HIV感染者的其他类型淋巴瘤可采用标准化疗和放射治疗方案。

人乳头瘤病毒相关癌症

宫颈癌和肛门癌在HIV感染者中的发病率越来越高，这与HPV的持续存在和免疫缺陷程度有关。抗逆转录病毒治疗可以降低宫颈HPV的持续感染率和侵袭性宫颈癌的发病率。根据宫颈癌指南，通过巴氏涂片和高危HPV筛查宫颈癌，对于HIV阳性女性的一生都是非常重要的措施（见后文）。感染HIV的男性和女性患肛门癌的风险也会升高。目前，尽管美国传染病学会（IDSA）的*HIV初级护理指南*建议进行肛门巴氏涂片检查，但还没有关于肛门癌筛查的全国性建议。如果发现宫颈癌和肛门癌，可根据指南进行治疗，对HIV感染者的治疗并无不同。与吸烟和人乳头瘤病毒有关的口咽癌发病率在HIV感染者中也有所增加。

非艾滋病标志性癌症

非艾滋病标志性癌症（NADC）包括肺癌、肝癌、肾癌、结直肠癌、口咽癌以及霍奇金病。其中，许多恶性肿瘤的发病率在HIV感染者中呈持续上升趋势，虽然最近随着抗逆转录病毒治疗的使用，发病率有所下降，但仍有许多恶性肿瘤的发病率高于普通人群。

- 与普通人群相比，肺癌在HIV感染者中的发病率增加了2~3倍，主要原因是吸烟率高（42%~59%），不过即使控制了吸烟，HIV感染者患肺癌的风险也会增加。与普通人群一样，非小细胞肺癌是HIV感染者最常见的类型。治疗遵循普通人群的指导原则，但需要注意的是，肺癌治疗的病例统计常不包括HIV感染者，因此没有专门针对这一人

survival for PLWH and lung cancer is poorer than the general population.
- *Colorectal cancer* is the third leading cause of cancer death in the United States in the general population. HIV has historically not been associated with increased rates of colorectal cancer, but of concern, the rates of colorectal cancer in PLWH appear to be increasing and occurring at a younger age. Both screening rates for colorectal cancer, and as a result survival rates, are lower for PLWH. Future efforts will need to focus on appropriate screening and treatment for this increasingly common and lethal malignancy, particularly as the population ages.
- Rates of *liver cancer*, particularly hepatocellular carcinoma, are increased in PLWH in part due to the increased rates of hepatitis B and C virus coinfection and increased alcohol use leading to cirrhosis. In addition, with increasing rates of obesity in people living with HIV, the risk for cirrhosis due to nonalcoholic steatohepatitis (NASH) and subsequent malignancy will rise as well. Treatments for viral hepatitides are now available and treatment is recommended for all PLWH. Similarly, identifying and then treating NASH remains a priority.
- Rates of *skin cancer*, including squamous cell carcinoma and malignant melanoma, are increased in PLWH and skin screening is an important part of primary care.
- Rates of *prostate and breast cancer* are not increased in PLWH. Screening recommendations and treatment guidelines do not differ for this population.

As the population of PLWH ages, rates of all malignancies will increase. Unfortunately, cancer-related mortality is predicted to increase along with increased rates. Screening and appropriate treatment for both AIDS-defining malignancies and NADC are essential in this at-risk population.

Immune Reconstitution Inflammatory Syndrome

The immune reconstitution inflammatory syndrome (IRIS) is a syndrome strongly associated with HIV, though the phenomenon is not specific to HIV and has been seen in association with other conditions, most notably tuberculosis. HIV-associated IRIS occurs after initiation of ART, usually in patients with low CD4 counts, and manifests as either a paradoxical worsening of treated opportunistic infections, called paradoxical IRIS, or an unmasking of a previously subclinical (untreated) infections, called unmasking IRIS. In both of these syndromes, patients are initiated on ART but subsequently develop a clinical decline, generally 2 weeks to several months later. Fever is extremely common with IRIS. Paradoxical IRIS will often present with fever and a clinical worsening of a known OI that is being treated. Unmasking IRIS usually presents as new-onset fevers and tachycardia, sometimes with localizing symptoms suggestive of a previously undiagnosed OI (e.g., headache and obtundation in the setting of cryptococcal disease, or abdominal pain in the setting of MAC). The frequency of IRIS in patients with HIV disease demonstrates a broad range; a meta-analysis found a rate in the published literature of around 13%, with differences by disease process: highest with CMV retinitis, cryptococcal meningitis, PML, and tuberculosis. IRIS is a clinical diagnosis, and there is no specific diagnostic test. Clinicians should have a suspicion for IRIS in the setting of recent ART initiation, particularly in patients with baseline low CD4 counts in which either a known OI appears to worsen, or a patient appears to worsen clinically despite evidence of immune reconstitution. There is significant morbidity to IRIS; up to 50% of IRIS cases require hospitalization, and patients often require extensive testing and both diagnostic and therapeutic procedures. Diagnostic work-up is driven by clinical presentation but generally would involve blood cultures, mycobacterial isolators on serum, sputum for bacterial and AFB staining and culture if respiratory symptoms or radiographic findings are suggestive, imaging such as CT abdomen and pelvis or brain imaging if symptoms are suggestive, a retinal exam if any eye symptoms are present, a lymph node biopsy if any lymphadenopathy is notable, and further additional work-up as dictated by symptoms. Management of IRIS focuses on management of the identified opportunistic infection and use of corticosteroids and/or NSAIDs to calm the immunologic response. In all but life-threatening cases, ART should be continued. Steroid treatment is often prolonged, generally for 4 weeks or more, with gradual tapering as symptom management tolerates.

CO-OCCURRING DISEASE AND MULTIMORBIDITY WITH HIV

Neurologic Disease in HIV

Nervous system complications ultimately occur in most persons with untreated HIV infection. They range from mild cognitive disturbances or peripheral neuropathy to severe dementia and life-threatening central nervous system (CNS) infections. As with other lentiviruses, HIV enters microglial cells of the CNS early in the course of infection. Both direct neuronal destruction and effects of viral proteins on neuronal cell function may contribute to nervous system disease in AIDS. Infection in the CNS can be documented by CSF viral load and elevated immune markers. ART generally suppresses viral load in the CNS as well as the peripheral blood, although rarely elevated viral loads can occur in the CSF while the PVL remains suppressed; this is termed "CSF viral escape." CNS penetration by ART is variable depending on the drug, and treatment of CNS HIV infection is an area of active research.

Before effective ART therapy, a variety of severe neurologic complications were noted in patients with AIDS, including progressive dementia (termed the AIDS dementia complex), focal CNS disease, and peripheral neuropathy. ART has dramatically decreased the incidence of neurocognitive complications of HIV but has led to recognition of more subtle neurologic manifestations on the spectrum of what is now described as HIV-associated neurocognitive disorder (HAND), which includes asymptomatic neurologic impairment (ANI), mild cognitive dysfunction (MCD), and HIV-associated dementia (HAD). Approximately 40% of people living with HIV will have some abnormalities based on careful neuropsychological testing. Most of these patients will be asymptomatic (ANI), but 12% will have minor manifestations (MCD), and 2% severe disorders (HAD). Patients may have memory deficits, decreased executive function, and flattened affect, all of which may markedly affect quality of life. Screening tools such as the Montreal Cognitive Assessment (MoCA) test and the Frontal Assessment Battery test can be used to diagnose HAND. MRI findings may show diffuse cerebral atrophy, which correlates with symptoms. Risk factors for developing HAND include age at seroconversion, low CD4 count, comorbidities such as hepatitis C virus, other CNS infections, and trauma. Neurologic manifestations in PLWH on ART generally seem to be nonprogressive or very slowly progressive, and thus adherence to ART is critical. Interestingly, therapy early after initial infection may lower the CNS reservoir for the virus and result in less immune activation compared to those initiated on treatment later in chronic infection.

Focal Lesions of the Central Nervous System

A large variety of neurologic problems can occur in patients with low CD4 T-cell counts. A neuroanatomic classification of these manifestations is presented in Table 16.4. Some of the more frequent or treatable problems are discussed here and in the next section.

群的数据。抗逆转录病毒治疗对肺癌风险或预后的影响尚不明确，肺癌患者的生存率低于普通人群。
- 在美国，结直肠癌是导致普通人群癌症死亡的第三大原因。HIV 感染历来与结直肠癌发病率的增加无关，但 HIV 感染者的结直肠癌发病率似乎在增加，而且发病年龄越来越小。HIV 感染者的结直肠癌筛查率和存活率都较低。随着人口老龄化趋势，今后的工作重点将是对这种常见和致命的恶性肿瘤进行及时筛查和治疗。
- HIV 携带者罹患肝癌（尤其是肝细胞癌）的比例增加，部分原因是乙型肝炎和丙型肝炎病毒合并感染的比例增加，以及酗酒导致肝硬化的比例增加。此外，随着 HIV 感染者肥胖率的增加，非酒精性脂肪性肝炎（NASH）导致肝硬化及恶性肿瘤的风险也会增加。目前已有治疗病毒性肝炎的治疗方案，并建议所有 HIV 感染者都接受相应治疗。同样，非酒精性脂肪性肝炎的诊治也十分重要。
- HIV 感染者的皮肤癌（包括鳞状细胞癌和恶性黑色素瘤）发病率增加，皮肤筛查是基础医疗的重要组成部分。
- 前列腺癌和乳腺癌的发病率在 HIV 感染者中并没有增加。针对这一人群的筛查建议和治疗指南同一般人群。

随着 HIV 感染者人口的老龄化，所有恶性肿瘤的发病率都将上升。不幸的是，与癌症相关的死亡率预计也会随之而上升。针对艾滋病标志性恶性肿瘤和 NADC 的筛查及治疗，对这一高危人群至关重要。

免疫重建炎症综合征

免疫重建炎症综合征（IRIS）是一种与 HIV 密切相关的综合征，但这种现象并非 HIV 所特有，也见于其他疾病，尤其是结核病。与 HIV 相关的 IRIS 发生在开始接受抗逆转录病毒治疗之后，通常发生在 CD4$^+$ T 细胞计数较低的患者，表现为已治疗的机会性感染恶化，称为矛盾性 IRIS；或以前的亚临床（未治疗）感染被掩盖，而称为掩盖性 IRIS。表现为患者开始接受抗逆转录病毒治疗后，在两周至数月后出现临床症状恶化。发热在 IRIS 中极为常见。矛盾型 IRIS 通常表现为发热和正在治疗的已知机会性感染的临床恶化。未掩盖的 IRIS 通常表现为发热和心动过速，有时会伴有局部症状，这提示先前未确诊的机会性感染（如隐球菌病时的头痛和钝痛，或 MAC 时的腹痛）。HIV 感染者发生 IRIS 的频率及范围很广，一项荟萃分析发现，已发表的研究中 IRIS 的发生率约为 13%；不同疾病过程的发生率也有所不同：CMV 视网膜炎、隐球菌脑膜炎、PML 和结核病的发生率最高。IRIS 是一种临床诊断，没有专门的诊断用的检测方法。以下情况下，临床医生应怀疑 IRIS：近期开始接受抗逆转录病毒治疗的患者，尤其是基线 CD4$^+$ T 细胞计数较低，出现已知的机会性感染恶化；或者尽管有免疫恢复的证据，但临床症状仍出现恶化。IRIS 的发病率很高，且高达 50% 的 IRIS 病例需要住院治疗。诊断由临床表现决定，但一般需要进行血液检查、血清分枝杆菌检查和痰液细菌检查等。如果有呼吸道症状或放射学检查结果，则进行病原学染色和培养；如果有症状，则进行腹部和骨盆 CT 或脑部影像学检查；如果有眼部症状，则进行视网膜检查；如果有明显的淋巴结肿大，则需进行淋巴结活检；并根据症状进一步进行其他检查。IRIS 的治疗重点是控制已确定的机会性感染，并使用激素和（或）非甾体抗炎药来缓解免疫反应。除危及生命的病例外，其他病例均应继续抗逆转录病毒治疗。激素治疗通常需要序贯治疗，一般为 4 周或更长时间，并在症状控制后逐渐减量。

HIV 并发症与合并疾病

HIV 神经系统疾病

大多数未经治疗的 HIV 感染者，最终都会出现神经系统并发症，从轻微的认知障碍或周围神经病变，到严重的痴呆和危及生命的中枢神经系统感染。与其他慢病毒一样，HIV 也会在感染早期进入中枢神经系统的小胶质细胞，导致直接的神经元破坏以及导致病毒蛋白对神经元细胞功能的影响，从而出现 HIV 相关神经系统疾病。中枢神经系统感染可通过脑脊液病毒载量和免疫标志物升高来确诊。抗逆转录病毒治疗通常会抑制中枢神经系统和外周血中的病毒载量，但在极少数情况下，当血浆病毒载量抑制时，反而会出现中枢神经系统病毒载量升高，这种情况被称为"中枢神经系统病毒逃逸"。抗逆转录病毒治疗对中枢神经系统的穿透力因药物而异，中枢神经系统 HIV 感染仍是一个需积极研究的领域。

在接受有效的治疗前，HIV 感染者会出现各种严重的神经系统并发症，包括渐进性痴呆（称为艾滋病痴呆综合征）、局灶性中枢神经系统疾病和周围神经病变。抗逆转录病毒治疗大大降低了艾滋病神经认知并发症的发病率，但也使人们逐渐扩展了艾滋病相关神经认知障碍（HAND）的疾病谱，其中包括无症状神经系统损害（ANI）、轻度认知功能障碍（MCD）和艾滋病相关痴呆（HAD）。根据神经心理学测试，大约 40% 的 HIV 感染者会出现一些神经系统异常，其中大多数患者无症状（ANI），但 12% 的患者有轻微表现（MCD），2% 的患者有严重失调（HAD）。患者可能会出现记忆障碍、执行功能下降和情感平淡，这些都会明显影响生活质量。蒙特利尔认知评估（MoCA）测试和额叶评估电池测试等筛查工具，均可用于诊断艾滋病相关神经认知障碍。MRI 结果可能会显示症状相关性弥漫性脑萎缩。艾滋病相关神经认知障碍的易患因素包括血清转换年龄、低 CD4$^+$ T 细胞计数、合并症（如丙型肝炎病毒）、其他中枢神经系统感染及外伤。接受抗逆转录病毒治疗的 HIV 感染者的神经系统表现似乎通常进展非常缓慢，因此坚持治疗至关重要。与感染后期开始治疗的患者相比，早期治疗有助于降低中枢神经系统的病毒库，并导致较低的免疫激活水平。

中枢神经系统局灶性病变

低 CD4$^+$ T 细胞计数的患者可能会出现多种神经系

Several opportunistic complications of HIV infection produce focal CNS lesions, as mentioned previously. Patients with focal neurologic signs, seizures of new onset, or recent onset of rapidly progressive cognitive impairment should undergo magnetic resonance imaging (MRI) or CT of the brain. Toxoplasmosis, CNS lymphoma, and PML are the most common causes of CNS focal lesions in this setting (Table 16.5). A more detailed review of these opportunistic diseases was discussed previously.

Central Nervous System Diseases Without Prominent Focal Signs

Evaluation of PLWH with fever and headache is difficult because of the often subtle manifestations of serious CNS lesions in immunocompromised patients. Bacterial meningitis management is the same as for non-immunocompromised patients. Meningeal diseases in PLWH fall into the broad categories of aseptic meningitis, chronic meningitis, and meningoencephalitis.

A brief review of these conditions is as follows:
- *Aseptic Meningitis:* Patients with aseptic meningitis, which can be a manifestation of the acute retroviral syndrome, complain most often of headache. Their sensorium is generally intact, and findings on neurologic examination are normal. In the individual with established HIV infection, aseptic meningitis may result from several potentially treatable causes.
- *Chronic Meningitis:* As discussed previously, *Cryptococcus* followed by tuberculosis are the most common causes of chronic meningitis in PLWH. Patients with an AIDS diagnosis with chronic meningitis characteristically have headache, fever, difficulty in concentrating, or changes in sensorium. Neurosyphilis in PLWH is more common than in uninfected patients and may manifest earlier after infection.
- *Meningoencephalitis:* Patients with meningoencephalitis manifest alterations in sensorium varying from mild lethargy to coma. Patients may be febrile, and neurologic examination often shows evidence of diffuse CNS involvement. MRI may show only nonspecific abnormalities, whereas electroencephalography often is consistent with diffuse disease of the brain. CMV, HSV, and HIV itself are possible causes.

Distal symmetrical peripheral neuropathy (PN) is a common neurological complication of HIV. In addition to the direct effect of the virus itself, older ART drugs, particularly stavudine and didanosine, were associated with PN. Distressing pain, hyperesthesia, or hypesthesia, occurring most commonly in the lower extremities and worse at night, were previously common and were difficult to treat. With newer drugs and earlier treatment of all patients with HIV, new diagnoses of PN are becoming less common. Treatment consists of removing potentially neurotoxic drugs and, depending on symptoms, typically initiating gabapentin therapy.

Gastrointestinal Diseases

Patients with advanced HIV disease have a variety of potential gastrointestinal complications, whereas those with elevated CD4 counts and suppressed viral loads on ART have far less risk. Thus, in the pre-ART era, gastrointestinal complications ranging from severe oral stomatitis and esophagitis caused by *Candida* infections, to acalculous cholecystitis, severe chronic hepatitis, and chronic diarrhea caused by protozoal parasites, were common. In the ART era, these complications in diagnosed and treated patients are far rarer.

Mouth and Esophagus

Thrush, or *Candida* pharyngitis, and *Candida* esophagitis have been some of the historic markers of HIV, although many other causes of immunodeficiency can also put people at risk for these infections (see prior section on *Candida* disease). Other causes of ulcerations in the mouth and esophagus include aphthous ulcers and herpes virus reactivation, including HSV-1 and CMV. In patients with AIDS, KS frequently occurs in the mouth and may also occur in the stomach and liver.

Large and Small Intestines

The lower GI tract was previously the site of chronic infection due to a variety of microorganisms, including *Cryptosporidium, Cystoisospora*

TABLE 16.4 Neuroanatomic Classification of Neurologic Complications of HIV Infection

Category	Condition
Meningitis and headache	Aseptic meningitis
	Cryptococcal meningitis
	Tuberculous meningitis
	Neurosyphilis
Diffuse brain diseases	
With preservation of consciousness	AIDS dementia complex
	Neurosyphilis
With decreased arousal	*Toxoplasma* encephalitis
	Cytomegalovirus encephalitis
Focal brain diseases	Tuberculous brain abscess
	Primary central nervous system lymphoma
	Progressive multifocal leukoencephalopathy
	Cerebral toxoplasmosis
	Neurosyphilis
Myelopathies	Subacute or chronic progressive vacuolar myelopathy
	Cytomegalovirus myelopathy
Peripheral neuropathies	Predominantly sensory polyneuropathy
	Toxic neuropathies
	Autonomic neuropathy
	Cytomegalovirus polyradiculopathy
Myopathies	Noninflammatory myopathy
	Zidovudine myopathy

TABLE 16.5 Neurologic Complications of HIV Infection

	CLINICAL ONSET			NEURORADIOLOGIC FEATURES		
Condition	Time	Alertness	Fever	Number of Lesions	Characteristics of Lesions	Location of Lesions
Cerebral toxoplasmosis	Days	Reduced	Common	Usually multiple	Spherical, ring enhancing	Basal ganglia, cortex
Primary CNS lymphoma	Days to weeks	Variable	Absent	One or few	Irregular, weakly ring enhancing	Periventricular
PML	Weeks to months	Variable	Absent	Often multiple	Multiple lesions visible on MRI	White matter

MRI, Magnetic resonance imaging; *PML,* progressive multifocal lymphoma.

统问题。表 16.4 以神经解剖学分类总结了这些症状。这里和下一节将共同讨论一些常见问题。如前所述，HIV 感染的几种机会性并发症会产生中枢神经系统局灶性病变。对于出现局灶性神经系统体征、新发癫痫或近期出现快速进展性认知障碍的患者，应进行脑部 MRI 或 CT 检查。弓形虫病、中枢神经系统淋巴瘤和 PML 是导致中枢神经系统局灶性病变的最常见原因（表 16.5）。有关这些机会性疾病的更多详情已在前文讨论。

无明显的局灶性体征的中枢神经系统疾病

对发热和头痛症状的 HIV 感染者进行评估非常困难，因为免疫力低下患者的严重中枢神经系统病变往往表现不明显。细菌性脑膜炎的治疗与一般人群相同。HIV 感染者的脑膜疾病可大致分为无菌性脑膜炎、慢性脑膜炎和脑膜脑炎。简要总结如下：

- **无菌性脑膜炎**：无菌性脑膜炎可能是急性逆转录病毒综合征的一种表现形式，患者的主诉大多是头痛。他们的感觉通常完好无损，神经系统检查结果正常。对于已确诊的 HIV 感染者，无菌性脑膜炎可能由多种潜在的原因引起。

- **慢性脑膜炎**：如前所述，隐球菌和结核病是 HIV 感染者慢性脑膜炎最常见的病因。通常会出现头痛、发热、注意力难以集中或感觉改变等症状。与未感染者相比，神经梅毒在 HIV 感染者中更为常见，而且可能在感染后更早地出现症状。

- **脑膜脑炎**：脑膜脑炎患者表现出从轻度嗜睡到昏迷不等的感觉改变，可能会出现发热，神经系统检查常显示弥漫性中枢神经系统受累的证据。MRI 可能只显示非特异性征象，而脑电图通常与大脑弥漫性改变一致。CMV、HSV 和 HIV 本身都可能是病因。

- **远端对称性周围神经病变（PN）**：是一种常见的 HIV 相关神经系统并发症。除了病毒本身的直接影响外，早期的抗逆转录病毒治疗药物，尤其是司坦夫定和地达诺辛，也与 PN 有关。常见症状包括下肢疼痛、感觉过敏或感觉减退，常在夜间加重，而且难以治疗。随着药物的更新换代和对 HIV 感染者的早期治疗，新诊断 PN 患者越来越少。治疗包括停用潜在的神经毒性药物，并根据症状加用加巴喷丁治疗。

消化道疾病

晚期 HIV 疾病患者有各种潜在的胃肠道并发症，而 $CD4^+$ T 细胞计数升高、接受抗逆转录病毒治疗使病毒载量受到抑制的患者的风险要小得多。因此，在前抗逆转录病毒治疗时代，胃肠道并发症很常见，从念珠菌感染引起的严重口腔炎和食管炎，到原虫寄生引起的结石性胆囊炎、严重慢性肝炎和慢性腹泻。在抗逆转录病毒治疗时代，这些并发症在确诊和治疗的患者中已少见。

口腔和食管

鹅口疮（或念珠菌性咽炎）和念珠菌性食管炎一直是 HIV 感染的经典标志，尽管许多其他免疫缺陷状态也会使人们出现相应感染的风险增加（见前面关于念珠菌病的章节）。导致口腔和食管溃疡的其他原因包括阿弗他溃疡和疱疹病毒反应，包括 HSV-1 和 CMV。在艾滋病患者中，KS 经常发生在口腔，也可发生在胃和肝。

大肠和小肠

下消化道以前是各种微生物造成慢性感染的场所，包括隐孢子虫、贝氏等孢子球虫、小孢子虫属、巨细胞病毒和分枝杆菌。这些感染会引起慢性腹泻，导致厌食和消瘦。随着抗逆转录病毒治疗药物出现，这些感染已不常见，但

表 16.4　以神经解剖学分类的 HIV 感染并发症

类别	疾病
脑膜炎和头痛	无菌性脑膜炎 隐球菌性脑膜炎 结核性脑膜炎 神经梅毒
弥漫性脑部疾病 　有自主意识 　唤醒减少	艾滋病痴呆综合征 神经梅毒 弓形虫脑炎 巨细胞病毒脑炎
局灶性脑部疾病	结核性脑脓肿 原发性中枢神经系统淋巴瘤 进行性多灶性白质脑病 脑弓形虫病 神经梅毒
脊髓病变	亚急性或慢性进行性空泡性脊髓病 巨细胞病毒脊髓病
周围神经病	感觉性多发性神经病 中毒性神经病 自律神经病 巨细胞病毒多发性神经病
肌病	非炎症性肌病 齐多夫定肌病

表 16.5　HIV 感染的神经系统并发症

	临床表现			神经影像学特征		
疾病	时间	觉醒程度	发热	病变数量	病变特征	病变位置
脑弓形虫病	数天	下降	常见	通常多个	球形、环状增强	基底节、皮质
原发性中枢神经系统肿瘤	数天至数周	不定	无	一个或几个	不规则、弱环状增强	脑室周围
进行性多灶性白质脑病	数周至数月	不定	无	通常多个	磁共振成像可见多个病灶	白质

belli, *Microsporidia* spp, CMV, and mycobacteria. These infections caused chronic diarrhea leading to inanition and wasting. In the era of ART, these infections are much less common and have been superseded in frequency by *Clostridioides difficile* infection due to frequent antibiotic exposure in PLWH. Additionally, increased risk of anal cancer has been recognized in PLWH. With the aging population of PLWH, colon cancer risk is also on the rise (see prior section on HIV and malignancy).

Hepatobiliary Disease

Abnormalities on liver function testing are common in HIV disease and often are nonspecific. Elevations of serum alanine aminotransferase and aspartate aminotransferase may represent chronic active viral hepatitis B or C but may also reflect hepatic inflammation caused by alcohol or medications, including trimethoprim-sulfamethoxazole or antiretroviral agents. Alcohol use is highly prevalent among PLWH and may contribute, as can use of other drugs such as MDMA ("ecstasy"). Marked elevations in serum alkaline phosphatase levels may reflect infiltrative disease of the liver (e.g., MAC, CMV, tuberculosis, tumor) but also may occur in patients with acalculous cholecystitis, cryptosporidiosis, AIDS-associated sclerosing cholangitis, or syphilitic hepatitis.

Viral hepatitides, particularly hepatitis C, are an important cause of morbidity and mortality among PLWH. More than 80% of persons with HIV who have a history of injection drug use are coinfected with hepatitis C, and the risk of progression to end-stage liver disease is greater for those with HIV and hepatitis C coinfection. Recently, therapy of hepatitis C has been revolutionized by combination directly acting agents (DAAs), which achieve hepatitis C cure rates of over 95%. Response rates among PLWH appear to be similar to those among HIV-negative persons. In contrast, treatment of hepatitis B is rarely curative; however, very effective suppression can be achieved utilizing combination therapy. Common agents used for HIV ART, such as tenofovir, emtricitabine, and lamivudine, have potent hepatitis B antiviral activity, and an ART regimen that treats both HIV and hepatitis B coinfection is easily possible. Occult hepatitis infections (antibody negative but with detectable virus on RNA/DNA testing) have been described for both hepatitis C and hepatitis B, particularly in the context of advanced immunodeficiency. Hepatocellular carcinoma is a complication of both hepatitis B and C infection. Regular screening with liver imaging is indicated for all patients with hepatitis C and known cirrhosis, all patients with hepatitis B who are at increased risk, namely those with active hepatitis (elevated serum ALT) and/or high viral load (>20,000 IU/mL), those with a family history of hepatocellular carcinoma, Asian males over 40, Asian females over 50, and all Africans and African Americans.

Cardiovascular Disease

Before ART, patients with HIV with low CD4 counts were at risk for myocarditis, pericardial effusion, and dilated cardiomyopathy, but at present these conditions are markedly less common. What has become apparent, however, is an increased risk for cardiovascular disease, including both myocardial infarction and stroke. In a landmark study from the US Veteran Affairs system in 2013, PLWH were found to have a 50% increase in acute myocardial infarction compared to HIV-uninfected patients, even after controlling for traditional risk factors such as smoking and diabetes. In a more recent review in 2018, a relative risk of 2.16 for cardiovascular (CV) disease in PLWH was noted. Unlike HIV-negative patients, there is an increased rate (up to 50%) of type II myocardial infarction (vasospasm, endothelial dysfunction) compared to type I (thromboembolic) infarction, suggesting different etiologic processes. Longitudinal studies have shown that the risk for stroke and, more recently, congestive heart failure are similarly elevated.

Several additional features of CV disease are worth noting. Long-term studies from the Kaiser Permanente system in California and from Europe initially demonstrated increased rates of CV disease in PLWH but found that more recent data in selected populations saw a convergence of rates with HIV-negative patients, perhaps due to improvements in CV prevention, such as the widespread use of HMG co-A reductase inhibitors ("statins"). It is also worth noting that PLWH do have a higher prevalence of some risk factors for CV disease, particularly smoking, diabetes mellitus, renal disease, metabolic syndrome, and hypertension. The risk conveyed by these factors in total is of a much larger magnitude than that contributed by HIV itself. Thus, addressing these risk factors is particularly important in this population that has a baseline elevated CV risk due to HIV. Proven interventions include smoking cessation and the use of antihypertensives and statins, which should be prescribed following American College of Cardiology/American Heart Association guidelines. Improving diet and exercise also are important, especially for patients as they age.

The effect of certain antiretrovirals on CV risk remains an area of controversy. Protease inhibitors (PIs) are known to have an adverse effect on the metabolic profile, including inducing hyperlipidemia, when compared to newer classes of ART drugs such as integrase inhibitors. Risk is not necessarily uniform across the class; a recent cohort analysis specifically identified darunavir to be associated with increased risk when compared to atazanavir. In addition, several studies have shown that abacavir increases CV risk, but these findings have not been confirmed in others. Integrase inhibitors and newer reverse transcriptase inhibitors have a lesser effect on patients' lipid profiles, although integrase inhibitors have been associated with more weight gain than other classes, which itself may raise the risk of other diseases that raise CV risk (e.g., diabetes, hypertension).

Renal Disease

In the early years of the HIV epidemic, a new form of progressive renal disease was identified, termed HIV-associated nephropathy (HIVAN). It was characterized by rapidly progressive renal failure and nephrotic-range proteinuria. This disease was found to be more common in African Americans. The incidence of HIVAN rose until the mid-1990s and then fell with the advent of effective ART. Although HIVAN has become uncommon, the incidence of chronic renal disease in PWHV remains significantly higher than in the general population. The prevalence of stage III chronic kidney disease (glomerular filtration rate of 30 to 59 mL/min) has ranged from 3.5% to 9.7%. PLWH are more than 16 times more likely to need renal replacement therapy.

The etiology of renal disease in PLWH is multifactorial; risk factors include low CD4 counts, high viral loads, hypertension, diabetes mellitus, cardiovascular disease, African American race, hepatitis C coinfection, and prior exposure to certain ART drugs such as tenofovir. Patients are also at risk of acute kidney injury, particularly in the setting of dehydration, infection, and polypharmacy. In addition, patients may develop immune complex kidney disease and thrombotic microangiopathy. Most important in prevention and treatment of renal disease is the use of effective ART and consistent monitoring of renal function. Controlling both hypertension and diabetes are also essential in preventing the progression of renal disease.

Osteoporosis and Bone Disease

PLWH have increased rates of osteopenia and osteoporosis and consequently longitudinal controlled studies have shown an almost 3-fold rate of fractures compared to that of the general population. Risk factors for decreased bone density are usually multiple and include effects of ART, particularly protease inhibitor– and tenofovir disoproxil fumarate–containing regimens; low body weight; vitamin D deficiency;

由于HIV感染者经常应用抗生素，目前艰难梭菌感染成为更常见的感染疾病。此外，还发现HIV感染者患有肛门癌的风险增加。随着HIV感染人群的老龄化，结肠癌的发病风险也在上升（参见前文"HIV与恶性肿瘤"部分）。

肝胆疾病

非特异性的肝功能指标异常在艾滋病患者中很常见。血清谷丙转氨酶和天冬氨酸氨基转移酶升高可能代表慢性活动性乙型或丙型病毒性肝炎，但也可能反映酒精或药物（包括甲氧苄啶-磺胺甲噁唑或抗逆转录病毒药物）引起的肝炎。饮酒、使用摇头丸（MDMA）等其他药物等都可能导致肝炎。血清碱性磷酸酶水平明显升高，可能提示肝浸润性疾病（如MAC、CMV、结核病、肿瘤），也可能发生在无结石性胆囊炎、隐孢子虫病、艾滋病相关硬化性胆管炎或梅毒性肝炎患者中。

病毒性肝炎，尤其是丙型肝炎，是导致HIV感染者发病和死亡的重要原因。在有注射吸毒史的HIV感染者中，超过80%的人同时感染了丙型肝炎，而HIV感染者和HCV合并感染者发展为终末期肝病的风险更高。最近，丙型肝炎的治疗因使用直接抗病毒药物（DAA）方案而发生了革命性的变化，其治愈率超过95%。丙型肝炎感染者的应答率似乎与HIV阴性者相似。相比之下，乙型肝炎的治疗很难达到治愈，但在联合治疗下可以达到非常有效的抑制效果。用于HIV抗逆转录病毒治疗的常用药物（如替诺福韦、恩曲他滨和拉米夫定）具有很强的抗乙型肝炎抗病毒活性，因此通常采用同时治疗HIV和HBV合并感染的抗逆转录病毒方案。丙型肝炎和乙型肝炎都有隐匿性肝炎感染的病例（抗体阴性，但在RNA/DNA检测中可检测到病毒），尤其是在重度免疫缺陷的情况下更易出现。肝细胞癌是HBV及HCV感染的并发症之一。对于所有HCV合并肝硬化及所有HBV感染的肝癌高危患者，应定期进行肝影像学筛查。HBV肝癌危险因素包括：活动性肝炎（血清谷丙转氨酶升高）或高HBV病毒载量（> 20 000 IU/ml）、有肝细胞癌家族史者、40岁以上的亚洲男性、50岁以上的亚洲女性以及所有非洲人及非裔美国人。

心血管疾病

在出现抗逆转录病毒治疗药物前，低$CD4^+$ T细胞计数的HIV感染者患有心肌炎、心包积液和扩张型心肌病等疾病的风险较高，而目前这些病症的发病率已明显减少。然而，HIV感染者心血管疾病（包括心肌梗死和卒中）的患病风险增加，这已成为显而易见的事实。在美国退伍军人事务系统于2013年进行的一项重要研究中发现，与未感染HIV的患者相比，HIV感染者发生急性心肌梗死的风险增加了50%，即使在控制了吸烟和糖尿病等传统危险因素之后仍明显高于非感染者。在2018年的一篇综述中指出，HIV感染者患心血管疾病的为非感染者的2.16倍。与HIV阴性者不同的是，与Ⅰ型（血栓栓塞性）心肌梗死相比，Ⅱ型心肌梗死（血管痉挛、内皮功能障碍）的发生率更高，可高达50%，这表明HIV感染者中发病机制不同。纵向研究表明，卒中以及充血性心力衰竭的风险也同样升高。

心血管疾病的另外几个特点也值得注意。加利福尼亚州的Kaiser Permanente体系及欧洲的长期研究表明，HIV感染者心血管疾病的患病率比例较一般人群更高；但最近在部分调研中发现，与非感染者相比，HIV感染者心血管疾病的发病比例趋于一致，这可能是由于心血管疾病预防治疗的推动，如他汀类药物的广泛使用。此外，HIV携带者确实有更多的心血管疾病危险因素，尤其是吸烟、糖尿病、肾病、代谢综合征和高血压。这些因素所带来的风险总和远远大于HIV本身所带来的风险。因此，对于因HIV而导致心血管风险升高的人群来说，预防这些危险因素尤为重要。行之有效的干预措施包括戒烟、使用降压药和他汀类药物，处方应遵循美国心脏病学会/美国心脏协会指南。改善饮食和加强锻炼，尤其是对于高龄患者，是非常重要的措施。

某些抗逆转录病毒药物对心血管风险的影响仍然是一个存在争议。众所周知，与整合酶抑制剂等新型抗逆转录病毒治疗药物相比，蛋白酶抑制剂（PIs）会对代谢产生不利影响，如导致高脂血症。最近的一项队列研究发现，与阿扎那韦相比，达茹那韦会增加心血管疾病风险。此外，一些研究显示阿巴卡韦增加了心血管疾病的风险，但这些发现尚未在其他研究中得到证实。整合酶抑制剂和较新的逆转录酶抑制剂对患者血脂的影响较小，但整合酶抑制剂比其他类药物更易导致体重增加，而体重增加本身可能会增加其他疾病（如糖尿病、高血压）的风险，从而增加心血管疾病的风险。

肾病

在HIV流行的早期，发现了一种新的进行性肾病，称为HIV相关性肾病（HIVAN）。它的特点是快速进展性肾衰竭和肾性蛋白尿，常见于非裔美国人。HIVAN的发病率在20世纪90年代中期前持续上升，后续随着有效抗逆转录病毒药物的出现转而下降。尽管HIVAN已再不常见，但HIV感染者中慢性肾病的发病率仍明显高于普通人群。慢性肾病Ⅲ期（肾小球滤过率为30～59 ml/min）的患病率在HIV感染者中的比例为3.5%～9.7%不等。HIV感染者需要接受肾替代治疗的概率是普通人的16倍以上。

HIV导致肾病的病因是多种多样的，其中包括：低$CD4^+$ T细胞计数、高病毒载量、高血压、糖尿病、心血管疾病、非裔美国人、HCV合并感染以及某些抗逆转录病毒治疗药物治疗史（如替诺福韦）。部分患者还存在急性肾损伤的风险，尤其是在脱水、感染和使用多种药物的情况下。此外，患者还可能出现免疫复合物肾病及血栓性微血管病。预防和治疗肾病，最重要的是使用有效的抗逆转录病毒治疗，以及持续监测肾功能。同时，控制高血压和糖尿病也是预防肾病恶化的关键。

骨质疏松症和骨病

HIV感染者的骨质疏松症和骨质疏松症发病率升高，既往研究显示，与普通人群相比，HIV感染者的骨折发病率几乎是普通人群的3倍。导致骨密度下降

alcohol use; hypogonadism; opiate exposure; smoking; and effects of HIV itself. Patients should be assessed for vitamin D deficiency and other risk factors and treated and counseled appropriately. Bone density assessment by dual-energy x-ray absorptiometry (DXA) is recommended for all men with HIV who are over 50, all postmenopausal women, those with a history of fragility fractures, patients on chronic corticosteroids, and patients at high risk for fall. Risk of fragility fracture should be assessed primarily using the Fracture Risk Assessment Tool (FRAX). ART regimens should be reviewed for osteopenia and osteoporosis risk. Patients diagnosed with osteopenia or osteoporosis should be treated following established guidelines.

Endocrine Disorders
Metabolic Syndrome

PLWH are at increased risk for metabolic syndrome, which includes central obesity, insulin resistance, hypertension, and hypertriglyceridemia. Some classes of ART such as protease inhibitors seem to increase the risk for metabolic syndrome, and this risk translates into increased risk for CV disease. Treatment with weight loss and exercise, anti-hypertensives, and diabetic medications if diabetes is diagnosed, are recommended.

Diabetes Mellitus

The risk for diabetes mellitus (DM) in PLWH patients was not initially appreciated but has become apparent in more recent years. One estimate is that the relative risk for DM in PLWH is 2.4 when compared to the general population. This risk is compounded by the rates of metabolic syndrome, obesity, and adverse lifestyle (such as poor diet and low rates of exercise). In addition, a diagnosis of DM markedly increases the risk for CV disease, including stroke and peripheral vascular disease, as well as renal disease. Screening PLWH with a hemoglobin A_{1c} or fasting blood sugar on an annual basis is important, particularly as the population ages. Treatment for patients at risk for DM and those with DM should follow established guidelines for management of diabetes.

Other Endocrine Disorders

Other endocrine disorders that disproportionately affect PLWH, particularly those with low CD4 counts, include adrenal insufficiency (AI), hypogonadism, and male gynecomastia. In the pre-ART era, adrenal gland pathology caused by CMV and mycobacteria was frequent, but clinical AI characterized by malaise, orthostatic hypotension, weight loss, hyponatremia, and hypoglycemia, was uncommon. Clinical AI remains rare. Hypogonadism is common in men with HIV and may manifest as erectile dysfunction and loss of libido but may also occur more subtly with low energy, depression, or inability to gain muscle mass. Screening with serum testosterone may indicate hypogonadism that can be treated with androgen replacement therapy. Gynecomastia in men with HIV may also occur and be due to hypoandrogenism, liver disease, medication side effects, or as a part of normal aging.

Nonalcoholic Fatty Liver Disease

Nonalcoholic fatty liver disease (NFLD) ranges from simple hepatic steatosis (or fatty liver) to NASH and hepatic fibrosis that can lead to cirrhosis. The rates of steatosis and NASH in PLWH are increasing and appear to be greater than in the general population, perhaps because of the increased rates of obesity, metabolic syndrome, and diabetes mellitus. NASH and subsequent cirrhosis pose a significant risk for PLWH and emphasize the importance of preventative measures including weight control.

Obesity

In the early years of the HIV epidemic, advanced AIDS was associated with low weight, and in fact one of the characteristics of the disease was wasting and inanition. Effective ART prevented and even reversed this manifestation of infection, even in end-stage AIDS. Now with PLWH on ART, a new problem has arisen—obesity. In countries like the United States, the rates of obesity in PLWH (20% to 31%) match the rates in the general population. Rates of complications related to obesity in PLWH, such as diabetes mellitus and cardiovascular disease, are nearly twice the rates in uninfected patients. Rates of obesity in PLWH may be related to a combination of factors including poor diet quality, greater food insecurity, lack of exercise, and genetics. Perhaps most important, however, has been the lack of awareness of the consequences of obesity and also the best approaches to losing weight. Although there has been a dearth of research in the treatment of obesity in PLWH, behavioral weight loss programs focusing on behavior change, diet, and exercise have been shown to be effective for this population. In addition, bariatric surgery for morbidly obese patients has been an effective strategy in individual cases.

Aging and HIV

The average age of the first 1000 cases of HIV reported in 1983 was 34 years. With the advent of effective ART, the age of PLWH has steadily increased so that by the year 2015, it was estimated that 50% of PLWH were over the age of 50, and by the year 2030 it is estimated that 70% will be over the age of 50. Similar trends, although delayed, are being observed worldwide in low- to medium-income countries. Despite this increase in the age of PLWH, mortality remains elevated compared to the general population, although there is great heterogeneity. Individuals with risk factors such as low CD4 count, elevated viral loads, drug use, hepatitis coinfections, and other comorbidities have increased mortality rates, whereas subgroup analysis of population studies have shown that individuals with CD4 counts greater than 350 cells/microliter at diagnosis, consistent viral suppression, and an absence of other risk factors have a life expectancy similar to uninfected individuals. Nonetheless, most population studies comparing PLWH to the general population, controlling for risk factors, have shown a decrease in life expectancy of anywhere from 2 to 13 years depending on the subpopulation.

Whether HIV infection accelerates the aging process has been a controversial subject and continues to be investigated. It is known, however, that HIV is associated with chronic inflammation at levels that are similar to older individuals. Inflammation is presumed to be driven by ongoing low-level viral replication, even in virally suppressed individuals, and by the effect of the initial damage to the immune system during acute HIV infection (e.g., injury to gut immune tissue). Elevated markers of inflammation include elevated levels of IL-6, elevated markers of microbial translocation, and elevated levels of macrophage activation. In addition, immune dysregulation and immune senescence as evidenced by decreased pools of CD4 T cells, increased senescent CD8 T cells that secrete cytokines, and an inability to respond robustly to new antigens, all occur in PLWH as well as elderly noninfected people. Increased inflammation and immune dysregulation are part of the normal aging process but appear to occur earlier in PLWH. In addition, as discussed previously, PLWH are at increased risk for a variety of comorbidities, some of which are associated with increased inflammation, such as cardiovascular disease.

Compared to age-matched controls, PLWH have higher rates of geriatric syndromes including falls, urinary incontinence, difficulty with activities of daily living, slow gait, decreased vision and hearing, and frailty. As a result, they are at increased risk for associated morbidity. In addition, PLWH are more likely to develop frailty early. Frailty is defined several ways, but Fried's criteria are commonly used and include decreased strength, endurance, activity, and walking speed, as well as weight loss. Patients with frailty are at significant risk for poor outcomes including hospitalization and death. Risks for frailty

有多种危险因素,包括:抗逆转录病毒治疗药物的影响(尤其是蛋白酶抑制剂和含富马酸替诺福韦二吡呋酯的方案)、低体重、维生素 D 缺乏、酗酒、性腺功能减退、接触阿片类制剂、吸烟以及 HIV 本身的影响。应评估患者是否缺乏维生素 D 及其他危险因素,并给予适当的治疗和指导。建议所有 50 岁以上的男性 HIV 感染者、所有绝经后女性、有脆性骨折病史者、长期服用激素的患者以及跌倒高风险的患者,通过双能 X 射线吸收法(DXA)进行骨密度评估。脆性骨折风险应主要通过骨折风险评估工具(FRAX)进行评估。同时,应注意抗逆转录病毒药物是否存在骨质疏松症副作用。确诊患有骨质疏松症的患者应按照指南进行治疗。

内分泌疾病

代谢综合征

HIV 感染者代谢综合征的发病风险也会增加。代谢综合征包括向心性肥胖、胰岛素抵抗、高血压和高甘油三酯血症。蛋白酶抑制剂等一些抗逆转录病毒治疗可能导致代谢综合征的风险增加,继而出现心血管疾病风险的增加。建议采取减重和运动、抗高血压及糖尿病药物等治疗措施。

糖尿病

HIV 感染者的糖尿病发病风险最初未得到关注,但近年来逐渐得以显现。根据一项研究显示,HIV 感染者糖尿病发病风险是一般人群的 2.4 倍。这种风险因代谢综合征、肥胖和不良生活方式(如饮食不规律和运动量少)而加剧。此外,糖尿病会显著增加心血管疾病(包括卒中和外周血管疾病)以及肾病的风险。HIV 感染者每年进行糖化血红蛋白或空腹血糖筛查是非常重要的措施。糖尿病患者及高危人群的治疗应遵循糖尿病管理指南。

其他内分泌疾病

影响 HIV 感染者(尤其是低 $CD4^+$ T 细胞计数者)的其他内分泌疾病包括肾上腺功能减退症、性腺功能减退症和男性乳腺发育症。在前 ART 时代,由 CMV 和分枝杆菌引起的肾上腺病变很常见,但以乏力、体位性低血压、体重减轻、低钠血症和低血糖为特征的临床肾上腺功能减退症并不常见,目前仍较罕见。性腺功能减退症在 HIV 男性感染者中很常见,可表现为勃起功能障碍和性欲减退,但也可能更隐蔽地表现为精力不足、抑郁或无法提高肌肉质量。通过血清睾酮筛查有助于发现性腺功能减退症,并可给予雄激素替代治疗。HIV 男性感染者可能出现男性乳腺发育症,原因可能是雄激素水平过低、肝病、药物副作用或衰老。

非酒精性脂肪性肝病

非酒精性脂肪性肝病(NFLD)包括从单纯的肝脂肪变性(或脂肪肝)到非酒精性脂肪性肝炎(NASH)以及可能导致肝硬化的肝纤维化。在 HIV 感染者中,脂肪变性和 NASH 的发病率正在增加,而且高于普通人群,这可能是基于肥胖、代谢综合征和糖尿病的发病率的增加。NASH 和后续导致的肝硬化对 HIV 感染者的远期预后构成了巨大风险,更体现了包括控制体重在内的预防措施的重要性。

肥胖症

在 HIV 流行的最初几年,疾病进展至 AIDS 期常与低体重相关,该疾病的特征之一即消瘦和营养不良,而有效的抗逆转录病毒治疗可以预防甚至逆转这种表现。现在,随着 HIV 感染者进行抗逆转录病毒治疗的趋势,肥胖逐渐成了一个日益严重的新问题。在美国等国家,报告 HIV 感染者的肥胖率(20%~31%)可与普通人群的肥胖率相当。HIV 感染与肥胖有关的合并症,如糖尿病和心血管疾病,其发病率可达未感染者的 2 倍。HIV 感染者的肥胖发生与多种因素有关,包括饮食不健康、食品安全欠佳、缺乏锻炼和遗传因素等。然而,最重要的原因可能是人们对肥胖的后果以及最佳减肥方法缺乏认知。虽然治疗 HIV 合并肥胖症的证据尚不足,但行为改变、饮食和运动为重点的行为计划都是有效的干预措施。此外,在个别病例中,对病理性肥胖患者进行减重手术也是一种有效的策略。

HIV 与老化

1983 年,首批报告的 1000 例 HIV 感染者的平均年龄为 34 岁。随着 ART 治疗的出现,HIV 感染者的寿命稳步上升;到 2015 年,估计 50% 的 HIV 感染者年龄超过 50 岁,到 2030 年,估计 70% 的 HIV 感染者年龄超过 50 岁。全球中低收入国家也逐渐出现了类似的趋势。尽管 HIV 感染者的寿命有所延长,但死亡率仍高于一般人群。死亡率升高的影响因素包括:低 $CD4^+$ T 细胞计数、高病毒载量、吸毒、肝炎合并感染和其他合并症等。而人口研究的亚组分析表明,确诊时 $CD4^+$ T 细胞计数大于 $350/mm^3$、病毒持续抑制且无其他危险因素,此类患者的预期寿命与未感染者相似。然而,大多数将 HIV 感染者与一般人群的对照研究显示,根据人群亚组的不同,HIV 感染者的预期寿命会缩短 2~13 年不等。

HIV 感染是否会加速衰老过程,也一直是一个争议性话题。但目前已知的是,HIV 与慢性炎症相关,其炎症反应程度与老年人相当。据推测,炎症反应是由持续的低水平病毒复制(即使在病毒被抑制的个体)以及急性 HIV 感染期对免疫系统造成的最初损害(如对肠道免疫组织的损伤)所驱动的。炎症标志物升高包括 IL-6 水平升高、微生物转运标志物升高和巨噬细胞活化水平升高。此外,免疫失调和免疫衰老表现为 $CD4^+$ T 细胞池减少、分泌细胞因子的衰老、$CD8^+$ T 细胞增多,以及无法对新抗原做出强有力的反应。炎症反应加剧和免疫失调是正常衰老过程的一部分,但似乎在 HIV 感染者中发生得更早。此外,如前所述,HIV 感染者出现各种合并症的风险也较非感染者增加,其中一些疾病可能与炎症反应加重有关,如心血管疾病。

与年龄匹配的对照组相比,HIV 感染者更易出现老年综合征,包括跌倒、尿失禁、日常生活活动困难、步态缓慢、视力和听力下降以及体弱,他们发生相关疾病的风险更高。此外,HIV 感染者更有可能早期出现衰弱。衰弱的诊断最常应用的是 Fried 标准,包括体力、耐力、活动能力、行走速度下降,以及体重减轻

in PLWH include low current and nadir CD4 counts as well as other comorbidities and geriatric syndromes. As the population of PLWH ages, recognizing and addressing both geriatric syndromes and frailty will be increasingly important in their care.

Finally, aging patients in general face a number of challenges to their health and well-being including comorbidities, increasing physical impairments, loss of partners, and family and social isolation. PLWH are particularly at risk for some of these challenges and in addition many face challenges such as poverty, housing and/or food insecurity, and concern for safety. The loss of friends and community is particularly stressful and has been described by one aging PLWH as "a shrinking kind of life." It is important for physicians caring for PLWH to be aware of these issues.

Mental Health

As HIV has changed to a chronic and manageable illness, the emphasis of mental health treatment has shifted from managing acute syndromes to helping patients live well. Depression and anxiety, as well as other mental illnesses, are very common among PLWH. Often patients will not feel comfortable acknowledging the need for mental health care. For many PLWH, their HIV physician may be their only health care provider, and therefore it is crucial for providers to offer routine screenings for mental health concerns such as depression and anxiety. Screenings will also offer opportunities for physicians to facilitate referrals for additional mental health evaluation and appropriate behavioral and psychiatric care. Trauma is not uncommon and treatment of PTSD can be very helpful.

Substance Use Disorder

Substance/alcohol use and substance/alcohol use disorders are common among PLWH. Alcohol use (e.g., problematic and binge drinking) may also co-occur with the use of substances (e.g., cocaine, methamphetamine). Both alcohol use and substance use have been associated with higher rates of risk-taking behaviors (e.g., condomless sex with multiple partners) and have also been associated with decreased adherence to ART. It is also important to note that many individuals who use substances maintain high levels of adherence to ART; thus, the existence of substance or alcohol use should not prevent physicians from prescribing ART. There are many factors that contribute to or exacerbate substance and alcohol use. For instance, among methamphetamine users, there exists a high correlation between methamphetamine use and chemsex behaviors. Other common factors that may perpetuate continued use include co-occurring mental health diagnoses (e.g., PTSD, anxiety, ADHD), minority stress, and environmental instability. Many studies have shown that treatment of opiate use disorders with medication assisted therapy, such as buprenorphine, can be done in conjunction with HIV treatment. Likewise, treatment of alcohol use disorders can be done in conjunction with HIV treatment. Whereas pharmacotherapy for stimulant use disorders is lacking, the patient-physician relationship can still play an important role in facilitating referral for evidence-based behavioral care for stimulant use. Importantly, patient-centered HIV care cannot focus solely on HIV viral suppression but must proactively address mental health and substance use concerns to promote the goal of patients living meaningful lives with the chronic disease of HIV. Routine screening for substance abuse treatment (i.e., at regular follow-up visits) is recommended. Co-locating substance abuse treatment with HIV care (i.e., one stop shopping) is preferred.

Sexually Transmitted Infections

Rates of sexually transmitted infections (STIs) continue to rise in the United States, reaching an all-time high in 2018 (the last available reported data at the time of this publishing), with no sign of leveling off in the coming years. The presence of STIs increases the risk of HIV transmission from partner to partner, particularly syphilis and herpes simplex disease. In people living with HIV, rates of STIs have also increased. As "undetectable = untransmittable" becomes a more commonly understood concept among patients, education about protecting themselves from acquiring STIs is important as patients make informed decisions about condom use. Annual STI screening, or more frequent depending on risk behavior, is important in sexually active patients. Treatment of these STIs is the same in HIV-negative as in HIV-positive persons and the response to treatment is good.

HIV MANAGEMENT AND TREATMENT

Initial Counseling and Ambulatory Evaluation

Once HIV is diagnosed, the health care provider should talk to the patient about the clinical course and treatment of HIV infection and the use of immunologic and virologic studies (e.g., CD4 counts, PVL assays) to guide therapy. Stigma related to HIV remains an important concern and a key barrier to engagement in care. Addressing this as part of post-test counseling and intake to care is key to retention in care for persons newly diagnosed. The patient should be educated about modes of HIV transmission through unprotected sex or sharing of needles. The benefit of "U=U" (undetectable = untransmittable) should be discussed with patients so they understand that initiating treatment and achieving an undetectable viral load is both important for their own health as well as their partners.

The initial evaluation should include both an HIV-oriented review of systems and a complete physical examination. In particular, the skin must be examined for HIV-associated rashes and Kaposi's sarcoma. Examination of the oral cavity may reveal thrush, gingivitis, hairy leukoplakia, superficial ulcers caused by HSV, aphthous ulcers, or lesions characteristic of Kaposi's sarcoma. In persons with very advanced disease, the optic fundi may have hemorrhagic lesions characteristic of CMV retinitis. Lymph node enlargement, hepatomegaly, splenomegaly, and any genital lesions should be carefully noted. Neurologic examination for both peripheral neuropathy and decreased global cognition deserves close attention.

Laboratory Monitoring

The CD4 count and the PVL should be measured at the first visit, and the patient should be shown the results. Graphic illustrations of the interaction between PVL and CD4 can be useful to increase patient understanding. HIV genotyping to assess for drug resistance should also be performed. The PVL is a key measure of treatment adherence and is repeated at regular intervals, generally 2 to 8 weeks after initiation of therapy and every 3 to 6 months once patients are stably on treatment. Once a patient is stable on treatment with suppressed virus (<200 copies) and CD4 counts higher than 200 cells/mL, the value of CD4 monitoring is less clear, and guidelines allow for extending the monitoring interval to yearly. If a patient's count is greater than 500 for greater than 1 year, CD4 monitoring becomes optional, as long as the PVL remains undetectable.

An initial assessment of basic chemistries (including a creatinine), hepatic function testing, a complete blood count with differential, a random or fasting glucose, and a urinalysis should be performed to establish a baseline. Women should have a pregnancy test. Once patients are initiated on ART, they should have a basic chemistry panel and hepatic function testing (along with a PVL as noted previously) repeated between 2 to 8 weeks after starting therapy. Patients stably on ART should have these same labs repeated every 6 months, to monitor for toxicity and changes that might affect dosing. A yearly complete

衰弱患者面临住院和死亡等不良预后的风险极高。HIV 感染者出现衰弱的危险因素包括：当前及最低 $CD4^+$ T 细胞计数偏低、有其他合并症及老年综合征。随着 HIV 感染者的老龄化进展，认知及处理老年综合征和衰弱问题，在这类患者的护理中将变得越来越重要。

最后，维持老年患者的健康和生活质量面临着诸多挑战，包括合并症、身体退化、失去伴侣以及家庭和社会孤立，而 HIV 感染者更加容易受到这些因素影响。此外，许多感染者还面临贫困、住房和（或）食物无保障以及人身安全等挑战。一位年迈的 HIV 感染者曾形容失去朋友和社区的生活为"一种萎缩的生活"。照顾感染者的医护人员必须意识到这些问题。

心理健康

由于艾滋病已转变为一种可控制的慢性疾病，心理治疗的重点也从急性综合征的管理转向了帮助患者健康生活。抑郁和焦虑以及其他精神疾病在 HIV 感染者中很常见，而患者常不愿意承认自己需要心理健康护理。对于许多 HIV 感染者来说，他们的医生可能是他们唯一接触的医护人员，因此，医护人员进行抑郁、焦虑等心理健康问题的常规筛查具有重要的意义。心理问题筛查还将会帮助医生对患者进行更多的心理健康评估，并将需要的患者转至适宜的行为治疗及精神治疗。对于心理创伤的患者，创伤后应激障碍的治疗也非常有帮助。

药物滥用

吸毒及饮酒 / 酗酒在 HIV 感染者中也十分常见，且饮酒或酗酒也可能与使用药物或毒品（如可卡因、甲基苯丙胺等）同时发生。酗酒和使用药物，常与追求冒险的行为（如与多个性伴侣发生无保护性行为）有关，也与抗逆转录病毒治疗的依从性下降有关。不过，同时仍有许多应用吸毒者对抗病毒治疗依从性较好，故吸毒或酗酒不应影响医生开具 ART 治疗药物。导致或加剧药物和酒精使用的因素有很多，例如，甲基苯丙胺的使用者往往喜欢在性行为中也使用药物。其他常见因素包括合并精神疾患（如创伤后应激障碍、焦虑、多动症）、少数群体压力和环境不稳定。许多研究表明，使用药物辅助疗法（如丁丙诺啡）治疗阿片类药物成瘾，可与 ART 治疗同时进行；酒精滥用者的治疗也可以与 ART 治疗同时进行。虽然缺乏针对兴奋剂使用障碍的药物治疗，但患者与医生之间的良好关系，仍可在循证行为治疗方面发挥重要作用。以患者为中心的 HIV 护理不能仅仅关注 HIV 病毒的抑制，还必须积极主动地解决心理健康和副作用问题，以促进患者拥有更好的生活质量。建议对药物滥用者治疗时进行常规筛查，并最好能够一站式将药物滥用治疗与 HIV 护理同时进行。

性传播感染

美国的性传播感染（STI）发病率持续上升，在 2018 年（本报告发布时的最新报告数据）达到历史新高，且在未来的几年里没有放缓的趋势。性传播感染会增加伴侣间传播 HIV 的风险，尤其是梅毒和单纯疱疹。在 HIV 感染者中，性传播感染的发病率也有所上升。随着"检测不到＝不会传播"这一概念在患者中得到普及，教育患者如何保护自己免于性传播感染变得很重要，因为患者需要在知情的情况下做出关于安全套使用的决定。对性活跃的患者来说，每年进行一次性传播感染筛查或根据风险行为更频繁地进行筛查是非常重要的措施。性传播感染的治疗对于 HIV 阴性和阳性患者没有差异，而且治疗效果良好。

HIV 管理和治疗

初次咨询和门诊评估

一旦确诊为 HIV，医护人员应向患者介绍 HIV 感染的临床病程和治疗方案，以及如何使用免疫学和病毒学指标（如 $CD4^+$ T 细胞计数、血浆病毒载量检测）来指导治疗。与 HIV 相关的污名化仍然是一个重要的问题，也是参与医疗的主要障碍，解决这一问题是新确诊者能够长期随访及治疗的关键。应向患者讲解，无保护性行为或共用针头都是 HIV 传播的方式。应与患者讨论"U＝U"（检测不到＝不会传播）的益处，让他们明白控制并达到不可检测的病毒载量对他们自己及其伴侣的健康都很重要。

初步评估应包括以 HIV 为导向的系统检查和全面的体格检查。特别是，必须检查皮肤是否出现与 HIV 相关的皮疹和卡波西肉瘤。口腔检查可能会发现鹅口疮、牙龈炎、多毛白斑、HSV 引起的浅表溃疡、阿弗他溃疡或卡波西肉瘤的特征性病变。晚期患者的眼底可能出现 CMV 视网膜炎特有的出血性病变。应仔细注意淋巴结肿大、肝大、脾大和任何生殖器病变。神经系统检查应密切注意周围神经病变和周身感觉减退。

实验室监测

首次就诊时应测量 $CD4^+$ T 细胞计数及血浆病毒载量检测，并告知患者。病毒载量和 $CD4^+$ T 细胞计数之间相互作用的图解有助于加深患者的理解。还应进行 HIV 基因分型以耐药性的评估。病毒载量是衡量治疗依从性的关键指标，应定期重复检测，一般在开始治疗后 2～8 周进行一次，在患者稳定接受治疗后每 3～6 个月进行一次。一旦患者稳定治疗，病毒得到抑制（＜200 拷贝 / 毫升），$CD4^+$ T 细胞计数高于 $200/mm^3$，指南允许将监测间隔延长至每年一次。如果患者的 $CD4^+$ T 细胞计数大于 500 且持续时间超过 1 年，那么只要病毒载量保持在检测不到的水平，CD4 监测可不必须进行。

应进行血常规、生化指标（包括肌酐）、肝功能检测、随机或空腹血糖以及尿液分析，以确定患者基线化验水平。女性应进行妊娠检查。一旦患者开始接受抗逆转录病毒治疗，就应在开始治疗后 2～8 周重复进行生化、肝功能、病毒载量检测。稳定接受抗逆转录病毒治疗的患者应每 6 个月重复同样的实验室检查，

TABLE 16.6 Recommended Vaccinations in Adults With HIV

Vaccine	Recommendation
Influenza vaccination (inactivated or recombinant)	Recommended annually
Influenza vaccination (live attenuated)	Not recommended
Tdap (tetanus, diphtheria, pertussis) or Td	Recommended primary series then every 10 years
MMR (measles, mumps, rubella)	Not recommended if CD4 <200; recommended if nonimmune and CD4 >200
Varicella primary vaccination (Varivax)	Not recommended if CD4 <200; recommended if nonimmune and CD4 >200
Recombinant zoster vaccination (RZV; Shingrix)	No recommendation at this time[a]
Live attenuated varicella vaccination (ZVL; Zostavax)	Not recommended if CD4 <200; no recommendation at this time[a] if CD4 >200
Human papillomavirus (HPV) vaccination	Three-dose series recommended through age 26
PCV-13 (pneumococcal conjugate)	One lifetime dose recommended, at least 8 weeks prior to, or 1 year following PPS-23
PPS-23 (pneumococcal polysaccharide)	Recommended once, with a repeat dose at least 5 years later, and 1 dose after age 65
Hepatitis A	Recommended two-dose series, or three-dose HAV/HBV combined vaccine for all patients
Hepatitis B	Recommended two- or three-dose series for all patients
Meningitis ACYW135	Recommended two-dose series at least 8 weeks apart; repeat every 5 years
Meningitis B	Recommended only if additional risk factors exist (e.g., asplenia, complement deficiency)
Hib	Recommended only if additional risk factors exist (e.g., asplenia, hematopoietic stem cell transplant)

[a]Current ACIP guidelines do not recommend for or against RZV due to limited data. DHHS guidelines state that "given that risk of herpes zoster is high among persons with HIV, and the vaccine appears safe, experts recommend administration of RZV to persons with HIV aged ≥50 years following the FDA-approved schedule for persons without HIV (IM dose at 0 and 2 months)."

blood count is recommended in all patients. A urinalysis every 6 months is also recommended in patients on tenofovir-based regimens.

Screening for Associated Infections
Tuberculosis
Tuberculin skin test (TST) or blood interferon-γ release assays (IGRA) testing should be performed early in the course of HIV management. Induration of 5 mm or more on the TST should be considered positive. IGRA testing will provide an interpretation based on patient results. Any patient with a positive tuberculous test result should be evaluated for the presence of active tuberculosis with a thorough physical exam, chest radiograph, and symptom screen. If no active disease is present, the patient should receive 9 months of prophylaxis with isoniazid or combination drug therapy for a shorter period (see Chapter 7). If active tuberculosis is identified, multidrug therapy should be initiated after careful consideration of possible interactions with ART. It is important to remember that false-negative TB testing, both TSTs and IGRAs, can occur in patients with HIV, especially those with CD4 count less than 200.

STIs
Serologic testing for syphilis should be followed by prompt treatment if the patient is confirmed to be positive. Syphilis infections are common within many populations highly impacted by HIV, and coinfection with syphilis increases the risk of transmission of HIV to others. Gonorrhea and chlamydia testing of any potentially exposed orifice is recommended, and "triple-point testing" (oral, rectal, and urine PCR testing) should be offered whenever appropriate. All women should be tested for vaginal trichomonas as well. Following initial screening, annual STI screening is recommended. (See Chapter 15.)

Viral Hepatitis
Liver disease is an important cause of morbidity and mortality for PLWH. Screening for hepatitis B and C at baseline is recommended and vaccination offered if appropriate. Hepatitis C is highly prevalent among persons who acquired HIV from injection drug use, and MSM populations are also at higher risk due to sexual transmission. Given the lack of an effective vaccine for hepatitis C, regular screening is recommended for persons with ongoing risk of exposure.

Other Infections
Screening for antibodies to *Toxoplasma gondii* should be considered for persons with low CD4 counts who are potentially in need of prophylaxis. Persons from endemic areas may be screened for histoplasmosis and coccidiomycosis and considered for prophylaxis if positive.

Immunization
Antibody responses to polysaccharides are better among patients with higher CD4 counts, though the optimal timing of immunization is uncertain. For persons with low CD4 counts, many physicians provide initial immunization and reimmunization for certain vaccines after immune reconstitution occurs. Live vaccines should be avoided in persons with CD4 counts lower than 200 cells/mm^3. The US Centers for Disease Control and Prevention (CDC) recommends ensuring routine childhood vaccination (e.g., tetanus series, measles, mumps, rubella, varicella vaccination or reported history of disease). The following vaccines are additionally recommended in PLWH (Table 16.6).

Streptococcus pneumoniae Vaccination
All persons with HIV should receive a single lifetime dose of PCV13 (Prevnar13), followed by a dose of PPV23 (Pneumovax) at least 8 weeks later. If previously vaccinated with PPV23, the patients should receive PCV13 at least 1 year after PPV23. Patients should have a CD4 cell count greater than or equal to 200/microliter. A second PPV23 dose is recommended 5 years after the first PPV23, and again after the age of 65.

Influenza Virus Vaccination
PLWH have excess morbidity and mortality associated with influenza and its complications. They should receive seasonal influenza vaccination yearly.

Human Papillomavirus Vaccination
The CDC recommends use of the human papillomavirus (HPV) vaccine in boys or girls at age 11 or 12 regardless of HIV status, in MSM, and in persons with immune compromise, including those with HIV, up to the age of 26 if not previously vaccinated. Vaccination is now FDA-approved through age 45.

表 16.6 成人 HIV 感染者的疫苗接种建议

疫苗	建议
流感疫苗（灭活疫苗或重组疫苗）	每年接种
流感疫苗（减毒活疫苗）	不推荐
Tdap（破伤风、白喉、百日咳）或 Td	建议每 10 年进行一次接种
麻疹、腮腺炎、风疹三联疫苗（MMR）	如果 $CD4^+$ T 细胞计数小于 200，则不推荐使用；如果无免疫力且 $CD4^+$ T 细胞计数大于 200，则推荐使用
水痘初级疫苗接种（Varivax）	如果 $CD4^+$ T 细胞计数小于 200，则不推荐使用；如果无免疫力且 $CD4^+$ T 细胞计数大于 200，则推荐使用
重组带状疱疹疫苗（RZV；Shingrix）	目前无相关推荐 [a]
水痘减毒活疫苗（ZVL；Zostavax）	如果 $CD4^+$ T 细胞计数小于 200，则不建议使用；如果 $CD4^+$ T 细胞计数大于 200，目前无相关推荐 [a]
人类乳头瘤病毒（HPV）疫苗	建议在 26 岁之前进行三剂系列注射
PCV-13（肺炎球菌结合疫苗）	建议终身至少接种一次，时间在接种 PPS-23 之前至少 8 周或之后 1 年
PPS-23（肺炎球菌多糖疫苗）	接种一次后，至少 5 年后重复接种，65 岁时再接种 1 次
甲型肝炎疫苗	建议所有患者接种两剂疫苗接种，或三剂 HAV/HBV 联合疫苗
乙型肝炎疫苗	建议对所有患者进行两剂或三剂疫苗接种
脑膜炎 ACYW135	建议接种两剂疫苗，至少间隔 8 周；每 5 年重复一次
乙型脑炎疫苗	仅在存在其他危险因素（如无脾、补体缺乏症）时才建议使用
B 型流感嗜血杆菌疫苗	仅在存在其他危险因素（如无脾、造血干细胞移植）时才建议使用

[a] 由于数据有限，目前的 ACIP 指南并未建议是否接种 RZV；DHHS 指南指出，"鉴于 HIV 感染者中带状疱疹的风险很高，而且疫苗相对安全，专家建议按照 FDA 批准的非 HIV 感染者接种计划（0 个月和 2 个月时接种肌内注射剂量），为年龄 ≥ 50 岁的 HIV 感染者接种 RZV"。

以监测药物毒性和其他变化。建议每年进行一次包含血常规的全面复查；还建议使用替诺福韦治疗方案的患者每 6 个月进行一次尿检。

相关感染筛查

肺结核

在 HIV 管理过程中，应尽早进行结核菌素皮肤试验（TST）或血液 γ 干扰素释放试验（IGRA）。TST 显示 5 mm 或更大的压痕应视为阳性；IGRA 检测根据结果有助于进一步诊断。对于结核菌素检测结果呈阳性的患者，应通过全面体检、胸部 X 线片和症状筛查来评估是否存在活动性结核。若无，患者应接受 9 个月的异烟肼预防治疗或更短时间的联合药物治疗（见第 7 章）；若有，应在仔细考虑与抗逆转录病毒药物可能产生的相互作用后，再开始多种药物联合治疗。重要的是，HIV 感染者，尤其是 $CD4^+$ T 细胞计数低于 200 的患者，可能会出现 TST 和 IGRA 等结核病检测假阴性的情况。

性传播感染

如果梅毒血清学检测结果呈阳性，患者应立即接受治疗。梅毒在许多艾滋病高发人群中同样易患，同时感染梅毒会增加向他人传播艾滋病的风险。建议对任何可能出现口腔黏膜暴露（接触病原）的人群，进行淋病奈瑟球菌和衣原体检测，并在适当的时候提供"三点检测"（口腔、直肠和尿液 PCR 检测）。所有女性还应接受阴道滴虫检测。初次筛查后，建议每年进行一次性传播感染筛查（见第 15 章）。

病毒性肝炎

肝病是 HIV 感染者发病和死亡的重要原因。建议在基线时筛查乙型肝炎和丙型肝炎，并酌情提供疫苗接种。丙型肝炎在因注射毒品而感染 HIV 的人群中具有较高发病率，男男性行为者因性传播而感染丙型肝炎的风险也较高。鉴于缺乏有效的丙型肝炎疫苗，建议对有持续暴露风险的人群进行定期筛查。

其他感染

低 $CD4^+$ T 细胞计数且可能需要预防性治疗的患者，应考虑弓形虫抗体筛查。来自地方病流行地区的人，可进行组织胞浆菌病和球孢子菌病筛查，如果结果呈阳性，则应考虑进行预防。

免疫接种

$CD4^+$ T 细胞计数较高的患者，对病毒多糖的抗体反应应答更明显，但最佳免疫时机尚不确定。对于 $CD4^+$ T 细胞计数较低的患者，许多医生会建议初次疫苗接种，并在免疫重建后对某些疫苗进行再次免疫接种。$CD4^+$ T 细胞计数低于 $200/mm^3$ 的人群应避免接种活疫苗。美国 CDC 建议确保常规儿童疫苗接种（如破伤风、麻疹、腮腺炎、风疹、水痘疫苗接种或有既往史的其他疾病）。此外，还建议 HIV 感染者接种以下疫苗（表 16.6）。

肺炎链球菌疫苗接种

所有 HIV 感染者一生中应接种一剂 PCV13（肺炎球菌结合疫苗），至少 8 周后再接种一剂 PPV23（肺炎球菌多糖疫苗）。如果之前接种过 PPV23，患者应在 PPV23 接种至少 1 年后再接种 PCV13。患者的 $CD4^+$ T 细胞计数应大于或等于 $200/\mu l$。建议在接种第一针 PPV23 疫苗 5 年后再接种第二针 PPV23，并在 65 岁后再次接种。

流感病毒疫苗接种

HIV 感染者中，流感及其并发症相关的发病率和死亡率都很高，应每年接种季节性流感疫苗。

人类乳头瘤病毒疫苗

美国 CDC 建议，不论是否感染 HIV，11 或 12 岁

Hepatitis A and B Viruses Vaccination

PLWH should be assessed by serology for prior exposure to hepatitis B. All PLWH who are not immune to hepatitis B should receive immunization. All PLWH should receive immunization against hepatitis A. Antibody testing prior to vaccination is reasonable in patients likely to have had childhood exposure (e.g., immigrants from endemic countries).

Neisseria meningitidis Vaccination

Due to a higher incidence of meningococcal meningitis in PLWH, the CDC recommends all PLWH receive the quadrivalent conjugate meningitis A, C, Y, W-135 vaccine (MCV4). This vaccine can be administered as two doses spaced 8 weeks apart, with boosters given every 5 years.

Other Health Screening
Cervical Cancer

Women living with HIV should be screened for cervical cancer with a Pap smear. Due to the increased risk for cervical cancer in PLWH, screening guidelines are more aggressive for women living with HIV. Women with normal cytology with no high-risk HPV on Pap smear are recommended to have repeat screening in 3 years (whereas HIV-negative women undergo repeat screening at 5 years).

Anal Cancer

As discussed previously, HPV is associated with an increased risk of anal cancer in both men and women living with HIV. At this time, no national recommendations exist for routine screening for anal cancer, though the IDSA HIV Primary Care Guidelines do recommend anal Pap smear testing in MSM, women with a history of receptive anal intercourse or abnormal cervical Pap smears, and all patients with genital warts. The quality of supporting evidence is low and no specific timing interval for repeat testing is suggested. Despite clear national guidelines, anal Pap smear testing is commonly performed in clinical practice due to an acknowledgement of the increased risk of anal cancer in PLWH.

ANTIRETROVIRAL TREATMENT

The goal of ART is to ensure that all PLWH can lead symptom-free, productive lives. Currently available therapy makes achieving this goal possible in almost all individuals. Treatment guidelines in the United States and worldwide recommend that all patients be offered ART regardless of CD4 count, as early treatment has been demonstrated to have significant health benefit to the individual regardless of CD4 count; further, treatment is prevention because patients who are undetectable are do not transmit to others ("U=U"). This confers a significant public health benefit in addition to the benefit to the health of the individual.

Current Antiretrovirals

Currently available antiretrovirals fall into five classes:
1. **The nucleotide/nucleoside reverse transcriptase inhibitors (NRTIs):** These are nucleotide or nucleoside analogs that lack a 3′-hydroxyl group on the deoxyribose moiety, causing chain termination of viral DNA and inhibition of viral reverse transcriptase. Examples include tenofovir alafenamide, tenofovir disoproxil fumarate, lamivudine, emtricitabine, abacavir, and zidovudine.
2. **Non-nucleotide reverse transcription inhibitors (NNRTIs):** NNRTIs are also inhibitors of the reverse transcriptase enzyme, but they are not nucleotide analogs and do not bind at the nucleotide binding site of the enzyme. These agents have "-vir-" in their names. Agents available in this class include efavirenz, nevirapine, etravirine, rilpivirine, and doravirine.
3. **PIs:** PIs are inhibitors of the virally encoded protease, an enzyme necessary for proteolytic cleavage of protein precursors necessary for the production of an infectious viral particle. These agents end with the suffix "-navir." Examples include darunavir, atazanavir, and lopinavir.
4. **Entry Inhibitors:** "Entry inhibitors" is an "umbrella" grouping of agents that block viral entry into $CD4^+$ cells through a variety of mechanisms. This grouping includes attachment inhibitors (fostemsavir), fusion inhibitors (enfuvirtide), entry inhibitors (ibalizumab, a monoclonal antibody that binds to CD4), and CCR5 antagonists (maraviroc); none of these agents is first-line, and all are only used in salvage regimens.
5. **Integrase Inhibitors *or* Integrase Strand Transfer Inhibitors (InSTIs):** InSTIs are drugs that inhibit the viral integrase, which is responsible for integrating reverse-transcribed viral DNA into the host genome of infected cells. These agents end with the suffix "-tegravir." Agents in this class are raltegravir, elvitegravir, dolutegravir, and bictegravir.

Some agents, including all protease inhibitors and the integrase inhibitor elvitegravir, are paired with "boosters," agents that serve as cytochrome P450 3A4 enzymatic inhibitors. This inhibition slows the metabolism of the antiviral drug to decrease the needed dose and lower toxicity and slow metabolism to allow once-daily dosing. The two boosters utilized today are ritonavir and cobicistat. Both can be given independently or co-formulated into combination tablets. Boosting agents must be used with caution as they also affect the metabolism of a number of other drugs as well.

Treatment Guidelines

Since 1996, treatment of HIV has utilized the concept of "combination antiretroviral therapy," which involves treating patients with multiple agents targeting multiple steps in the viral replication cycle. This multitargeted approach overcomes the virus' ability to mutate and evolve resistance to single agents. A complete regimen is generally composed of three active agents (three drugs to which the virus is not believed to harbor resistance), though there are clinical situations in which fewer (two) or more agents are used. Co-formulations are common, as they are simpler for patients and improve adherence. The US Department of Health and Human Services (DHHS) and the International AIDS Society-USA (IAS-USA) both issue HIV treatment guidelines that are considered standard-of-care for HIV providers in the United States. They are available online at https://aidsinfo.nih.gov/guidelines and https://www.iasusa.org/resources/guidelines/, respectively. Both are updated frequently. The World Health Organization (WHO) also publishes treatment recommendations for resource-limited settings, which delineate first- and second-line regimen recommendations. The last decade has seen a major shift in recommended treatment guidelines such that a combination of NRTIs plus an InSTI are now recommended as the components of all first-line therapies for patients initiating HIV treatment.

Tables 16.7A and 16.7B review the current first-line recommended regimens of the DHHS and IAS-USA. Decisions on which regimen to recommend to patients should be made in cooperation with the patient and should take into consideration any known resistance, drug/drug interactions, coexisting conditions (e.g., hepatitis B, cardiovascular disease, renal disease), patient preference about time of day and taking the medication with or without food, and insurance coverage.

Resistance Testing

Approximately 16% of treatment-naïve patients have detectable baseline mutations that confer resistance in the genome of their HIV.

的男孩或女孩都应接种 HPV 疫苗；男男性行为、免疫力低下（包括 HIV 感染者）的未接种过疫苗者，26 岁以内均可接种。目前，美国 FDA 批准的疫苗接种年龄为 45 岁以内。

甲型肝炎和乙型肝炎病毒疫苗接种

所有对乙型肝炎没有免疫力的 HIV 感染者都应接受免疫接种，且所有感染者都应接种甲型肝炎疫苗。对于可能在童年时期有甲型肝炎接触史的患者（如来自流行国家的移民），接种疫苗前应进行抗体检测。

脑膜炎奈瑟球菌疫苗接种

由于 HIV 感染者的脑膜炎的发病率较高，美国疾病预防控制中心建议所有患者接种四价 A、C、Y、W-135 型结合型脑膜炎疫苗（MCV4）。这种疫苗可分两次接种，每次间隔 8 周，每 5 年加强一次。

其他健康检查

宫颈癌

女性 HIV 感染者应通过巴氏涂片进行宫颈癌筛查。由于 HIV 感染者罹患宫颈癌的风险更高，因此筛查指南对感染 HIV 的女性更加严格。建议细胞学检查正常且巴氏涂片检查未发现高危 HPV 的女性，在 3 年后进行重复筛查（而 HIV 阴性的女性则在 5 年后进行重复筛查）。

肛门癌

如前所述，HPV 与感染 HIV 的男性和女性罹患肛门癌的风险增加有关。尽管 IDSA HIV 初级医疗指南建议对男男性行为者、有肛交史或宫颈巴氏涂片异常的女性以及所有尖锐湿疣患者进行肛门巴氏涂片检测，但目前还没有国家指南推荐肛门癌进行常规筛查。目前的支持性证据的质量较低，也没有提出重复检测的具体时间间隔。但由于 HIV 感染者中，感染肛门尖锐湿疣的风险增加，临床实践中通常会进行肛门巴氏涂片检测。

抗逆转录病毒治疗

抗逆转录病毒治疗的目标是确保所有 HIV 感染者都能过上无症状、高质量的生活。目前可用的治疗，已使患者的生活质量得到极大提升。美国和全世界的治疗指南都建议，无论 $CD4^+$ T 细胞计数多少，都应为所有患者提供抗逆转录病毒治疗，因为事实证明，无论 $CD4^+$ T 细胞计数水平如何，早期启动治疗都能为患者带来显著获益；此外，治疗还能起到预防作用，因为无法治疗的患者不会传染给其他人（"U = U"）。这除了对个人健康有益外，还对公共卫生大有益处。

当前的抗逆转录病毒药物

目前可用的抗逆转录病毒药物分为五类：

1. 核苷类反转录酶抑制剂（NRTI）：它们是核苷酸或核苷类似物，在脱氧核糖分子上缺少一个 3′-羟基，从而导致病毒 DNA 连锁变性并抑制病毒逆转录酶。例如，丙酚替诺福韦、富马酸替诺福韦二吡呋酯、拉米夫定、恩曲他滨、阿巴卡韦和齐多夫定。

2. 非核苷类反转录酶抑制剂（NNRTI）：NNRTI 也是逆转录酶的抑制剂，但它们不是核苷酸类似物，不与酶的核苷酸结合位点结合。该类药物包括依非韦伦、奈韦拉平、依曲韦林、利匹韦林和多拉韦林。

3. 蛋白酶抑制剂（PI）：蛋白酶抑制剂是病毒编码蛋白酶的抑制剂，蛋白酶是产生传染性病毒粒子所必需的蛋白水解蛋白质前体酶。这些药物以后缀"-navir"结尾。例如达茹那韦（darunavir）、阿扎那韦（atazanavir）和洛匹那韦（lopinavir）。

4. 进入抑制剂：这是一个"伞形"分组，包括通过各种机制阻止病毒进入 $CD4^+$ 细胞的药物。这一组药物包括附着抑制剂、融合抑制剂（恩夫韦肽）、后附着抑制剂（伊巴珠单抗，一种与 $CD4^+$ T 细胞结合的单克隆抗体）和 CCR5 拮抗剂（马拉韦罗）。这些药物不属于一线治疗药物，多用于治疗失败患者。

5. 整合酶抑制剂或整合酶链转移抑制剂（InSTI）：InSTIs 是抑制病毒整合酶的药物，整合酶负责将逆转录的病毒 DNA 整合到感染细胞的宿主基因组中。这些药物以后缀"-tegravir"结尾。这类药物包括拉替拉韦（raltegravir）、艾维雷韦（elvitegravir）、多替拉韦（dolutegravir）和比克替拉韦（bictegravir）。

一些药物，包括所有蛋白酶抑制剂和整合酶抑制剂艾维雷韦，需要与"增强剂"（作为细胞色素 P450 3A4 酶抑制剂的药物）配伍以达到疗效。这种结合作用会减缓抗病毒药物的代谢，从而减少所需剂量，降低毒性，实现每日一次用药。目前使用的两种增强剂是利托那韦和考比司他。这两种药物可单独使用，也可与 PI 或 EVG 共同配制成复方片剂。必须谨慎使用增强剂，因为它们也会影响其他一些药物的代谢。

治疗指南

自 1996 年以来，艾滋病的治疗一直采用"联合抗逆转录病毒治疗"的概念，即用针对病毒复制周期中多个步骤的多种药物来联合治疗患者。这种多靶点治疗方法克服了病毒变异和对单一药物产生抗药性的问题。一个完整的治疗方案通常由三种活性药物组成，但临床上也有使用较少（两种）或更多药物的情况。复合制剂的应用对患者来说更加便利，并能提高依从性。美国卫生与人类服务部（DHHS）和美国国际艾滋病协会（IAS-USA）都发布了艾滋病治疗指南，这些指南被认为是美国艾滋病服务提供者的标准护理指南。可分别从 https://aidsinfo.nih.gov/guidelines 和 https://www.iasusa.org/resources/guidelines/ 在线获取，两者都在不断更新。WHO 也发布了针对资源有限环境的治疗建议，制定了一线和二线治疗方案建议。过去的十年，推荐的指南发生了重大变化，现建议将 NRTI 和 InSTI 的组合作为 HIV 初治患者一线治疗的组成。

表 16.7A 和 16.7B 回顾了目前 DHHS 和 IAS-USA 推荐的一线治疗方案。在决定向患者推荐哪种治疗方案时，应与患者充分沟通，并考虑任何已知的耐药性、

TABLE 16.7A Recommended Initial Regimens for Most People With HIV (DHHS)

Drug Combination	Restrictions	Strength
Bictegravir/tenofovir alafenamide/emtricitabine (Biktarvy)		AI
Dolutegravir/abacavir/lamivudine (Triumeq)	Only for patients who are HLA-B*5701 negative and without chronic hepatitis B coinfection	AI
Dolutegravir (Tivicay) plus emtricitabine or lamivudine plus tenofovir alafenamide or tenofovir disoproxil fumarate		AI
Dolutegravir/lamivudine (Dovato)	Except for individuals with HIV RNA >500,000 copies/mL, HBV coinfection, or in whom ART is to be started before the results of HIV genotypic resistance testing for reverse transcriptase or HBV testing are available	AI
Raltegravir (Isentress) plus emtricitabine or lamivudine plus tenofovir alafenamide or tenofovir disoproxil fumarate		BI for TDF / BII for TAF

TABLE 16.7B Generally Recommended Initial Regimens (IAS-USA)

Drug Combination	Details	Strength
Bictegravir/tenofovir alafenamide/emtricitabine (Biktarvy)		AIa
Dolutegravir/abacavir/lamivudine (Triumeq)	Testing for HLA-B*5701 allele should be performed before abacavir use (evidence rating AIa); patients who test positive should not be given abacavir (evidence rating AIa). Because it typically takes several days or longer to obtain results for HLA-B*5701 testing, tenofovir-containing regimens should be used when starting ART on the same day as HIV diagnosis or until HLA-B*5701 testing results are available. In patients with or at high risk for cardiovascular disease, a tenofovir-containing regimen, rather than an abacavir-containing regimen, should be used if possible.	AIa
Dolutegravir (Tivicay) plus emtricitabine/tenofovir alafenamide (Descovy)	In settings in which TAF/emtricitabine is not available or if there is a substantial cost difference, TDF (with emtricitabine or lamivudine) is effective and generally well tolerated, particularly if the patient does not have, or is not at high risk for, kidney or bone disease	AIa

Because of this, baseline resistance testing is recommended prior to initiation of ART. Treatment does not necessarily need to be delayed until results are available, as resistance testing can take several weeks to result. If treatment is initiated empirically, adjustments should be made promptly if resistance is discovered. Repeat resistance testing should be considered in the setting of treatment failure to help determine whether the patient's virus has developed resistance to the current regimen, or whether medication adherence, drug/drug interactions, absorption, or another issue is the reason for virologic failure.

Resistance testing can be performed in three major ways. The most common method is HIV-1 RNA genotyping. This involves direct sequencing of viral genes that encode the drug target proteins (i.e., reverse transcriptase, protease, and integrase). Genes are sequenced and compared to the wild-type genotype and previously determined resistance mutations. A second method for identifying resistance is by performing HIV-1 phenotype testing. This involves replication of the virus in culture when exposed to various antivirals. This provides a direct measure of viral resistance in vitro; growth would be expected to occur in the presence of a drug if the virus harbors resistance mutations to that agent. Finally, cellular-associated DNA genotyping allows for resistance testing even in the setting of patients with undetectable PVLs. This testing involves sequencing of archived HIV-1 proviral DNA that has been integrated into infected host cells during virus replication. The choice of a resistance test depends on the patient's viral load and the desired information.

In patients determined to have resistance, several resources are available to help choose a new regimen. The IAS-USA has developed a useful catalog of resistance mutations that is available online at https://www.iasusa.org/resources/hiv-drug-resistance-mutations/. Stanford University also maintains an interactive web-based database of known HIV resistance mutations, which is also freely available online at https://hivdb.stanford.edu. Its interactive format allows the user to input specific mutations and it will generate a predicted susceptibility profile of all available drugs. Use of these resources and expert consultation with an HIV specialist experienced in treatment of resistant virus is recommended.

Future Directions of Antiretroviral Treatment

Current antiretroviral therapy has made leaps and bounds from the early regimens, which involved multiple drugs with high toxicity given multiple times per day. Today, most patients can be treated with a small number of pills—usually one—dosed once or twice a day. Still, treatment is advancing. Several new regimens are challenging the "triple-therapy" paradigm, including two-drug combinations that demonstrate noninferiority when compared to traditional three-drug first-line regimens. More are sure to come. A few other treatment options that are likely close on the horizon include the following:

1. **Injectable regimens:** Clinical trials of injectable therapy have been completed, showing high efficacy and patient acceptance of once-monthly injectable treatments. Some issues of concern with these regimens include the need for more frequent appointments, how to provide oral "bridge" therapy to patients missing an appointment, how to deal with adverse reactions of medications with long half-lives, and concern over the subtherapeutic tail that follows discontinuation of an injectable depot-type regimen. Even so, these regimens present an exciting new direction for therapy.

表 16.7A 对于大多数 HIV 感染者的初治方案推荐（DHHS）

药物方案	限制	推荐等级
BIC/TAF/FTC		AⅠ
DTG/ABC/3TC	仅适用于 HLA-B*5701 阴性且无合并慢性 HBV 感染的患者	AⅠ
DTG + FTC/3TC + TAF/TDF		AⅠ
DTG/3TC	不建议用于 HIV-RNA > 500 000 拷贝/毫升及合并 HBV 感染患者；在 HIV 基因型耐药检测或 HBV 检测结果回报前不建议应用	AⅠ
RAL + FTC/3TC + TAF/TDF		BⅠ（含 TDF 方案） BⅡ（含 TAF 方案）

表 16.7B 常规初治方案推荐（IAS-USA）

药物方案	备注	推荐等级
BIC/TAF/FTC		AⅠa
DTG/ABC/3TC	在使用阿巴卡韦之前，应进行 HLA-B*5701 等位基因检测（AⅠa）；检测呈阳性的患者不应使用阿巴卡韦（AⅠb）；由于获得 HLA-B*5701 检测结果通常需要几天或更长的时间，因此在确诊 HIV 的同一天或获得 HLA-B*5701 检测结果之前开始 ART 时，应使用含 TDF 的方案；对于心血管疾病患者或高危患者，应尽可能使用不含阿巴卡韦的方案	AⅠa
DTG + TAF/FTC	在无法获得 TAF/FTC，或在费用相差较大的情况下，TDF（与 FTC 或 3TC 合用）疗效及耐受性良好，尤其是在患者没有肾病或骨病，或没有高风险的情况下，可以替换 TAF 应用	AⅠa

译者注：两者均为 2018 年及之前指南推荐情况。BIC，比克替拉韦；TAF，丙酚替诺福韦；FTC，恩曲他滨；DTG，多替拉韦；ABC，阿巴卡韦；3TC，拉米夫定；TDF，替诺福韦；RAL，拉替拉韦。

药物/药物相互作用、并存疾病（如乙型肝炎、心血管疾病、肾病）、患者对每天服药时间和进食偏好以及医疗保险情况。

耐药检测

约有 16% 的初治 HIV 感染者可检测到基线耐药突变，因此建议在开始抗逆转录病毒治疗之前进行基线耐药检测。由于耐药检测需要数周时间才能得出结果，因此治疗并不一定需要迟到结果回报之后。如果根据经验开始治疗，一旦发现耐药，应立即进行调整。在治疗失败的情况下，应考虑复查耐药检测，以确定患者的病毒是否对当前的治疗方案产生了耐药性，或者是否因为服药依从性、药物相互作用、吸收不良或其他问题导致了病毒学失败。

耐药检测主要通过三种方法进行。最常见的方法是 HIV-1 RNA 测序。该方法是对编码药物靶蛋白（即逆转录酶、蛋白酶和整合酶）的病毒核酸进行直接测序，并与野生型病毒的基因型以及和先前确定的耐药突变进行比较。第二种方法是进行 HIV-1 表型检测。该方法通过观察病毒在培养基中接触各种抗病毒药物后的复制情况进行，是一种体外检测方法；如果病毒对某种药物产生耐药突变，则病毒在药物暴露的情况下仍会生长。最后，通过细胞内 DNA 基因测序技术，甚至可以对检测不到病毒载量的患者进行耐药检测。这种检测涉及对存档的 HIV-1 前病毒 DNA 进行测序，前病毒 DNA 已在病毒复制过程中整合到受感染的宿主细胞中。耐药检测方式的选择取决于患者的病毒感染情况和需要了解的信息。

对于确定存在耐药突变的患者，一些资源有助于选择新的治疗方案。IAS-USA 编写了一份耐药突变目录，在线查阅网址为：https://www.iasusa.org/resources/hiv-drug-resistance-mutations/。斯坦福大学还运营着一个已知 HIV 耐药突变的网络数据库，该数据库也可在 https://hivdb.stanford.edu 免费在线获取。该数据库采用互动形式，用户可以输入特定的基因突变，它将生成所有可用药物的敏感性预测图谱。建议使用这些可及的资源，并向在耐药方面经验丰富的 HIV 专家咨询。

抗逆转录病毒治疗的未来方向

目前的抗逆转录病毒治疗与早期的治疗方案相比取得了飞跃性的进步，早期的治疗方案常须每天多次服用多种高毒性药物。如今，大多数患者只需服用少量药片，通常是每天服用 1~2 次，且治疗仍在不断进步。一些新的治疗方案挑战了经典"三联疗法"的模式，包括与传统的三联一线治疗方案相比并不逊色的两联疗法。未来肯定还会有更多新药问世。其他即将问世的治疗方案包括以下几类：

1. 注射方案：注射方案的临床试验已经完成，结果显示，每月一次的注射方案疗效显著，且患者接受度很高。但这些疗法也有令人担忧的问题，包括：需要更频繁就诊，如何为错过预约的患者提供口服"桥接"疗法，如何处理半衰期长的药物的不良反应，以及对中断注射治疗后拖尾效应的担忧。尽管如此，这些治疗方案还是提供了一个令人兴奋的新方向。

2. **Implantable slow-release medications:** Similar to implantable contraceptive devices, implantable antiretroviral-delivery devices offer an attractive approach to infrequent (once-monthly or even longer) dosing. The minor surgery needed for placement of the device is a concern, as is any complication of removal.
3. **Oral agents with longer half-lives:** Several oral agents are in development that might be able to be dosed once weekly or longer. As with injectable regimens, concerns remain about how to deal with adverse reactions of medications with long half-lives and the subtherapeutic tail that follows discontinuation.
4. **New drug classes:** Several new drug classes with novel mechanisms of action are in development and provide hope for patients with complex resistance patterns, patients who struggle with side effects of current regimens, and those seeking new delivery methods or dosing intervals. Classes currently in development include attachment inhibitors, nucleoside reverse transcriptase translocation inhibitors (NRTTIs), maturation inhibitors, monoclonal antibodies to CCR5, capsid inhibitors, and broadly neutralizing antibodies.

HIV CURE RESEARCH

Thus far, there have only been two documented cases of HIV cure. The first case, described as the "Berlin patient," was reported in 2009. He was a man with refractory AML who had HIV infection with a CCR5-tropic virus. He received two hematopoietic stem cell transplants, the second from a CCR5-negative donor. He also received total body irradiation and anti-thymocyte globulin. The second case, the "London patient," was reported in 2019. This patient had refractory Hodgkin's lymphoma and HIV with CCR5-tropic virus and received a stem cell transplant from a CCR5-negative donor. The patient did not receive irradiation, and T-cell depletion was achieved with an anti-CD52 agent. Both patients had mild graft-versus-host disease (GVHD). Both patients have had no recurrence of HIV viremia and no isolation of active virus from any tissue samples despite remaining off of antiretroviral therapy. These cases both illustrate extreme examples of potential routes to a cure—stem cell transplants carry a very high mortality, and GVHD is a lifelong disease that can have significant morbidity. However, the cases do demonstrate that the possibility of a cure is more than just theoretical, and ongoing studies for a cure to HIV is an area of intense research.

As a retrovirus, HIV integrates into the host genome, and latently infected cells are the primary reason that ART is not curative. All current ART targets viral proteins involved in viral replication; therefore, they are ineffective at removing the viral reservoir of latent disease, as the target viral proteins are not active in latently infected cells. Stopping ART always results in a recurrence of viremia over time in PLWH, as latent cells awaken and replication resumes. Thus the problem of finding a cure for HIV is largely a problem of determining how to cure latently infected cells. Further, currently ART is highly effective and very well tolerated, resulting in an essentially normal life expectancy. Ethically, the "cure" cannot be worse than treatment; this poses a high bar for researchers. A safe, effective, scalable, well-tolerated, and cost-effective intervention that is fully curative, or that allows for long-term viral control without the use of ART, is still many years away, but the groundwork has now been laid.

HIV PREVENTION, PEP AND PREP

Three broad approaches have had a major impact on reducing HIV transmission: harm reduction and behavioral modification, ART for "treatment as prevention," and the use of medications for pre- and postexposure prophylaxis. All of these activities are supported by expanded testing and improved linkage to care.

Harm reduction and behavior modification are broad categories of public health interventions to prevent HIV transmission. An example is the adoption of safer sexual practices, especially the use of condoms during sexual activity to prevent HIV transmission. Other interventions, such as those targeted toward people who inject drugs, including syringe exchange programs, safe injection facilities, and community methadone and buprenorphine programs, have also had a marked effect on reducing risk of HIV transmission. Many other approaches in the appropriate clinical and societal context can also have significant impact, such as male circumcision in highly impacted communities.

Treatment as prevention is the cornerstone of efforts to control the worldwide HIV epidemic, and widespread access to ART is a key goal of HIV prevention efforts today. Antiretroviral treatment of HIV-infected pregnant women and their infants in the peripartum period has decreased maternal-child transmission from 25% to less than 5% in North America. If a pregnant woman maintains viral suppression during pregnancy and during breast-feeding, the risk of transmission to her infant is less than 1%. Among sexually active individuals, a number of studies across thousands of individuals have demonstrated that patients who are on treatment and undetectable cannot transmit HIV to their sexual partners, regardless of condom use. The strength of these data are robust and results are consistent across multiple large studies in different populations across multiple countries, including in both heterosexual and MSM populations. In fact, none of the studies demonstrated a single case of transmission from an undetectable patient to their partner. The power of treatment as prevention has led to the popular educational campaign of "U=U" or "undetectable = untransmittable."

The use of ART has also been shown to be an effective tool for HIV prevention as postexposure prophylaxis after both occupational exposures to HIV (termed "PEP") and after unprotected sexual exposures (termed "nPEP"). Guidelines for PEP and nPEP recommend treatment as early as possible, within 72 hours at the most after an exposure. The treatment regimen should be based on the source patient's resistance pattern, if known, or if unknown, is generally with two NRTIs (tenofovir disoproxil fumarate and emtricitabine) and an integrase inhibitor (either raltegravir or dolutegravir) for 28 days. Occupational PEP is highly effective, and post exposure seroconversion of health care workers is virtually nonexistent since implementation of PEP. Guidelines for both PEP and nPEP are available through the CDC at: https://www.cdc.gov/hiv/risk/pep/index.html.

The use of ART for PrEP in HIV-negative individuals at high risk for HIV exposure has demonstrated excellent efficacy across multiple studies and populations. In individuals at high risk for sexual exposure, including MSM, individuals in serodiscordant relationships, sex workers, and individuals with multiple sexual partners, the daily use of either tenofovir disoproxil fumarate with emtricitabine (the combination tablet Truvada) or tenofovir alafenamide with emtricitabine (Descovy) has been shown to reduce risk of HIV transmission by 99% if taken with consistent adherence. PrEP has also been shown to be effective in people who inject drugs, with a 74% reduction with consistent daily use. Studies have been performed and others are ongoing to evaluate more risk-based, intermittent dosing. Additionally, studies are underway to look at other potential medications and delivery methods (e.g., injectable drugs, implantable devices).

Universal linkage, retention, and access to high-quality, culturally appropriate, and affordable HIV treatment should be the central goals of both HIV treatment and prevention, because effective treatment *is* effective prevention. Individuals should also be supported to protect themselves, and harm reduction techniques and behavior modification

2. 植入式缓释药物：与植入式避孕装置类似，植入式抗逆转录病毒给药装置也是一种极具吸引力的非频繁给药（每月一次甚至更长时间）的方法。植入装置需要进行小手术，故可能出现移除时的并发症，这也是一个令人担忧的问题。

3. 半衰期更长的口服药物：有几种口服药物正在开发中，可能达到每周一次或更长时间给药。与注射方案一样，如何处理半衰期较长的药物的不良反应以及停药后的拖尾效应仍令人担忧。

4. 新机制药物：目前正在开发几类具有新型作用机制的新药，它们为复合耐药、现有治疗不耐受以及寻求新给药方法或给药间隔的患者带来了希望。目前正在开发的药物包括附着抑制剂、核苷类逆转录酶转运抑制剂（NRTTI）、成熟抑制剂、CCR5 单克隆抗体、衣壳抑制剂和广谱中和抗体。

HIV 治愈研究

迄今为止，仅有两例 HIV 感染治愈的记录在案。第一个病例被称为"柏林病人"，于 2009 年报道。他是一名患有难治性急性髓细胞白血病的男性患者，感染了 CCR5 受体亲和性病毒；他接受了两次造血干细胞移植，第二次来自 CCR5 阴性捐赠者，他还接受了全身放疗和抗胸腺细胞球蛋白治疗。第二例"伦敦病人"于 2019 年报告。该患者患有难治性霍奇金淋巴瘤和 HIV，携带 CCR5 受体亲和性病毒，并接受了一位 CCR5 阴性供体的造血干细胞移植。患者没有接受放疗，而是通过抗 CD52 药物实现了 T 细胞去除。两名患者都有轻微的移植物抗宿主疾病（GVHD）。尽管仍在接受抗逆转录病毒治疗，但两名患者的 HIV 血症均未复发，也未从任何组织样本中分离出活性病毒。这些病例都是潜在治愈途径的极端例子，因为造血干细胞移植的死亡率非常高，极可能出现后续 GVHD 的发生，而 GVHD 是一种终身性疾病。不过，这些病例确实表明，治愈并不仅是理论上的可能性，目前这一研究领域也得到极大关注。

作为一种逆转录病毒，HIV 会整合到宿主基因组中，潜伏感染的细胞是抗逆转录病毒治疗无法治愈的主要原因。目前所有的抗逆转录病毒治疗都只针对参与病毒复制的病毒蛋白，因此，它们无法有效清除潜伏的病毒库，因为目标病毒蛋白在潜伏感染细胞中并不活跃。随着时间的推移、潜伏细胞的苏醒、病毒复制的恢复，停止药物治疗往往导致患者病毒血症的复发。因此，找到 HIV 临床治愈的方法，很大程度上取决于如何治愈潜伏感染细胞。此外，目前抗逆转录病毒治疗非常有效，耐受性也非常好，因此患者的寿命逐渐接近一般人群。从伦理上讲，"治愈"的效果不应差异于治疗，因此这对研究人员提出了更高的要求。寻找安全、有效、可推广、耐受性好且经济的干预措施，能够完全治愈，或能够在不使用抗逆转录病毒治疗的情况下长期控制病毒，虽然还有许多年的路要走，但现在已经奠定了基础。

HIV 暴露前及暴露后预防

有三大方法对减少 HIV 传播产生了重大影响：降低危害和行为改变、ART "治疗即预防"，以及通过药物进行 HIV 暴露前及暴露后预防。所有这些方法都得到了大范围实践证实，和医疗及护理体系的支持。

降低危害和行为改变是预防 HIV 传播的两大类公共卫生干预措施。例如，采取更安全的性行为方式，特别是在性行为中使用安全套来预防 HIV 传播。其他干预措施，如针对注射毒品者的干预措施，包括注射器交换计划、安全注射设施、社区美沙酮和丁丙诺啡计划等，这些措施也对降低 HIV 传播风险产生了显著效果。在适当的临床和社会背景下，还有许多重要措施，例如在流行严重的社区开展包皮环切手术。

治疗即预防是控制全球艾滋病疫情的基石，普及抗逆转录病毒治疗是当今艾滋病预防工作的关键目标。在北美，对感染 HIV 的孕妇及其围产期的婴儿进行母婴阻断治疗，已将母婴传播率从 25% 降至 5% 以下。如果孕妇在妊娠期和哺乳期保持病毒抑制状态，其婴儿感染 HIV 的风险低于 1%。在性活跃的人群中，数以千计的研究表明，无论是否使用安全套，接受治疗且检测不到病毒的患者都不会将 HIV 传染给其性伴侣。这些数据具有很强的证据等级，在多个国家的同性乃至异性人群中进行的多项大型研究也得到一致的结果。"治疗即预防"的力量促使"U = U"或"检测不到＝不会传播"的教育活动流行起来。

抗逆转录病毒治疗作为职业暴露（称为"PEP"）和无保护性暴露（称为"nPEP"）后的暴露后预防，也被证明是预防 HIV 感染的有效工具。预防相关指南建议该类人群尽早治疗，最晚应在暴露后 72 h 内启动预防药物。如传染源患者的耐药情况已知，药物的使用应基于传染源患者的情况；如果未知，则一般使用两种 NRTI（富马酸替诺福韦二吡呋酯和恩曲他滨）和一种整合酶抑制剂（拉替拉韦或多替拉韦），疗程为 28 天。职业性 PEP 非常有效，自实施 PEP 以来，医护人员暴露后血清转换的情况几乎未有发生。有关 PEP 和 nPEP 的指南可以从美国 CDC 网站获取：https://www.cdc.gov/hiv/risk/pep/index.html。

将抗逆转录病毒药物用于 HIV 阴性的 HIV 暴露高危人群的暴露前预防（PrEP）措施，已在多项研究和人群中证实了疗效。对于性暴露高危人群，包括男男性行为者、HIV 阳性者的性伴侣、性工作者和有多个性伴侣的人群，如果坚持每天服用 TAF/FTC（Truvada 复方片剂）或 TDF/FTC（Descovy），可降低 99% 的 HIV 传播风险。PrEP 对注射吸毒者也有效果，坚持每天使用可降低 74% 的传播风险。目前还在进行其他研究，以评估更多基于不同风险水平的间歇性用药疗效。此外，有关其他新型机制药物和新的给药方法（如注射药物、植入式设备）的研究也在进行中。

通用性、高依从性、高可及性、文化适宜和可负担的 HIV 药物治疗，应是 HIV 治疗和预防的共同核

interventions play an ongoing important role in HIV prevention for at-risk populations, with both PEP and PrEP offering additional pharmacologic aids to the universal goal of bringing an end to new HIV infections.

SUGGESTED READINGS

Aberg JA, Gallant JE, Ghanem KG, et al: Primary care guidelines for the management of persons infected with HIV: 2013 update by the HIV Medicine Association of the Infectious Diseases Society of America, Clin Infect Dis 58:e1–34, 2014.

International Antiviral Society–USA: Antiretroviral Drugs for Treatment and Prevention of HIV Infection in Adults: 2018 Recommendations of the International Antiviral Society–USA Panel. Available at: https://www.iasusa.org/resources/guidelines/. Accessed January 2020.

International Antiviral Society–USA: HIV Drug Resistance Mutations. Available at: https://www.iasusa.org/resources/hiv-drug-resistance-mutations/. Accessed January 2020.

Stanford University: HIV Drug Resistance Database. Available at: https://hivdb.stanford.edu. Accessed January 2020.

U.S. Center for Disease Control and Prevention: Post-Exposure Prophylaxis. Available at: https://www.cdc.gov/hiv/risk/pep/index.html. Accessed January 2020.

U.S. Department of Health and Human Services: Guidelines for the Prevention and Treatment of Opportunistic Infections in Adults and Adolescents with HIV. Available at: https://aidsinfo.nih.gov/guidelines/html/4/adult-and-adolescent-opportunistic-infection/0. Accessed January 2020.

U.S. Department of Health and Human Services: Guidelines for the Use of Antiretroviral Agents in Adults and Adolescents with HIV. Available at: https://aidsinfo.nih.gov/guidelines. Accessed January 2020.

心目标，因为有效的治疗即是有效的预防。应该鼓励患者自我保护，进行降低危害及行为改变措施，同时PEP和PrEP的应用，也为实现杜绝HIV新感染的普遍目标提供了更多的药物辅助手段。

推荐阅读

Aberg JA, Gallant JE, Ghanem KG, et al: Primary care guidelines for the management of persons infected with HIV: 2013 update by the HIV Medicine Association of the Infectious Diseases Society of America, Clin Infect Dis 58:e1–34, 2014.

International Antiviral Society–USA: Antiretroviral Drugs for Treatment and Prevention of HIV Infection in Adults: 2018 Recommendations of the International Antiviral Society–USA Panel. Available at: https://www.iasusa.org/resources/guidelines/. Accessed January 2020.

International Antiviral Society–USA: HIV Drug Resistance Mutations. Available at: https://www.iasusa.org/resources/hiv-drug-resistance-mutations/. Accessed January 2020.

Stanford University: HIV Drug Resistance Database. Available at: https://hivdb.stanford.edu. Accessed January 2020.

U.S. Center for Disease Control and Prevention: Post-Exposure Prophylaxis. Available at: https://www.cdc.gov/hiv/risk/pep/index.html. Accessed January 2020.

U.S. Department of Health and Human Services: Guidelines for the Prevention and Treatment of Opportunistic Infections in Adults and Adolescents with HIV. Available at: https://aidsinfo.nih.gov/guidelines/html/4/adult-and-adolescent-opportunistic-infection/0. Accessed January 2020.

U.S. Department of Health and Human Services: Guidelines for the Use of Antiretroviral Agents in Adults and Adolescents with HIV. Available at: https://aidsinfo.nih.gov/guidelines. Accessed January 2020.

17

Infections in the Immunocompromised Host

Dimitrios Farmakiotis, Ralph Rogers

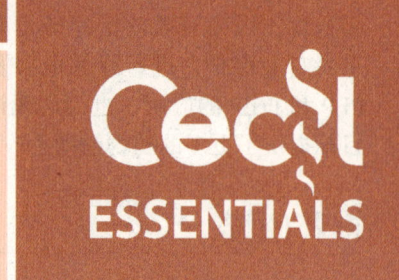

INTRODUCTION

Individuals with an impaired immune system are at risk for infections due to typical pathogens and less virulent organisms that usually do not cause illness. Diagnosis can be challenging due to atypical disease manifestations. The pace and severity of illness in tenuous patients demands that complicated treatment decisions are made early, despite lack of diagnostic certainty. This chapter aims to provide a clinically oriented framework for diagnosis and management of infections in immunocompromised hosts, excluding patients with HIV/AIDS (Figs. 17.1 and 17.2).

EPIDEMIOLOGY

The population of immunocompromised individuals is rapidly growing and becoming more diverse, including patients with primary (congenital) immunodeficiencies, some of which are newly recognized; individuals with hematologic malignancies (HM), who are now surviving longer; solid organ (SOT) and hematopoietic cell transplant (HCT) recipients; and finally, patients being treated with newly developed immunomodulatory medications (TNF-α inhibitors, monoclonal antibodies, ibrutinib) that expose more and more individuals to potential infectious complications.

PATHOGENESIS

Not all immunocompromised individuals are at equal risk for every possible infection. Instead, "immunocompromised hosts" are a heterogenous group, in which specific immune deficits come with distinct risks (see Fig. 17.1 and Tables 17.1 and 17.2).

Neutropenia

Neutrophils are the primary defense against bacterial and fungal infections. Neutropenia associated with increased risk for infection is defined as absolute neutrophil count less than 500/μL. Primary immunodeficiency syndromes such as congenital neutropenia (inadequate production), chronic granulomatous disease (ineffective microbial killing), and leukocyte adhesion deficiency (ineffective recruitment to sites of infection) are associated with increased number and severity of infections, usually caused by typical bacterial (e.g., *Staphylococcus*, *Streptococcus*, Enterobacteriaceae) and fungal (e.g., *Candida*) colonizers of skin, gastrointestinal, genitourinary, and respiratory tracts.

Neutropenia is common with HM, due to decreased neutrophil production from both bone marrow infiltration and cytotoxic chemotherapy. Cytotoxic chemotherapy acts primarily on rapidly dividing cells, thus in addition to its desired effect it also has negative impact on the rapidly dividing cells of the gastrointestinal tract lining (mucositis). This decrease in an anatomic barrier in combination with decreased neutrophil defense can lead to rapidly progressive infections from microbial translocation. Therefore, "neutropenic fever" is a medical emergency, and such patients need prompt and broad antimicrobial therapy against typical enteric pathogens and *Pseudomonas* (which is associated with high mortality).

Cell-Mediated and Humoral Immune Deficits

The adaptive immune response provided by the cell-mediated and humoral components of the immune system allows for effective intracellular and extracellular microbial killing and is critical against viral infections, while also contributing to antibacterial and antifungal defenses. Many primary immunodeficiency syndromes affect cellular and humoral immunity, each causing increased susceptibility to various bacterial, fungal, and viral infections. Severe combined immunodeficiency (underdevelopment of both T cells and B cells) predisposes infants to serious infections from common viruses (e.g., Herpesviridae), bacteria, and fungi (e.g., *Pneumocystis*). DiGeorge syndrome (thymic hypoplasia leading to underdevelopment of T cells) and hyperimmunoglobulin-E syndrome (impaired T cell differentiation and function) predispose individuals to recurrent bacterial skin or sinopulmonary infections. X-linked agammaglobulinemia (underdevelopment of B cells) predisposes patients to bacterial infections with encapsulated organisms (pneumococcus, *Haemophilus influenza*, *Neisseria meningitidis*) and common viral pathogens (e.g., Enteroviridae). Secondary causes of hypogammaglobulinemia (e.g., chronic lymphocytic leukemia [CLL], protein-losing enteropathy, nephrotic syndrome) may also lead to increased risk for viral and bacterial infections.

Asplenia and Complement Deficits

Functional or anatomic asplenia leads to increased risk for severe infections due to encapsulated bacteria and blood-borne parasites (e.g., *Plasmodium*, *Babesia*) since the spleen is the primary site that filters out parasitized red blood cells. The complement system acts by opsonization of pathogens allowing for subsequent phagocytosis and can also act on its own to eliminate pathogens via the membrane attack complex. Complement deficiencies lead to an increased risk for infections due to encapsulated bacteria, especially *N. meningitidis*. They can be congenital or from eculizumab, a monoclonal antibody that is effective treatment for atypical hemolytic uremic syndrome by inhibiting terminal complement.

免疫妥协宿主的感染

阮巧玲　张文宏　译　肖江　张福杰　审校　张福杰　通审

引言

免疫系统受损的个体处于典型病原体和通常不致病的低毒力生物体的感染风险中。由于疾病表现不典型，诊断可能具有挑战性。即使在诊断尚未确定时，因这些脆弱患者的病情严重且发展迅速，往往需要尽早做出复杂的治疗决定。本章旨在为免疫妥协宿主（不包括 HIV/AIDS 患者）的感染诊断和管理提供一个临床导向的框架（图 17.1 和图 17.2）

流行病学

免疫妥协的人群正在迅速增长，并变得更加多样化，包括原发性（先天性）免疫缺陷患者，其中一些是新近了解的；恶性血液病（HM）患者，他们现在生存的时间更长；最后，还包括使用新近开发使用的免疫调节剂（TNF-α 抑制剂、单克隆抗体、伊布替尼）治疗的患者，这些药物使越来越多的人面临潜在的感染并发症。

发病机制

并非所有免疫妥协的人都会有同样的感染风险。相反，"免疫妥协宿主"是一个异质性群体，其中特定的免疫缺陷会带来不同的风险（图 17.1、表 17.1 和表 17.2）。

中性粒细胞减少症

中性粒细胞是抵御细菌和真菌感染的主要防御细胞。与感染风险增加相关的中性粒细胞减少症定义为绝对中性粒细胞计数小于 $500/\mu l$。先天性中性粒细胞减少症（中性粒细胞生成不足）、慢性肉芽肿病（不能有效杀死微生物）和白细胞黏附缺陷（不能有效聚集到感染部位）等原发性免疫缺陷综合征与感染的次数和严重程度增加有关，通常由皮肤、胃肠道、泌尿生殖道和呼吸道的典型细菌（如金黄色葡萄球菌、链球菌、肠杆菌科）和真菌（如念珠菌）定植菌引起。

由于骨髓浸润和细胞毒性化疗导致中性粒细胞生成减少，中性粒细胞减少症在 HM 中很常见。细胞毒性化疗主要作用于快速分裂的细胞，因此除了预期效果外，它还会对胃肠道内壁快速分裂的细胞产生负面影响（黏膜炎）。解剖屏障作用降低与中性粒细胞防御能力的下降两相结合，可导致微生物易位引起的快速进展性感染。因此，"中性粒细胞减少性发热"是一种医学急症，这类患者需要及时接受广泛的抗菌治疗，以抗击典型的肠道病原体和铜绿假单胞菌（与高死亡率相关）感染。

细胞介导免疫和体液免疫缺陷

免疫系统中的细胞免疫和体液免疫所提供的适应性免疫反应可有效杀死细胞内和细胞外的微生物，对病毒感染至关重要，同时也有助于抗细菌和抗真菌防御。许多原发性免疫缺陷综合征都会影响细胞免疫和体液免疫，从而导致对各种细菌、真菌和病毒感染的易感性增加。重症联合免疫缺陷病（T 细胞和 B 细胞发育不全）使婴儿容易受到常见病毒（如疱疹病毒科）、细菌和真菌（如肺孢子虫）的严重感染。迪格奥尔格综合征（胸腺发育不全导致 T 细胞发育不全）和高免疫球蛋白 E 综合征（T 细胞分化和功能受损）易导致反复的皮肤或鼻窦肺部细菌感染。X 连锁无丙种球蛋白血症（B 细胞发育不全）使患者容易受到荚膜细菌（肺炎球菌、流感嗜血杆菌、脑膜炎奈瑟球菌）和常见病毒病原体（如肠道病毒）的感染。继发性低丙种球蛋白血症［如慢性淋巴细胞白血病（CLL）、蛋白丢失性肠病、肾病综合征］也可能导致病毒和细菌感染的风险增加。

无脾及补体缺陷

功能性或解剖性无脾会增加因荚膜细菌和血液寄生虫（如疟原虫、巴贝斯虫）而导致严重感染的风险，因为脾是过滤寄生红细胞的主要部位。补体系统通过包被病原体起作用，从而易于随后的吞噬作用，并且还可以通过膜攻击复合物自行消除病原体。补体缺陷会导致有荚膜细菌（尤其是脑膜炎奈瑟球菌）感染的风险增加。这可能是先天性的，也可能来自依库珠单抗使用后引起，这是一种单克隆抗体，通过抑制末端补体来有效治疗非典型溶血性尿毒综合征。

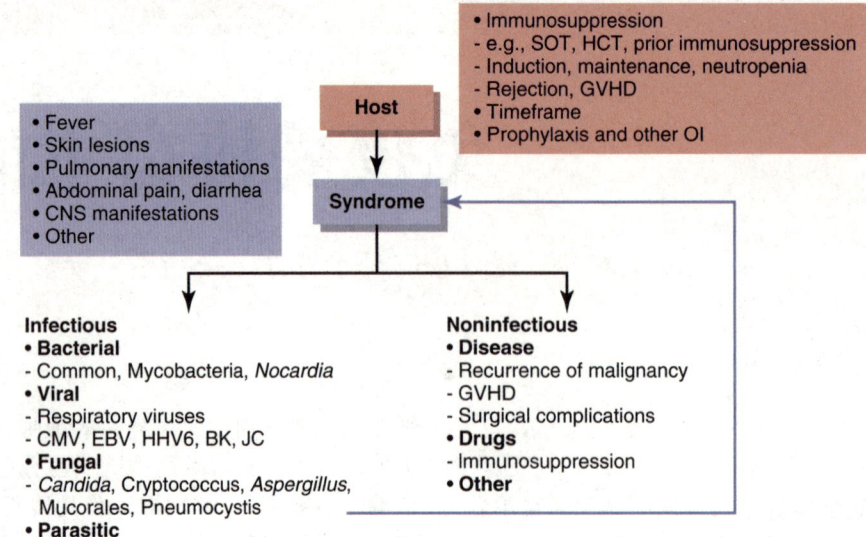

Fig. 17.1 Algorithmic approach to the diagnosis of syndromes suspicious for infection in the immunocompromised host. Continuous reassessment is paramount. For a discussion of abbreviations and specific pathogens see "Specific Pathogens" section below.

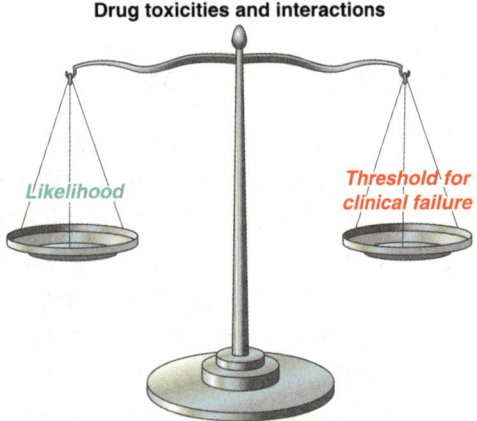

Fig. 17.2 Management decisions should be based on the balance between the likelihood of a diagnosis and the clinical consequences of not treating immediately, given the toxicities and drug-drug interactions of antimicrobials.

Hematologic Malignancies

Neutropenia is the main risk factor for infection in patients with acute leukemia. At the time of diagnosis, an individual may have already been neutropenic for an extended time and thus at risk for infection by environmental molds, such as *Aspergillus* or the Mucorales. After induction chemotherapy, patients stay profoundly neutropenic for several weeks, leading to increased risk for infection as outlined previously. Lymphoma patients usually do not experience extended periods of neutropenia from chemotherapy, which is, nonetheless, profoundly lymphocyte-depleting. Risk for infection sometimes depends on dosing (e.g., there is increased risk for *Pneumocystis* with R-CHOP-14, i.e., bi-weekly, due to more frequent administration of steroids). CLL is a chronic leukemia that is often monitored but not treated given its indolent course. However, these patients frequently have hypogammaglobulinemia and may be at increased risk for bacterial or viral sinopulmonary infections.

TABLE 17.1 Primary Immunodeficiency Syndromes

Syndrome	Description
Defects in Phagocytes	
Congenital neutropenia	Inadequate neutrophil production
Chronic granulomatous disease	Ineffective microbial killing by phagocytes due to decreased NADPH oxidase activity
Leukocyte adhesion deficiency	Ineffective recruitment of phagocytes to sites of infection
Defects in Cellular and Humoral Immunity	
Severe combined immunodeficiency	T- and/or B-cell deficiency or absence
ZAP-70 deficiency	Defects in T-cell proliferation and activation
DiGeorge syndrome	Thymic hypoplasia leading to defects in T-cell maturation
Idiopathic CD4 lymphopenia	Inadequate CD4$^+$ T-cell production
Hyper-IgE syndrome	Defect in JAK/STAT signaling pathway leading to multiple immune deficits
Hyper-IgM syndrome	Defect in class-switch recombination leading to inadequate IgG/IgA/IgE production
X-linked agammaglobulinemia	Defect in B-cell maturation leading to decreased or absent immunoglobulin production
Common variable immunodeficiency	Defective immunoglobulin production
Defects in Innate Immunity	
NK cell deficiency	Absent or defective NK cells
Complement deficiencies	Absent or defective complement components

Solid Organ Transplantation

SOT is a life-saving procedure, but unless the transplanted organ (allograft) is coming from the recipient's identical twin, the transplant recipient must take immunosuppressive medications in order to prevent their immune system from rejecting the allograft as "nonself."

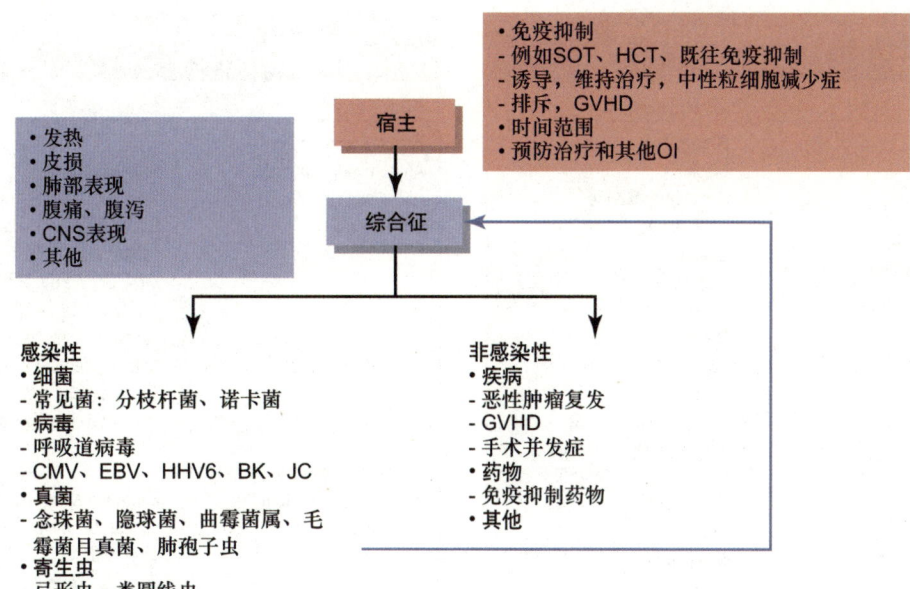

图 17.1 诊断免疫妥协宿主疑似感染综合征的流程。持续的重新评估至关重要。有关缩写和特定病原体的讨论，参阅下文"特定病原体"部分

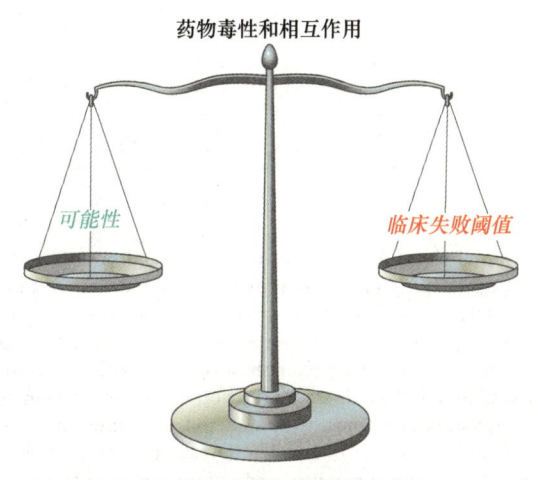

图 17.2 考虑到抗菌药物的毒性和药物间的相互作用，治疗决定应基于诊断的可能性和不立即治疗的临床后果之间的平衡

恶性血液病

中性粒细胞减少症是急性白血病患者感染的主要危险因素。在诊断时，患者可能已经处于中性粒细胞减少症很长时间，因此有被环境霉菌（如曲霉菌或毛霉菌目真菌）感染的风险。诱导化疗后，患者会持续数周处于严重的中性粒细胞减少症，导致感染风险增加，如前所述。淋巴瘤患者通常不会因化疗而出现长时间的中性粒细胞减少症，尽管如此，化疗会严重消耗淋巴细胞。感染风险有时取决于剂量（例如，由于更频繁地使用类固醇激素，即每 2 周一次使用 R-CHOP-14 会增加肺孢子菌感染的风险）。慢性淋巴细胞白血病是一种慢性白血病，由于其惰性进程，因此通常需要监测但不实施治疗。然而，这些患者经常患有低丙种球蛋白血症，并且可能面临细菌或病毒性鼻窦肺感染风险增加。

表 17.1 原发性免疫缺陷综合征

综合征	描述
吞噬细胞缺陷	
先天性中性粒细胞减少症	中性粒细胞生成不足
慢性肉芽肿病	由于 NADPH 氧化酶活性降低，吞噬细胞无法有效杀死微生物
白细胞黏附缺陷症	无法有效地将吞噬细胞募集到感染部位
细胞和体液免疫缺陷	
重症联合免疫缺陷病	T 细胞和（或）B 细胞缺乏或缺失
ZAP-70 缺陷	T 细胞增殖和活化缺陷
迪格奥尔格综合征	胸腺发育不全导致 T 细胞成熟缺陷
特发性 $CD4^+$ T 细胞减少症	$CD4^+$ T 细胞生成不足
高免疫球蛋白 E 综合征	JAK/STAT 信号通路缺陷导致多种免疫缺陷
X 连锁无丙种球蛋白血症	B 细胞成熟缺陷导致免疫球蛋白生成减少或缺失
普通变异型免疫缺陷病	免疫球蛋白生成缺陷
先天免疫缺陷	
NK 细胞缺陷	NK 细胞缺失或有缺陷
补体缺陷	补体成分缺失或有缺陷

实质器官移植

实质器官移植（SOT）是一种挽救生命的手术，但除非移植的器官（同种异体移植）来自受体的同卵双胞胎，否则接受移植器官必须服用免疫抑制药物，以防止其免疫系统将同种异体移植视为"非自身"器官而排斥。SOT 患者在移植时（诱导）接受强效免疫

TABLE 17.2 Immunosuppressive Medications	
Class	Examples
Cytotoxic agents	Bleomycin
	Cisplatin
	Cyclophosphamide
	Cytarabine
	Doxorubicin
	Etoposide
	Fluorouracil
	Methotrexate
	Paclitaxel
	Vincristine
Lymphocyte depleting agents	Alemtuzumab
	Anti-thymocyte globulin
	Basiliximab
	Belatacept
	Rituximab
TNF-α inhibitors	Adalimumab
	Etanercept
	Infliximab
Corticosteroids	Prednisone
Common antirejection medications	Azathioprine
	Cyclosporine
	Mycophenolate
	Sirolimus
	Tacrolimus
Other monoclonal antibodies and signal transduction inhibitors associated with increased risk for infection	Eculizumab
	Ibrutinib
	Idelalisib
	Natalizumab
	Ruxolitinib
	Tocilizumab

TABLE 17.3 Infections After Solid Organ Transplantation	
Risk Category	Examples
Early Infections	
Anatomic disruption	Anastomotic leak
	Surgical site infection
Donor derived	Bacterial: *Mycobacterium tuberculosis*
	Fungal: *Aspergillus*
	Viral: CMV, EBV, HBV, HCV, HIV, HSV, LCMV, VZV
	Parasite: *Toxoplasma*
Hospital acquired	Catheter-related infection
	Clostridioides difficile colitis
	Ventilator-associated pneumonia
Middle Infections	
Reactivation of latent pathogens	Bacterial: *M. tuberculosis*
	Fungal: *Candida*
	Viral: BKPyV, CMV, HBV, HCV, HSV, VZV
	Parasite: *Strongyloides, Toxoplasma*
Opportunistic infections	Bacterial: *Nocardia*
	Fungal: *Aspergillus, Pneumocystis*
	Parasite: *Microsporidia*
Late Infections	
Community acquired	Pneumonia
	Urinary tract infection
Post-prophylaxis reactivation	CMV
	HSV
	VZV

SOT recipients are given potent immunosuppressive medications to prevent acute rejection at the time of their transplant (induction) and thereafter stay on two to three immunosuppressants (maintenance). The risks for specific types of infection differ, depending on the time since transplantation (Table 17.3). Infections early on are related to the transplant surgery itself (anastomotic leak, surgical site infection) or are hospital acquired (catheter infection, *C. difficile* colitis); early infections can also be donor derived (i.e., present in the donor at the time of transplant, then transferred to the recipient with the allograft). Infections in the "middle period" are often due to reactivation of pre-existing latent infections (CMV, hepatitis B or C, *Toxoplasma*) or to opportunistic pathogens (*Pneumocystis, Aspergillus*). Late infections are usually community acquired (e.g., pneumonia) and organ specific (recurrent urinary tract infections in kidney transplant recipients, cholangitis in liver transplant recipients, late aspergillosis in lung transplant recipients). Augmented immunosuppression for rejection increases the risk for infection. So does "immunosenescence," and elderly SOT recipients sometimes present with opportunistic infections many years after transplantation.

Hematopoietic Cell Transplantation

Hematopoietic (stem) cell transplantation (HCT) involves replacing the bone marrow and immune system with a new, healthier one. This life-saving procedure is associated with many infectious and noninfectious post-transplantation complications. HCT recipients are given high doses of cytotoxic medications and/or radiation therapy to destroy their old immune system (conditioning) and thus are at risk for many infections while waiting for their new hematopoietic cells to populate the bone marrow and begin functioning (engraftment). A common complication after HCT is graft-versus-host disease (GVHD), where the donor immune system recognizes recipient organs (mostly the skin and gastrointestinal tract) as "nonself" and mounts a potentially devastating immune response. Additional immunosuppressive medications are given to prevent or treat GVHD, adding to the risk for infection. Further, GVHD is itself an immunosuppressive condition given that it acts to slow immune expansion after HCT.

As in individuals receiving SOT, risks for specific types of infection differ depending on the time since transplantation and presence of GVHD (Table 17.4). Early on, infections are related to profound neutropenia and mucositis from the conditioning regimen. Functional neutrophils are newly present after engraftment, but other arms of adaptive and innate immunity are slowly reconstituted thereafter, first NK-cells, then CD8+ T cells, and finally B cells and CD4+ T cells, sometimes years later. This process can be delayed by both GVHD and immunosuppressive medications for it (see Table 17.4).

Novel Immunomodulatory Medications

The number and variety of immunomodulatory medications has dramatically increased in recent years, leading to newly recognized syndromes. Examples are invasive fungal infections with ibrutinib (a tyrosine kinase inhibitor used to treat lymphoid malignancies),

表 17.2 免疫抑制药物

类别	示例
细胞毒性药物	博来霉素 顺铂 环磷酰胺 阿糖胞苷 阿霉素 依托泊苷 氟尿嘧啶 氨甲蝶呤 紫杉醇 长春新碱
淋巴细胞耗竭剂	阿仑单抗 抗胸腺细胞球蛋白 巴利昔单抗 贝拉西普 利妥昔单抗
TNF-α 抑制剂	阿达木单抗 依那西普 英夫利西单抗
皮质类固醇	泼尼松
常用抗排斥药物	硫唑嘌呤 环孢素 霉酚酸 西罗莫司 他克莫司
其他与感染风险增加有关的单克隆抗体和信号转导抑制剂	依库珠单抗 伊布替尼 艾代拉里斯 那他珠单抗 鲁索替尼 托珠单抗

表 17.3 实体器官移植后的感染

风险分类	示例
早期感染	
解剖破坏	吻合口渗漏 手术部位感染
供体来源	细菌：结核分枝杆菌 真菌：曲霉菌属 病毒：CMV、EBV、HBV、HCV、HIV、HSV、LCMV、VZV 寄生虫：弓形虫
医院获得	导管相关感染 艰难梭菌结肠炎 呼吸机相关肺炎
中期感染	
潜伏病原体的重新激活	细菌：结核分枝杆菌 真菌：念珠菌 病毒：BKPyV、CMV、HBV、HCV、HSV、VZV 寄生虫：类圆线虫、弓形虫
机会性感染	细菌：诺卡菌 真菌：曲霉菌、肺孢子虫 寄生虫：微孢子虫
晚期感染	
社区获得	肺炎 尿路感染
预防治疗后再激活	CMV HSV VZV

抑制药物以防止急性排斥，此后继续服用2～3种免疫抑制剂（维持）。具体类型的感染风险因移植时间而异（表17.3）。早期感染与移植手术本身有关（吻合口渗漏、手术部位感染）或医院获得性感染（导管感染、艰难梭菌结肠炎）；早期感染也可能来自供体（即在移植时存在于供体中，然后通过同种异体移植物转移到受体身上）。"中期"感染通常是由于先前存在的潜伏感染（CMV、乙型或丙型肝炎、弓形虫）或机会性病原体（肺孢子虫、曲霉菌）的重新激活所致。晚期感染通常是社区获得性感染（例如肺炎）和器官特异性感染（肾移植患者的复发性尿路感染、肝移植患者的胆管炎、肺移植患者的晚期曲霉病）。增强免疫抑制以抵抗排斥会增加感染风险。"免疫衰老"也是如此，老年SOT患者有时会在移植多年后出现机会性感染。

造血细胞移植

造血（干）细胞移植（HCT）对患者的骨髓和免疫系统进行了替换。这种挽救生命的手术与许多感染性和非感染性移植后并发症的发生有关。HCT患者会接受高剂量的细胞毒性药物和(或)放射治疗来破坏其旧有的免疫系统（调节），因此在等待新的造血细胞进入骨髓并开始发挥作用（植入）时，他们面临着多种感染的风险。HCT后常见的并发症是移植物抗宿主病（GVHD），供体的免疫系统将接受者的器官（主要是皮肤和胃肠道）识别为"非自身"，并产生可能具有破坏性的免疫反应。还会使用其他免疫抑制药物来预防或治疗GVHD，这进一步增加了感染风险。此外，GVHD本身就是一种免疫抑制疾病，因为它会减缓HCT后的免疫扩增。

与接受SOT的个体一样，特定类型感染的风险因移植后的时间和GVHD的存在而异（表17.4）。早期感染与严重的中性粒细胞减少症和预处理方案引起的黏膜炎有关。功能性中性粒细胞是在移植后新出现的，但适应性免疫和先天性免疫的其他器官随后会慢慢重建，首先是NK细胞，然后是CD8$^+$ T细胞，最后是B细胞和CD4$^+$ T细胞，有时甚至是在数年之后。该过程可以通过GVHD和免疫抑制药物来延缓（表17.4）。

新型免疫调节剂

近年来，免疫调节剂的数量和种类急剧增加，导致一些新综合征的发现。例如，伊布替尼（一种用于治疗淋巴系统恶性肿瘤的酪氨酸激酶抑制剂）导致侵袭性真菌感染，那他珠单抗（用于治疗多发性硬化症

TABLE 17.4 Infections After Hematopoietic Cell Transplant

Risk Category	Examples
Pre-engraftment	
Neutropenia	Bacterial: skin/GI/GU flora
Mucositis	Fungal: *Candida, Aspergillus*
	Viral: HSV, VZV
Hospital acquired	Catheter-related infection
	Clostridioides difficile colitis
	Ventilator-associated pneumonia
Early Post-engraftment	
Reactivation of latent pathogens	Bacterial: *Mycobacterium tuberculosis*
	Fungal: *Candida*
	Viral: adenovirus, BKPyV, CMV, HBV, HCV, HHV-6, HHV-8, HSV, JCPyV, VZV
	Parasite: *Strongyloides, Toxoplasma*
Opportunistic infections	Bacterial: *Nocardia*
	Fungal: *Aspergillus, Mucorales, Pneumocystis*
	Parasite: *Microsporidia*
Late Post-engraftment	
Community acquired	Pneumonia
	Sinusitis
	Urinary tract infection
Post-prophylaxis reactivation	CMV
	HSV
	VZV

progressive multifocal encephalopathy (PML) with natalizumab (selective adhesion molecule inhibitor used to treat multiple sclerosis), hepatitis B reactivation or rituximab (anti-CD20+ monoclonal antibody used for treatment of B-cell lymphomas), and mycobacterial infections and histoplasmosis with TNF-α inhibitors (see Table 17.2).

CLINICAL PRESENTATION

Central Nervous System Infection

Headache, neck stiffness, photophobia, encephalopathy, or new focal neurologic deficits, with or without fever, may be indicative of central nervous system (CNS) infection. Clinical symptoms of meningitis and cerebrospinal fluid (CSF) pleocytosis may be dampened in the setting of immunosuppression. In addition to typical pathogens (pneumococcus, enterovirus, herpes simplex virus [HSV]), one should consider other bacterial *(Listeria, Nocardia)*, viral (e.g., arbovirus, astrovirus, CMV, Epstein-Barr virus [EBV], lymphocytic choriomeningitis [LCMV], varicella zoster virus [VZV]), fungal (e.g., *Cryptococcus*), and parasitic *(Toxoplasma)* etiologies. CNS infection can be part of a systemic syndrome, and dysfunction of other organs may give a clue to the etiology (e.g., severe pneumonia with adenovirus meningitis, *Nocardia* lung nodules). CNS imaging is paramount and can aid in diagnosis (e.g., multiple ring-enhancing lesions with *Toxoplasma* encephalitis, multifocal white matter changes with PML [Fig. 17.3]).

Pneumonia

Although fever and productive cough are the hallmark sign and symptom of pneumonia, both may be muted in immunocompromised hosts. Alternatively, pneumonia may be rapidly progressive and fulminant. Beyond typical bacterial and viral etiologies, pneumonia in immunocompromised patients can be caused by atypical bacterial (*Legionella, Nocardia, Mycobacterium tuberculosis* or nontuberculous mycobacteria), viral (adenovirus, CMV, HSV, VZV), fungal (*Aspergillus, Cryptococcus*, dimorphic fungi, non-*Aspergillus* molds, *Pneumocystis*), and parasitic (*Toxoplasma, Strongyloides* hyperinfection) etiologies. Associated nonpulmonary manifestations (e.g., cryptococcal meningitis) can help make the diagnosis. Computed tomography (CT) and bronchoscopy are often necessary to better define the infectious process.

Diarrhea

Clinicians should consider bacterial (*Clostridioides difficile, Salmonella*), viral (adenovirus, CMV, enterovirus, norovirus), and parasitic *(Cryptosporidium, Giardia)* etiologies. Stool PCR panels can be useful but sometimes cannot differentiate between colonization and infection for some organisms, such as enteropathogenic *E. coli*. A careful exposure history can help narrow the possible diagnoses, especially for infections with regional endemicity. Colonoscopy with tissue biopsy may be necessary to make a definite diagnosis. At our institution, multiplex PCR, *C. difficile* toxin in the stool, and CMV viral load in the blood are standard protocol for SOT recipients with diarrhea. Leading noninfectious causes are medications, especially mycophenolate (an antimetabolite used for maintenance immunosuppression), and GVHD.

Skin Manifestations

Skin lesions in the immunocompromised patient can be a sign of localized ("outside-in") or disseminated ("inside-out") infection. Necrotic lesions raise concern for angioinvasive mold, although they can also be seen with severe bacterial infections and neutropenia, due to toxin effect with minimal inflammation. The most classic lesion is ecthyma gangrenosum, a painful eschar in neutropenic sepsis caused by *Pseudomonas*, but also other gram-negative or gram-positive (*S. aureus*) bacteria. Disseminated candidiasis can present with diffuse maculopapular rash and *Fusarium* sepsis with painful nodules. Vesicular lesions always raise concern for herpetic infection, although HSV (especially resistant or HSV2) can also cause large ulcerated lesions. "Sporotrichoid lesions" (cordlike clusters of inflammatory nodules) can be due to *Sporothrix, S. aureus, Nocardia* or atypical mycobacteria. Noninfectious causes are very common, such as drug rash, primary skin cancer (the most common malignancy after SOT), skin metastases and leukemia cutis, GVHD, neutrophilic eccrine hidradenitis, and Sweet syndrome (febrile neutrophilic dermatosis, an inflammatory reaction to tumors and chemotherapy that is best treated with corticosteroids). For accurate diagnosis, a skin biopsy with cultures is often necessary.

Fever of Unknown Origin

Persistent fever in an immunocompromised host without a clear etiology or any focal signs or symptoms is a relatively common clinical scenario. History and physical examination will often reveal subtle signs or symptoms integral to steering further diagnostic efforts. Careful attention to the mouth (Fig. 17.4), skin, and perineal area is imperative, because each may provide easily overlooked clues. Perineal infection can manifest with rectal pain alone. Beyond typical screening studies such as blood and urine cultures and a chest radiograph, an algorithmic approach to further investigation may involve stepwise additional testing including fungal markers, PCR-based testing for viruses (CMV, EBV, HHV-6), and cross-sectional imaging of the chest, abdomen, and pelvis. Advanced laboratory tests (e.g., cell-free DNA sequencing, an emerging technology that detects and identifies nonhuman DNA fragments in a clinical sample) and

表 17.4　造血干细胞移植后的感染	
风险分类	示例
移植前期	
中性粒细胞减少症	细菌：皮肤 /GI/GU 菌群
黏膜炎	真菌：念珠菌，曲霉菌
	病毒：HSV、VZV
医院获得	导管相关感染
	艰难梭菌肠炎
	呼吸机相关肺炎
移植后早期	
潜伏病原体的重新激活	细菌：结核分枝杆菌
	真菌：念珠菌
	病毒：腺病毒、BKPyV、CMV、HBV、HCV、HHV-6、HHV-8、HSV、JCPyV、VZV
	寄生虫：类圆线虫、弓形虫
机会性感染	细菌：诺卡菌
	真菌：曲霉菌、毛霉菌目真菌、肺孢子菌
	寄生虫：小孢子虫
移植后晚期	
社区获得	肺炎
	鼻窦炎
	尿路感染
预防治疗后再激活	CMV
	HSV
	VZV

的选择性黏附分子抑制剂）导致进行性多灶性白质脑病（PML）、利妥昔单抗（用于治疗 B 细胞淋巴瘤的抗 CD20 ＋单克隆抗体）导致乙型肝炎再激活，以及 TNF-α 抑制剂导致霉菌感染和组织胞浆菌病（表 17.2）。

临床表现

中枢神经系统感染

头痛、颈强直、畏光、脑病或新的局灶性神经功能障碍、伴或不伴发热可能提示中枢神经系统（CNS）感染。在免疫抑制的情况下，脑膜炎和脑脊液（CSF）细胞增多的临床表现可能不明显。除了典型的病原体（肺炎球菌、肠道病毒、单纯疱疹病毒）外，还应考虑其他细菌（李斯特菌、诺卡菌）、病毒（例如虫媒病毒、星状病毒、CMV、EBV、淋巴细胞脉络丛脑膜炎病毒、VZV）、真菌（例如隐球菌属）和寄生虫（弓形虫）病因。CNS 感染可能是全身综合征的一部分，其他器官的功能障碍可能为病因提供线索（例如，腺病毒脑膜炎引起的严重肺炎、诺卡菌肺结节）。CNS 影像至关重要，可帮助诊断［例如，弓形虫脑炎的多发性环状增强病变、PML 的多灶性白质改变（图 17.3）］。

肺炎

虽然发热和咳嗽是肺炎的典型症状，但在免疫妥协宿主中，这两种症状都可能不明显。另外，肺炎也可能会迅速进展和恶化。除了典型的细菌和病毒病因外，免疫妥协患者的肺炎还可能由非典型细菌（军团菌、诺卡菌、结核分枝杆菌或非结核分枝杆菌）、病毒（腺病毒、CMV、HSV、VZV）、真菌（曲霉菌属、隐球菌属、双态性真菌、非曲霉菌霉菌、肺孢菌）和寄生虫（弓形虫、类圆线虫重度感染）病因引起。相关的非肺部表现（例如隐球菌性脑膜炎）有助于诊断。通常需要进行 CT 和支气管镜检查，以更好地确定感染性病变。

腹泻

临床医生应考虑细菌（艰难梭菌、沙门菌）、病毒（腺病毒、CMV、肠道病毒、诺如病毒）和寄生虫（隐孢子虫属、贾第鞭毛虫）病因。粪便 PCR 很有用，但有时无法区分某些微生物的定植和感染，例如肠致病性大肠埃希菌。仔细了解接触史有助于缩小可能的诊断范围，尤其是区域性流行的感染。可能需要进行结肠镜检查和组织活检来明确诊断。在我们的机构，多重 PCR、粪便中的艰难梭菌毒素和血液中的 CMV 病毒载量是诊断 SOT 患者腹泻的标准方案。主要的非感染性病因是药物，尤其是霉酚酸（一种用于维持免疫抑制的抗代谢药）和 GVHD 所致。

皮肤表现

免疫妥协患者的皮肤病变可能是局部（"由外而内"）或播散性（"由内而外"）感染的征兆。坏死性病变需警惕血管侵袭性霉菌感染所致，尽管这类病变也可见于严重的细菌感染和中性粒细胞减少症患者，病变由于毒素作用引起，但炎症反应轻微。最典型的病变是坏疽性深脓疱，这是一种由假单胞菌引起的中性粒细胞感染中毒症中的疼痛性焦痂，但也可能是其他革兰氏阴性或革兰氏阳性（金黄色葡萄球菌）细菌引起。播散性念珠菌病可表现为弥漫性斑丘疹，镰刀菌感染中毒症可伴有疼痛性结节。水疱性病变常被怀疑为疱疹病毒感染，尽管 HSV（尤其是耐药 HSV 或 HSV2）也会导致大面积溃疡病变。"孢子丝菌病样病变"（绳索状炎症结节群）可能是由孢子丝菌、金黄色葡萄球菌、诺卡菌或非典型分枝杆菌引起的。非感染性病因也很常见，如药疹、原发性皮肤癌（SOT 之后的最常见恶性肿瘤）、皮肤转移和白血病性皮肤病、GVHD、嗜中性小汗腺炎和 Sweet 综合征（发热性嗜中性细胞皮肤病，是肿瘤和化疗的一种炎症反应，最好用皮质类固醇治疗）。为了准确诊断，通常需要进行皮肤组织活检和培养。

不明原因发热

免疫妥协宿主出现持续发热且无明确病因或任何局部体征或症状，是一种相对常见的临床情况。病史和体格检查通常会发现一些细微的体征或症状，这些体征或症状是进一步诊断不可或缺的依据。密切关注口腔（图 17.4）、皮肤和会阴区域至关重要，因为每个部位都可能提供容易被忽视的线索。先进的实验室检测（如细胞外游离 DNA 测序，这是一种新兴技术，可检测和识别临

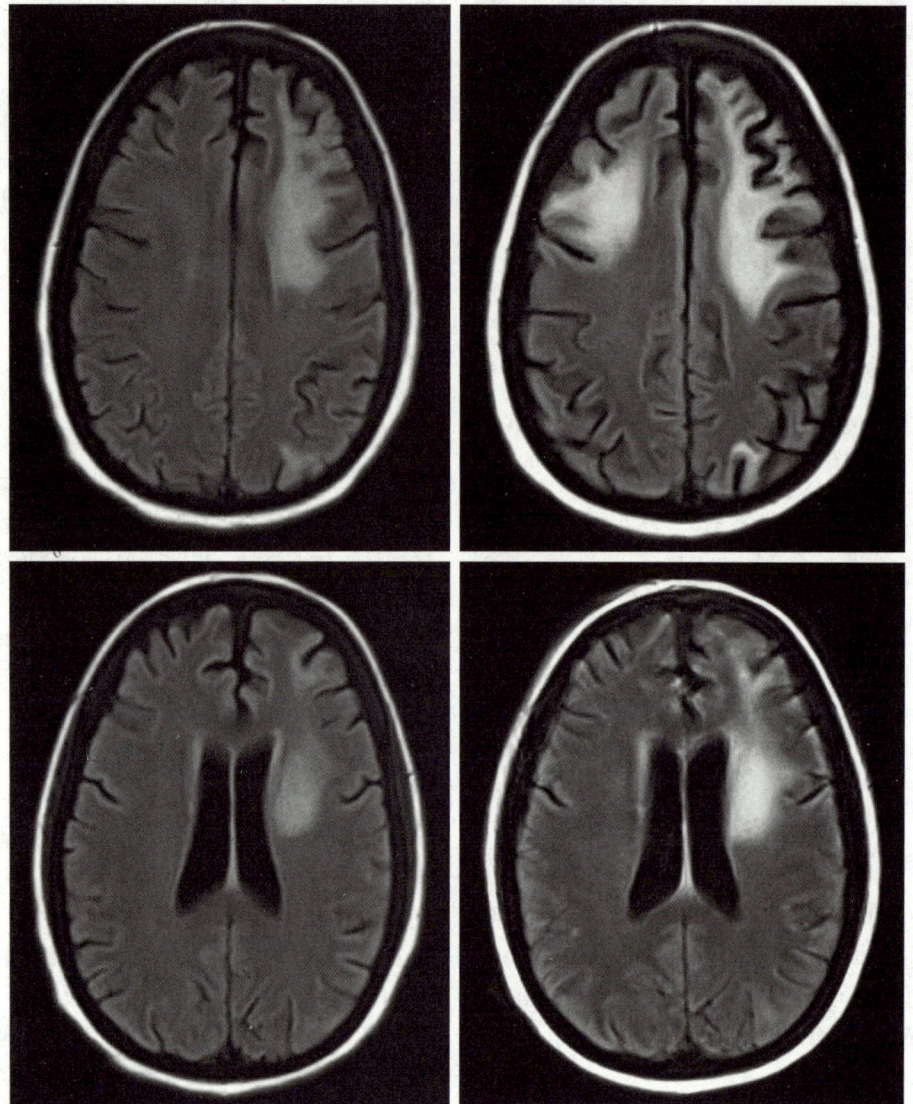

Fig. 17.3 Progressive multifocal encephalopathy (PML) in an immunocompromised patient with severe combined immunodeficiency (SCID) and autoimmune hemolytic anemia requiring many cycles of rituximab and high-dose corticosteroids. MRI shows significant progression of white matter abnormalities after 3 months.

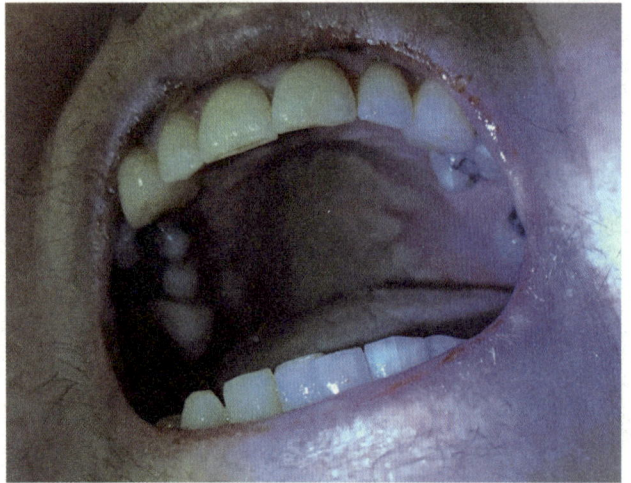

Fig. 17.4 Oral lesions in an HCT recipient with GVHD on high-dose steroids who developed disseminated HSV1 infection with fulminant hepatitis.

imaging studies (positron emission tomography-PET) may be useful adjuncts depending on the clinical scenario.

DIAGNOSIS

The pace and breadth of diagnostic testing is best driven by the pace and severity of a patient's underlying illness. Although there is a vast number of potential pathogens that may be the cause of an individual's presenting illness, the history the patient gives along with their physical examination is usually enough to dramatically narrow the differential diagnosis. Although most patients present with a single unifying diagnosis, it is not uncommon for immunocompromised patients to present with multiple ongoing processes. Therefore, we favor a structured approach, frequently revisiting the initial or new clinical manifestations (see Fig. 17.1).

Host Considerations

First, one should understand the host, mainly the immune deficits specific to the individual patient: How long has the patient been

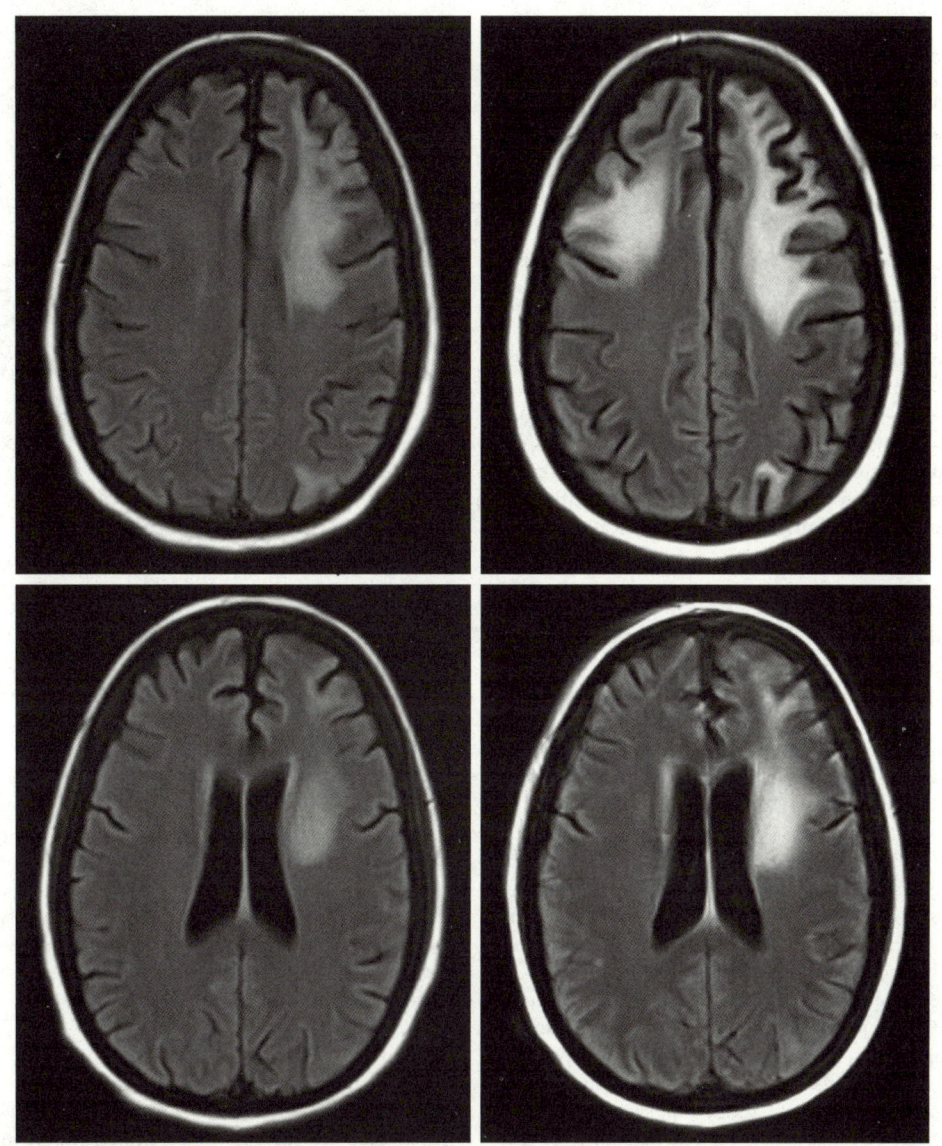

图 17.3 一名患有重症联合免疫缺陷（SCID）和自身免疫性溶血性贫血的免疫妥协患者出现进行性多灶性脑病（PML），需要接受多个周期的利妥昔单抗和大剂量皮质类固醇治疗。3 个月后，MRI 显示白质异常明显恶化

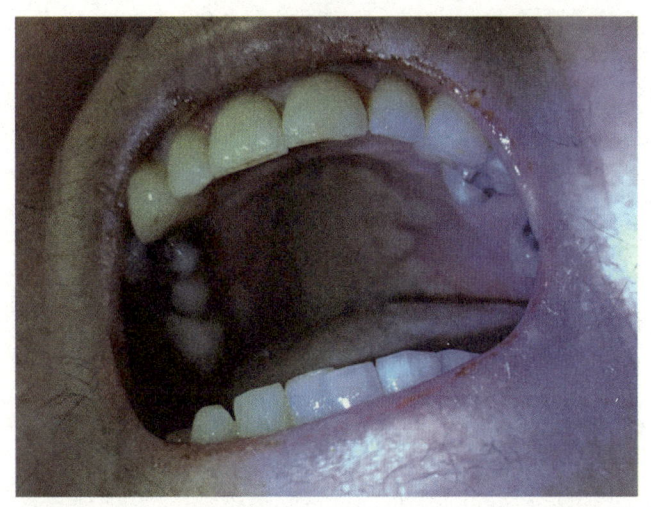

图 17.4 一名 HCT 患者的口腔病变。该患者因 GVHD 接受大剂量类固醇治疗后出现了播散性 HSV1 感染合并暴发性肝炎

床样本中的非人类 DNA 片段）和影像学检查（PET）可能是有用的辅助手段，具体应取决于临床情况。

诊断

诊断检测的速度和广度最好取决于患者潜在疾病的进展速度和严重程度。虽然有大量的潜在病原体可能是导致患者发病的原因，但患者提供的病史和体格检查通常足以大大缩小鉴别诊断的范围。虽然大多数患者只有单一的诊断，但免疫妥协的患者出现多种持续性病变的情况并不少见。因此，我们倾向于采用结构化方法，经常重新审视最初或新出现的临床表现（图 17.1）。

宿主注意事项

首先，应该了解宿主，主要是患者个体特有的免疫缺陷：患者中性粒细胞减少持续多久了？在中性粒细胞减少期间接触过哪些潜在病原体？多久前进行的

neutropenic and what potential pathogens has the patient been exposed to while neutropenic? How long has it been since SOT and what is the immunosuppression? For HCT recipients, are they pre- or post-engraftment, do they have GVHD, and what immunosuppressive medications are they on? What prophylactic antimicrobials are they taking, and for how long? What previous chemotherapy have they received? Previous and concomitant opportunistic infections often speak for the host.

Syndrome Considerations

Next, one identifies the syndrome using presenting complaints. Often there is a single clinical syndrome such as pneumonia or diarrhea. At other times, the signs and symptoms are less focal, and instead the presenting syndrome may simply be fever and fatigue; more than one clinical syndrome can be present. One structured way to construct a broad differential diagnosis for the host and the syndrome is to first consider infectious versus noninfectious causes and then build a differential diagnosis by pathogen kingdom (bacterial, fungal, viral, parasitic) and noninfectious causes (underlying disease, GVHD, medication toxicities, unusual causes) (see Fig. 17.1).

Laboratory Testing

In immunocompromised hosts, direct tests for pathogens (antigen or PCR-based testing) are much more useful than antibody assays, which mainly indicate past exposure, and because the measured immune response may be absent. Fungal markers are components of the fungal cell wall that can be detected in blood or other body fluids and help make the diagnosis of fungal infections. The most commonly used are serum and CSF cryptococcal antigen, serum, bronchoalveolar lavage (BAL) or CSF *Aspergillus* galactomannan, and serum or CSF 1,3-β-D-glucan, which is a broad fungal marker that can aid in the diagnosis of invasive aspergillosis, candidiasis, and pneumocystis pneumonia. However, fungal markers can be falsely elevated (e.g., false-positive 1,3-β-D-glucan in patients receiving hemodialysis or intravenous immunoglobulin [IVIG]) and should be interpreted in context. Peripheral blood cultures (including standard bacterial cultures and those facilitating growth of acid-fast bacilli and fungi) and cultures from more invasive procedures (BAL) may provide a diagnosis and also give a measure of antimicrobial susceptibility. Invasive tissue biopsy may at times be necessary for a definitive diagnosis and to help differentiate between colonization and infection.

Diagnostic Imaging

Imaging studies are also important in the diagnostic process. As with laboratory testing, the lack of inflammation can lead to misleading imaging findings (e.g., relatively normal abdominal imaging despite ongoing acalculous cholecystitis). Some findings can be suggestive of specific diagnoses when interpreted in the context of a specific syndrome in an at-risk immunocompromised host (e.g., the halo sign [ground-glass opacities surrounding a pulmonary nodule] suggestive of invasive pulmonary aspergillosis [Fig. 17.5] versus the reversed halo sign [ground-glass opacity surrounded by a ring of consolidation] suggestive of mucormycosis).

TREATMENT

General Principles

Choosing an appropriate empiric treatment regimen for an immunocompromised patient can be challenging. Waiting for test results may not be wise given the potentially rapid progression of infection in this population. Medication toxicities and drug-drug interactions

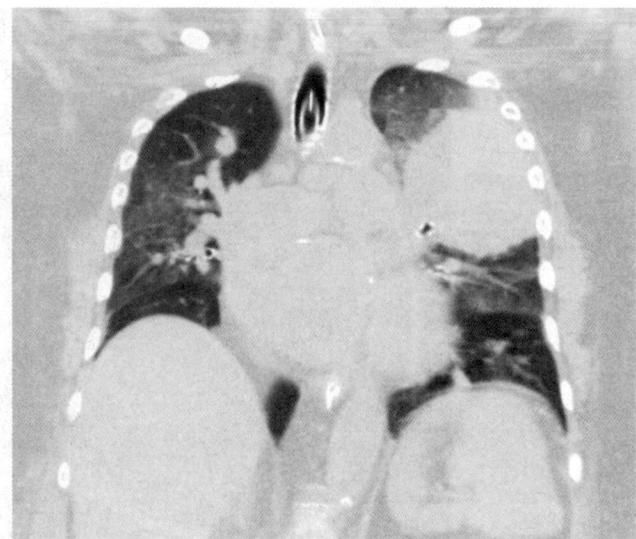

Fig. 17.5 Invasive aspergillosis in a patient receiving high-dose corticosteroids. Chest CT shows dense consolidation and surrounding "halo sign" (i.e., hazy, ground-glass-like opacities surrounding a nodule or mass), which represents hemorrhage and is typically seen in invasive aspergillosis. Blood and BAL cultures grew *A. fumigatus*; the value of *Aspergillus* antigen (galactomannan) in the blood was great than the assay cut off.

(DDI) are often a determining factor in the clinical outcome. Early and aggressive treatment is often necessary, though given the breadth of potential infectious etiologies, treating every possible pathogen is not feasible. Instead, when considering empiric treatment, the unlikeliness of a specific diagnosis should be balanced against the potential consequences of not treating. As a rule, broad coverage is in order while the patient's clinical presentation is unfolding, with de-escalation of therapy to prevent toxicities after further diagnoses are ruled out and as the patient improves (see Fig. 17.2).

Source Control

Control of the source of infection is imperative. In immunosuppressed patients, antimicrobials alone are often insufficient to combat infection. Given the diminished clinical reserve and lack of expected immune response, an undrained abscess or an infection due to a biofilm-forming agent on a blood stream or unremoved intravascular catheter or urinary catheter can be devastating.

Adjusting Immunosuppression

Reducing immunosuppression can be life-saving. With neutropenia in particular, granulocyte colony-stimulating factor (G-CSF) administration can help early ANC recovery. In SOT, acute rejection can develop after reducing immunosuppression, but it is very unusual to have simultaneous acute rejection and overwhelming infection given the polarization of an already impaired immune system towards fighting infection. There is also the possibility of developing immune reconstitution inflammatory syndrome (IRIS) (i.e., increased inflammation from reduction of immunosuppression), which often needs to be treated with corticosteroids. Further, some immunosuppressive medications have desirable adjuvant properties (e.g., antifungal effect of calcineurin inhibitors [CNI]). Specifically, in cryptococcal infections, CNI discontinuation leads to increased risk for IRIS and unfavorable outcomes. Immunosuppression adjustments are thus individualized. Reinstitution of immunosuppressive therapy may be indicated as infection resolves.

SOT？免疫抑制情况如何？对于 HCT 患者，他们处于移植前还是移植后状态？是否患有 GVHD？正在服用哪些免疫抑制药物？正在使用哪些预防性抗菌药物？使用了多长时间？既往接受过哪些化疗？既往和并发的机会性感染往往代表了宿主的病情。

综合征注意事项

其次，根据出现的主诉确定综合征。通常只有一种临床综合征，如肺炎或腹泻。有时，症状和体征不那么集中，而表现出的综合征可能仅仅是发热和乏力；临床综合征可能不止一种。对宿主和综合征进行广泛鉴别诊断的一种结构化方法是首先考虑是感染性还是非感染性病因，然后根据病原体种类（细菌、真菌、病毒、寄生虫）和非感染性病因（基础疾病、GVHD、药物毒性、少见病因）进行鉴别诊断（见图 17.1）。

实验室检查

在免疫妥协宿主中，直接检测病原体（抗原或基于 PCR 的检测）要比抗体检测有用得多，因为抗体检测主要反映既往暴露情况，而且其检测的免疫反应可能缺失。真菌标志物是指可在血液或其他体液中检测到并有助于诊断真菌感染的真菌细胞壁成分。最常用的真菌标志物有血清和 CSF 的隐球菌抗原，血清、支气管肺泡灌洗液（BAL）或 CSF 的曲霉菌半乳甘露聚糖，以及血清或 CSF 的 1,3-β-D- 葡聚糖。1,3-β-D- 葡聚糖是一种广泛的真菌标志物，有助于诊断侵袭性曲霉菌病、念珠菌病和肺孢子虫肺炎。然而，真菌标志物可能会出现假性升高［例如，接受血液透析或静脉注射免疫球蛋白（IVIg）的患者会出现 1,3-β-D- 葡聚糖假阳性］，因此应根据具体情况进行解释。外周血培养（包括标准细菌培养、抗酸分枝杆菌培养和真菌培养）和更具侵入性操作所得标本（如 BAL）的培养可提供诊断依据，也可用于检测病原体的抗菌药物敏感性。有时，侵入性组织活检可能是确诊和帮助区分定植与感染所必需的。

诊断性影像学检查

影像学检查在诊断过程中也很重要。与实验室检查一样，缺乏炎症也会导致误导性的影像学检查结果（例如，腹部影像学检查结果无明显异常而无结石胆囊炎持续存在）。如果结合高危免疫妥协宿主的特定综合征进行分析，一些影像学检查结果可能提示特定诊断，例如晕征（围绕在一肺部结节周围的磨玻璃影）提示侵袭性肺曲霉病（图17.5），而反晕征（磨玻璃影被一实性环包绕）提示毛霉病。

治疗

一般原则

为免疫妥协患者选择适当的经验性治疗方案可能颇具挑战性。鉴于该人群的感染可能进展迅速，等待

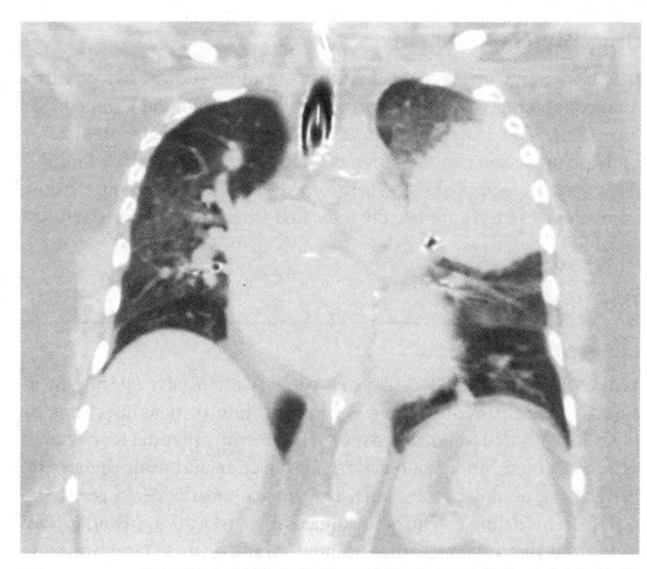

图 17.5　一名接受大剂量皮质类固醇治疗的患者发生侵袭性曲霉病。胸部 CT 显示致密实变影，周围有"晕征"（即围绕在一结节或肿块周围的模糊磨玻璃影）。该征象表明存在出血，是侵袭性曲霉病的典型表现。血液和 BAL 培养均检出曲霉菌，血液中曲霉菌抗原（半乳糖甘露聚糖）含量高于检测临界值

检测结果可能不是明智之举。药物毒性和药物相互作用（DDI）通常是影响临床结局的决定性因素。鉴于潜在感染性致病因素广泛，早期、积极的治疗通常是有必要的，但是覆盖每一种可能的病原体并不可行。在考虑经验性治疗方案时，实则应权衡某一病原体排除诊断的把握度和不治疗的潜在后果。一般来说，当患者逐渐出现临床表现时，应采用广谱治疗方案，然后随着进一步排除诊断、患者病情好转，治疗方案应降阶梯以防止药物毒副反应（见图 17.2）。

感染源控制

控制感染源是当务之急。对于免疫妥协患者，仅靠抗菌药物往往不足以对抗感染。由于临床储备减少且缺乏预期免疫应答，一处未引流的脓肿，或由血流中生物膜形成介质或未拔除的血管内导管、导尿管导致的感染对于免疫妥协患者均可能是毁灭性的。

调整免疫抑制

减少免疫抑制可以挽救生命。尤其是在中性粒细胞减少的情况下，使用粒细胞集落刺激因子（G-CSF）有助于 ANC 尽早恢复。在 SOT 中，减少免疫抑制后可能会出现急性排斥反应，但急性排斥反应和严重感染同时出现的情况非常罕见，因为受损的免疫系统的极化方向有利于对抗感染。这种情况下还有可能出现免疫重建炎症综合征（IRIS）（即因免疫抑制减少而导致炎症加重），通常需要使用皮质类固醇进行治疗。此外，部分免疫抑制剂具有一些理想的辅助作用，如钙调磷酸酶抑制剂（CNI）的抗真菌作用。具体来说，在隐球菌感染中，停用 CNI 会导致 IRIS 风险增加和预后不良。因此，免疫抑制的调整需要因人而异。随着感染的缓解，可能需要恢复免疫抑制治疗。

Drug-Drug Interactions

It is imperative to check for DDI with immunosuppressive or other medications every time any antimicrobial is started and stopped (see Fig. 17.2). For instance, triazole antifungal medications predictably increase the serum concentration of CNI (via triazole-mediated inhibition of their metabolism by cytochrome P-450), and thus empiric dose adjustments of CNI are usually indicated when stopping or starting a triazole.

PREVENTION

Lifestyle Precautions

While in the hospital, neutropenic patients often have specific measures in place to reduce the risk of acquisition of new infections by ingestion (bottled water, avoidance of foods with potential for bacterial or fungal colonization), inhalation (air filtration and positive pressure ventilation, no flowers or plants, avoidance of nearby heavy construction or remodeling activities), or mucosal translocation (avoidance of hard food that can cause oral trauma). Many of these commonsense precautions can also be implemented at home. For immunocompromised patients, close contact with other individuals with viral infection should be avoided, and thorough evaluations before travel are advised.

Immunizations

The best time to give immunizations is prior to the onset of immunosuppression, which allows for the most robust immune response. Otherwise, most vaccines are administered 1 year post-transplant. Live vaccines are generally contraindicated in immunocompromised individuals, out of concern for clinical illness caused by the vaccine strain. Immunization of household contacts and health care workers is mandated.

Antimicrobial Prophylaxis

At many centers, individuals with acute leukemia undergoing induction chemotherapy and patients receiving HCT are given a fluoroquinolone (levofloxacin) and a yeast-only (fluconazole) or mold-active (voriconazole, posaconazole) triazole. Antiviral prophylaxis with acyclovir protects against reactivation of latent herpesviruses (e.g., HSV, VZV).

Fluconazole is used sometimes in liver transplant recipients and anti-*Aspergillus* prophylaxis in lung transplant recipients. Antiviral prophylaxis active against CMV ([val]ganciclovir) is given to many SOT patients. Given the potential myelotoxicity of (val)ganciclovir, alternative strategies are used to prevent CMV infection in HCT (close monitoring of viral load or alternative antivirals such as letermovir). Prophylaxis against *Pneumocystis* is indicated in SOT and HCT recipients for 6 to 12 months after transplant and in patients receiving prolonged high-dose corticosteroids. Some HCT recipients with severe GVHD receive antibacterial prophylaxis active against encapsulated bacteria and antifungal prophylaxis.

SPECIFIC PATHOGENS

HSV and VZV

HSV1/2 cause mainly mucocutaneous disease (oral or genital lesions), but in immunocompromised patients they can more frequently disseminate, cause CNS infection, multiorgan failure, predominantly fulminant hepatitis, and protean manifestations (e.g., pneumonia) (see Fig. 17.4). VZV can also cause disseminated disease and various CNS syndromes, including vasculitis. The treatment of choice for severe infections is intravenous acyclovir. (Val)acyclovir and (val)ganciclovir are effective prophylaxis; (val)acyclovir administration in very immunosuppressed patients can lead to resistance, mostly in HSV1. Resistant herpetic infections are treated with foscarnet.

CMV

Similar to other herpesviruses, CMV remains dormant after primary infection and can reactivate, causing disease. The highest-risk patients are SOT recipients who are not immune to CMV and receive it from the donor (D+/R−), as well as lymphocyte-depleted and D−/R+ HCT recipients (because they adopt the immune system of their donor). CMV causes fever and infectious mononucleosis-like symptoms and signs, gastrointestinal disease (esophagitis, gastritis, colitis) and pneumonia (mostly in lung and HC transplant recipients). Retinitis is rare in HIV-negative patients. Treatment of choice is (val)ganciclovir and foscarnet for resistant CMV. Multidrug-resistant CMV is rare but an emerging threat. Prophylaxis with (val)ganciclovir is used in most SOT recipients for the first few months after transplant. The main toxicity of (val)ganciclovir is bone marrow suppression, whereas foscarnet can cause nephrotoxicity and electrolyte abnormalities.

Other Herpesviruses

EBV can manifest as lytic infection (directly caused by proliferating virus, such as infectious mononucleosis or CNS infection). However, it is mainly associated with post-transplant lymphoproliferative disorder (PTLD) (progressive transformation of EBV-infected B-lymphocytes to lymphoma). Treatment is reduction of immunosuppression to allow for cytotoxic T-cell surveillance of the abnormal EBV-infected B cells. For the same reason, rituximab is often used early on, even preemptively with rising EBV viremia in HCT recipients.

Other pathogenic human herpesviruses include HHV-6, which typically causes CNS infection in HCT recipients (PALE: Post-transplant acute limbic encephalopathy) treated with ganciclovir or foscarnet, and HHV-8, which causes Kaposi's sarcoma.

Polyomaviruses

In addition to patients with AIDS, JC virus causes PML in a variety of hosts (SOT, HCT recipients, and patients with HM) (see Fig. 17.3). PML manifests with progressive cognitive decline, focal neurologic deficits, and characteristic MRI findings; it overall has poor prognosis. BK virus causes renal allograft dysfunction in kidney transplant recipients, hemorrhagic cystitis in HCT or (less commonly) other severely T-cell depleted individuals; BK can rarely cause PML and disseminated infection. The cornerstone of management for polyomavirus infections is decrease in immunosuppression. A promising recent approach to the management of PML and other refractory viral infections is infusion of virus-specific active T cells (adoptive immunity).

As a rule, laboratory diagnosis of viral infections in immunocompromised patients is based on detection of the virus by quantitative PCR and, sometimes, histopathology.

Candida

Candida albicans is the most common fungal pathogen in the Western world and an important commensal of the normal skin, oral, gastrointestinal, and vaginal flora. Non-albicans *Candida* species can be resistant to antifungal drugs, therefore an important threat with rising frequency in patients receiving antifungal prophylaxis. *Candida auris* has recently emerged as the first virulent fungus that exhibits multidrug resistance and the potential for nosocomial transmission, which is considered a public health emergency.

Candida species cause mucocutaneous (dermatitis, thrush, esophagitis or vaginitis) and invasive candidiasis. Neutropenia, corticosteroids, and abdominal pathology are the main risk factors. Indwelling catheters are an important source of candidemia, given the strong propensity of this organism to form biofilms (Fig. 17.6). Therefore, central line removal is strongly advised for the successful management of candidemia. Echinocandins (caspo/mica/anidulafungin) are the

药物相互作用

每次启用和停用任何抗菌药物时，都必须检查是否与免疫抑制剂或其他药物存在 DDI（见图 17.2）。例如，三唑类抗真菌药物会使 CNI 的血药浓度增加（三唑类会抑制 CNI 经细胞色素 P450 代谢），因此在停用或启用三唑类药物时，经常需要根据经验调整 CNI 的剂量。

预防

生活方式注意事项

住院期间，中性粒细胞减少症患者通常会采取特定措施降低通过摄入（饮用瓶装水、避免食用可能有细菌或真菌定植的食物）、吸入（空气过滤和正压通风、不养花种草、远离大型施工场所）或黏膜移位（避免可能损伤口腔的硬质食物）发生感染的风险。这些常识性预防措施多数也可以在家里实施。对于免疫妥协患者，应避免与其他病毒感染者密切接触，并建议在旅行前进行全面评估。

免疫接种

免疫接种的最佳时机是在免疫抑制开始之前，这样可以最大限度增强免疫反应。否则，大多数疫苗应在移植后 1 年接种。出于对疫苗株引发疾病的担忧，免疫妥协者一般禁用活疫苗。免疫妥协者的家庭接触者和医护人员也必须接种疫苗。

预防性抗菌治疗

在许多医疗机构，接受诱导化疗的急性白血病患者和接受 HCT 的患者会服用氟喹诺酮类药物（如左氧氟沙星）和针对酵母菌（如氟康唑）或针对霉菌（如伏立康唑、泊沙康唑）的三唑类药物。预防性使用抗病毒药物阿昔洛韦，防止潜伏的疱疹病毒（如 HSV、VZV）感染再激活。

肝移植患者有时会使用氟康唑，肺移植患者则会使用预防性抗曲霉。许多 SOT 患者会预防性使用对 CMV 有活性的抗病毒药物［如（缬）更昔洛韦］。鉴于（缬）更昔洛韦具有潜在骨髓毒性，因此使用其他方案预防 HCT 患者发生 CMV 感染（密切监测病毒载量，或使用其他抗病毒药物，如来特莫韦）。SOT 和 HCT 患者移植后 6～12 个月，以及长期接受大剂量皮质类固醇治疗的患者应预防肺孢子虫感染。一些发生严重 GVHD 的 HCT 患者应接受针对有荚膜菌的抗菌药物预防治疗和抗真菌预防治疗。

特定病原体

HSV 和 VZV

HSV1/2 主要引起皮肤黏膜疾病（口腔或生殖器病变），但在免疫妥协患者中，HSV1/2 感染通常更为播散，可引起 CNS 感染、以暴发性肝炎为主的多器官功能衰竭，以及多变的表现（如肺炎）（见图 17.4）。VZV 也可引起播散性疾病和各种中枢神经系统 CNS 综合征，包括血管炎。严重感染的首选治疗方法是静脉注射阿昔洛韦。（缬）阿昔洛韦和（缬）更昔洛韦是有效的预防药物；在免疫抑制非常严重的患者中使用（缬）阿昔洛韦会导致耐药，以 HSV1 为主。耐药的疱疹病毒感染可使用膦甲酸治疗。

CMV

与其他疱疹病毒类似，原发感染后 CMV 会保持休眠状态，并可重新激活导致疾病。风险最高的患者是对 CMV 没有免疫力并从供者（D+/R−）获得 CMV 的 SOT 受者，以及去除淋巴细胞且 D−/R+ 的 HCT 受者（因为他们接受了供者的免疫系统）。CMV 会导致发热、传染性单核细胞增多症样症状和体征、胃肠道疾病（食管炎、胃炎、结肠炎）和肺炎（主要发生在肺移植和 HC 移植受者中）。HIV 阴性的患者很少发生视网膜炎。耐药 CMV 的首选治疗药物有（缬）更昔洛韦和膦甲酸。耐多药 CMV 虽然罕见，但却是一种新出现的威胁。大多数 SOT 受者在移植后的头几个月都要使用（缬）更昔洛韦进行预防。（缬）更昔洛韦的主要毒性是骨髓抑制，而膦甲酸可引起肾毒性和电解质紊乱。

其他疱疹病毒

EBV 可表现为裂解性感染（直接由增殖的病毒引起，如传染性单核细胞增多症或 CNS 感染）。但是，EBV 主要与移植后淋巴增殖性疾病（PTLD）（受 EBV 感染的 B 淋巴细胞进行性转化为淋巴瘤）相关。治疗方法是减少免疫抑制，让细胞毒性 T 细胞对异常的 EBV 感染 B 细胞进行监控。出于同样的原因，通常会在早期使用利妥昔单抗，甚至在 HCT 受者的 EBV 病毒血症上升期预先使用。

其他致病性的人类疱疹病毒包括 HHV-6，它通常会导致接受更昔洛韦或膦甲酸治疗的 HCT 受者出现 CNS 感染，如移植后急性边缘系统脑病（PALE）；还有会导致卡波西肉瘤的 HHV-8。

多瘤病毒

除了 AIDS 患者，JC 病毒还会导致多种宿主（SOT、HCT 受者和 HM 患者）出现 PML（见图 17.3）。PML 表现为进行性认知能力下降、局灶性神经功能障碍，并有特征性 MRI 表现，总体预后不良。BK 病毒会导致肾移植患者出现同种异基因移植肾功能障碍，以及 HCT 或（较少见）其他严重 T 细胞去除者出现出血性膀胱炎。BK 病毒很少会导致 PML 和播散性感染。治疗多瘤病毒感染的基础是减少免疫抑制。通过输注活化的病毒特异性 T 细胞（过继免疫）治疗 PML 和其他难治性病毒感染是一种新晋、颇具前景的疗法。通常，免疫妥协患者病毒感染的实验室诊断是通过定量 PCR，有时通过组织病理学，检出病毒。

念珠菌

白念珠菌是西方世界最常见的真菌病原体，也是正常皮肤、口腔、胃肠道和阴道菌群的重要共生菌。非白念珠菌可对抗真菌药物产生耐药性，因此成为接受预防性抗真菌治疗的患者中日益常见的重要威胁。最近出现的耳念珠菌是第一种表现出多重耐药性，并可能造成院内传播的烈性真菌，被视为公共卫生紧急事件。

treatment of choice for severe invasive candidiasis, except for urinary, eye or CNS infections given their poor penetration in these compartments. Amphotericin-B and azoles have activity against most *Candida* species; the latter can be used for mild infections and as step-down oral therapy.

Cryptococcus

Cryptococcus can cause meningitis, encephalitis, pneumonia, sepsis-like syndrome, and atypical infections (such as cellulitis) in patients with significant T-cell immunosuppression (SOT or HCT recipients, lymphoma patients). Diagnosis is made by culture, detection of cryptococcal antigen in blood or CSF, and histopathology. Severe infections, including meningitis, are treated with amphotericin-B and flucytosine, followed by many months of fluconazole. Decrease in immunosuppression without discontinuation of CNI should be individualized. Fluconazole and other azoles, often used as antifungal prophylaxis in immunosuppressed patients, decrease the risk for cryptococcosis.

Aspergillus

Unlike *Candida*, molds such as *Aspergillus* and the Mucorales are not part of normal flora but inhaled from the environment. In the setting of impaired immune (especially neutrophil) defenses, they grow and invade tissues, causing invasive sinopulmonary or even disseminated mold infections. Individuals with prolonged neutropenia, those receiving high-dose corticosteroids, and lung transplant recipients are the highest risk groups, especially with exposure to high inocula (e.g., construction). *Aspergillus* can often be a colonizer (saprophytic aspergillosis), without causing invasive disease, such as in the absence of radiographic abnormalities, or as an isolated aspergilloma (Fig. 17.7). Fungal markers (*Aspergillus* galactomannan, 1,3-β-D-glucan), with careful review of imaging findings (see Fig. 17.5), host factors, and clinical presentation, can help differentiate between colonization and infection.

An interesting entity at the intersection of saprophytic and invasive disease is chronic necrotizing (also known as cavitary or semi-invasive) aspergillosis. It affects "immunomodulated" patients, such as elderly patients with chronic obstructive pulmonary disease (COPD), often with negative fungal markers but positive anti-*Aspergillus* antibodies, and warrants antifungal treatment (Fig. 17.8).

The treatment for the majority of aspergilloses is voriconazole, with close follow-up of drug levels and dose adjustments of other medications that have significant DDI. Alternative agents include isavuconazole, amphotericin, or the echinocandins; the latter are static and not preferred as monotherapy.

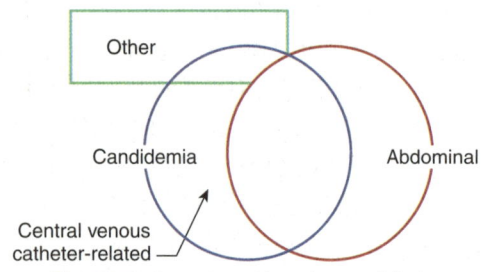

Fig. 17.6 Spectrum of invasive candidiasis.

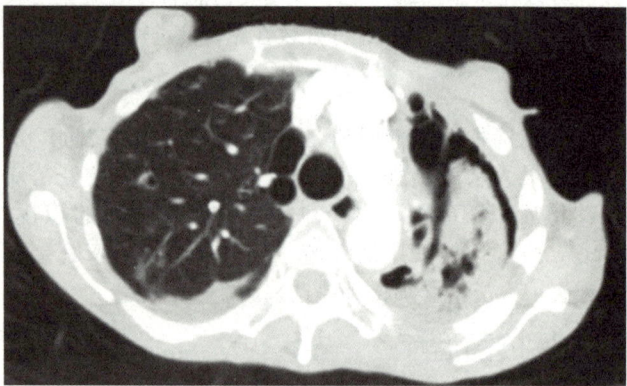

Fig. 17.8 Chronic cavitary aspergillosis of the left lung in a patient with severe COPD. *A. fumigatus* antibodies were positive, galactomannan negative, BAL cultures grew *A. fumigatus*. The lesions on CT progressed over months.

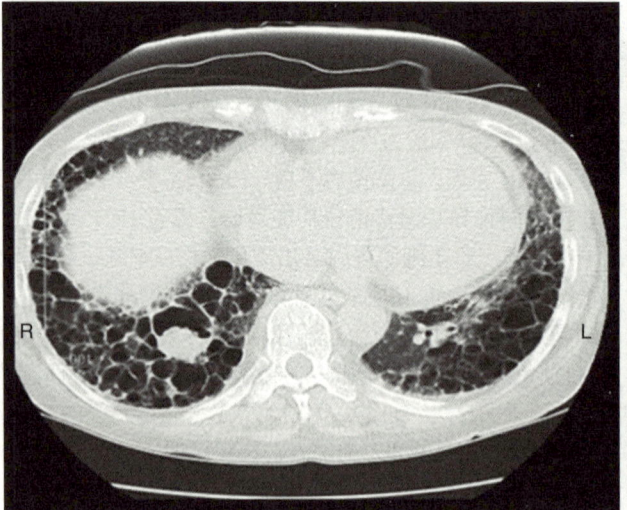
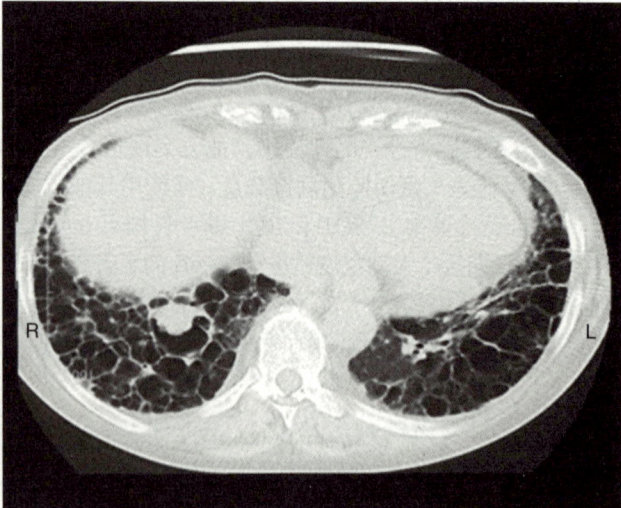

Fig. 17.7 Aspergilloma (saprophytic aspergillosis) in a patient with emphysema. Chest CT shows a mobile mass (*Left:* supine, *right:* prone) within a small cavity.

念珠菌可引起皮肤黏膜（皮炎、鹅口疮、食管炎或阴道炎）和侵袭性念珠菌病。中性粒细胞减少症、皮质类固醇和腹部病变是主要的危险因素。留置导管是念珠菌血症的重要来源，因为这种病原体极易形成生物膜（图17.6）。因此，为了成功治疗念珠菌血症，强烈建议拔除中心静脉导管。棘白菌素类药物（卡泊芬净/米卡芬净/阿尼芬净）是治疗严重侵袭性念珠菌病的首选药物，但泌尿系统、眼部或CNS感染除外，因为这些药物在这些部位的渗透性较差。两性霉素B和唑类药物对大多数念珠菌属都有疗效；后者可用于轻度感染和口服降级治疗。

隐球菌

在T细胞免疫严重抑制的患者（SOT或HCT患者、淋巴瘤患者）中，隐球菌可引起脑膜炎、脑炎、肺炎、感染中毒症样综合征和非典型感染（如蜂窝织炎）。可通过培养、检测血液或CSF中隐球菌抗原以及组织病理学诊断。严重感染（包括脑膜炎）可使用两性霉素B和氟胞嘧啶治疗，然后使用氟康唑治疗数月。在不停用CNI的情况下减少免疫抑制应因人而异。氟康唑和其他唑类药物常用于免疫妥协患者的预防性抗真菌治疗，可降低隐球菌病的风险。

曲霉菌

与念珠菌不同，曲霉菌和毛霉菌等霉菌不是正常菌群的一部分，而是从环境中吸入的。在免疫（尤其是中性粒细胞）防御功能受损的情况下，它们会生长并侵入组织，引起侵袭性鼻窦肺感染或甚至播散性霉菌感染。长期中性粒细胞减少症患者、接受大剂量皮质类固醇治疗的患者和肺移植患者是高危人群，尤其是暴露于高接种量的人群（如建筑工人）。曲霉菌通常可成为定植菌（腐生曲霉病），而不引起侵袭性疾病，例如没有影像学异常，或表现为孤立的肺曲霉球（图17.7）。真菌标志物（曲霉菌半乳甘露聚糖、1,3-β-D-葡聚糖）以及对影像学检查结果（见图17.5）、宿主因素和临床表现的仔细审查有助于鉴别定植和感染。

慢性坏死性（也称为空洞性或半侵袭性）曲霉病是一种介于腐生性和侵袭性疾病之间的特殊疾病。它影响"免疫调节"患者，例如患有慢性阻塞性肺疾病（COPD）的老年患者。这些患者的真菌标志物常为阴性，而抗曲霉菌抗体为阳性，需要抗真菌治疗（图17.8）。

大多数曲霉病的治疗方法是用伏立康唑，同时密切随访血药浓度，并调整具有明显DDI的其他药物的剂量。替代药物包括艾沙康唑、两性霉素或棘白菌素；后者静态抑菌，不宜单用。

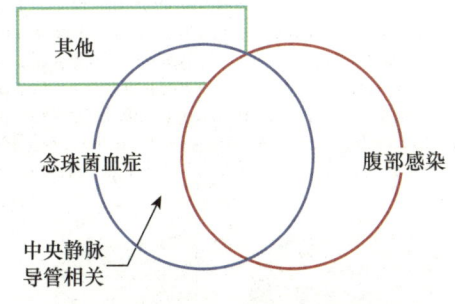

图17.6 侵袭性念珠菌病疾病谱

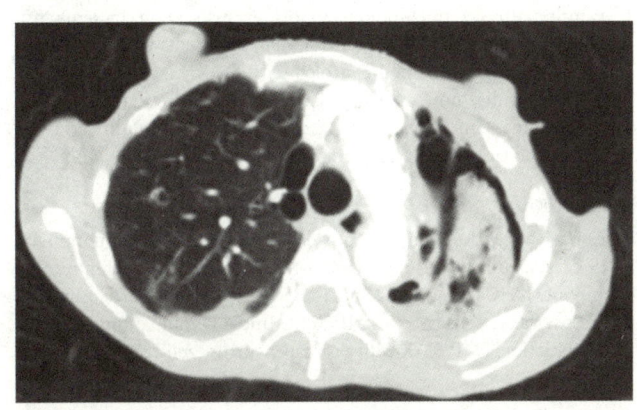

图17.8 一名严重COPD的患者左肺出现慢性空洞性曲霉病。该患者烟曲霉抗体呈阳性，半乳甘露聚糖呈阴性，BAL培养检出烟曲霉。CT示病灶在数月内不断进展

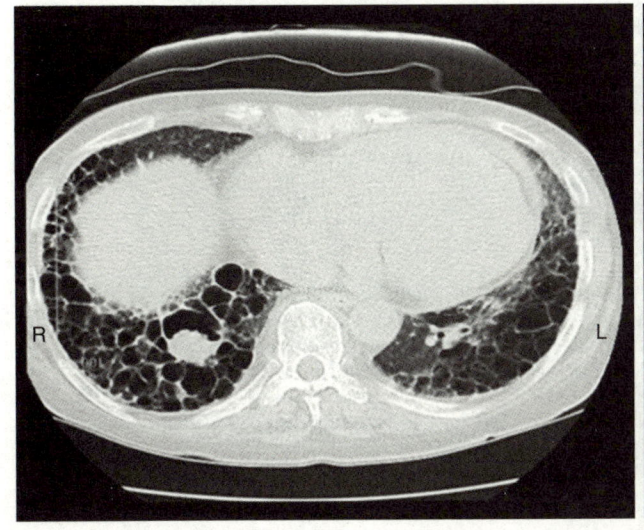

图17.7 一名肺气肿患者的肺曲菌球（腐生曲菌病）。胸部CT显示小空洞内一个可移动的肿块（左图：仰卧位，右图：俯卧位）

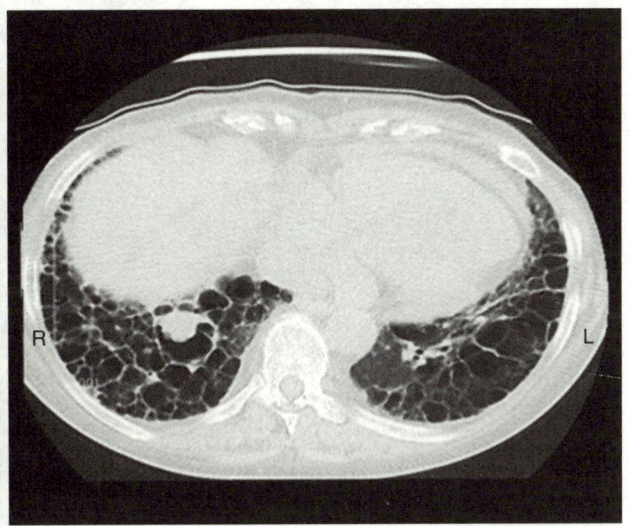

Mucorales and Other Fungi

Clinical syndromes caused by molds of the order Mucorales (e.g., *Rhizopus, Mucor, Rhizomucor, Cunninghamella, Lichtheimia,* and *Apophysomyces* spp) are rare, aggressive infections with the potential for rapid progression and high mortality. The most common manifestations are sinus and pulmonary infections in neutropenic patients, those receiving high-dose corticosteroids, diabetics, and even immunocompetent individuals when there is high inoculum exposure (e.g., in natural disasters and trauma with significant soil inhalation or contamination of deep wounds). These organisms are highly angio-invasive, and necrotic tissue is an important clue on physical exam. The "reversed halo" sign on CT is considered suggestive of pulmonary mucormycosis. The Mucorales do not have significant amounts of 1,3-β-D-glucan or galactomannan, therefore fungal markers will typically be negative. In vitro culture can be challenging. Therefore, the diagnosis of mucormycoses is elusive and often made by tissue histopathology with visualization of aseptate, broad-angled hyphae. In contrast, *Aspergillus* hyphae are narrow branching at 45° angles and septate (Fig. 17.9). Surgical débridement, when possible, and timely initiation of appropriate treatment with amphotericin-B are paramount. Posaconazole and isavuconazole have activity against the Mucorales, but voriconazole and the echinocandins do not.

Immunocompromised patients are at risk for endemic infections from dimorphic fungi (histoplasmosis, blastomycosis, and coccidiomycosis); preemptive testing and/or prophylaxis might be indicated in certain geographic areas. Histoplasmosis in particular has been associated with TNF-α inhibition.

Pneumocystis infection can manifest as typical interstitial or focal ("granulomatous") pneumonia, almost exclusively in patients not receiving prophylaxis. Treatment is similar to patients with AIDS (first line: trimethoprim/sulfamethoxazole [TMP/SMX]).

Microsporidia, now classified as fungi, can cause diarrhea, CNS, and multiorgan infections (including donor-derived outbreaks), for which albendazole is the treatment of choice.

Nocardia

Nocardia species are abundant in soil and cause subacute pulmonary, CNS or skin infections in patients with impaired cellular immunity, mainly SOT/HCT recipients and those on high-dose corticosteroids. Most species are sensitive to TMP/SMX. Initial combination of at least two antibiotics (TMP/SMX with a carbapenem, linezolid or minocycline) is usually indicated given distinct susceptibilities of different *Nocardia* species. Targeted treatment should be continued for many months.

Mycobacteria

Individuals with latent tuberculosis (LTB) are at high risk for reactivation after TNF-α inhibition or T-cell immunosuppression, such as SOT/HCT. In immunosuppressed patients, active TB is often disseminated and its treatment challenging due to medication toxicities and DDI. Therefore, candidates for SOT, HCT, or TNF-α inhibitors are tested for LTB by protocol and if positive treated with isoniazid or an alternative regimen, prior to or shortly after onset of immunosuppression.

Atypical (nontuberculous) mycobacteria (NTM) cause diverse clinical syndromes, mainly pulmonary, skin, and catheter-related infections. The immune deficits predisposing to such infections are similar to TB. NTM are frequent colonizers of the respiratory tract. Treatment regimens are often complicated, with multiple toxicities and DDI; therefore, it is important to differentiate infection from colonization and treat, when indicated, in a timely manner, especially lung transplant candidates and recipients.

Parasites

Immunocompromised patients (especially heart transplant recipients) are at risk for donor-derived or reactivation of toxoplasmosis. TMP/SMX is effective prophylaxis. Toxoplasmosis can manifest as CNS lesions, pneumonia, or fever of unknown origin (FUO) and severe sepsis, the latter mainly in HCT recipients who are not on prophylaxis prior to engraftment, given concern for bone marrow suppression from TMP/SMX. Sulfamethoxazole with pyrimethamine or high-dose TMP/SMX are effective treatments.

Strongyloides hyperinfection is rare but devastating and can be recipient- or donor-derived. It develops usually weeks after onset of T-cell immunosuppression (e.g., transplant, high-dose steroids) with diarrhea, and, as the larvae translocate from the bowel and disseminate to different organs, ileus, pulmonary infiltrates, skin lesions, and gram-negative sepsis from intestinal bacterial co-translocation. Diagnosis is made by visualization of *Strongyloides* larvae in the stool, BAL or tissue. The treatment for hyperinfection is oral or parenteral veterinary ivermectin for days. Mortality is very high. Transplant candidates and donors from endemic areas are typically screened by serology (antibody) and, if positive, receive 1 to 2 days of ivermectin.

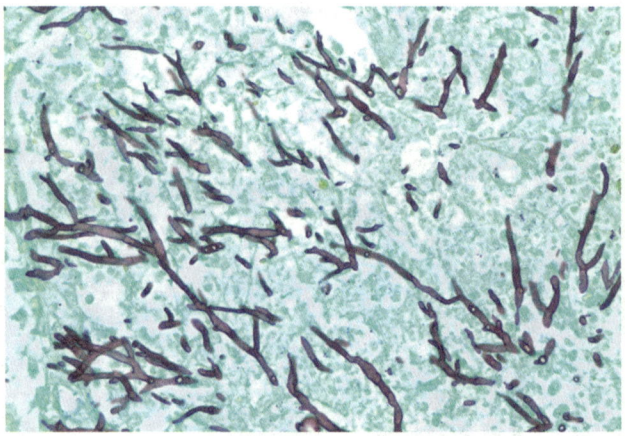 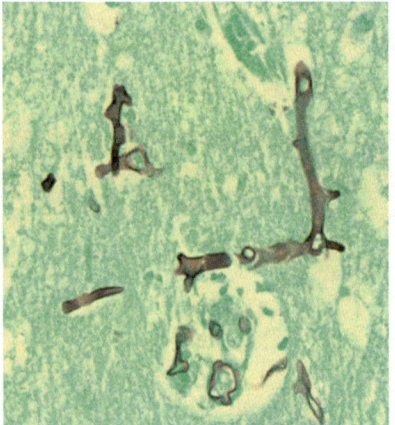

Fig. 17.9 *Aspergillus* (*left:* narrow-angled, septate) and *Lichtheimia* (*right:* wide-angled, aseptate) hyphae on Gomori-methenamine silver (GMS) stains of lung and heart tissue, respectively, from the autopsy of a patient with CLL on high-dose steroids. In immunocompromised patients, Ockham's razor doesn't always apply and multiple infections can coexist. (Tsikala-Vafea M, Weibiao C, Olszewski AJ, et al. Fatal mucormycosis and aspergillosis in an atypical host: What do we know about mixed invasive mold infections? Case Rep Infect Dis 2020:8812528, 2020.)

毛霉菌和其他真菌

由毛霉菌目真菌（例如，根霉、毛霉、根毛霉、小克银汉霉、横梗霉和节顶霉）引起的临床综合征是一种罕见的侵袭性感染，病情发展迅速，死亡率高。最常见的表现是中性粒细胞减少患者、接受大剂量皮质类固醇治疗患者、糖尿病患者，甚至免疫健全个体在大剂量暴露时（如自然灾害和创伤中大量吸入土壤或深部伤口污染）发生鼻窦和肺部感染。这些微生物具有高度血管侵袭性，坏死组织是体格检查的重要线索。CT上的"反晕"征被认为提示肺毛霉菌病。毛霉菌并不富含1,3-β-D-葡聚糖或半乳甘露聚糖，因此真菌标志物通常呈阴性。其体外培养也具有挑战性。因此，毛霉的诊断较为困难，通常通过组织病理学检查观察到无隔、钝角菌丝诊断。与此相反，曲霉菌的菌丝呈45°锐角分叉且有隔（图17.9）。有条件时进行手术清创，并及时应用适量两性霉素B进行治疗至关重要。泊沙康唑和艾沙康唑对毛霉有活性，但伏立康唑和棘白菌素对其无效。

免疫妥协患者有发生双相真菌造成的地方性感染（组织胞浆菌病、芽生菌病和球孢子菌病）的风险；在某些地区可能需要进行优先检测和（或）预防。组织胞浆菌病尤其与TNF-α抑制有关。

肺孢子菌感染可表现为典型的间质性或局灶性（"肉芽肿性"）肺炎，几乎只发生在未接受预防的患者身上。治疗方法与AIDS患者所用方案类似（一线治疗：TMP/SMX）。

微孢子虫现在被归类为真菌，可引起腹泻、CNS和多器官感染（包括供体源性暴发感染），阿苯达唑是治疗这些疾病的首选药物。

诺卡菌

诺卡菌在土壤中含量丰富，可导致细胞免疫受损患者发生亚急性肺部、CNS或皮肤感染，其中以SOT/HCT患者和使用大剂量皮质类固醇的患者为主。大多数诺卡菌种对TMP/SMX敏感。鉴于不同诺卡菌种的药物敏感性存在差异，初始治疗通常需要联合使用至少两种抗生素（TMP/SMX联合一种碳青霉烯类、利奈唑胺或米诺环素）。针对性治疗应持续数月。

分枝杆菌

进行TNF-α抑制或T细胞免疫抑制（如SOT/HCT）后，潜伏性结核（LTB）感染者有很高的再激活风险。在免疫抑制患者中，活动性TB往往会播散，而且由于药物毒性和DDI，其治疗具有挑战性。因此，即将进行SOT、HCT或使用TNF-α抑制剂的患者都要按照规范进行LTB检测，如果检测结果呈阳性，则应在免疫抑制开始之前或开始后不久使用异烟肼或替代方案进行治疗。

非典型（非结核）分枝杆菌（NTM）会引起多种临床综合征，主要是肺部、皮肤和导管相关感染。导致此类感染的免疫缺陷与导致TB的类似。NTM是呼吸道的常见定植菌。NTM感染的治疗方案通常比较复杂，并具有多种药物毒性作用和DDI；因此，必须鉴别感染和定植，并在必要时及时治疗，尤其对于肺移植候选者和受者。

寄生虫

免疫妥协患者（尤其是心脏移植受者）有从供体中感染弓形虫或弓形虫病再活化的风险。TMP/SMX是有效的预防药物。弓形虫病可表现为CNS病变、肺炎、不明原因发热（FUO）和严重感染中毒症，后者主要发生在移植前出于对TMP/SMX骨髓抑制副作用的顾虑而未进行预防治疗的HCT患者中。磺胺甲噁唑联合乙胺嘧啶或大剂量TMP/SMX是有效的治疗方法。

类圆线虫超感染虽然罕见，但却颇具破坏性，受者直接感染或供者来源感染均可见。该疾病通常发生于T细胞免疫抑制（如移植、使用大剂量类固醇）数周后，伴有腹泻。并且，随着幼虫从肠道迁移、播散至其他器官，患者会出现回肠、肺部浸润、皮肤病变以及因肠道菌群易位而引起的革兰氏阴性菌感染中毒症。可通过在粪便、BAL或组织中观察到类圆线虫幼虫进行诊断。治疗超感染的方法是口服或注射兽用伊维菌素，疗程为数天。该疾病死亡率非常高。来自流行地区的移植候选者和供者通常要接受血清学（抗体）筛查，如果呈阳性，则要接受1～2天的伊维菌素治疗。

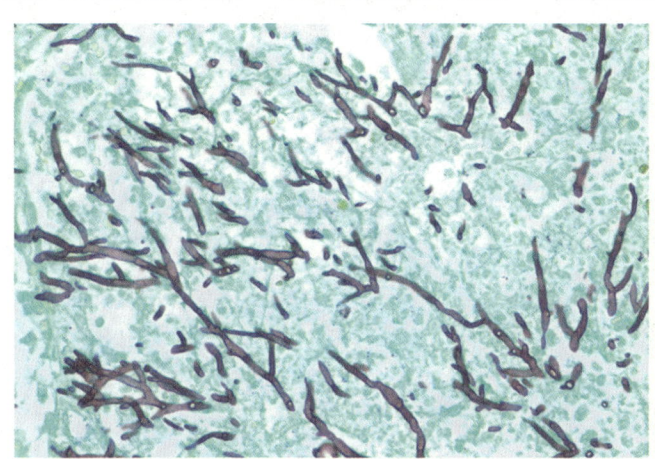
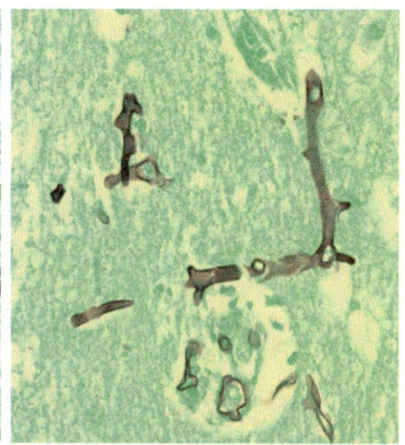

图17.9 一名接受大剂量类固醇治疗的CLL患者的尸检结果。肺组织和心脏组织的嗜银染色（GMS）结果中分别可见曲霉菌（左图：锐角，有隔）和横梗霉（右图：钝角，无隔）菌丝。在免疫妥协患者中，奥卡姆剃刀定律有时并不适用，多种病原体感染可能同时存在（Tsikala-Vafea M, Weibiao C, Olszewski AJ, et al. Fatal mucormycosis and aspergillosis in an atypical host: What do we know about mixed invasive mold infections? Case Rep Infect Dis 2020；8812528，2020.）

Intestinal parasites *(Giardia lamblia, Entamoeba histolytica, Cryptosporidium parvum)* can cause acute or chronic diarrhea in immunocompromised patients. *Giardia* in particular affects patients with IgA deficiency. Free-living amoebas can cause severe meningoencephalitis with almost 100% mortality.

SUGGESTED READINGS

Bousfiha A, Jeddane L, Picard C, et al: The 2017 IUIS phenotypic classification for primary immunodeficiencies, J Clin Immunol (38):129–143, 2018.

Denning DW, Cadranel J, Beigelman-Aubry C, et al: Chronic pulmonary aspergillosis: rationale and clinical guidelines for diagnosis and management, Eur Respir J 47(1):45–68, 2016.

ESCMID Study Group for Infections in Compromised Hosts (ESGICH) Consensus Document on the safety of targeted and biologic therapies: an infectious diseases perspective, Clin Microbiol Infect (24), 2018, Supplement 2.

Farmakiotis D, Kontoyiannis DP: Emerging issues with diagnosis and management of fungal infections in solid organ transplant recipients, Am J Transplant 15(5):1141–1147, 2015.

Farmakiotis D, Ross J, Koo S: Chapter 201: Candida and Aspergillus. In McKean SC, Ross JJ, Dressler DD, Scheurer DB, editors: Principles and practice of hospital medicine, ed 2, McGraw-Hill, 2017, pp 1618–1624.

GarciaCadenas I, Rivera I, Martino R, et al: Patterns of infection and infection-related mortality in patients with steroid-refractory acute graft versus host disease, Bone Marrow Transplant 52(1):107–113, 2017.

Guidelines from the American Society of Transplantation Infectious Diseases Community of Practice, Clin Transplant, 2019.

Li X, Jevnikar A: Transplant immunology, West Sussex, 2016, John Wiley & Sons.

Mehta H, Malandra M, Corey S: G-CSF and GM-CSF in neutropenia, J Immunol 195(4):1341–1349, 2015.

Pizzo P: Management of patients with fever and neutropenia through the arc of time: a narrative review, Ann Intern Med 170(6):389–397, 2019.

Qian C, Wang Y, Reppel L, et al: Viral-specific T-cell transfer from HSCT donor for the treatment of viral infections or diseases after HSCT, Bone Marrow Transplant 53(2):114–122, 2018.

Simner P, Miller S, Carroll K: Understanding the promises and hurdles of metagenomic next-generation sequencing as a diagnostic tool for infectious diseases, Clin Infect Dis 66(5):778–788, 2018.

Taplitz R, Kennedy E, Bow E, et al: Antimicrobial prophylaxis for adult patients with cancer related immunosuppression: ASCO and IDSA clinical practice guideline update, J Clin Oncol 36(30):3043–3054, 2018.

肠道寄生虫（蓝氏贾第鞭毛虫、溶组织内阿米巴、小隐孢子虫）可导致免疫妥协患者发生急性或慢性腹泻。贾第虫尤其影响 IgA 缺乏患者。自由生活的阿米巴原虫可引起严重的脑膜脑炎，死亡率几乎为 100%。

推荐阅读

Bousfiha A, Jeddane L, Picard C, et al: The 2017 IUIS phenotypic classification for primary immunodeficiencies, J Clin Immunol (38):129–143, 2018.

Denning DW, Cadranel J, Beigelman-Aubry C, et al: Chronic pulmonary aspergillosis: rationale and clinical guidelines for diagnosis and management, Eur Respir J 47(1):45–68, 2016.

ESCMID Study Group for Infections in Compromised Hosts (ESGICH) Consensus Document on the safety of targeted and biologic therapies: an infectious diseases perspective, Clin Microbiol Infect (24), 2018, Supplement 2.

Farmakiotis D, Kontoyiannis DP: Emerging issues with diagnosis and management of fungal infections in solid organ transplant recipients, Am J Transplant 15(5):1141–1147, 2015.

Farmakiotis D, Ross J, Koo S: Chapter 201: Candida and Aspergillus. In McKean SC, Ross JJ, Dressler DD, Scheurer DB, editors: Principles and practice of hospital medicine, ed 2, McGraw-Hill, 2017, pp 1618–1624.

GarciaCadenas I, Rivera I, Martino R, et al: Patterns of infection and infection-related mortality in patients with steroid-refractory acute graft versus host disease, Bone Marrow Transplant 52(1):107–113, 2017.

Guidelines from the American Society of Transplantation Infectious Diseases Community of Practice, Clin Transplant, 2019.

Li X, Jevnikar A: Transplant immunology, West Sussex, 2016, John Wiley & Sons.

Mehta H, Malandra M, Corey S: G-CSF and GM-CSF in neutropenia, J Immunol 195(4):1341–1349, 2015.

Pizzo P: Management of patients with fever and neutropenia through the arc of time: a narrative review, Ann Intern Med 170(6):389–397, 2019.

Qian C, Wang Y, Reppel L, et al: Viral-specific T-cell transfer from HSCT donor for the treatment of viral infections or diseases after HSCT, Bone Marrow Transplant 53(2):114–122, 2018.

Simner P, Miller S, Carroll K: Understanding the promises and hurdles of metagenomic next-generation sequencing as a diagnostic tool for infectious diseases, Clin Infect Dis 66(5):778–788, 2018.

Taplitz R, Kennedy E, Bow E, et al: Antimicrobial prophylaxis for adult patients with cancer related immunosuppression: ASCO and IDSA clinical practice guideline update, J Clin Oncol 36(30):3043–3054, 2018.

18

Infectious Diseases of Travelers: Protozoal and Helminthic Infections

Jessica E. Johnson, Rebecca Reece

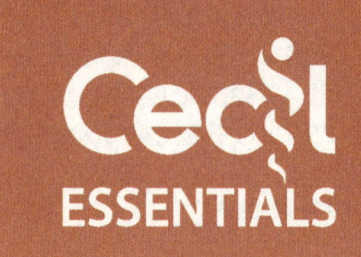

INTRODUCTION

Medical advice for overseas travelers, recommended protective measures, and the diagnosis and treatment of common parasitic diseases endemic in the United States and abroad are reviewed in this chapter.

PREPARATION OF TRAVELERS

Americans made more than 70 million international trips in 2015, and this number continues to increase every year. If we look at a breakdown of where these travels occur, 75% were to a malaria-endemic country. Increases in international travel are associated with exposures to infectious diseases worldwide and bring the issues of prevention and management of health problems in travelers into the office of every physician. The risk of becoming ill while traveling internationally depends on the destination and duration of the trip, the underlying health and age of the traveler, and activities/exposures that occur while abroad. Major issues to be addressed before traveling include required and recommended immunizations, malaria prophylaxis, and traveler's diarrhea, as well as measures to prevent tick and mosquito bites. Information about health risks in specific geographic areas, updated weekly, can be obtained from the US Centers for Disease Control and Prevention (CDC) through its publications or website (www.cdc.gov/travel/destinations/list).

Immunizations

All international travelers should ensure they are up-to-date on routine vaccinations. Only yellow fever vaccination may be required by law for international travel, but other immunizations are often strongly recommended, depending on the destination, type, and duration of travel. Before immunization, a thorough history should be obtained to determine the safety of immunizations and any allergies to eggs or chick embryo cells. Pregnant women and individuals who are immunocompromised by human immunodeficiency virus (HIV), malignancy, or chemotherapy pose specific and important concerns requiring review before receiving vaccinations.

Hepatitis A

In the United States, one of the most frequently identified risks for hepatitis A infection is travel. The risk varies with living conditions, length of stay, and incidence of hepatitis A in the area visited. In some areas, the disease affects an estimated 1 of every 500 to 1000 travelers on a 2- to 3-week trip. Therefore, hepatitis A vaccination is recommended for all susceptible persons traveling to or working in countries with intermediate or high endemicity of infection. Hepatitis A vaccine should be given at least 2 weeks before departure but remains effective if given up until the time of travel. A single dose provides protection for 1 to 2 years; a booster 6 to 18 months later is required for long-lasting immunity (at least 20 years and possibly lifelong).

Influenza

Although influenza is not necessarily considered a travel-related illness, it is the most common vaccine-preventable disease in travelers. The influenza vaccine should be considered in the panel of vaccines offered to the traveler. Influenza seasons can occur at different times of the year in different parts of the world. If a patient cannot be immunized, a course of the antiviral medication oseltamivir can be provided to take at the first sign of a flu-like illness.

Japanese Encephalitis

Japanese encephalitis (JE) virus is closely related to the West Nile and Saint Louis encephalitis viruses and is transmitted to humans through the bite of an infected mosquito. JE virus is the most common vaccine-preventable cause of encephalitis in Asia. It occurs throughout most of Asia and parts of the western Pacific. The overall incidence of JE among people from non-endemic countries traveling to Asia is estimated to be less than 1 case per 1 million travelers. However, expatriates and travelers who stay for prolonged periods in rural areas with active JE virus transmission are likely to be at similar risk as the susceptible resident population (i.e., 5 to 50 cases per 100,000 children per year). Even during brief trips, travelers might be at increased risk if they have extensive outdoor or nighttime exposure in rural areas during periods of active transmission. Short-term (<1 month) travelers whose visits are restricted to major urban areas are at minimal risk for JE. The inactivated JE vaccine, a two-dose series given 28 days apart, is approved for individuals 2 months old and up.

Measles

In the United States, most measles cases result from international travel, and measles remains a common disease in many parts of the world. A large outbreak in 2015 originating from Disney parks in California demonstrated how imported diseases can spread widely to unvaccinated individuals. Currently, measles vaccination is recommended at 15 months of age, with a second vaccination after age 5. Individuals born after 1956 who have no physician-documented record of immunization or who have not received a booster after early childhood should have a one-time booster before travel.

Meningococcal Meningitis

Vaccination for meningococcal disease is recommended to persons who travel to or reside in countries in which the bacterium *Neisseria meningitidis* is hyper-endemic or epidemic, particularly if they will be in close contact with the local population. Vaccination is recommended

旅行者感染性疾病：原虫和蠕虫感染

代丽丽 译　韩宁 肖江 张福杰 审校　张福杰 通审

引言

本章综述了针对海外旅行者的医学建议、防护措施，以及在美国和海外流行的常见寄生虫病的诊断和治疗。

旅行前准备

2015年，美国人进行了超过7000万次国际旅行，并且这一数字每年都在增加。从分布来看，75%是前往疟疾流行国家。国际旅行会增加全球传染病的风险，这使得预防传染病和管理旅行者健康的问题成为每位医生的职责。在国际旅行中患病的风险取决于旅行目的地和旅行时间的长短、旅行者的基础健康状况和年龄以及在国外的活动和暴露病原体的机会。旅行前需要完成的主要准备包括：必要的疫苗接种、疟疾预防，以及防止发生旅行者腹泻和避免蜱、蚊虫叮咬的措施。可以通过美国CDC的出版物或网站（www.cdc.gov/travel/destinations/ist）获取每周更新的特定地理区域的健康风险信息。

疫苗接种

所有国际旅行者都应确保按照规范接种了常规疫苗。唯一可能被国际旅行法定要求接种的疫苗是黄热病疫苗，但根据旅行目的地、旅行类型和持续时间的不同，有些疫苗也被强烈推荐在旅行前接种。在接种疫苗之前，应详细询问接种对象是否对鸡蛋或鸡胚细胞过敏，以确定疫苗接种的安全性。孕妇以及因感染人类免疫缺陷病毒（HIV）、罹患恶性肿瘤或接受化疗而导致免疫功能受损的个体在接种疫苗前需要特别关注适应证。

甲型肝炎

在美国，旅行是导致甲型肝炎感染的最常见原因之一。风险随旅行地卫生条件、停留时间和当地甲型肝炎发病率而异。在某些地区，每500～1000名旅行者中就有1人在2～3周的旅行中感染甲型肝炎。因此，建议所有易感者在前往中高流行地区旅行或者工作之前接种甲型肝炎疫苗。接种应在出发前至少2周完成，但即使在出发前接种仍然有效。单剂量疫苗可提供1～2年的保护作用，而6到18个月后的加强剂可提供长期免疫（至少20年，可能终身）。

流感

尽管流感不一定被看作是旅行相关的疾病，但它是旅行者中最常见的可通过疫苗接种预防的疾病。因此在旅行前，旅行者应考虑接种流感疫苗。需要注意的是，不同地区的流感流行季节可能不同。如果患者不能提前接种流感疫苗，也可以准备一个疗程的抗病毒药物奥司他韦，在出现流感样症状的第一时间服用。

乙型脑炎（日本脑炎）

乙型脑炎（日本脑炎）（JE）病毒与西尼罗病毒和圣路易脑炎病毒密切相关，通过受感染的蚊子叮咬而传播。JE病毒是亚洲最常见的可通过疫苗预防的脑炎病原体。它遍布亚洲大部分地区及西太平洋部分地区。来自非流行地区的旅行者在亚洲旅行罹患JE总体几率估计低于百万分之一。然而，对于长时间居留在JE病毒流行的农村地区的外籍人士和旅行者，其感染风险可能与当地易感居民相似（每年每10万名儿童中有5～50例感染）。即使是短期旅行，如果旅行者在病毒流行期间在农村地区进行大量户外或夜间活动，感染风险也会增加。短期（<1个月）且仅在城市地区活动的旅行者感染JE的风险最小。灭活JE疫苗需要间隔28天接种两剂，适用于2个月及以上的儿童和成人。

麻疹

在美国，大多数麻疹病例是由国际旅行引起的，并且麻疹在世界许多地方仍然是一种常见病。2015年，在加利福尼亚州迪士尼乐园暴发的一次大规模麻疹疫情显示了输入麻疹如何广泛传播给未接种疫苗的人。目前，建议在儿童15月龄时第一次接种麻疹疫苗，并在5岁以后进行第二次接种。1956年以后出生且没有麻疹免疫接种记录或在幼儿期后未接种加强疫苗的个体，应在旅行前进行一次性加强接种。

脑膜炎球菌性脑膜炎

建议前往或长期居住在脑膜炎奈瑟球菌高流行区或疫情暴发区的人，特别是会与当地人密切接触的时候，应该提前接种脑膜炎球菌疫苗。建议前往沙特阿拉伯参加朝觐的旅行者、前往撒哈拉以南非洲"脑膜

for travelers to Saudi Arabia during the Hajj, along the "meningitis belt" of sub-Saharan Africa, and in other locations for which travel advisories have been issued (information available on the CDC website). The meningococcal conjugate vaccine (MCV4) is preferred for people age 9 months through 55 years, and the meningococcal polysaccharide vaccine (MPSV4) is the recommended vaccine for persons older than 55. Serogroup B vaccine was approved in the United States in 2015; however, there are no specific recommendations for travelers because serogroup B is rare internationally. It should be considered in the setting of a reported outbreak or in those with certain risk factors.

Polio

Polio remains endemic in only three countries since 2016: Nigeria, Pakistan, and Afghanistan. Before traveling to areas where poliomyelitis cases are still occurring, travelers should ensure that they have completed the recommended age-appropriate polio vaccine series and have received a booster dose with the inactivated polio vaccine as an adult.

Typhoid

International travelers are at greatest risk for contracting typhoid in the Indian subcontinent, Central America, western South America, and sub-Saharan Africa. Vaccination is recommended for travel to endemic areas where exposure to contaminated food and water is likely. Both a live oral vaccine (four enteric-coated capsules given over 7 days) and an injectable vaccine (single-dose) are available; they are essentially equivalent in effectiveness, which ranges from 50% to 70%.

Yellow Fever

The yellow fever vaccine is a live, attenuated virus vaccine that is recommended for persons traveling to areas in South America and Africa where yellow fever is endemic. Proof of vaccination is required for entry into several countries in these regions unless the traveler meets medically exempt criteria. Since 2016, the World Health Organization (WHO) has lifted the recommendation of a booster every 10 years, stating that a single vaccination is protective for life except in three situations: pregnancy, bone marrow transplant, and HIV infection. Severe adverse events are rare and include yellow fever vaccine–associated viscerotropic and neurologic disease, both of which are more common in elderly persons and in those with thymus disease. Because the adverse events occur more commonly in people older than 60 years of age, a careful assessment of risks and benefits for these travelers should be made before vaccination.

Other Vaccines

Some individuals live for prolonged periods in developing countries or are at special risk for contracting certain highly contagious diseases. Consideration should be given to immunization against hepatitis B, cholera, plague (not commercially available in United States), and rabies. Tetanus vaccinations should be up to date: for travel, a tetanus booster within the previous 5 years is recommended. The cholera vaccine became approved in the United States as of 2016 as a single-dose oral vaccine. Immunity is not long-lasting, with protection less than 80% at 3 months. Given this and limited travel to areas of active cholera transmission, it is not routinely recommended for travelers in the United States, but standard cholera prevention and control measures are emphasized.

Malaria Prophylaxis

Malaria infection is associated with significant morbidity and mortality, particularly if the causative agent is *Plasmodium falciparum*. Worldwide, over 200 million cases occur per year, with increasing numbers of cases among travelers. The need for, as well as the type of, malaria prophylaxis depends on known resistance patterns and the exact itinerary within a given country because the risk of transmission is regional. In general, travelers to areas where chloroquine-sensitive *P. falciparum* strains are exclusively found (i.e., parts of Central America, the Caribbean, and some countries in the Middle East) should take chloroquine phosphate (300 mg base or 500 mg salt) weekly, starting 1 week before travel to malarious areas and continuing during the trip and for 4 weeks after leaving the area.

Travelers to Southeast Asia, sub-Saharan Africa, South America, and South Asia, where chloroquine-resistant *P. falciparum* is common, may take mefloquine (Lariam), atovaquone-proguanil (Malarone), or doxycycline. Mefloquine may be associated with neurologic side effects (dizziness, tinnitus, and vivid dreams) and, rarely, with significant neuropsychiatric side effects. A US Food and Drug Administration (FDA) black box warning issued in 2013 indicated that the neurologic side effects can occur at any time and persist indefinitely; this has lent some caution to the prescription of mefloquine. Mefloquine is also not completely effective in Myanmar, rural Thailand, or some parts of East Africa, where resistance is a growing problem. Mefloquine is taken once weekly for prophylaxis, so is an attractive option for long-term travelers, but must be taken for 4 additional weeks on return. Atovaquone-proguanil and doxycycline are effective in Southeast Asia and may be used in other areas of chloroquine resistance. Atovaquone-proguanil is well tolerated but must be taken every day and extended for 1 week on return. Daily doxycycline can be associated with photosensitivity, esophagitis, and, occasionally, vaginal candidiasis. Doxycycline must also be taken for 4 additional weeks on return from travel.

Where it is approved, primaquine can be used for primary prophylaxis in areas with higher rates of *Plasmodium vivax* or *Plasmodium ovale* infection. It has the advantage of both preventing acute infection from all malaria parasites and preventing the later recurrent infections of *P. vivax* and *P. ovale*. This is taken as a daily dose and continued for 4 weeks on return. It cannot be used in individuals with glucose-6-phosphate dehydrogenase (G6PD) deficiency. Tafenoquine is a newer agent that also prevents acute infection and the later recurrent disease of *P. vivax* and *P. ovale*, as in primaquine, but must be avoided in those with G6PD deficiency. Emphasis must also be given to the use of mosquito bite prevention measures, including netting, screens, permethrin for clothing, and insect repellents, because this can help prevent malaria as well as other vector-borne diseases.

Traveler's Diarrhea

Each year between 30% and 75% of international travelers develop diarrhea. Bacterial infections such as enterotoxigenic *Escherichia coli* are most common, causing more than 80% of traveler's diarrhea; other causes include parasites (i.e., *Giardia*) and viruses (i.e., Norovirus). The average duration of an episode of traveler's diarrhea is 3 to 6 days, but about 10% of episodes last longer than 1 week. The diarrhea may be accompanied by abdominal cramping, nausea, headache, low-grade fever, vomiting, or bloating. Travelers with fever greater than 101° F (38° C), bloody stools, or both should see a physician at once (see Chapter 11).

Diarrheal illness can be avoided by taking precautions with regard to food and beverages. All water and ice should be presumed to be unsafe. Salads are often contaminated by protozoal cysts; along with street vendor foods, they are the most dangerous foods encountered by most travelers. Food should be well cooked, and unpasteurized dairy products should be avoided.

Prophylactic antibiotics are not generally recommended. Diphenoxylate (Lomotil) and loperamide (Imodium) may provide symptomatic relief of mild diarrhea. Oral rehydration is recommended in all cases regardless of severity and serves as an adjunct to antibiotics

炎带"地区的旅行者，以及前往已发布预防脑膜炎奈瑟球菌相关旅行建议的其他地区的旅行者（相关信息可在 CDC 网站上获取）提前接种脑膜炎球菌疫苗。对于 9 个月至 55 岁的人群，优先推荐接种脑膜炎球菌结合疫苗（MCV4），而对于 55 岁以上的人群，推荐接种脑膜炎球菌多糖疫苗（MPSV4）。2015 年，美国批准了 B 型脑膜炎球菌疫苗，但由于 B 型脑膜炎球菌在国际上很少见，因此没有针对旅行者的具体建议。在报告暴发的情况下或在某些高风险人群中应考虑接种。

脊髓灰质炎

自 2016 年以来，脊髓灰质炎仍仅在尼日利亚、巴基斯坦和阿富汗三个国家流行。前往仍有脊髓灰质炎病例地区的旅行者，应确保已完成推荐的适龄脊髓灰质炎疫苗接种程序，并在成年后接种一剂灭活脊髓灰质炎疫苗作为加强剂。

伤寒

国际旅行者在印度次大陆、中美、南美洲西部和撒哈拉以南非洲地区感染伤寒的风险最高。建议前往这些高流行地区且可能接触到受污染食品和水的旅行者接种疫苗。目前有口服活疫苗（7 天内服用 4 个肠溶胶囊）和注射疫苗（单剂）两种选择；两者在有效性方面基本相当，有效率为 50%～70%。

黄热病

黄热病疫苗是一种减毒活病毒疫苗，推荐前往南美和非洲黄热病流行地区的旅行者接种。除非符合医学豁免标准，否则这些地区的多个国家均需持有接种证明才能进入。自 2016 年以来，世界卫生组织（WHO）取消了每 10 年接种一次加强针的建议，声明除孕妇、骨髓移植受者和 HIV 感染者外，单次接种疫苗即可终身保护。严重不良事件罕见，包括与黄热病疫苗相关的内脏型和神经型疾病，主要发生在老年人和胸腺疾病患者。由于不良事件在 60 岁以上人群中更为常见，因此在为这些旅行者接种疫苗前应仔细评估风险和收益。

其他疫苗

有些长期居住在发展中国家或面临感染某些高度传染性疾病风险的旅行者，应考虑接种乙型肝炎、霍乱、鼠疫（在美国尚无商业可用疫苗）和狂犬病疫苗。破伤风疫苗应保持最新：建议在旅行前 5 年内接种破伤风加强针。霍乱疫苗自 2016 年起在美国被批准为单剂量口服疫苗，其免疫效果不持久，3 个月后保护率低于 80%，并且考虑到前往霍乱流行地区旅行者有限，美国不推荐旅行者常规接种，但强调标准的霍乱预防和控制措施。

疟疾预防

疟原虫感染会导致很高的疟疾发病率和死亡率，特别是当病原体是恶性疟原虫时。全球每年报告超过 2 亿例的疟疾病例，旅行者中的病例数不断增加。疟疾的传播风险具有区域性，因此，是否需要以及该采取哪种方式预防疟疾取决于旅行目的地的耐药疟疾流行情况以及旅行者的具体行程。一般来说，旅行目的地只发现对氯喹敏感的恶性疟原虫（即中美洲部分地区、加勒比地区和中东一些国家），旅行者应从旅行前 1 周开始，每周服用磷酸氯喹（300 mg 的氯喹活性成分或 500 mg 的磷酸氯喹盐），直至离开该地区后 4 周。

东南亚、撒哈拉以南非洲、南美洲和南亚常见氯喹耐药的恶性疟原虫，去这些地方的旅行者可以服用甲氟喹、阿托伐醌-氯胍（商品名 Malarone）或多西环素预防。甲氟喹可能导致神经系统副作用（头晕、耳鸣和生动梦境），以及罕见显著的神经精神副作用。2013 年美国 FDA 发布的黑框警告表明，甲氟喹神经系统副作用可能在任何时候发生，并可能无限期持续，这对甲氟喹的使用提出了一些警示。甲氟喹在缅甸、泰国农村或东非部分地区也不完全有效，因为耐药问题日益严重。甲氟喹适合长期旅行者，每周服用一次，持续至返回后 4 周。阿托伐醌-氯胍和多西环素在东南亚有效，也可用于其他氯喹耐药的地区。阿托伐醌-氯胍耐受性良好，但必须每天服用，并持续至返回后 1 周。每天服用多西环素，可能导致光敏感疾病、食管炎，有时还会导致阴道念珠菌病，同样也必须持续至返回后 4 周。

在批准的地区，伯氨喹可用于预防间日疟原虫或卵形疟原虫感染。其优点在于既能预防疟疾急性感染，又能预防间日疟原虫和卵形疟原虫的复发。伯氨喹需每日服用，并持续至返回后 4 周。伯氨喹禁用于葡萄糖-6-磷酸脱氢酶（G6PD）缺乏的个体。他非诺喹是一种较新的药物，像伯氨喹一样，可以同时预防疟原虫急性感染和间日疟原虫及卵形疟原虫的复发，G6PD 缺乏者避免使用。除此以外，还必须强调防蚊措施，包括使用蚊帐、纱窗、衣物上喷洒氯菊酯和驱蚊剂，除了疟疾还可以预防其他虫媒传播疾病。

旅行者腹泻

每年有 30%～75% 的国际旅行者会发生腹泻。最常见的病因是细菌感染，如产肠毒素大肠埃希菌，占病原体的 80% 以上；其他病因包括寄生虫（如贾第鞭毛虫）和病毒（如诺如病毒）。旅行者腹泻的平均持续时间为 3～6 天，但大约 10% 的病例持续超过 1 周。腹泻可能伴有腹部痉挛、恶心、头痛、低热、呕吐或腹胀。发热超过 101 ℉（38 ℃）、伴有血便或者同时出现这两种情况的旅行者应立即就医（见第 11 章）。

注意饮食卫生可以避免腹泻。所有当地的水和冰块都应被视为不清洁的。沙拉通常被寄生虫包囊污染，与街头小吃一样，是引起旅行者腹泻最常见的食物。所有食物都应煮熟，避免食用未经巴氏消毒法消毒的乳制品。

通常不推荐预防性使用抗生素。地芬诺酯（商品名 Lomoti）和洛哌丁胺（商品名 Imodium）可以缓解轻度腹泻的症状。无论病情轻重，都推荐使用口服补

in moderate and severe disease. First-line treatment includes fluoroquinolones, although increasing resistance is being seen in South and Southeast Asia, as well as other destinations. Alternative to quinolones is azithromycin. Updated guidelines by the International Society of Travel Medicine recommends a single-dose antibiotic regimen (of either choice above) as treatment for traveler's diarrhea.

Special Problems
Pregnant Women
Although travel is rarely contraindicated during a normal pregnancy, complicated pregnancies require special consideration and may warrant a recommendation that travel be delayed. The risk of obstetric complications is highest during the first and third trimesters.

Most live-virus vaccines are contraindicated during pregnancy. Yellow fever vaccine, for which pregnancy is considered a precaution by the Advisory Committee on Immunization Practices (ACIP), should be avoided if possible. If travel is unavoidable and the risks for yellow fever virus exposure are believed to outweigh the risks of vaccination, a pregnant woman should be vaccinated. Pregnant women should avoid or delay travel to malaria-endemic areas because no prophylactic measures provide complete protection. If travel is unavoidable, pregnant women should take utmost precautions to avoid mosquito bites; for chemoprophylaxis, chloroquine and mefloquine are the drugs of choice for destinations with chloroquine-sensitive and chloroquine-resistant malaria, respectively.

Zika virus has been shown to cause congenital brain abnormalities including microcephaly as seen in the 2015-2016 outbreak throughout the Americas and Pacific Islands. Though WHO declared an end of the epidemic in November 2016, pregnant women should be counseled to avoid travel to areas with active local transmission. If travel is unavoidable, pregnant women should be counseled on mosquito prevention methods to reduce their risk. Zika virus can also be sexually transmitted, and barrier precaution with condoms, or abstinence, should be advised throughout pregnancy.

Acquired Immunodeficiency Syndrome
Several countries continue to have policies that bar entry to persons with human immunodeficiency virus (HIV)/acquired immunodeficiency syndrome (AIDS). Several countries require serologic testing for HIV from all travelers applying for visas lasting longer than 3 months; official documentation is required well in advance of travel. Patients with HIV infection need special preparation before travel to developing countries because of their increased susceptibility to certain illnesses (e.g., pneumococcal infection, tuberculosis). Risk of HIV infection and other sexually transmitted diseases should be discussed, especially with young, sexually active adults.

The Returning Traveler
The most common medical problems encountered by travelers after their return home are diarrhea, fever, respiratory illnesses, and skin lesions. A detailed history should focus on the traveler's exact itinerary, including dates of travel, exposure history (e.g., food indiscretions, drinking-water sources, freshwater contact, sexual activity, animal contact, insect bites), style of travel (urban vs. rural), immunization history, and use of antimalarial chemoprophylaxis.

Diarrhea
Traveler's diarrhea is an acute condition that usually resolves within 2 weeks. If the traveler's diarrhea is not responsive to empiric antibiotic treatment, a work-up should be performed to evaluate for *Giardia lamblia* (see later discussion). Three stool specimens for ova and parasites and a stool culture are indicated. If *Giardia* tests are negative, an empirical trial of metronidazole for treatment of a possible infection with *Giardia* or other protozoan (e.g., amebiasis) should be considered. Noninfectious causes such as temporary lactose intolerance, irritable bowel syndrome, and, less commonly, inflammatory bowel disease should also be in the differential diagnosis.

Fever
Malaria should be the first diagnosis considered in a febrile traveler who has returned from a malarious area. *P. falciparum* malaria can be fatal if it is not diagnosed and treated promptly. Detection of the *Plasmodium* species on Giemsa-stained blood smears by light microscopy is the standard tool for diagnosis of malaria. Rapid diagnostic tests for detection of malaria parasite antigens are becoming increasingly important tools in resource-limited endemic settings because of their accuracy and ease of use.

Travelers with chloroquine-sensitive *P. falciparum* malaria should be treated with chloroquine. Reasonable agents for uncomplicated malaria caused by chloroquine-resistant *P. falciparum* include atovaquone-proguanil, artemisinin derivative combinations (if available) and mefloquine- or quinine-based regimens. Quinine- and mefloquine-based regimens are more frequently associated with adverse effects, and mefloquine should not be used to treat *P. falciparum* malaria acquired in the Thai-Myanmar-Cambodia area because of high resistance rates.

Severe malaria is defined as acute malaria with major signs of organ dysfunction or a high level of parasitemia (>5%) or both. It should be treated with intravenous quinidine for 7 days with close monitoring of the QTc interval. In many parts of the world, intravenous artesunate is used, but it may be associated with high rates of relapse.

Other important causes of fever after travel include viral hepatitis (hepatitis A and E), typhoid fever, bacterial enteritis, arboviral infections (e.g., dengue, chikungunya, Zika), rickettsial infections, and, in rare instances, leptospirosis, acute HIV infection, and amebic liver abscess (see also Chapter 3).

Skin Diseases
Sunburn, insect bites, skin ulcers, and cutaneous larva migrans are the most common skin conditions affecting travelers after their return home. Persistent skin ulcers should prompt a work-up for cutaneous leishmaniasis, mycobacterial infection, or fungal infection. Careful, complete inspection of the skin is important in detecting the rickettsial eschar in a febrile patient or the central breathing hole in a "boil" caused by myiasis.

PROTOZOAL INFECTIONS

Protozoal infections, though endemic to certain regions, can be encountered all around the world, partly because of the increase in travel and migration (Table 18.1). They cause a tremendous burden of disease in the tropics and subtropics as well as more temperate climates. Immunosuppression associated with various conditions, particularly HIV infection, leads to more severe manifestations. Of all protozoal diseases, malaria causes the most deaths globally, approximately 1 million people each year.

Protozoal Infections in the United States
Giardiasis
Giardiasis is a common cause of nonbloody diarrhea in returning travelers. *G. lamblia* and *G. intestinalis* are found worldwide, including in the United States. However, giardiasis is most commonly diagnosed in travelers returning from Latin America, Southeast Asia, or the Middle East. Transmission is by the fecal-oral route in the setting of contaminated

液，中度和重度腹泻应同时使用抗生素治疗。氟喹诺酮类抗生素属于一线治疗抗生素，但在南亚和东南亚及其他地区，其耐药性日益增加。氟喹诺酮类的替代药物是阿奇霉素。国际旅行医学会更新的指南建议使用单剂量抗生素（上述任何一种）治疗旅行者腹泻。

特殊问题
妊娠女性

虽然正常妊娠几乎不存在旅行禁忌，但复杂妊娠需要慎重对待，可能需要推迟旅行。产科并发症的风险在孕早期和孕晚期最高。大多数活病毒疫苗在妊娠期间是禁忌的。根据免疫实践咨询委员会（ACIP）的建议，在妊娠期间应尽可能避免接种黄热病疫苗。只有在旅行不可避免且黄热病毒暴露的风险被认为超过接种疫苗的风险的情况下为孕妇接种。孕妇应避免或推迟前往疟疾流行地区，因为没有预防措施能提供完全的保护。如果旅行不可避免，孕妇应采取一切措施避免蚊虫叮咬；对于化学预防，氯喹和甲氟喹分别是对氯喹敏感和对甲氟喹耐药的疟疾患者的首选药物。

寨卡病毒已被证明会导致先天性大脑异常，包括在2015—2016年美洲和太平洋岛屿暴发中出现的小头畸形。尽管WHO在2016年11月宣布疫情结束，但仍建议孕妇避免前往该病毒活跃传播的地区。如果旅行不可避免，应建议孕妇采取蚊虫预防措施以降低感染风险。寨卡病毒还可以通过性传播，建议孕妇在整个怀孕期间使用避孕套或禁欲。

获得性免疫缺陷综合征

一些国家禁止人类免疫缺陷病毒（HIV）感染者或获得性免疫缺陷综合征（AIDS）患者入境。一些国家要求所有申请超过3个月签证的旅行者进行HIV血清学检测；需要在旅行前很长时间内准备好正式文件。HIV感染者在前往发展中国家前更需要做好充分准备，因为他们更容易感染某些疾病（如肺炎球菌感染、结核病）。建议医生在进行旅行前咨询时，与年轻的、性活跃的成年人讨论HIV感染和其他性传播疾病的风险。

返程旅行者

旅行者回国后遇到的最常见医疗问题是腹泻、发热、呼吸道疾病和皮肤病变。详细的病史应重点关注旅行者的确切行程，包括旅行日期、可能的病原暴露史（如饮食情况、饮用水源、淡水接触、性活动、动物接触、昆虫叮咬）、旅行方式（城市或农村）、免疫接种史和是否使用疟疾化学预防等。

腹泻

旅行者腹泻是一种急性病症，通常在2周内缓解。如果旅行者腹泻对经验性抗生素治疗没有反应，应进行贾第鞭毛虫相关检查（参见后续讨论）。收集3份粪便标本进行虫卵和寄生虫检查以及粪便培养。如果贾第鞭毛虫检测呈阴性，可以考虑进行甲硝唑的经验性治疗。甲硝唑对贾第鞭毛虫或其他寄生虫感染（如阿米巴病）有效。非感染性原因如暂时性乳糖不耐受、肠易激综合征和不常见的炎症性肠病也应在鉴别诊断范围内。

发热

在从疟疾流行区返回且发热的旅行者中，应首要考虑疟疾诊断。如果不及时诊断和治疗，恶性疟疾可能致命。利用光学显微镜在吉姆萨染色的血涂片上查找疟原虫，是确诊疟疾的标准方法。在资源有限的疟疾流行区，使用快速诊断试剂筛查疟原虫抗原具有较高的准确性和便捷性，因而日显重要。

对氯喹敏感的恶性疟应使用氯喹治疗。对于氯喹耐药的恶性疟原虫引起的无并发症疟疾，合理的治疗药物包括阿托伐醌-盐酸氯胍组合、青蒿素衍生物联合用药（如果可以获得），以及基于甲氟喹或奎宁的治疗方案。基于奎宁和甲氟喹的方案不良反应更多见。因为耐药率高，甲氟喹不应用于治疗自泰国-缅甸-柬埔寨地区获得的恶性疟。

重症疟疾定义为伴有主要器官功能障碍或高水平疟疾血症（＞5%）或两者兼有的急性疟疾。应静脉注射奎尼丁治疗7天，并密切监测QTc间期。在许多地方，使用静脉注射青蒿琥酯，但可能与高复发率有关。

旅行后发热的其他重要原因包括病毒性肝炎（甲型和戊型肝炎）、伤寒、细菌性肠炎、虫媒病毒感染（例如登革病毒、基孔肯亚病毒、寨卡病毒）、立克次体感染，以及在极少数情况下的钩端螺旋体病、急性HIV感染和阿米巴肝脓肿（见第3章）。

皮肤病变

晒伤、虫咬、皮肤溃疡和皮肤幼虫移行症是返程旅行者最常见的皮肤病。持续性皮肤溃疡应进行皮肤利什曼病、分枝杆菌感染或真菌感染的检查。对皮肤进行仔细、全面的检查对于发现发热患者的立克次体焦痂或由蝇蛆病引起的"疖"中央呼吸孔非常重要。

原虫感染

尽管原虫感染主要在某些地区流行，但由于旅行和移民的增加，在世界各地都可能遇到（表18.1）。它们在热带和亚热带地区以及更温暖的地区造成了巨大的疾病负担。各种原因的免疫抑制，特别是HIV感染，会导致更严重的临床表现。在所有原生病原体感染中，疟疾在全球导致的死亡人数最多，每年大约有100万人因此死亡。

美国的原虫感染
贾第虫病

贾第虫病是旅行者回国后发生的非血性腹泻的常见原因。蓝氏贾第鞭毛虫和肠贾第虫在全球范围内分布，包括美国。然而，贾第虫病最常见于从拉丁美

TABLE 18.1 Protozoal Infections

Protozoan	Setting	Vectors	Diagnosis	Special Considerations	Treatment
Endemic in the United States					
Babesia microti	New England	Ixodid ticks, transfusions	Thick or thin blood smear	Severe disease in asplenic persons	Quinine and clindamycin
Giardia lamblia	Mountain states	Humans, small mammals	Microscopic examination of stool or duodenal fluid	Common in homosexual men, travelers, children in daycare centers	Quinacrine, nitazoxanide, or metronidazole
Toxoplasma gondii	Ubiquitous	Domestic cats, raw meat	Clinical; serologic confirmation	Pregnant women, immunosuppressed host (AIDS)	Pyrimethamine and sulfadiazine
Entamoeba histolytica	Southeast	Human	Microscopic examination of stool or touch preparation from ulcer	Common in homosexual men, travelers, institutionalized persons	Metronidazole
Cryptosporidium species	Ubiquitous	Human	Acid-fast stain of stool	Severe in immunosuppressed hosts (AIDS)	Nitazoxanide
Trichomonas vaginalis	Ubiquitous	Human	Wet preparation of genital secretions	Common cause of vaginitis	Metronidazole
Primarily Seen in Travelers and Immigrants					
Plasmodium species	Africa, Asia, South America	*Anopheles* mosquito	Thick and thin blood smears	Consider in returning travelers with fever	Dependent on regional resistance pattern (see text)
Leishmania donovani	Middle East	Sandfly	Tissue biopsy	Consider in immigrants with fever and splenomegaly	Sodium stibogluconate
Trypanosoma species	Africa, South America	Reduviid bugs, transfusion	Direct examination of blood or CSF	Very rare in travelers, transfusion associated	Dependent on species and stage of disease

AIDS, Acquired immunodeficiency syndrome; *CSF*, cerebrospinal fluid.

food or water or public swimming areas, or by person-to-person contact in certain risk populations such as men who have sex with men. It is usually a self-limited diarrheal illness that lasts 2 to 4 weeks but may persist longer. Rarely, individuals have associated fevers, nausea, or vomiting. The diagnosis is made by microscopic examination of stool for cysts or trophozoites or by an antigen detection test. Treatment options include metronidazole, tinidazole, or nitazoxanide.

Amebiasis

Amebiasis is another diarrheal illness that occurs in travelers. Like *Giardia*, *Entamoeba histolytica* is found worldwide, and transmission is by the fecal-oral route. However, most infected individuals (80%) are asymptomatic. The presentation in those acutely infected includes bloody or watery diarrhea with abdominal cramping lasting up to 4 weeks. In immunocompromised individuals, a severe invasive infection can occur with risk of necrotizing colitis or bowel perforation. Extraintestinal amebiasis can occur as well, particularly liver abscesses. The diagnosis can be made by microscopic examination of stool for ova and parasites or by antigen detection tests of stool or serum. Treatment is with metronidazole or tinidazole in symptomatic individuals, followed by paromomycin or iodoquinol. Asymptomatic patients should also be treated with iodoquinol or paromomycin to prevent spread or later disease development.

Protozoal Infections Common in Travelers and Immigrants

Leishmaniasis

Leishmaniasis is transmitted by the sandfly and can manifest with cutaneous, mucocutaneous, or visceral involvement. The skin finding is a persistent ulcer with raised edges in a traveler returning from the Middle East (Old World: *Leishmania major*, *Leishmania tropica*) or Latin America (New World: *Leishmania braziliensis*, *Leishmania peruviana*, others). Diagnosis is by tissue biopsy. Visceral leishmaniasis can have hepatic, splenic, or bone marrow involvement and is more commonly identified in immigrants from Asia (*Leishmania donovani*) or South America (*Leishmania chagasi*). Diagnosis is by tissue biopsy or culture of the involved organ.

Treatment varies based on severity of presentation and resistance characteristics. Most cutaneous lesions are self-limited, but treatment options include sodium stibogluconate (Pentostam) or paromomycin. For visceral involvement, treatment includes sodium stibogluconate, amphotericin B, or a combination of these two agents.

African Trypanosomiasis

African trypanosomiasis, or African sleeping sickness, is a protozoal infection caused by *Trypanosoma rhodesiense* (East Africa) or *Trypanosoma gambiense* (Central and West Africa), which is transmitted by the tsetse fly. Presenting symptoms include fever, headache, and central nervous system involvement. The disease is rarely reported in travelers returning from sub-Saharan Africa but should be considered in immigrants from these areas. Frequently, the patient remembers a chancre at the site of the insect bite. The diagnosis is made by microscopic examination of blood, lymph, or cerebrospinal fluid for the parasite. Treatment varies by species and is highly toxic. Consultation with an expert in infectious disease or tropical medicine is recommended.

American Trypanosomiasis

American trypanosomiasis, or Chagas' disease, is caused by *Trypanosoma cruzi* and is endemic in Central and South America. Transmitted by contact with feces of reduviid bugs (kissing bugs), it can also be acquired through blood transfusion or organ transplantation from an infected individual. The risk to travelers is extremely low but increases with prolonged stays in poor-quality

表 18.1 原虫感染

原虫	传染环境	传播媒介	诊断	特殊考虑	治疗
美国本土流行的原虫感染					
微小巴贝虫	美国新英格兰地区	硬蜱，输血	厚血涂片或薄血涂片	严重病情见于无脾功能者	奎宁和克林霉素
蓝氏贾第鞭毛虫	山区	人类，小型哺乳动物	粪便或十二指肠液的显微镜检查	常见于男同性恋者、旅行者、日托中心的儿童	奎纳克林，硝唑尼特或甲硝唑
弓形虫	普遍存在	家猫，生肉	临床；血清学确认	孕妇，免疫抑制宿主（AIDS）	乙胺嘧啶和磺胺嘧啶
溶组织内阿米巴	东南亚	人类	粪便显微镜检查或溃疡触片	常见于男同性恋者、旅行者、被收容者	甲硝唑
隐孢子虫	普遍存在	人类	粪便抗酸染色	免疫抑制宿主病情严重（AIDS）	硝唑尼特
阴道毛滴虫	普遍存在	人类	生殖道分泌物涂片检查	常见阴道炎的病因	甲硝唑
主要见于旅行者和移民中的原虫感染					
疟原虫	非洲、亚洲和南美洲	按蚊	厚血涂片或薄血涂片	伴有发热症状的旅行返回人员	需要考虑特定地区的病原体抗药性
杜氏利什曼原虫	中东	白蛉	组织活检	考虑发热和脾大的移民	钠锑葡萄糖酸盐
锥虫属	非洲、南美洲	锥蝽，输血	直接检查血液或脑脊液	旅行者中非常罕见，输血相关	取决于种类和疾病阶段

洲、东南亚或中东返回的旅行者。其传播途径为粪-口途径，在受污染的食物或水或公共游泳区环境中传播，或通过某些高风险人群（如男男性行为者）的人际接触传播。这通常是一种自限性腹泻性疾病，持续 2~4 周，或更长时间。罕见情况下，可能伴有发热、恶心或呕吐。通过显微镜检查粪便中的包囊或滋养体，或通过抗原检测来诊断。治疗药物包括甲硝唑、替硝唑或硝唑尼特。

阿米巴病

阿米巴病是旅行者中另一种腹泻疾病。与贾第鞭毛虫相似，溶组织内阿米巴在全球范围内分布，通过粪-口途径传播。然而，大多数感染者（80%）是无症状的。急性感染表现为伴有腹部痉挛的血性或水样腹泻，持续时间可达 4 周。在免疫功能受损的个体中，可能发生严重的侵袭性感染，存在坏死性结肠炎或肠穿孔的风险。还可能发生肠外阿米巴病，特别是肝脓肿。诊断可以通过显微镜检查寻找粪便中的虫卵和病原体，或通过粪便或血清的抗原检测。对有症状的个体，使用甲硝唑或替硝唑治疗，随后使用巴龙霉素或替硝唑。无症状患者也应使用碘奎诺或巴龙霉素治疗，以防止传播或后期疾病的发展。

旅行者和移民中常见的原虫感染

利什曼病

利什曼病通过白蛉传播，临床表现可分为皮肤型、黏膜皮肤型或内脏型。从中东（旧世界/东半球：主要利什曼原虫、热带利什曼原虫），或者在从拉丁美洲（新世界/西半球：巴西利什曼原虫、秘鲁利什曼原虫等）返回的旅行者，皮肤表现为边缘隆起的持续性溃疡，通过组织活检进行诊断。内脏利什曼病可能累及肝、脾或骨髓，更常见于来自亚洲（杜氏利什曼原虫）或南美（恰氏利什曼原虫）的移民。通过受累器官的组织活检或培养诊断。

治疗根据病情严重程度和病原体耐药性而有所不同。大多数皮肤损伤是自限性的，但治疗选择包括葡萄糖锑酸钠（商品名 Pentostam）或巴龙霉素。对于内脏型利什曼病，治疗包括葡萄糖锑酸钠、两性霉素 B，或这两种药物的组合。

非洲锥虫病

非洲锥虫病，或称非洲睡眠病，是由罗得西亚锥虫（东非）或冈比亚锥虫（中非和西非）引起的原虫感染，通过采采蝇传播。主要症状包括发热、头痛和中枢神经系统受累的表现。这种疾病在从撒哈拉以南非洲返回的旅行者中少有报告，但在来自这些地区的移民中应予考虑。患者通常记得在昆虫叮咬处有一个硬节。通过显微镜查找血液、淋巴或脑脊液中的锥虫进行诊断。治疗药物因锥虫种类而异，且毒性很大，建议咨询传染病或热带医学专家。

美洲锥虫病

美洲锥虫病，或称查加斯病，由克氏锥虫引起，流行于中美洲和南美洲，通过接触锥蝽（又称亲吻虫）的粪便传播，也可以通过接受感染者的血或器官移植获得。旅行者感染风险极低，但长期居住在条件简陋

housing. The presentation has an acute phase of 3 months followed by a chronic infection for life. The classic acute presentation involves swelling and erythema of the eyelid and ocular tissue at the entry site of infection, known as the Romaña sign. However, most individuals are asymptomatic throughout the infection and are identified only at the time of blood donation. Between 20% and 30% of individuals develop manifestations of chronic infection decades later that can include cardiomegaly and heart failure, megaesophagus, or megacolon.

Diagnosis in the acute phase is by microscopic examination of peripheral blood. In the chronic phase, various serologic analyses are available to aid in diagnosis. Treatment is recommended early because it may prevent chronic manifestations. In the United States, antitrypanosomal drugs are available through the CDC in consultation with an expert in the field. For most chronic manifestations, however, treatment is supportive.

HELMINTHIC INFECTIONS

Infestation by nematodes, or roundworms, is the most common parasitic infection in the world. The intestinal nematodes *Ascaris* and *Trichuris* are the two most prevalent types. Other important helminths include *Strongyloides*, *Enterobius*, schistosomes, and tapeworms (see later discussion). Although most helminths are found worldwide, they disproportionately affect the developing world and pose potential risk to travelers to those areas (Table 18.2).

Helminthic Infections Common in the United States
Pinworm
Enterobiasis is common in the United States and worldwide. Children are predominantly infected, and transmission is by the fecal-oral route. The clinical presentation is perianal pruritus. Diagnosis is made by the tape test, in which transparent tape is applied to the perianal skin overnight and then examined microscopically for ova on the tape. Treatment is with mebendazole or albendazole.

Roundworm
Ascaris lumbricoides is found worldwide, including in the United States, but mostly affects people in the developing world. Although affected individuals are usually asymptomatic, some develop pulmonary infiltrates during the migration phase of the worm or obstruction of the biliary, pancreatic, or intestinal tract. These manifestations usually occur in the setting of high worm burden. Diagnosis is by stool examination for ova and parasites. Treatment is with mebendazole or albendazole.

Whipworm
Trichuris trichiura are called whipworms because of their characteristic shape in the adult form. Like *Ascaris*, this is an intestinal nematode that infects mostly children. It is usually asymptomatic except in the setting of heavy worm burden, which can lead to rectal prolapse and bloody diarrhea among children in the developing world. Diagnosis is made by stool examination for ova and parasites or by endoscopy revealing colitis and the presence of adult worms. The treatment of choice is mebendazole or albendazole.

Hookworm
Ancylostoma duodenale and *Necator americanus* (hookworms) are similar to roundworms in their worldwide distribution and are common among immigrants from Asia and sub-Saharan Africa. Infection occurs through direct penetration of the skin by the larvae, which travel through the lymphatics and the bloodstream to the lungs and are then swallowed. Infected individuals may be asymptomatic, or they may develop pruritic dermatitis at the site of entry. As with the roundworm, pulmonary infiltrates can occur during the migration phase; this is known as Löffler syndrome. Chronic iron deficiency anemia associated with heavy hookworm infection can be severe and debilitating. Eosinophilia is common. The diagnosis is made by stool examination for ova and parasites. The treatment is mebendazole or albendazole.

Helminth Infections Common in Travelers and Immigrants
Strongyloidosis
Strongyloides stercoralis is a helminthic parasite that is found worldwide, although more commonly in the tropics. Infection occurs from contact with contaminated soil; the larva penetrates the skin, migrates to the lungs, and is then swallowed by the individual. The infection is usually asymptomatic, but infection can persist into the chronic phase decades later. Those with symptoms usually have gastrointestinal complaints of bloating, diarrhea, and abdominal pain. Eosinophilia is a common finding in these individuals. In immunocompromised individuals, a hyperinfection syndrome with dissemination of the organism can occur. Hyperinfection syndrome has a higher mortality rate and occurs usually in immigrants who become immunosuppressed as a result of chemotherapy, use of steroids, or illness. Diagnosis is made by stool examination (approximately 30% to 50% sensitivity) or by serology but this does not distinguish between chronic and acute disease. Treatment is with ivermectin for 2 days; in the setting of hyperinfection, a longer course is required.

Schistosomiasis
Schistosomiasis is found throughout the tropics and the developing world. Also known as blood flukes, schistosomes use freshwater mollusks as their intermediate host and penetrate the skin of individuals, leading to infection. The three major species are: *Schistosoma mansoni* (Africa, Middle East, South America), *Schistosoma haematobium* (Africa, Middle East), and *Schistosoma japonicum* (China, Philippines, and Southeast Asia). Acute infection can manifest with dermatitis, although most cases are asymptomatic. Chronic infection develops from the immune response to egg deposition. *S. haematobium* can lead to urinary obstruction or hematuria and is associated with an increased risk of bladder cancer. *S. mansoni* and *S. japonicum* can lead to hepatosplenomegaly, hepatic fibrosis, obstruction of portal blood flow, and varices. *S. japonicum* can infect the central nervous system causing ring enhancing lesions and seizures. Diagnosis is by examination of stool or urine for schistosome eggs in individuals from endemic areas, who have a high egg burden; among travelers, in whom the egg burden is usually low, serology is used for diagnosis. The treatment of choice is praziquantel.

Lymphatic Filariasis (Elephantiasis)
Wuchereria bancrofti and *Brugia malayi* are found throughout the tropics; they are lymph-dwelling filariae that cause elephantiasis. The presentation can vary from acute lymphadenitis, to asymptomatic microfilaremia, filarial fevers, or tropical pulmonary eosinophilia. Lymphadenitis can involve both upper and lower extremities with both of these filarial species, but scrotal involvement only occurs with *W. bancrofti*. The diagnosis is made by examination of a peripheral blood smear for microfilariae obtained between 10 PM and 4 AM because these organisms are nocturnally periodic.

Diethylcarbamazine is used for lymphatic filariasis to eradicate the microfilariae and the adult worms. However, the management of chronic lymphatic obstruction remains a challenge because it is not fully reversible and requires supportive therapy.

的住所会增加感染风险。该病先经过3个月的急性期，随后是终身的慢性感染。经典的急性期表现包括感染部位和眼睑、眼部组织的肿胀和红斑，称为罗曼纳征。然而，大多数个体在感染期间无症状，通常在献血时被发现。20%～30%的个体在几十年后出现慢性感染的表现，包括心脏肥大、心力衰竭、食管扩张或巨结肠。

急性期通过显微镜外周血查找病原体诊断，在慢性期，可通过各种血清学检查来帮助诊断。建议早期治疗，因为其可能会预防慢性感染的症状。在美国，抗锥虫药物通过与专业领域专家讨论后从CDC获得。然而，大多数慢性期的治疗是仅支持性的。

蠕虫感染

线虫，或称圆虫感染是世界上最常见的寄生虫感染。肠道线虫中的蛔虫和鞭虫是两种最常见的类型。其他重要的蠕虫包括粪类圆线虫、蛲虫、血吸虫和绦虫（参见后续讨论）。尽管大多数蠕虫在全球范围内分布，但它们对发展中国家的影响尤为严重，并对前往这些地区的旅行者构成潜在风险（表18.2）。

美国常见蠕虫感染
蛲虫

蛲虫感染在美国和全球范围内常见。主要见于儿童，通过粪-口途径传播。临床表现为肛周瘙痒。透明胶带试验可以用于诊断，透明胶带贴在肛门皮肤上过夜，然后显微镜检查胶带上的虫卵。治疗方法是使用甲苯达唑或阿苯达唑。

蛔虫

似蚓蛔线虫在全球范围内分布，包括美国，但主要影响发展中国家。虽然感染者通常无症状，但一些人在虫体迁移阶段会出现肺部浸润，或者出现胆道、胰腺、肠道阻塞。这些表现通常发生在高虫负荷的情况下。通过粪便显微镜检查虫卵和查找寄生虫诊断。治疗方法是使用甲苯咪唑或阿苯达唑。

鞭虫

毛首鞭形线虫因其成虫形态特征而得名。与蛔虫类似，这是一种主要感染儿童的肠道线虫。除非在高虫负荷情况下，否则通常无症状，高虫负荷可导致儿童出现直肠脱垂和血性腹泻。通过粪便检查虫卵和寄生虫或内镜检查显示结肠炎及存在成虫诊断。首选治疗方法是使用甲苯咪唑或阿苯达唑。

钩虫

十二指肠钩虫和美洲钩虫在全球范围内分布，常见于来自亚洲和撒哈拉以南非洲的移民。感染通过幼虫直接穿透皮肤进入，幼虫通过淋巴系统和血流到达肺部，然后被吞咽。感染者可能无症状，或者在进入部位出现瘙痒性皮炎。与蛔虫类似，在迁移阶段可能出现肺部浸润，这被称为Löffler综合征（劳氏综合征）。与严重钩虫感染相关的慢性缺铁性贫血可能很严重，并导致患者虚弱。嗜酸性粒细胞增多很常见。通过粪便检查虫卵和寄生虫诊断。治疗方法是使用甲苯咪唑或阿苯达唑。

旅行者和移民中常见的蠕虫感染
粪类圆线虫病

粪类圆线虫是一种蠕虫，分布于全球，尤其在热带地区更常见。通过接触受污染的土壤感染；幼虫穿透皮肤，迁移到肺部，然后被个人吞咽。感染通常无症状，但可持续几十年。症状通常有胃肠道不适，如腹胀、腹泻和腹痛。嗜酸性粒细胞增多很常见。在免疫功能低下的个体中，可能发生伴随病原体播散的高感染综合征。高感染综合征的死亡率较高，通常发生在因化疗、类固醇使用或疾病而免疫抑制的移民中。通过粪便检查（敏感性30%～50%）或血清学检测诊断，但血清学检测无法区分慢性和急性疾病。治疗方案是使用伊维菌素2天；在高感染情况下，需要更长时间的治疗。

血吸虫病

血吸虫病在热带和发展中国家广泛存在。血吸虫利用淡水软体动物作为中间宿主，通过皮肤进入人体，引起感染。主要有三种血吸虫：曼氏血吸虫（分布于非洲、中东和南美洲）、埃及血吸虫（分布于非洲和中东）和日本血吸虫（分布于中国、菲律宾和东南亚）。急性感染可表现为皮肤炎症，但大多数病例无症状。慢性感染源于对虫卵沉积的免疫反应。埃及血吸虫可导致尿路梗阻或血尿，并与膀胱癌风险增加相关。曼氏血吸虫和日本血吸虫可导致肝脾大、肝纤维化、门静脉血流阻塞和静脉曲张。日本血吸虫可感染中枢神经系统，导致环形增强病变和癫痫发作。来自流行区的高虫卵负荷者，可以通过检查粪便或尿液中的血吸虫卵诊断；对于旅行者，由于虫卵负荷通常较低，通常通过血清学诊断。首选治疗药物是吡喹酮。

淋巴性丝虫病（象皮肿）

班氏丝虫和马来丝虫在热带地区广泛分布；它们是寄生于淋巴系统的丝虫，可引起象皮肿。表现可以从急性淋巴结炎、无症状的微丝蚴血症、丝虫热到热带肺嗜酸性粒细胞增多症不等。两种丝虫感染都可以发生淋巴结炎，累及上下肢，但阴囊累及仅发生在班氏丝虫感染中。通过在晚上10点至凌晨4点之间获取的外周血涂片检查微丝蚴可以诊断，丝虫是夜间周期性活动的。

使用乙胺嗪可以消灭微丝蚴和成虫，治疗淋巴性丝虫病。然而，慢性淋巴阻塞不能完全逆转，缺乏有效治疗手段，以支持性治疗为主。

TABLE 18.2 Helminthic Infections

Helminth	Setting	Vectors	Diagnosis	Treatment
Endemic in the United States				
Pinworm (enterobiasis)	Ubiquitous	Human	Direct examination for ova	Mebendazole, albendazole
Ascaris lumbricoides	Southeast	Human	Stool examination for ova	Mebendazole, albendazole
Trichuris trichiura	Southeast	Human	Stool examination for ova	Mebendazole, albendazole
Hookworm	Southeast	Human	Stool examination for ova	Mebendazole, albendazole
Common in Travelers and Immigrants				
Strongyloides stercoralis	Developing world	Human	Stool examination for larvae	Thiabendazole, ivermectin
Schistosoma species	Developing world	Snails	Stool or urine examination for ova	Praziquantel
Wuchereria and *Brugia* species	Asia, some parts of Africa	Mosquitoes	Nocturnal blood examination	Ivermectin
Onchocerca volvulus	Africa, South and Central America	Black flies	Biopsy	Ivermectin
Loa loa	Africa	Tabanid flies	Blood examination, clinical setting	Diethylcarbamazine or ivermectin
Clonorchis sinensis	Asia	Undercooked fish and snails	Stool examination for ova, radiology	Praziquantel
Echinococcus species	Worldwide	Canines and livestock	Radiology, serology, biopsy	Surgery, supportive therapy
Taenia solium (cysticercosis)	Developing world	Humans, pigs	Radiology, serology	Surgery, albendazole
T. solium, *Taenia saginata*, *Diphyllobothrium latum* (tapeworms)	Worldwide	Pigs, bovine, fish	Stool examination for ova or proglottids	Praziquantel

Loa loa (Eyeworm)

Loiasis is caused by the eyeworm *(Loa loa)* and is found in West and Central Africa. Presentation can vary and may include pruritus, subcutaneous swellings, joint manifestations, or neurologic symptoms. In the rarest presentation, the adult worm can be seen in the anterior chamber of the individual's eye. Diagnosis is confirmed by the presence of microfilariae in blood samples or isolation of the adult worm. Treatment is as for lymphatic filariasis, with diethylcarbamazine.

River Blindness

Onchocerca volvulus infection mostly occurs in regions of West and Central Africa but also in South and Central America. Pruritic dermatitis is the most common presentation; but involvement of the eye is the most serious presentation. Ocular involvement occurs in endemic areas in individuals with heavy worm burden. The complications can begin with conjunctivitis and photophobia. Corneal involvement with the microfilariae causes an inflammatory reaction leading to sclerosing keratitis and blindness. River blindness is the most common cause of blindness in Africa. The diagnosis is made by examination of skin snips for microfilariae. Ivermectin is the drug of choice; an initial single dose is followed by a repeat dose at 3 or 6 months to suppress any further microfilariae because this does not eliminate the adult worm.

Clonorchiasis

Clonorchis sinensis is the Chinese liver fluke. This is an important infection to consider in Asian immigrants who have symptoms consistent with biliary tract disease, including right upper quadrant pain, anorexia, and weight loss. Though the disease is uncommon, untreated infections can lead to cholangiocarcinoma. Treatment is curative with praziquantel in 85% of cases.

Cysticercosis

Cysticercosis is caused by the pork tapeworm, *Taenia solium*. Individuals report new-onset seizures or headaches. Head computed tomographic (CT) scans show ring enhancing lesions. The diagnosis is usually based on the history and imaging findings, and confirmation can be made by immunoblot assay. Treatment depends on the site of infection and symptoms. It may include antiparasitic treatment, antiseizure medications, and surgical removal. The antiparasitic drug of choice is praziquantel or albendazole. Expert consultation before treatment is recommended because of the risk of increasing focal cerebral edema and seizure activity.

Intestinal Tapeworms

Tapeworms that commonly infect humans include *Taenia solium* (from raw pork), *Taenia saginata* (raw beef), and *Diphyllobothrium latum* (raw fish). Most infections are asymptomatic except in the case of invasive disease with *T. solium*, as discussed earlier (see Cysticercosis). Praziquantel is the treatment of choice for all three tapeworms.

Echinococcus

The tapeworm *Echinococcus granulosus* causes hydatid disease with production of a cystic liver mass. This occurs in immigrants from sheep-raising parts of the world such as South America, Central Asia, and the Middle East. The characteristic appearance of the cyst includes a calcified wall with a dependent hydatid on CT scans. This appearance and the supporting history help to make the diagnosis; the serologic testing available can be falsely negative. Treatment often includes percutaneous drainage or surgical removal. Care must be taken to avoid rupture or spillage of the contents, which can result in life threatening anaphylaxis. Albendazole is usually given before surgical removal.

Less common is *Echinococcus multilocularis*, which causes alveolar cyst disease. This more aggressive infection leads to liver lesions as well as brain and lung involvement. Treatment includes resection of liver lesions in combination with antiparasitic therapy with mebendazole or albendazole. However, these agents are not parasiticidal, so the mortality rate remains high. Other potential therapies, such as amphotericin B and nitazoxanide, are being explored.

表 18.2 蠕虫感染

蠕虫种类	传染环境	传播媒介	诊断	治疗
美国本土流行的蠕虫感染				
蛲虫	普遍流行	人	粪便显微镜检查虫卵	甲苯达唑或阿苯达唑
蛔虫	东南地区	人	粪便显微镜检查虫卵	甲苯达唑或阿苯达唑
鞭虫	东南地区	人	粪便显微镜检查虫卵	甲苯达唑或阿苯达唑
钩虫	东南地区	人	粪便显微镜检查虫卵	甲苯达唑或阿苯达唑
主要见于旅行者和移民中的蠕虫感染				
粪类圆线虫	发展中国家	人	粪便显微镜检查幼虫	硫苯唑，伊维菌素
血吸虫属	发展中国家	钉螺	粪便或尿中查找虫卵	吡喹酮
班氏丝虫和马来丝虫属	亚洲及非洲部分地区	蚊子	夜间血检	伊维菌素
盘尾丝虫	非洲、南美洲和中美洲	黑蝇	活检	伊维菌素
罗阿丝虫	非洲	虻	血检、临床检查	乙胺嗪或伊维菌素
华支睾吸虫	亚洲	未煮熟的鱼和钉螺	粪便检查虫卵，放射学检查	吡喹酮
包虫属	普遍流行	犬，牲畜	放射学，血清学，活检	手术、支持疗法
猪带绦虫（囊虫病）	发展中国家	人，猪	放射学，血清学	手术，阿苯达唑
猪带绦虫，牛带绦虫，阔节裂头绦虫（或称为鱼带绦虫）	普遍流行	猪，牛，鱼	粪检虫卵或节片	吡喹酮

罗阿丝虫（眼丝虫）

罗阿丝虫病是由眼丝虫（罗阿丝虫）引起的，主要分布在西非和中非。临床表现多样，包括瘙痒、皮下肿块、关节症状或神经系统症状。最罕见的表现是成虫出现在患者眼睛的前房中。通过血液样本中找到微丝蚴或成虫分离来诊断。治疗方法与淋巴性丝虫病相同，使用乙胺嗪。

河盲

盘尾丝虫感染主要在西非和中非地区发生，也见于南美和中美。最常见的表现是瘙痒性皮炎，但眼部受累是最严重的表现。在流行区的重度感染者中，眼部表现可能从结膜炎和畏光开始。微丝蚴引起的角膜炎症反应会导致硬化性角膜炎和失明。河盲是非洲最常见的失明原因。通过皮肤活检检查微丝蚴诊断。首选药物是伊维菌素；初次单剂量治疗后，在3个月或6个月时重复一次以进一步杀死残余微丝蚴，这种药物不能消灭成虫。

华支睾吸虫病

华支睾吸虫是中国肝吸虫。在伴有胆道疾病症状（如右上腹痛、厌食和体重减轻）的亚洲移民中要重点考虑的一种感染性疾病。尽管不常见，但不进行治疗可导致胆管癌。吡喹酮治疗在85%的病例中是有效的。

囊尾蚴病

囊尾蚴病是由猪带绦虫引起的。患者通常有新发的癫痫发作或头痛。头部CT扫描显示环形增强病变。通常需结合病史和影像学诊断，确诊可以通过免疫印迹试验进行。治疗取决于感染部位和症状，可能包括抗寄生虫治疗、抗癫痫药物和手术切除。首选抗寄生虫药物是吡喹酮或阿苯达唑。由于驱虫治疗可能增加局部脑水肿和癫痫活动的风险，建议在治疗前咨询专家。

肠道绦虫

常见的感染人类的绦虫包括猪带绦虫（来自生猪肉）、牛带绦虫（来自生牛肉）和阔节裂头绦虫（来自生鱼）。除先前讨论的囊尾蚴病（见囊尾蚴病）外，大多数感染者无症状。三种绦虫的首选治疗方法都是吡喹酮。

棘球蚴

细粒棘球绦虫引起包虫病，形成肝囊肿，主要发生于来自绵羊饲养地区（如南美、中亚和中东）的移民中。CT扫描显示的囊肿特征表现包括：钙化壁及包虫囊肿。结合影像学和相关病史有助于诊断；血清学检测可能出现假阴性。治疗通常包括经皮囊肿引流或手术切除。必须小心避免囊肿破裂或溢出内容物，否则可能导致危及生命的过敏反应。通常在手术切除前给予阿苯达唑。

较少见的是多房棘球绦虫，引起泡型棘球蚴病。这种更具侵袭性的感染导致肝病以及脑和肺的受累。治疗包括切除肝病并结合使用甲苯咪唑或阿苯达唑进行抗寄生虫治疗。然而，这些药物并不敏感，死亡率仍然很高。其他潜在疗法，如两性霉素B和硝唑尼特，正在探索中。

FUTURE DIRECTIONS

The field of travel medicine is constantly changing as infectious diseases do not always follow a historical pattern. With the increasing globalization of travel, we can see outbreaks and epidemics develop in new areas such as the West Africa Ebola outbreak in 2014-2015, the Zika epidemic 2015-2016, and the ongoing MERS-CoV outbreak in the Middle East that alter our guidance to patients and our management of returning travelers from these areas. As a physician caring for travelers, we must stay informed of the changing landscape of infectious diseases across the world.

SUGGESTED READINGS

Arguin P: Approach to the patient before and after travel. In Goldman L, Schafer A, editors: Cecil textbook of medicine, ed 24, Philadelphia, 2012, Saunders, pp 1800–1803.

Centers for Disease Control and Prevention: CDC health information for international travel 2018, New York, 2017, Oxford University Press2017.

Freedman DO, Chen LH, Kzoarsky PE: Medical considerations before international travel, N Eng J Med 375:247–260, 2016.

Jeronimo S, de Queiroz Sousa A, Pearson R: Leishmaniasis. In Guerrant RL, Walker DH, Weller PF, editors: Tropical infectious diseases: principles, pathogens, and practices, ed 3, Philadelphia, 2011, Saunders, pp 696–706.

Kirchoff L: Trypanosoma species (American trypanosomiasis, Chagas' disease): biology of trypanosomes. In Mandell GL, Bennett JE, Dolin R, editors: Principles and practice of infectious diseases, ed 7, Philadelphia, 2010, Churchill Livingstone, pp 3481–3488.

Leder K, Torresi J, Libman M, et al: GeoSentinel surveillance of illness in returned travelers, 2007-2011, Ann Intern Med 158:456–468, 2013.

未来方向

旅行医学领域不断变化,因为传染病并不总是遵循历史模式。随着旅行全球化的增加,我们可以看到疾病暴发和流行区域变化,例如2014—2015年的西非埃博拉疫情、2015—2016年的寨卡病毒流行以及中东持续的MERS-CoV疫情,这些都改变了我们既往对这些地区旅行者的指导和管理意见。作为致力于旅行性疾病治疗的医生,我们必须了解全球传染病不断变化的形势。

推荐阅读

Arguin P: Approach to the patient before and after travel. In Goldman L, Schafer A, editors: Cecil textbook of medicine, ed 24, Philadelphia, 2012, Saunders, pp 1800–1803.

Centers for Disease Control and Prevention: CDC health information for international travel 2018, New York, 2017, Oxford University Press2017.

Freedman DO, Chen LH, Kzoarsky PE: Medical considerations before international travel, N Eng J Med 375:247–260, 2016.

Jeronimo S, de Queiroz Sousa A, Pearson R: Leishmaniasis. In Guerrant RL, Walker DH, Weller PF, editors: Tropical infectious diseases: principles, pathogens, and practices, ed 3, Philadelphia, 2011, Saunders, pp 696–706.

Kirchoff L: Trypanosoma species (American trypanosomiasis, Chagas' disease): biology of trypanosomes. In Mandell GL, Bennett JE, Dolin R, editors: Principles and practice of infectious diseases, ed 7, Philadelphia, 2010, Churchill Livingstone, pp 3481–3488.

Leder K, Torresi J, Libman M, et al: GeoSentinel surveillance of illness in returned travelers, 2007-2011, Ann Intern Med 158:456–468, 2013.

APPENDIX

Coronavirus Disease 2019 (COVID-19)

Edward J. Wing

The Coronavirus Disease 2019 (COVID-19) pandemic occurred after the initial deadline for this book had passed, and as a result I have written this appendix to reflect our knowledge of COVID-19 as of October 2020. The COVID-19 pandemic burst on the world as a totally new viral respiratory infection at the end of 2019 and the beginning of 2020. Initially the virology, epidemiology, transmission, diagnosis, clinical aspects, treatment, and prevention were largely unknown. Since then the amount of scientific focus and effort on all aspects of the disease from its molecular virology to clinical understanding to vaccine and drug development has been extraordinary.

While we know much more now about the infection than initially, our knowledge and hence this appendix is still largely incomplete. The ability to recognize, diagnose, care for our patients, and prevent this virus will undoubtedly change and evolve over time. Therefore, all physicians and health care workers need to continue to update their knowledge of COVID-19 to become long-term learners concerning all aspects of the infection.

COVID-19 PANDEMIC

Infectious pandemics, usually associated with animal–human contact, have afflicted mankind for millennia. Although some infections such as malaria have probably infected primates for millions of years, most pandemic infections have occurred since the beginning of agriculture. Pandemics such as the bubonic plague, which killed from one third to one half of the population of Europe and devastated other parts of the world, and the 1918 to 1919 influenza H1N1 pandemic that killed 675,000 people in the United States and at least 50 million people worldwide, have been catastrophic. More recent pandemics have included HIV, cholera, Zika virus and other influenza strains (1957, H2N2; 1968, H3N2; 2009, H1N1pdm09). The majority of recent pandemics in this century have been due to viral infections in which animals have been either the primary or intermediate host or the vectors of the diseases. RNA viruses such as the influenza and coronaviruses that have inherent genetic instability have been particularly prominent.

Coronaviruses have been known to have natural animal reservoirs, particularly in bat populations, and to cause mild, seasonal upper respiratory disease. Four human coronaviruses—OC43, 229E, HKU1 and NL63 viral strains—have been shown to have a predilection for children under the age of 5, to cause respiratory illness, and to be transmitted similarly to influenza virus. In 2002 to 2003, a new coronavirus, SARS-CoV, derived from bat strains, was identified in China. It caused severe respiratory infection infecting more than 8000 people in 29 countries with a mortality of approximately 10%. Because of limited transmissibility, the pandemic was controlled and then eliminated with strict public health measures. In 2012, a second coronavirus, Middle East respiratory syndrome (MERS-CoV), was first recognized in Saudi Arabia and subsequently in other Middle Eastern countries. Evidence indicates that its source is camels and that close contact with these animals is a risk for contracting the disease. Gastrointestinal and pulmonary symptoms occur. To date there have been approximately 2500 cases with a mortality rate of 34%.

In early December 2019, cases of pneumonia of unknown cause were identified in the city of Wuhan, capital city of Hubei province, China. Many of the initial cases had worked in or had close contact with wet markets that sell fresh meat, fish, and other perishable produce. The outbreak increased during December, and on December 31 the WHO was informed of an outbreak of a new cause of pneumonia. With remarkable speed, the cause was identified as a new coronavirus and the gene sequence reported from China and the WHO on January 9, 2020. The virus was named SARS-CoV-2, and the infection is referred to as COVID-19. The epidemic continued to increase in Wuhan during January 2020 and peaked in late January and early February. The high population density in Wuhan, population movements, and the lack of clarity regarding human-to-human transmission drove the epidemic. Severe overcrowding of medical facilities occurred, prompting draconian public health measures including the imposition of a *cordon sanitaire* that prevented movement in or out of Wuhan, universal and compulsory home restriction with drastic penalties for violations, suspension of public transportation, closure of entertainment venues, closure of the implicated wet markets, and compulsory mask wearing. Subsequently, the number of new cases decreased steadily so that few cases were reported after March 1 in Wuhan although cases continued to be reported in other areas of China including Beijing. The total number of confirmed cases in Mainland China as of February 11 was reported as over 72,000 although this may represent a low estimate. The overall fatality rate was reported as 2.3%, but it was soon understood that mortality rate varies based on age group, testing availability, and other factors. Vigorous public health measures as described appear to have been effective in at least limiting the number of cases in China.

Cases of COVID-19 were reported outside of China as early as January 13 in persons who had traveled from Wuhan. The first case in the United States occurred on January 19, 2020, in Snohomish County, Washington, in an individual who had recently returned from visiting family in Wuhan. The patient had gastrointestinal and respiratory symptoms with fever that persisted for 8 days, requiring treatment with oxygen and remdesivir, an experimental antiviral agent. The patient recovered without incidence. Notably, future studies demonstrated that the virus circulated on both coasts for many weeks before it was recognized.

On January 30 with cases in Asia including Japan, South Korea, Vietnam, and Singapore; in Europe including France; and in the United States, the WHO declared a global emergency. Cases were reported from Africa (first in Egypt) but remained relatively low. By March the number of cases in Europe exploded, with particularly devastating effects in Italy, Spain, France, and the United Kingdom, and the WHO labeled COVID-19 a pandemic. Health care systems were overwhelmed in northern Italy as well as other areas, and mortality

附录

2019 冠状病毒病（COVID-19）

刘智博 译　崔晓敬 葛瑛 审校　曹彬 通审

2019冠状病毒病（COVID-19）大流行发生在本书最初成书日期之后，因此我以附录形式来反映截至2020年10月我们对COVID-19的了解。2019年底到2020年初，COVID-19大流行作为一种新发病毒性呼吸道感染在全球暴发。最初，从病毒学、流行病学、传播、诊断、临床特点到治疗和预防，该疾病在很大程度上是未知的。从那时起，从分子病毒学到临床理解，再到疫苗和药物开发，科学界对该疾病各方面的关注和努力探索都是非同寻常的。

虽然我们现在对这种感染的了解比最初多了很多，但我们的认识以及本附录仍是不完整的。随着时间的推移，对该疾病识别、诊断、患者照护和预防的能力无疑会继续变化和发展。因此，所有医生和卫生保健工作者都需要继续更新他们对COVID-19的知识并成为长期的学习者。

COVID-19 大流行

传染性流行病通常和动物与人类的接触有关，近千年来一直困扰着人类。虽然一些传染病，如疟疾，可能已经感染了灵长类动物数百万年，但大流行大多是从农耕开始后发生的。鼠疫大流行杀死了欧洲1/3～1/2的人口，也摧毁了世界其他地区，1918—1919年的H1N1流感大流行导致美国67.5万人死亡，全球至少5000万人死亡，这些流行病都是灾难性的。新近的大流行包括HIV、霍乱、寨卡病毒和其他流感毒株（1957年，H2N2；1968年，H3N2；2009年，H1N1pdm09）。本世纪最近的大多数大流行病都是由病毒感染引起的，其中动物是疾病的主要宿主或中间宿主或媒介。具有固有遗传不稳定性的RNA病毒，如流感病毒和冠状病毒，尤其突出。

已知冠状病毒具有天然动物宿主，特别是在蝙蝠种群中，并可引起轻症季节性上呼吸道疾病。四种人类冠状病毒——OC43、229E、HKU1和NL63病毒株——已被证明更易感染5岁以下儿童，引起呼吸道疾病，传播上与流感病毒类似。2002—2003年中国发现了一种新的冠状病毒SARS-CoV，来源于蝙蝠株。它造成了严重的呼吸道感染，导致29个国家8000多人感染，死亡率约为10%。由于其传播能力有限，通过严格的公共卫生措施，SARS-CoV大流行得到控制并随即被消除。2012年，又一种冠状病毒——中东呼吸综合征病毒（MERS-CoV）首先在沙特阿拉伯、随后在其他中东国家被发现。有证据表明，其来源是骆驼，与这些动物密切接触可能感染该病。该病会出现胃肠道和肺部症状。到目前为止，大约有2500个病例，死亡率为34%。

2019年12月初，中国湖北省会武汉市发现不明原因肺炎病例。许多最初的病例曾在出售鲜肉、鱼和其他易腐农产品的生鲜市场工作或有过密切接触。疫情在12月加剧，12月31日，WHO获悉一种新病因的肺炎暴发。2020年1月9日，中国和WHO以非凡的速度确定病因为新型冠状病毒并报告了基因序列。该病毒被命名为SARS-CoV-2，这种感染被称为COVID-19。2020年1月，武汉疫情继续加剧，并在1月底和2月初达到高峰。武汉的高人口密度、人员流动、对人际传播缺乏清醒认识等因素推动了疫情蔓延。医疗资源负荷加重，促使政府采取了严厉的公共卫生措施，包括实施阻止人员进出武汉的防疫封控，居家隔离并对违规者采取严格的措施，暂停公共交通，关闭娱乐场所，关闭相关生鲜市场，佩戴口罩。随后，新发病例数稳步下降，3月1日以后虽然包括北京在内的中国其他地区仍有报告病例，但武汉仅有很少的病例报告。中国内地共报告72 314例病例，其中确诊病例44 672例（61.8%）；在确诊病例中，死亡1023例，粗病死率为2.3%（译者注：以上数据摘自《中华流行病学杂志》2020年2月第41卷第2期，新型冠状病毒肺炎流行病学特征分析一文）。但人们很快认识到，死亡率因年龄、检测可及性和其他因素而波动。上述有力的公共卫生措施有效地控制了中国的病例数量。

早在1月13日，中国境外就报告了有武汉旅居史的COVID-19病例。美国首例病例于2020年1月19日出现在华盛顿州斯诺霍米什县，患者由武汉探亲归来。患者有胃肠道和呼吸道症状，持续发热8天，在接受了吸氧和瑞德西韦试验性抗病毒治疗后痊愈。值得注意的是，之后的研究表明，在被发现前，该病毒已在东西海岸传播了数周。

1月30日，包括日本、韩国、越南和新加坡在内的亚洲国家，包括法国在内的欧洲国家，以及美国都报告了病例，WHO宣布进入全球紧急状态。非洲报告了病例（首例在埃及），但数量仍然相对较低。到3月，欧洲的病例数量激增，对意大利、西班牙、法国和英国造成了毁灭性的影响，WHO将COVID-19列为大流行。意大利北部和其他地区的卫生保健系统不堪重负，老

was particularly high among the elderly. By June 29 COVID-19 had occurred in over 200 countries with 10 million cases and over 500,000 confirmed deaths. By the fall of 2020 it was estimated that more than 30 million cases of COVID-19, with more than 1 million deaths, had occurred worldwide.

By the end of April 2020, the number of cases in the Americas, primarily the United States, had skyrocketed, reaching over 1 million cases with 58,000 deaths. As an early example in the United States, an outbreak of COVID-19 was identified in February 2020 in a long-term care skilled nursing facility in King County, Washington State. In the facility, 81 residents (median age 81), 48 health care workers (median age 42.5 years), and 14 visitors (median age 42.5 years) were infected. Twenty-two of the 81 residents (27%), 0 of the 48 (0%) health care workers, and 1 of the 14 visitors (7.1%) died. In addition to age and residence in a nursing home, residents had a high rate of chronic underlying conditions, including cardiovascular disease (including hypertension), renal disease, diabetes mellitus/obesity, and pulmonary disease.

By March, the epicenter in the United States was New York City and the surrounding counties where the number of cases exploded, overwhelming some medical centers and devastating nursing homes and their residents where the mortality was the greatest. By May widespread outbreaks were noted in Mid-Atlantic and New England states, Louisiana, Florida, and in West Coast states. The number of cases fell in May in the United States, most likely due to restrictive measures including school and business closings, restrictions on public events, quarantine regulations, and wearing masks. The incidence of COVID-19 began to rise again in June with outbreaks in states such as Florida and Arizona, perhaps due to relaxation of earlier restrictive public health measures. Unfortunately, in late August and September the number of deaths continued at greater than 1000/day and the number of deaths directly associated with COVID-19 in the United States reached 200,000. In the fall, with reopening schools, particularly colleges and universities, and relaxation of restrictions on businesses and entertainment venues such as restaurants and bars, the number of new cases continued to rise as did the rates of hospitalizations. Early data indicate that the age of persons infected has decreased and the severity and mortality is lower. The rise in rates among those 18 to 24 years old was particularly striking. In addition, the disproportionate impact of the pandemic on the Black and Latinx communities became apparent. As of October 15, 2020, 216,035 deaths were reported in the United States, although excess deaths possibly related to the effects of COVID-19 have been estimated to be higher.

Finally, the 2020 to 2021 influenza season will intersect with the COVID-19 pandemic in the United States this winter and spring with unknown severity. The effects of COVID-19 public health measures, vaccination rates for influenza, and the already devastating effects of COVID-19 on vulnerable populations will all influence the morbidity and mortality of the influenza season.

VIROLOGY

The COVID-19 virus is an enveloped single-stranded RNA virus with surface spike proteins, like other coronaviruses, that give the group its distinctive contour under electron microscope, hence its name "coronavirus" ("corona" means crown). COVID-19 has 79% similarity to SARS-CoV and 50% similarity to MERS-CoV based on genetic analysis. Bats are believed to be the original source of COVID-19 with perhaps an intermediate host such as the pangolin, sometimes called the spiny anteater, which is regarded as a delicacy in parts of China and sold in wet markets. Genetic mutations presumably allowed the virus to cross species and cause disease. However, the origins of the virus are not completely understood at this point.

The 180-kDa spike (S) protein binds to the peptidase angiotensin-converting enzyme 2 receptor (ACE2) on cell surfaces and mediates viral and cell membrane fusion for entry into cells. Membrane fusion also requires the interaction of other proteases, particularly transmembrane protease serine 2 (TMPRSS2), on cell surfaces. The presence of ACE2 determines cell tropism of COVID-19 and is found on epithelial cells of both the upper and lower respiratory tract. ACE2 also has a wide distribution in other tissues including vascular endothelial cells, the gastrointestinal tract, and kidney. SARS-CoV-2 virus enters cells by endocytosis, uses the cells' own machinery to reproduce, and then is released to infect other cells. Nasal epithelial cells are infected, which in early infection may result in initial upper respiratory symptoms and anosmia. Bronchial, alveolar, and endovascular epithelial cells are also infected early, causing an inflammatory response consisting of neutrophils, T lymphocytes, macrophages and the release of cytokines including TNF-α, and IL-6. As the infection and inflammation progresses in the lungs there is interstitial thickening, pulmonary edema, activation of the coagulation pathway, and lymphocyte depletion. Further inflammation can result in fibrosis with marked compromise of pulmonary function.

PATHOLOGY

Autopsy findings demonstrate high SARS-CoV-19 titers particularly in the lung, but also in blood, liver, kidney, brain, and heart. In individuals who died of COVID-19, autopsy shows diffuse alveolar damage in all lobes but with more pronounced findings in the lower lobes. During the early phase, signs of acute alveolar damage include edema, hyaline membrane formation, and thickened alveolar septa with perivascular lymphocytic infiltration. There is severe endothelial injury associated with disrupted cell membranes and the presence of virus. Pulmonary vessels including alveolar capillaries show widespread microthrombi and vascular angiogenesis, both of which distinguish it from the pathology of severe influenza infection. In later stages there is diffuse alveolar damage, fibroblastic proliferation leading to fibrosis, pneumocyte hyperplasia and interstitial thickening, and collapsed alveoli. In some areas of diffuse alveolar damage, metaplasia or widespread fibrosis is observed.

Other findings have included bronchopneumonia; lymphocytic myocarditis and epicarditis; periportal lymphocytic infiltration with hepatic congestion and steatosis, hepatic cell necrosis, and central vein thrombosis; acute tubular injury; and thrombotic features in multiple organs including lung, heart, and kidney. Also noted are focal pancreatitis, adrenocortical hyperplasia, and lymphocyte depletion in spleen and lymph nodes. In the brain, extensive inflammation has been noted in the olfactory bulbs and medulla oblongata. It was recognized early on that severe COVID-19 could result in activation of coagulation and consumption of clotting factors resulting in diffuse intravascular coagulation. Increased coagulation can result in deep venous thrombosis and unsuspected pulmonary embolism, myocardial infarction, stroke, and vascular compromise in other organs. Thrombosis of small and mid-sized pulmonary arteries with associated infarction is found in a high percentage of cases. In addition, neutrophilic plugs have been observed composed of neutrophil extracellular traps (NETS). NETS are composed of extracellular strands of DNA from neutrophils that trap pathogens. In an autopsy series NETS have been observed with platelets, which may induce thrombus formation.

HOST DEFENSES

Host defenses against coronaviruses consist of both innate and specific immunity, but the specific mechanisms and their relative importance

年人的死亡率特别高。截至 6 月 29 日，COVID-19 已在 200 多个国家出现，有 1000 万确诊病例和 50 余万例死亡。到 2020 年秋季，估计全球发生了超过 3000 万例 COVID-19 病例，死亡人数超过 100 万。

到 2020 年 4 月底，美洲（主要是美国）的病例数激增，达到 100 多万例，死亡 5.8 万人。2020 年 2 月华盛顿州金县一个长期专业护理机构中暴发的 COVID-19 疫情是美国疫情发生早期的一个例子。在该机构中，81 名居住者（中位年龄 81 岁）、48 名医护人员（中位年龄 42.5 岁）和 14 名访客（中位年龄 42.5 岁）被感染。22 名居住者死亡（27%），48 名医护人员中无人死亡（0%），1 名访客死亡（1%）。除了年龄和居住环境外，养老院居住者有较高的慢性病发病率，包括心血管疾病（包括高血压）、肾病、糖尿病/肥胖和肺部疾病。

到 3 月，美国的疫情中心是纽约市及其周边，病例数量激增，使一些医疗中心不堪重负，并严重影响养老院及其居住者，那里死亡率最高。到 5 月，疫情在大西洋中部和新英格兰州、路易斯安那州、佛罗里达州和西海岸各州都出现大范围暴发。由于学校和企业关闭、限制公共场所活动、隔离规定和佩戴口罩等限制措施，美国的病例数量在 5 月份下降。6 月，随着佛罗里达州和亚利桑那州等州暴发疫情，COVID-19 的发病率再次开始上升，这可能是由于先前的限制性公共卫生措施有所放松。不幸的是，在 8 月下旬和 9 月，死亡人数持续超过 1000 人/天，美国与 COVID-19 直接相关的死亡人数达到 20 万人。到了秋季，随着学校（尤其是学院和大学）重新开学，以及对餐馆和酒吧等商业和娱乐场所的限制放松，新增病例数量和住院率都在上升。早期数据表明，受感染者的年龄下降，严重程度和死亡率也降低。18～24 岁人群的患病比例上升尤为引人注目。此外，大流行对黑人和拉丁裔社区造成的过度影响也显而易见。截至 2020 年 10 月 15 日，美国报告的死亡人数为 216 035 人，但可能与 COVID-19 影响有关的超额死亡人数估计会更高。

最后，2020—2021 年的流感流行季节将与今年冬季和明年春季的 COVID-19 大流行交织在一起，其严重程度尚不得而知（译者注：2020—2021 年度我国流感呈低流行水平，2021—2022 年度及以后冬季，流感高峰复现）。COVID-19 公共卫生措施的影响、流感疫苗接种率以及 COVID-19 对易感人群已经造成的破坏性影响都将影响流感季节的发病率和死亡率。

病毒学

COVID-19 病毒是一种有包膜的单链 RNA 病毒，与其他冠状病毒一样具有表面刺突蛋白，这使该病毒在电子显微镜下具有独特的外形，因此被称为"冠状病毒"（"corona"的意思是冠）。根据遗传分析，COVID-19 与 SARS-CoV 的相似性为 79%，与 MERS-CoV 的相似性为 50%。蝙蝠被认为是 COVID-19 的原始来源。其中间宿主可能为穿山甲，有时被称为针鼹，在中国部分地区被视为美味佳肴并在潮湿的生鲜市场出售。基因突变可能导致病毒跨物种传播并引起疾病。然而，该病毒的起源目前还并不完全清楚。

180-kDa 刺突（S）蛋白与细胞表面的肽酶血管紧张素转换酶 2 受体（ACE2）结合，介导病毒和细胞膜融合进入细胞。膜融合还需要其他蛋白酶的相互作用，特别是细胞表面的跨膜蛋白酶丝氨酸 2（TMPRSS2）。ACE2 的存在决定了细胞对 COVID-19 的易感性，上呼吸道和下呼吸道的上皮细胞都有表达。ACE2 也广泛分布于其他组织，包括血管内皮细胞、胃肠道和肾。SARS-CoV-2 病毒通过内吞作用进入细胞，利用细胞自身的机制进行繁殖，然后释放出来感染其他细胞。鼻上皮细胞被感染，感染早期可导致最初的上呼吸道症状和嗅觉丧失。支气管、肺泡和血管内上皮细胞在感染早期引起中性粒细胞、T 淋巴细胞、巨噬细胞的炎症反应，并释放包括 TNF-α 和 IL-6 在内的细胞因子。随着肺内感染和炎症的发展，会出现肺间质增厚、肺水肿、凝血途径激活、淋巴细胞减少。进一步的炎症可导致纤维化，肺功能明显受损。

病理学

尸检结果显示，SARS-CoV-19 的检测滴度除在肺部尤其高外，在血液、肝、肾、大脑和心脏内也很高。在死于 COVID-19 的患者中，尸检显示所有肺叶都有弥漫性肺泡损伤，下叶更为明显。在早期，急性肺损伤的征象包括水肿、透明膜形成和肺泡间隔增厚伴血管周围淋巴细胞浸润。严重的内皮损伤与细胞膜破坏和病毒的存在有关。包括肺泡毛细血管在内的肺血管显示广泛的微血栓和血管生成，这两种情况都有别于严重流感病毒的感染病理变化。晚期出现弥漫性肺泡损伤，成纤维细胞增生导致的纤维化，肺细胞增生、间质增厚和肺泡塌陷。在弥漫性肺泡损伤的某些区域，可观察到化生或广泛纤维化。

其他发现包括支气管肺炎、淋巴细胞性心肌炎和心包炎；肝周淋巴细胞浸润，伴有肝充血和脂肪变性、肝细胞坏死和中心静脉血栓形成；急性肾小管损伤；以及包括肺、心脏、肾在内的多个器官血栓形成的特征。同样值得注意的是局灶性胰腺炎、肾上腺皮质增生、脾和淋巴结的淋巴细胞减少。在大脑中，嗅球和延髓可见广泛炎症。人们很早就认识到，严重的 COVID-19 可能导致凝血激活和凝血因子的消耗，从而导致弥散性血管内凝血。凝血增强可导致深静脉血栓形成和不易发现的肺栓塞、心肌梗死、卒中和其他器官血管受损。小、中肺动脉血栓形成与相关的梗死发生比例很高。此外，还观察到由中性粒细胞胞外诱捕网（NETS）组成的中性粒细胞栓子。NETS 由捕获病原体的中性粒细胞的细胞外 DNA 链组成。在一系列尸检中观察到 NETS 和血小板一起存在，这可能诱发血栓形成。

宿主防御

宿主对冠状病毒的防御包括先天免疫和特异性免疫，但是具体的机制和相对重要性还有待阐明。感染

have yet to be clarified. Sites of infection, particularly the lung with endothelial damage, attract immune cells including T and B lymphocytes, macrophages, and neutrophils. The immune response includes release of cytokines and inflammatory molecules including interleukins 1 and 6, interferons, TNF-α as well as antibody production of IgM and IgG, and activation of the coagulation system with increases in D-dimer and micro- and macro-thrombosis. Inflammatory markers include elevated erythrocyte sedimentation rate, C-reactive protein, ferritin, and lactic dehydrogenase. A characteristic of the inflammatory process is the destruction and apoptosis of both CD4 and CD8 T lymphocytes with resulting lymphopenia. Experimental data suggest that neutralizing antibodies directed towards the S protein afford protection after infection; thus, vaccine development has targeted the response against this protein. Recent data suggest that the specific immune response to SARS-CoV-2 consists of CD4, CD8, and antibody in a coordinated response. Lack of such a response and decreased number of T cells occur in persons over 65 and may account for greater susceptibility to the virus. It is not clear, however, whether infection itself provides long-lasting immunity, whether the presence of antibody after infection protects, whether antibody persists after infections, or what the relative importance of T-cell immunity is.

TRANSMISSION

Transmission of COVID-19 is an essential issue in determining risk for acquiring the virus. At the beginning of the pandemic, it was unclear whether transmission was airborne, through contact with infected animals or material in the wet markets of Wuhan, or by some other mechanism. The rapid spread of the infection within households, among health care workers, and the spread of the disease outside of Wuhan quickly indicated that human-to-human contact was the primary mode of transmission. It is apparent now that most transmission occurs within households, nursing homes, and other congregate settings. Within households, the greatest risk is among the elderly and spouses. Infected individuals appear to be most infectious just before or for several days after the beginning of symptoms when viral loads peak. However, patients who remain asymptomatic can also transmit the infection.

A major question has centered on the infectivity of individuals after contracting COVID-19. Reverse transcriptase-polymerase reaction (RT-PCR) tests usually become negative when an individual recovers from COVID-19 infection but may remain positive for prolonged periods. However, in the majority of cases recovery of viable virus has been shown to disappear 8 days after the onset of symptoms. Thus, in most protocols, the quarantine is stopped 10 to 14 days after the onset of symptoms.

Airborne transmission occurs when viable virus becomes airborne after an infected individual exhales, speaks, particularly in a loud voice, sings, coughs or sneezes. Infectious particles can be broadly classified as either large droplets, which are usually defined as larger than 5 micrometers, or aerosols, which are smaller particles of less than 5 micrometers. A mixture of large particles and aerosols are generated after a person coughs or sneezes. Certain medical procedures such as intubation or noninvasive positive-pressure ventilation potentially cause aerosol formation. After leaving the respiratory tract, large droplets rapidly fall to the ground—usually within 6 feet of an infected individual. Influenza is a typical pathogen transmitted primarily by large droplets. Close contact with someone who is coughing or sneezing maximizes the risk for acquiring influenza. The CDC has recently defined a close contact as "someone who was within six feet of an infected person for a cumulative time of 15 minutes or more over a 24-hour period starting from 2 days before illness onset (or for asymptomatic patients, 2 days prior to test specimen collection) until the time the patient is isolated."

In contrast, aerosols evaporate quickly, leaving infectious particles suspended in the air for a considerable period of time—usually hours—in closed and particularly in poorly ventilated spaces. Microbial pathogens such as tuberculosis or measles are typically spread by aerosol. These pathogens can potentially infect large numbers of people because of the airborne suspension of infectious particles. The difference between large droplet spread, such as found with influenza, and aerosols, such as found with measles, is indicated by the average number of people who are infected by an index case, which is termed the reproduction number. For COVID-19 the average reproduction number is 2 to 3, similar to influenza. Risk of transmission does vary with the type of exposure. For example, close contact exposure gives a risk of perhaps 5% whereas household contact can be as high as 40%. But brief interactions, such as while shopping, have a risk of less than 1%. For aerosol transmission, the reproduction number can be as high as 18. Thus, in an epidemic, each active measles case infects on average of 18 other individuals. Because the reproduction number for COVID-19 is low, as is the secondary attack rate, and because the evidence that masks and social distancing of 6 feet reduces incidence of disease, large droplet transmission seems the likely mode of most transmission. Also, a potential association between the size of the inoculum and the clinical presentations and outcome has been proposed and is under investigation.

Nonetheless, some data do support the possibility of aerosol transmission of SARS-CoV-2. Aerosols with SARS-CoV-2 RNA have been demonstrated experimentally and in hospitals. In addition, viable virus has been demonstrated in hospital settings. Furthermore, aerosol transmission has been suggested epidemiologically in certain situations. An outbreak in a nursing home in the Netherlands in June and July 2020 suggested aerosol transmission. In this outbreak 17 (81%) residents and 17 (50%) health care workers (who wore masks) from one of seven wards in a psychogeriatric nursing home were diagnosed with COVID-19 as confirmed by RT-PCR. All residents were diagnosed within 4 days of each other. None of the 95 residents or 106 health care workers in the six other wards was infected. Investigation of the ventilation system in this ward revealed the possibility that air was recirculated, rather than circulated to the outside, due to a recent renovation of the system. Thus, circumstantial evidence in this widespread, ward-specific outbreak over a short time suggests aerosol transmission. Other reports of short-term, extensive outbreaks in poorly ventilated venues suggest the possibility of occasional aerosol transmission. Finally, transmission by "super transmitters" has occurred when a single individual appears to infect a large number of people, well beyond the expected number of two (discussed previously). The frequency and the mechanism for transmission from these individuals remains to be clarified.

Therefore, at the time of this writing, the major route of transmission of COVID-19 during the pandemic appears to be by large droplets in situations where there is close contact without the protection of masks (see later) and over a sustained period, and not by aerosol. In certain circumstances, however, usually indoors in poorly ventilated venues, transmission by aerosols may occur.

Experimental conditions with large inocula of SARS-CoV-2 have demonstrated persistence of the virus on fomites for periods of up to 72 hours, depending on the surface and the conditions. Virus persists longer on impermeable surfaces such as steel or plastic than on permeable surfaces such as paper. More realistic conditions with lower inocula suggest survival of the viable virus for several hours. Virus has been found on numerous surfaces in hospital rooms of infected patients, although data from the United Kingdom indicate that the presence of virus as detected by RT-PCR in the air and on surfaces is

部位，特别是内皮损伤的肺组织，会吸引免疫细胞，包括 T 细胞、B 细胞、巨噬细胞和中性粒细胞。免疫反应有细胞因子和炎症分子的释放，包括白细胞介素 1 和白细胞介素 6、干扰素、TNF-α 和 IgM、IgG 抗体产生，以及凝血系统的激活，表现为 D- 二聚体升高、微血栓和大的血栓形成。炎症标志物如红细胞沉降率、C 反应蛋白、铁蛋白和乳酸脱氢酶升高。炎症过程的一个特征是 $CD4^+$ 和 $CD8^+$ T 淋巴细胞的破坏和凋亡，导致淋巴细胞减少。实验数据表明，针对 S 蛋白的中和抗体在感染后起保护作用；因此，疫苗开发的目标是针对这种蛋白质的反应。最近的数据表明，针对 SARS-CoV-2 的特异性免疫反应由 CD4、CD8 和抗体协同完成。65 岁以上的人群缺乏这种反应，T 细胞数量减少，这可能是更容易感染病毒的原因。然而，感染后是否产生持久的免疫力、感染后抗体能否持续存在、T 细胞免疫的相对重要性是什么，这些问题仍不清楚。

传播

COVID-19 的传播是判断感染该病毒风险的一个关键问题。在大流行开始时，尚不清楚病毒是通过空气、通过接触感染的动物或武汉生鲜市场的物品，还是通过其他途径传播。感染在家庭内、医护人员中迅速蔓延，并很快扩散到武汉以外的地区，这表明人际接触是主要的传播方式。现在已经很清楚，大多数传播发生在家庭、疗养院和其他聚集环境中。在家庭中，风险最高的是老年人和配偶之间。感染者似乎在出现症状的前后几天，病毒载量达到峰值时最具传染性，而无症状的患者也可以传播感染。

主要问题集中在感染 COVID-19 后的传染性上。当患者从 COVID-19 感染中恢复时，逆转录聚合酶链反应（RT-PCR）检测通常变为阴性，但也可能在较长时间内保持阳性。但在大多数恢复期患者中活病毒会在出现症状 8 天后消失。因此，在大多数方案中，在出现症状后 10～14 天可结束隔离。

当感染者呼气、说话（尤其是大声说话）、唱歌、咳嗽或打喷嚏后，活病毒就可以通过空气传播。传染性颗粒可大致分为大飞沫（通常定义为大于 5 μm）和气溶胶（小于 5 μm 的小颗粒）。一个人咳嗽或打喷嚏后会产生大颗粒和气溶胶的混合物。某些医疗措施，如插管或无创正压通气可能导致气溶胶的形成。离开呼吸道后，大飞沫迅速落到地面上——通常在距感染者 6 英尺之内的范围。流感病毒是主要通过大飞沫传播的典型病原体。与咳嗽或打喷嚏的人密切接触会增加流感感染的风险。美国 CDC 最近将"密切接触者"定义为"24 h 内在 6 英尺范围内接触感染者（从发病前 2 天到被隔离，无症状患者为采集检测标本前 2 天）累计达 15 min 或更长时间的人"。

相比之下，气溶胶蒸发得很快。在封闭的，特别是在通风不良的空间里，传染性颗粒在空气中悬浮相当长时间——通常是几个小时。肺结核或麻疹等疾病的微生物病原体通常通过气溶胶传播。由于传染性颗粒在空气中悬浮，这些病原体可能会感染大量人群。大飞沫传播（如流感）和气溶胶传播（如麻疹）间的差异由被指示病例感染的平均人数表示，即传染数。COVID-19 的平均传染数为 2～3，与流感相似。传播的风险因接触的类型而异。例如，密切接触暴露的风险可能为 5%，家庭接触的风险可能高达 40%。但短暂的互动，如购物，风险不到 1%。对于气溶胶传播，传染数可高达 18。因此，在流行期间，每个活动性麻疹病例平均感染 18 人。由于 COVID-19 的传染数低，二代传染率也低，而且有证据表明，佩戴口罩和保持 6 英尺的社交距离可以降低发病率，因此大飞沫传播似乎是其最可能的传播方式。此外，接触病毒量的大小与临床表现和预后之间可能存在关联，目前正在进行研究。

尽管如此，一些数据确实支持了 SARS-CoV-2 通过气溶胶传播的可能性。带有 SARS-CoV-2 RNA 的气溶胶在实验条件下和医院中被证实存在。在医院环境中也已证实存在活病毒。此外，从流行病学角度来看，在某些情况下存在气溶胶传播。2020 年 6～7 月在荷兰一家养老院暴发的疫情提示存在气溶胶传播。在这次疫情中，老年精神疗养院的 7 个病房中，一间病房内的 17 名（81%）居住者和 17 名（50%）医护人员（佩戴口罩）经 RT-PCR 检测被诊断为 COVID-19。所有居住者均在 4 天内被确诊。其他 6 个病房的 95 名居住者和 106 名医护人员均无人感染。对该病房通风系统的调查显示，由于近期对系统进行了翻新，空气可能是再循环的，而不是向外流通。因此，短时间在特定病房内广泛传播的疫情间接证明存在气溶胶传播。其他在通风条件差的场所内发生的短期大范围疫情报告表明，偶尔可能发生气溶胶传播。最后，"超级传播者"的传播指一个个体传播了很多人，远远超过了预期的两个人（如前所述）。这些患者传播的频率和机制仍有待阐明。

因此，在撰写本文时，COVID-19 大流行期间主要的传播途径似乎仍是在没有口罩保护（见下文）的情况下通过大飞沫进行持续密切接触，而非通过气溶胶传播。但是在特定情况下，通常是在通风不良的室内场所，可能发生气溶胶传播。

在实验条件下大量接触 SARS-CoV-2，根据物体表面和条件的不同，病毒在污染物上可持续存在长达 72 h。病毒在钢铁或塑料等不透水的物体表面上，比在纸张等透水表面上存在的时间更长。更现实的情况下，低接触量的活病毒可存在几个小时。在感染患者病房的许多物体表面上发现了病毒，但英国的数据表明，通过 RT-PCR 检测到的空气和物体表面上的病毒量很低，特别是在清洁后，而且活病毒的复苏率非常低。

low, particularly after cleaning, and that recovery of viable virus is very low. There is little epidemiologic or clinical data at this point suggesting significant transmission through fomites, although it is certainly reasonable to keep open the possibility and act on that assumption.

SARS-CoV-2 RNA has been found in stool as might be expected with a gastrointestinal tropic virus, but there is no evidence that transmission results from contaminated water or food.

COVID-19 is much less likely to be transmitted in outside venues because of rapid dispersal of droplets and aerosols. Sunlight and ultraviolet light have been shown to rapidly inactivate the virus.

Finally, epidemiologic data suggest that masks and social distancing reduce the risk of transmission. N-95 masks provide protection for both aerosols and large droplets. Surgical masks in hospital settings have been shown to reduce the risk of transmission. Experimental data showed that surgical masks and well-fitted homemade masks with multiple layers of quilting fabric were most effective in preventing droplet and even aerosol dispersal after a cough or loud singing. Bandana and folded handkerchief masks were less effective. Although epidemiologic and experimental data support mask wearing, to date, there are very limited controlled clinical data supporting the effectiveness of masks for COVID-2.

DIAGNOSIS

To date, RT-PCR testing for COVID-19 in nasopharyngeal swabs or nasal swabs is the most common diagnostic test. Samples from saliva may be as accurate. Different gene targets are used by different manufacturers. Viral RNA is measured by the number of polymerase chain reproductive cycles and expressed as threshold (Ct). Ct values less than 40 cycles indicate that a higher number of RNA copies are in the original sample and are regarded as positive. Specificity for most tests approaches 100%. RT-PCR positivity is highest for bronchoalveolar lavage specimens followed by nasopharyngeal, nasal, and oral specimens. False-negative results may occur due to improper specimen collection or due to collection too long before or after the onset of symptoms. RT-PCR may remain positive in some patients for 6 weeks or more. However, viable SARS-CoV-2 can be detected only for the first 8 days after symptoms begin. Therefore, infectivity is presumed to be low after that point. RT-PCR may remain positive in other sites such as sputum and stool for more prolonged periods but does not seem to have clinical relevance.

One important point to remember for any test is that accuracy depends on both the pretest probability, taking into account the symptomatology, history, and local infection rates of a patient, as well as the sensitivity and specificity of a test. The sensitivity for many of the available RT-PCR tests for COVID-19 varies from 71% to 98% and depends on a number of factors, including how the specimen was collected. With a low pretest probability that a patient has COVID-19 and with a relatively low-sensitivity test, a negative result would not assure lack of disease. Thus, depending on the clinical scenario, it is important not to rule out disease if the RT-PCR is negative.

In addition to RT-PCR technology, diagnostic tests are being rapidly developed and tested. They include assays based on the following technology: antigen based, isothermal amplification (LAMP), sequencing, and CRISPR/Cas. Potential advantages of these methodologies include reduced time for results, reduced resources necessary for the test, use of saliva rather than nasopharyngeal or nasal specimens, and more accuracy.

The antibody response of infected persons is usually measured by an ELISA (enzyme-linked immunoassay) test that detects the host's specific IgM and IgG antibodies to COVID-19 virus. Uses for antibody testing include aid in diagnosing acute disease and determining immunity after infection. Antibodies to the receptor-binding domain of S protein are the most specific and are expected to be a neutralizing antibody. IgM and IgG antibodies are usually not detected until the second or third week of illness, and conversion for most patients occurs by the third to fourth week. After that IgM antibodies begin to decline, usually disappearing by week 7, whereas IgG antibodies persist. The specificity of antibody testing may be compromised by immune responses to other coronaviruses that cause common respiratory illness. Although many serodiagnostic tests have been developed by different manufacturers, most have not undergone appropriate external validation. Therefore, the persistence of the antibody response and whether neutralizing antibodies protect and for how long are unknown at this point.

Most of the data on diagnostic tests for COVID-19 have derived from adults with symptomatic disease. It is not clear whether a similar pattern of RT-PCR and antigen positivity and antibody response will be found in other populations including immunocompromised patients, children, and asymptomatic patients.

CLINICAL ASPECTS

We don't know what percentage of patients who are infected with COVID-19 are asymptomatic. Numerous studies have suggested that a significant percentage of infected people remain asymptomatic. For example, all 217 passengers and crew members on an isolated cruise ship sailing in the South Atlantic Ocean were tested for COVID-19 and 128 (59%) tested positive. Of the positive patients, 24 (19%) were symptomatic, 8 (6%) required evacuation, and 1 patient died. The remaining 104 patients were asymptomatic. Similar data were obtained from analysis of asymptomatic infected patients in a well-publicized outbreak on a cruise ship named *Diamond Princess*. In another remarkable report in September 2020, point prevalence surveys in 33 nursing homes across Connecticut were done on 2117 residents. Six hundred and one were positive and of those 530 (88.2%) were asymptomatic at the time of testing. Sixty-two of 530 developed symptoms within 14 days of testing, and thus 468 of 601(78%) patients with positive tests remained asymptomatic. Furthermore, population-based antibody testing suggests that a significant percentage of patients who test positive for SARS-CoV-2 antibodies were asymptomatic.

A narrative review published in the *Annals of Internal Medicine* concluded that the asymptomatic rate may be as high as 40% to 45%, and a conservative estimate may be closer to 30%. CDC estimates of asymptomatic rates have been even higher. Similar to most clinical aspects of the infection, these numbers depend on the age and comorbidities of the population. Overall, the data are preliminary; however, since reports have been retrospective, presymptomatic or minimally symptomatic disease may have been underestimated, and patient selection was not random.

Initial studies from China indicate that of the symptomatic patients, 81% had mild symptoms, 14% had severe manifestations, and 5% were critically ill. Studies on COVID-19 symptoms initially focused on hospitalized patients, although most of these findings apply to patients with mild disease as well. The incubation period for COVID-19 averages 5 days but can range from 2 to 11 days. Rarely, the incubation period can extend to 14 days or even longer. For symptomatic patients early in the disease, upper respiratory tract symptoms including rhinorrhea and nasal congestion are frequent. Initial symptoms noted in hospitalized patients are fever (initially 50% but up to 90% later), dry cough (60% to 86%) and dyspnea (53% to 80%). Other common symptoms are fatigue, myalgias, and headache. Some patients initially have gastrointestinal symptoms including nausea and vomiting and/or diarrhea (15% to 39%). As in other respiratory viruses, anosmia is

目前几乎没有流行病学或临床数据表明通过污染物会造成严重传播，但保留这种可能性并根据这种假设采取行动当然还是合理的。

在粪便中也发现了 SARS-CoV-2 RNA，这是胃肠道致病病毒可能出现的情况，但没有证据表明传播是由受污染的水或食物引起的。

由于飞沫和气溶胶的迅速扩散，COVID-19 在室外传播的可能性要小得多。阳光和紫外线已被证明能迅速灭活病毒。

最后，流行病学数据表明，口罩和保持社交距离可降低传播风险。N-95 口罩对气溶胶和大飞沫都有防护作用。在医院环境中外科口罩已被证明可以降低传播风险。实验数据表明，外科口罩和密封良好的自制多层棉口罩对预防咳嗽或大声唱歌后的飞沫甚至气溶胶传播有效。头巾和折叠手帕口罩效果较差。尽管流行病学和实验数据支持佩戴口罩，但目前关于支持口罩对COVID-2 防护有效性的临床对照研究数据非常有限。

诊断

迄今为止，鼻咽拭子或鼻拭子中进行 COVID-19 的 RT-PCR 检测是最常用的诊断测试。唾液样本同样准确。不同的试剂盒使用不同的基因靶序列。病毒 RNA 通过聚合酶链增殖周期的数量来测量，并以阈值（Ct）表示。Ct 值小于 40 个周期表明原始样本中有较多的 RNA 拷贝数，结果认定为阳性。大多数检测的特异性接近 100%。RT-PCR 阳性率最高的标本是支气管肺泡灌洗液，其次是鼻咽、鼻腔和口腔标本。当标本采集不当、在症状出现之前或之后太久时采集，可能出现假阴性结果。一些患者在 6 周或更长时间内，RT-PCR 都可能为阳性。然而，只有在症状开始后的前 8 天才能检测到 SARS-CoV-2 活病毒。因此推测，在此之后传染性低。在痰和粪便等其他部位，RT-PCR 可能在更长时间内保持阳性，但可能并没有临床意义。

要记住的重要一点是，任何测试的准确性既取决于验前概率（考虑到症状、病史和当地感染率），也取决于该检测的敏感性和特异性。许多现有 COVID-19 RT-PCR 的敏感性为 71%~98% 不等，这取决于许多因素，包括标本的采集方式。当患者感染 COVID-19 的预测概率较低，且检测敏感性相对较低，那么阴性结果并不能保证没有疾病。因此，根据临床情况，如果 RT-PCR 是阴性的不能排除该病，这一点很重要。

除 RT-PCR 技术外的诊断检测也正在迅速开发和测试中。它们包括基于以下技术的检测：基于抗原、等温扩增（LAMP）、测序和 CRISPR/Cas。这些方法的潜在优势包括缩短获得结果的时间，减少测试所需的资源，使用唾液而不是鼻咽拭子或鼻拭子，以及更高的准确性。

感染者的抗体反应通常通过酶联免疫吸附试验（ELISA）来检测宿主对 COVID-19 病毒的特异性 IgM 和 IgG 抗体。抗体检测的用途包括帮助诊断急性疾病和确定感染后的免疫状态。针对 S 蛋白受体结合域的抗体是最特异的，被认为是中和抗体。IgM 和 IgG 抗体通常要到患病的第 2 或第 3 周才能检测到，大多数患者在第 3~4 周发生转化。之后 IgM 抗体开始下降，通常在第 7 周消失，而 IgG 抗体持续存在。抗体检测的特异性可能会因其他引起常见呼吸道感染的冠状病毒的免疫反应而受到影响。虽然不同的制造商开发了许多血清诊断检测，但大多数没有经过适当的外部验证。因此，目前尚不清楚抗体反应的持久性、中和抗体是否有保护作用以及保护时间。

关于 COVID-19 诊断检测的大多数数据来自有症状的成年人。目前尚不清楚在其他人群，包括免疫功能低下患者、儿童和无症状患者中，RT-PCR、抗原阳性和抗体反应的模式是否与此类似。

临床表现

我们不知道 COVID-19 感染者中有多少是无症状的。许多研究表明，相当大比例的感染者无症状。例如，在南大西洋航行的一艘与世隔绝的游轮上，所有 217 名乘客和船员都接受了 COVID-19 检测，128 人（59%）检测呈阳性。阳性患者中，24 例（19%）出现症状，8 例（6%）需要住院，1 例死亡。其余 104 例患者无症状。在"钻石公主号"游轮众所周知的疫情中，针对无症状感染者的分析也得到了类似的数据。在 2020 年 9 月另一份引人注目的报告中，对康涅狄格州 33 家养老院的 2117 名居住者进行了点状患病率调查。601 例呈阳性，其中 530 例（88.2%）在检测时无症状。530 名患者中有 62 名在检测后 14 天内出现症状，因此 601 名检测阳性患者中有 468 名（78%）一直无症状。此外，基于人群的抗体检测表明，在 SARS-CoV-2 抗体检测呈阳性的患者中，有很大一部分是无症状的。

发表在 *Annals of Internal Medicine* 上的一篇叙述性综述总结，无症状率可能高达 40%~45%，保守估计可能接近 30%。美国 CDC 估计的无症状率甚至更高。与该感染的大多数临床情况类似，这些数据取决于人群的年龄和合并症。总体来说，这些数据是初步的；由于报告是回顾性的，前驱症状或轻度症状可能被低估了，患者也不是随机选取的。

中国的最初研究表明，在有症状的患者中，81% 为轻症，14% 为重症，5% 为危重症。对 COVID-19 症状的研究最初聚焦在住院患者，但大多数研究结果也适用于轻症患者。COVID-19 的潜伏期平均为 5 天，从 2 天到 11 天不等。少数情况下，潜伏期可延长至 14 天甚至更长。对于疾病早期有症状的患者，上呼吸道症状常见，包括流涕和鼻塞。住院患者的初始症状为发热（最初为 50%，后期升至 90%）、干咳（60%~86%）和呼吸困难（53%~80%）。其他常见症状有疲劳、肌痛和头痛。一些患者最初有胃肠道症状，包括恶心、呕吐和（或）腹泻（15%~39%）。与

frequently reported by patients with COVID-19 (up to 64%), although it is not often the presenting symptom.

Respiratory symptoms predominate in most patients with COVID-19. Nonproductive cough, dyspnea, and at times chest pain predominate. Peripheral pulse oxygen levels are used to determine the degree of pulmonary involvement and the need for hospitalization. One phenomenon noted with some patients is lack of dyspnea despite low peripheral oxygen levels (<90). The respiratory symptoms are progressive, resulting in 17% to 35% of hospitalized patients requiring ICU care. In severe cases hypoxemia may increase in severity, requiring sequentially supplemental oxygen, noninvasive respiratory support (for example noninvasive high-flow nasal cannulas), invasive respiratory support with intubation, and in extreme cases extracorporeal membrane oxygenation (ECMO). The great majority of patients do not progress to invasive respiratory support. The entire topic of respiratory support has undergone re-evaluation and change and remains controversial.

Cough is usually nonproductive; the occurrence of productive cough, worsening respiratory function, and signs of localized pulmonary infection may indicate the onset of bacterial or in some cases fungal superinfection. However, the preemptive use of antimicrobial agents has not improved outcomes.

Chest imaging by plain radiographs and particularly chest CT typically show bilateral ground-glass opacification, consolidation, and peripheral distribution in the lower lobes that are characteristic of viral pneumonia. Plain chest films will often miss disease early. Of note, even patients with no symptoms but positive COVID-19 testing may have characteristic findings on chest CT. Laboratory investigations show blood lymphopenia and elevated erythrocyte sedimentation rate, C-reactive protein, D-dimer, lactate dehydrogenase, and ferritin. Elevated blood sugar, creatinine, and hepatic enzymes are common.

EXTRAPULMONARY MANIFESTATIONS

COVID-19 infection in severely ill patients may have protean extrapulmonary manifestations including cardiovascular, renal, gastrointestinal, neurologic, thromboembolic, and endocrine. Myocarditis, cardiomyopathy, and acute coronary syndrome with cardiac injury as detected by elevated troponin levels have been reported in as high as 20% to 30% of hospitalized patients, particularly critically ill patients. Cardiac injury may occur by direct infection of cardiac myocytes by the virus or by the inflammatory response, which can cause thrombosis and endothelialitis. Cardiac arrhythmias including new-onset atrial fibrillation and heart block have been reported in up to 17% of hospitalized patients. Congestive heart failure, especially with preserved ejection fraction and right ventricular dilation, occurs frequently in critically ill patients, complicating the interpretation of chest radiographs. Vascular instability, sepsis-like picture, and bleeding and coagulation abnormalities are also common in ICU patients. Thrombosis of both the venous and arterial systems occurs in up to one quarter of hospitalized patients and greater than one half in ICU patients.

Acute kidney injury (AKI) occurs in up to 37% of severely ill hospitalized patients with up to 14% requiring dialysis. Hematuria and proteinuria are common in severely ill patients. Pathologic studies have shown high rates of viral infection of kidney cells, presumably due to the high distribution of ACE2 in the kidney. In addition, high rates of microvascular and tubular dysfunction may contribute to AKI and impact the prognosis. Careful fluid management and use of scarce dialysis resources are particularly important. Patients who are already on dialysis before acquiring COVID-19 have a very high mortality rate.

Gastrointestinal symptoms including anorexia, diarrhea, and nausea can occur in up to one third of patients and range in series from 12% to 61%. A smaller percentage will develop vomiting and abdominal pain. Gastrointestinal manifestations including transaminitis, ileus, and mesenteric ischemia are more common in critically ill intubated patients with COVID-19 compared to matched uninfected patients.

In some patients, gastrointestinal symptoms may be the initial indications of COVID-19 and should prompt testing for the virus since delays in diagnosis have been reported. Although the virus infects gastric epithelial cells and glandular cells, which have ACE2 present, and viral shedding can be demonstrated, gastrointestinal bleeding is not common, and endoscopy should be avoided if possible in infected patients because of the risk of aerosolization of the virus.

Hepatocellular injury may occur in up to 20% of patients with severe COVID-19 but rarely results in significant hepatitis. Liver function abnormalities including bilirubin have been associated with disease severity. Abnormal liver studies may also be related to drugs, particularly certain antiviral medications, as well as severe disease-causing cytokine release and with vascular compromise. Diagnostic studies are not indicated in most cases.

Neurologic manifestations are common in hospitalized patients, including headache, dizziness, and anosmia. The nasal epithelium has a high frequency of ACE2 and is an early target for COVID-19, probably contributing to anosmia. Delirium occurs frequently, particularly in ICU patients. Acute vascular stroke, encephalopathy, and encephalitis occur in up to 8% of severely ill patients. The extent of direct viral tropism for the central nervous system has yet to be fully defined.

Endocrine abnormalities in COVID-19 center around glycemic control. Hyperglycemia is common in hospitalized patients. Patients with undiagnosed diabetes mellitus often present with hyperglycemia alone or ketoacidosis. Patients who have preexisting diabetes mellitus or obesity are at greater risk for severe disease.

Preliminary data indicate that many patients continue to have symptoms 2 to 3 months after acute infection and a syndrome of "long COVID" has been described. More recently, post-acute COVID-19 has been defined as symptoms extending beyond 3 weeks and chronic COVID-19 beyond 12 weeks. Fatigue, dyspnea, and joint and chest pain are common. Risk factors include age greater than 50 and three or more chronic medical conditions. In one study of hospitalized patients from the United Kingdom who had been discharged at least 2 to 3 months previously, 74% reported at least one symptom, including dyspnea, fatigue, and insomnia. Approximately 14% continued to have abnormal chest radiographs. Some patients who had had more severe disease continued to have abnormal pulmonary function tests. In other studies, myocarditis and myocardial injury by MRI have been described. Significant emotional health issues are not unusual.

RISK FACTORS FOR SEVERE DISEASE AND MORTALITY

Mortality rates for COVID-19 infection vary based on population characteristics, are impacted by testing availability, and have ranged from 0.1% to 2% to 3%. Calculations are complicated by estimating the number of asymptomatic infected individuals, the normal expected death rate, and the deaths due to COVID-19 not recorded. A more meaningful expression of mortality is the excess number of expected deaths, because the individuals most at risk for COVID-19 (elderly, frail, nursing home residents) have a high baseline mortality rate.

The major risk factors for acquisition of symptomatic disease, hospitalization, and mortality are advanced age, frailty, and residing in a nursing home or congregate living facility. In some series more than 90% of deaths occur in patients over the age of 65, particularly those who are frail and those living in nursing homes or the equivalent. Early

其他呼吸道病毒一样，COVID-19 患者经常有嗅觉缺失（高达 64%），尽管它通常不是首发症状。

大多数 COVID-19 患者以呼吸道症状为主。表现为干咳、呼吸困难，有时主要为胸痛。外周血氧水平用于确定肺部受累程度和是否需要住院治疗。一个值得注意的现象是，一些患者尽管外周血氧水平低（< 90%），但呼吸困难并不明显。呼吸系统症状会进行性进展，导致 17% ～ 35% 的住院患者需要入住 ICU。在重症病例中，低氧血症加重，需要持续吸氧，无创呼吸支持（如经鼻无创高流量氧疗）、气管插管有创呼吸支持，以及在极端情况下需要体外膜氧合（ECMO）。绝大多数患者不会进展到有需要创呼吸支持。整个呼吸支持的主题经历了重新评估和改变，仍然存在争议。

咳嗽通常是干咳，出现咳痰、呼吸功能恶化和出现局部肺部感染的迹象可能表明发生了细菌或真菌的继发感染。然而，抢先使用抗菌药物并不改善预后。

胸部 X 线片和胸部 CT 的影像学表现为双侧磨玻璃影、实变影，分布于下肺和外周，这是病毒性肺炎的特征。疾病早期胸部 X 线片往往会漏诊。值得注意的是，无症状但 COVID-19 检测阳性的患者胸部 CT 也可能有特征性表现。实验室检查显示血淋巴细胞减少，红细胞沉降率升高，C 反应蛋白、D- 二聚体、乳酸脱氢酶和铁蛋白升高。血糖、肌酐和肝酶升高很常见。

肺外表现

COVID-19 重症感染患者可能有多种肺外表现，包括心血管、肾、胃肠道、神经系统、血栓栓塞和内分泌等系统。据报道高达 20% ～ 1130% 的住院患者，特别是危重患者，可通过肌钙蛋白水平升高发现心脏损伤的心肌炎、心肌病和急性冠状动脉综合征。心脏损伤可由病毒直接感染心肌细胞或炎症反应引起，后者可引起血栓形成和内皮炎。已报道有高达 17% 的住院患者有心律失常，包括新发心房颤动和心脏传导阻滞。充血性心力衰竭，特别是保留射血分数的心力衰竭和右心室扩张，经常发生在危重患者，使胸部 X 线片的解读复杂化。血流动力学不稳定、感染中毒症样表现、出血和凝血异常在 ICU 患者中也很常见。多达 1/4 的住院患者和超过一半的 ICU 患者中出现静脉和动脉系统的血栓形成。

37% 的重症住院患者有急性肾损伤（AKI），14% 的患者需要透析。血尿和蛋白尿在重症患者中很常见。病理研究表明肾细胞的病毒感染率很高，可能是由于 ACE2 在肾的高分布。此外，高比例的微血管和小管功能障碍可能导致 AKI 并影响预后。精细的液体管理和对稀缺透析资源的使用尤为重要。在感染 COVID-19 之前就已透析的患者死亡率非常高。

多达 1/3 的患者可出现胃肠道症状，包括厌食、腹泻和呕吐，这一系列症状从 12% 到 61% 不等。一小部分人会出现呕吐和腹痛。转氨酶升高、肠梗阻和肠系膜缺血等胃肠道症状在插管的 COVID-19 危重患者中比未感染患者更常见。

在一些患者中，胃肠道症状可能是 COVID-19 的最初症状，可能使诊断延误，应及时进行病毒检测。虽然病毒感染有 ACE2 存在的胃上皮细胞和腺细胞，并可以证明病毒排放，但消化道出血并不常见。由于有病毒气溶胶播散的风险，感染患者应尽量避免内镜检查。

20% 的重症 COVID-19 患者可能出现肝细胞损伤，但很少导致肝炎。包括胆红素异常在内的肝功能异常与疾病严重程度有关。肝脏异常也可能与药物有关，特别是某些抗病毒药物，还可能由于严重的致病细胞因子释放和血管损伤。大多数病例不需要进行诊断性检查。

神经系统症状在住院患者中很常见，包括头痛、头晕和嗅觉丧失。鼻黏膜上皮高表达 ACE2，是 COVID-19 早期的靶点，可能导致嗅觉缺失。谵妄常见，特别是在 ICU 患者中。急性血管性中风、脑病和脑炎可出现在 8% 的重症患者中。病毒嗜中枢神经系统的程度仍不完全清楚。

COVID-19 的内分泌异常以血糖控制为中心。高血糖症在住院患者中很常见。未确诊的糖尿病患者常表现为高血糖或酮症酸中毒。既往患有糖尿病或肥胖的患者发生重症感染的风险更高。

初步数据显示，许多患者在急性感染后 2 ～ 3 个月仍有症状，被描述为"长 COVID"综合征。最近，后急性期 COVID-19 被定义为症状持续 3 周以上，慢性 COVID-19 为持续 12 周以上。疲劳、呼吸困难、关节痛和胸痛常见。危险因素包括年龄 > 50 岁和有 3 种或以上慢性疾病。在英国一项针对至少 2 ～ 3 个月前出院的住院患者的研究中，74% 报告有至少一种症状，包括呼吸困难、疲劳和失眠。约 14% 的患者胸部 X 线片仍有异常。一些病情更严重的患者肺功能检查仍然异常。在其他研究中描述了 MRI 检测到的心肌炎和心肌损伤。严重的心理健康问题并不罕见。

重症与死亡的危险因素

COVID-19 感染的死亡率因人群特征而异，受检测率影响，从 0.1%、2% 到 3% 不等。由于无法记录无症状感染者人数，正常预期死亡率和由于 COVID-19 死亡的人数，计算非常复杂。对死亡率更有意义的表达是超额死亡人数，因为 COVID-19 风险最高的个体（老年人、体弱者、养老院居住者）具有较高的基线死亡率。

有症状感染、住院和死亡的主要危险因素是高龄、衰弱、住养老院或康复机构。在一些系列报道中，90% 以上的死亡发生在 65 岁以上的住院患者身上，特别是那些衰弱和住在养老院或类似机构的人。表 A.1 中来

TABLE A.1	Hospitalization, Intensive Care Unit (ICU) Admission, and Case Fatality Percentages for COVID-19 Cases by Age Group of 2499 Cases: United States, February 12–March 16, 2020[a]			
Age	Hospitalization	ICU Admission	Case-Fatality	
0–19 (123)	1.6–2.5	0	0	
20–44 (705)	14.3–20.8	2.0–4.2	0.1–0.2	
45–54 (429)	21.2–28.3	5.4–10.4	0.5–0.8	
55–64 (429)	20.5–30.1	4.7–11.2	1.4–2.6	
65–74 (409)	28.6–43.5	8.1–18.8	2.7–4.9	
75–84 (201)	30.5–58.7	10.5–31.0	4.3–10.5	
>85 (144)	31.3–70.3	6.3–29	10.4–27.3	
Total (2449)	20.7–31.4	4.9–11.5	1.8–3.4	

[a]Lower bound of range = number of persons hospitalized, admitted to ICU, or who died among the total in the age group. Upper bound of range = number of persons hospitalized admitted to ICU, or who died among the total in age group.

data from the CDC in Table A.1 show the striking risk that age has for hospitalization, ICU admission, and fatality.

Large outbreaks of COVID-19 have occurred in nursing homes in which both staff and residents have been infected. In one CDC study from West Virginia, nursing homes with low quality ratings from Center for Medicare and Medicaid Services (CMS) were more at risk for outbreaks of COVID-19 than those with high ratings.

Early data from the CDC indicated that 37% of patients diagnosed with COVID-19 had at least one underlying health condition. In addition to age, frailty, and nursing home residence, the most common risk factors for severity and hospitalization are diabetes mellitus and obesity, cardiovascular disease (including hypertension), and chronic lung disease. Risk increases with established diabetes mellitus and increasing BMI and is also related to central obesity and metabolic syndrome. Undiagnosed diabetes mellitus is frequently uncovered and diagnosed when patients are hospitalized for COVID-19. Other chronic diseases associated with COVID-19 include immunocompromised conditions, chronic renal disease, and chronic neurologic and psychiatric disorders. Very weak data have suggested an increased risk for patients with type A blood type although this is controversial. There was initial concern that angiotensin-converting enzyme inhibitors or angiotensin-receptor blockers would increase susceptibility to COVID-19, but subsequent data indicate that use of these agents is not associated with more disease.

Minority populations in the United States have significantly greater risk for mortality from COVID-19 than other populations. For example, the age-adjusted rate for mortality for the Black population is 3.4 times and for the Latinx population is 3.3 times that of the white population. Minority populations also have increased rates of disease and hospitalization. There are multiple causes for this discrepancy including (1) workplace exposure; (2) use of public transportation; (3) poor and crowded housing; (4) underlying diabetes mellitus, obesity, and asthma; (5) congregate living settings; (6) delayed health care and lack of access to health care; and (7) distrust of the health care system. Addressing these issues is a critical priority for the equal care of all patients and for controlling the epidemic.

In addition, there is evidence that COVID-19 affects other populations at a greater rate, including those in prisons (people in prisons have 5.5 times the case rate of the general population), group homes, and those with HIV.

TREATMENT

Treatment for COVID-19 for the vast majority of patients is supportive, similar to other respiratory viral illnesses. For hospitalized patients the primary therapy is respiratory, consisting of conventional supplemental oxygen support. Heated, humidified, high-flow nasal canula oxygen treatment or other oxygen supplementation may be necessary if standard oxygen is inadequate. If invasive ventilation is necessary, low tidal volumes and low plateau pressure are recommended. One lesson from COVID-19 is that hypoxemia is often tolerated well with various modes of supplemental oxygen and without invasive endotracheal ventilation. ECMO has been used in patients who have progressive respiratory and/or cardiovascular failure, but its effectiveness is unknown at this point. Details of ICU care and further goals of ICU care are outlined in guidelines from the Society of Critical Care Medicine, the CDC, and the National Institutes of Health.

A number of drugs in different classes are in clinical trial at this point but few at this time have been shown to be effective. The only one on which there is persuasive data from prospective randomized clinical trials (RCT) is the anti-inflammatory drug dexamethasone. It was shown to reduce mortality in the Randomized Evaluation of COVID-19 Therapy (RECOVERY) trial. Compared to control patients, a significant decrease in mortality was noted in patients on mechanical ventilation (41% vs. 29%) and those on oxygen supplementation (26% vs. 23%). Those without oxygen requirement had no benefit, but even in this situation there could be a subgroup that would benefit, and further studies are ongoing.

Antiviral drugs including remdesivir, hydroxychloroquine, azithromycin, and lopinavir are being studied but none have shown a reduction in mortality. Remdesivir was recently approved by the FDA on the basis of a study in which patients assigned to a 10-day course of remdesivir had a recovery time that was 4 days shorter compared with placebo (median, 11 vs. 15 days).

Other therapies being actively investigated in clinical trials include anti–COVID-19 antibodies, such as convalescent plasma and monoclonal antibodies, and targeted immunomodulatory drugs such as anti-IL-6 (tocilizumab), anti-IL-1, JAK inhibitors, and tyrosine kinase inhibitors. Some of these immunomodulatory drugs may have antiviral properties as well. Likewise, antiviral interferon alpha2b therapy is under active investigation. Chloroquine/hydroxychloroquine has been controversial. A systemic review in August 2020 concluded that the evidence on the benefits and harms of this drug is very weak and conflicting. Future studies should clarify what if any drugs have a significant effect on morbidity and mortality.

It is recommended that all hospitalized patients receive subcutaneous low-molecular-weight heparin to prevent thrombotic complications. Which patients need therapeutic anticoagulation is under study,

表A.1 2020年2月12日至3月16日美国2499例按年龄组分列的COVID-19病例的住院、重症监护病房（ICU）入院和病死率[a]

年龄	住院（%）	ICU居留（%）	病死率（%）
0～19（123）	1.6～2.5	0	0
20～44（705）	14.3～20.8	2.0～4.2	0.1～0.2
45～54（429）	21.2～28.3	5.4～10.4	0.5～0.8
55～64（429）	20.5～30.1	4.7～11.2	1.4～2.6
65～74（409）	28.6～43.5	8.1～18.8	2.7～4.9
75～84（201）	30.5～58.7	10.5～31.0	4.3～10.5
>85（144）	31.3～70.3	6.3～29	10.4～27.3
总数（2449）	20.7～31.4	4.9～11.5	1.8～3.4

[a] 范围下界=该年龄组中住院、住ICU或死亡的总人数。范围上界=该年龄组中住ICU人数或死亡人数。

自美国CDC的早期数据显示，年龄是住院、入住ICU和死亡的高危因素。

COVID-19在养老院中会发生大规模暴发，工作人员和居住者都被感染。在西弗吉尼亚州一项疾病预防控制中心（CDC）的研究显示，在医疗保险和医疗补助服务中心（CMS）质量评级低的养老院中暴发COVID-19，比评级高的养老院风险大。

CDC的早期数据表明，37% COVID-19患者至少有一种基础疾病。除了年龄、衰弱和住在养老院之外，最常见的病重和住院的危险因素是糖尿病和肥胖、心血管疾病（包括高血压）和慢性肺部疾病。这种风险随着糖尿病确诊和BMI的增加而增加，也与中枢性肥胖和代谢综合征有关。在患者因COVID-19住院期间，经常发现并诊断出此前未诊断的糖尿病。与COVID-19相关的其他慢性疾病包括免疫功能低下、慢性肾病以及慢性神经和精神疾病。非常有限的数据提示A型血患者的风险增加，这存在争议。最初人们担心血管紧张素转换酶抑制剂或血管紧张素受体阻滞剂会增加对COVID-19的易感性，但随后的数据表明，使用这些药物与患病增加无关。

美国少数族裔因COVID-19死亡的风险明显高于其他人群。例如，黑人人口的年龄调整死亡率是白人人口的3.4倍，拉丁裔人口是白人人口的3.3倍。少数族裔人口的发病率和住院率也增高。造成这种差异的原因有很多，包括：①工作场所暴露；②公共交通工具的使用；③住房条件恶劣、拥挤；④糖尿病、肥胖症、哮喘；⑤聚集性生活环境；⑥医疗保健延误和缺乏获得医疗保健的机会；⑦对医疗体系的不信任。解决这些问题是为所有患者提供平等照顾和控制疾病流行的当务之急。

此外，有证据表明COVID-19对其他一些人群的影响也会更大，包括监狱中的人群（监狱中的人的发病率是一般人群的5.5倍）、集体之家和AIDS患者。

治疗

与其他呼吸道病毒感染类似，对绝大多数患者COVID-19的治疗是支持性的。住院患者的主要治疗是呼吸支持治疗，包括常规氧疗。如果标准氧气不足，可能需要加温、加湿的经鼻高流量氧疗或其他氧疗。如果需要有创通气，建议低潮气量和低平台压。COVID-19治疗的一个经验是，通过各种方式的氧疗和无创通气，通常可以很好地耐受低氧血症。ECMO已用于进行性进展的呼吸和（或）心力衰竭患者，但其有效性目前尚不清楚。重症监护室（ICU）照护的细节和进一步目标在重症监护医学学会、CDC和国家卫生研究院的指南中进行了概述。

目前，许多不同类别的药物正在进行临床试验，但很少有药物被证明有效。唯一从前瞻性随机临床试验（RCT）中获得了有说服力数据的是抗炎药物地塞米松。在"COVID-19治疗随机评估（RECOVERY）"试验中，地塞米松被证实可降低死亡率。与对照组患者相比，在机械通气患者（41% vs. 29%）和吸氧患者（26% vs. 23%）中，死亡率显著降低。不需吸氧者没有获益，但也可能其中一个亚组会受益，进一步的研究正在进行中。

目前正在研究的抗病毒药物包括瑞德西韦、羟氯喹、阿奇霉素和洛匹那韦，但无一显示可降低死亡率。瑞德西韦最近获得了FDA的批准，其依据是在一项研究中，接受瑞德西韦10天疗程患者的康复时间比安慰剂短4天（中位数，11天 vs. 15天）。

其他正在临床试验中积极研究的疗法包括抗COVID-19抗体，如恢复期血浆和单克隆抗体，以及靶向免疫调节药物，如抗IL-6（托珠单抗）、抗IL-1、JAK抑制剂和酪氨酸激酶抑制剂。其中一些免疫调节药物也可能具有抗病毒作用。同样，抗病毒干扰素α2b疗法也在积极研究中。氯喹/羟氯喹作用存在争议，2020年8月的一项系统综述得出结论，关于这种药物益处和危害的证据都非常有限且相互矛盾。未来的研究应阐明哪些药物对发病率和死亡率有显著影响。

建议所有住院患者接受低分子肝素皮下注射预防血栓并发症。哪些患者需要治疗剂量抗凝还在研究中，大

but in most centers use is based on clinical presentation, comorbidities, and D-dimer level.

Most patients hospitalized with COVID-19 have evidence of viral pneumonia but not bacterial superinfection and thus do not benefit from routine antimicrobial therapy that predisposes to bacterial and fungal superinfection from resistant pathogens.

Standard therapy for cardiac, renal, endocrinologic, hematologic, and neurologic complications is detailed in subspecialty guidelines.

VACCINES

Vaccine development is one of the highest priorities in COVID-19 research. Traditional vaccine development typically takes more than a decade to complete. The traditional process includes: discovery (2 to 5 years); preclinical including animal studies (2 years); clinical (phase 1: 2 years involving 10 to 50 people, phase 2: 2 to 3 years involving hundreds of people, and phase 3: protection studies involving thousands of subjects taking years); regulatory phase of 2 years; and manufacturing and delivery, which takes 1 to 2 years. With the COVID-19 pandemic the process was streamlined with rapid early phases producing as many candidates as possible, then clinical studies using sites across the globe, and eventually building global manufacturing capacity.

Vaccines have in general targeted the spike protein, but it is not clear what site on the molecule will be the most effective target. Types of vaccines include RNA/DNA, inactivated virus, live attenuated virus, nonreplicating vector, protein subunit, and replicating viral vector. Much attention and preliminary findings have focused on mRNA vaccines. At this writing at least eight potential vaccines are in phase 3 trials in various countries around the world.

Concerns about vaccines include the following:
1. Will the vaccine produce lasting immunity in all populations including those most at risk such as the elderly?
2. Are studies adequately addressing both short-term and long-term adverse effects?
3. Vaccines produced for other coronaviruses have shown lung toxicity, and therefore toxicity must be investigated first in animal models.
4. Will manufacturing capacity and clinical capacity be adequate and will distribution of the vaccine be equitable and target the most vulnerable populations?
5. Will people be willing to take the vaccine?
6. What will be the immune response of the vulnerable population to the vaccine? It is important to recognize that vaccines for respiratory illnesses such as influenza are only 40% to 80% effective at most.

Information about vaccines and their effectiveness and safety will be forthcoming rapidly in the next several years. Preliminary data from two phase 3 trials indicate remarkable efficacy and safety for two mRNA vaccines.

PREGNANCY AND CHILDREN

Preliminary experience from China indicated that pregnant women did not have increased risk from COVID-19 during the third trimester of pregnancy and that newborns were not at risk for infection. Data from the United States are accumulating but remain preliminary. Data from the CDC early in the epidemic indicate that pregnant women with COVID-19 may have fewer symptoms but are more likely to be hospitalized and have severe disease than pregnant women who are not infected. In a study among 598 hospitalized pregnant women with COVID-19, 55% were asymptomatic at admission. Severe illness occurred among symptomatic pregnant women including ICU admissions (16%), mechanical ventilation (8%), and death (1%). Pregnancy losses occurred for 2% of pregnancies completed during COVID 19–associated hospitalizations and were experienced by both symptomatic and asymptomatic women. Of concern, however, are women with increased risk factors in the United States, such as glucose intolerance, diabetes mellitus, obesity, hypertension, and minority status. Data from the CDC showed that women with obesity and/or gestational diabetes were at higher risk for severe disease. A later study (PRIORITY study) compared women who tested positive for COVID-19 0 to 14 days before delivery versus those who tested negative. COVID-19 was not associated with a difference in birthweight, difficulty breathing, apnea, or respiratory infection in the first 8 weeks of life. Women infected with COVID-19 delivered 1.5 weeks earlier on average. Guidelines for the care of pregnant women and delivery have been published by the CDC and the American Academy of Pediatrics, the American College of Obstetricians and Gynecologists and the Society for Maternal-Fetal Medicine, and the Society for Obstetric Anesthesia and Perinatology.

Data from the early phase of the pandemic indicate that children account for only a small portion of confirmed cases and that most cases of clinical COVID-19 in children are mild and self-limiting. Subsequent data indicate that a percentage of pediatric patients are asymptomatic. Symptomatic patients have fever and cough; a lower percentage have typical viral respiratory symptoms including nasal congestion, myalgia, fatigue, and sore throat. Less than 10% presented with gastrointestinal symptoms. Case fatality rates in children are less than 0.5% and are lower than those of seasonal influenza. Children with underlying respiratory/cardiac disease are most at risk.

Childhood multisystem inflammatory syndrome (MIS-C) was initially described in the United Kingdom as a disease having some characteristics of Kawasaki disease, a rare vasculitis of childhood that can cause coronary aneurysms, and subsequently was reported worldwide. As of mid-July 2020, approximately 1000 cases had been reported. The pathophysiology is still being defined, but most definitions include an inflammatory illness with fever and increased inflammatory markers that involve at least four organ systems including the gastrointestinal, cardiovascular, hematologic, skin, and respiratory systems and in most patients evidence of COVID-19 infection. The disease typically begins 2 to 4 weeks after COVID-19 symptoms. It occurs in previously healthy children who are older than 5 years of age, including adolescents, compared to patients with Kawasaki disease who are usually younger than 5 years. A relatively high percentage (10% to 20%) have evidence of cardiovascular involvement and coronary artery aneurysms. Treatment is anti-inflammatory agents. Most patients recover but mortality ranges as high as 2%. Further data on the epidemiology, clinical characteristics, and treatment of this rare condition are needed.

PREVENTION

It is beyond this Appendix to review the complex epidemiology and public health efforts to prevent and mitigate the COVID-19 pandemic. It was clear from the experience in Wuhan that draconian governmental action including preventing travel in and out of Wuhan, strict quarantine, wearing face masks, shutting down public transportation and public gatherings, closing businesses, and increasing medical care capacity halted the epidemic over several months. Less stringent measures have been instituted in Europe, the United States, and other parts of the world, although there has been wide variation in the extent of restrictions. Contact tracing has been practiced effectively in some countries such as South Korea, but lack of adequate testing and the high percentage of asymptomatic patients has made that impractical in many settings. What have become generally accepted as effective

多数中心是基于临床表现、合并症和 D- 二聚体水平。

大多数因 COVID-19 住院的患者有病毒性肺炎的证据，但没有继发细菌感染，因此无法从常规抗菌治疗中获益且易诱发耐药细菌和真菌的继发感染。

心脏、肾、内分泌、血液学和神经系统并发症的标准治疗详见亚专科指南。

疫苗

疫苗开发是 COVID-19 研究的重中之重。传统疫苗的开发通常需要 10 年以上。传统的过程包括：发现（2～5 年）；临床前包括动物研究（2 年）；临床（第一阶段：2 年，涉及 10～50 人；第二阶段：2～3 年，涉及数百人；第三阶段：保护性研究，涉及数千受试者，耗时数年）；监管阶段 2 年；制造和交付需要 1～2 年。随着 COVID-19 大流行这一过程被简化，在早期阶段快速生产尽可能多的候选疫苗，然后在全球各地进行临床研究，最终建立全球制造能力。

疫苗通常针对刺突蛋白，但尚不清楚分子上的哪个位点会是最有效的靶点。疫苗类型包括 RNA/DNA、灭活病毒、减毒活病毒、非复制性病毒载体、蛋白质亚基和复制性病毒载体。大量的注意力和初步发现都集中在 mRNA 疫苗上。在撰写本文时，至少有 8 种潜在疫苗正在世界各国进行 3 期试验。

对疫苗的担忧包括：

1. 疫苗能否在所有人群中产生持久的免疫力，包括那些风险最高的人群，如老年人？
2. 研究是否充分解决了短期和长期的副作用？
3. 针对其他冠状病毒的疫苗表现出肺毒性，因此必须首先在动物模型中研究毒性。
4. 生产能力和临床能力是否足够，疫苗的分配是否公平并以最脆弱的人群为目标？
5. 人们会愿意接种疫苗吗？
6. 易感人群对疫苗的免疫反应如何？重要的是要认识到，流感等呼吸道疾病的疫苗最多只有 40%～80% 的有效性。

关于疫苗及其有效性和安全性的信息将在今后几年内迅速公布。两项 3 期试验的初步数据表明，两种 mRNA 疫苗具有显著的有效性和安全性。

孕妇与儿童

中国的初步经验表明，孕妇在妊娠晚期感染 COVID-19 的风险没有增加，新生儿也没有被感染风险。来自美国的数据正在积累，仍处于初步阶段。CDC 在疫情早期的数据表明，与未感染的孕妇相比，感染 COVID-19 的孕妇可能症状较少，但更有可能住院并出现重症。在一项对 598 名 COVID-19 住院孕妇的研究中，55% 在入院时无症状。有症状的孕妇可发展为重症，包括入住 ICU（16%），机械通气（8%）和死亡（1%）。在与 COVID-19 相关的孕期住院中，有 2% 发生了流产，这在有症状和无症状的孕妇中均有发生。然而令人担忧的是，美国存在一些危险因素较高的妇女，如糖耐量异常、糖尿病、肥胖、高血压患者和少数族裔者。美国 CDC 数据显示，肥胖和（或）妊娠期糖尿病的女性重症风险更高。后来的一项研究（PRIORITY 研究）比较了分娩前 0～14 天 COVID-19 检测呈阳性的和阴性的妇女。COVID-19 与婴儿出生体重、呼吸困难、呼吸暂停或 8 周内呼吸道感染等差异无关。感染 COVID-19 的妇女平均提前 1.5 周分娩。美国 CDC 和美国儿科学会、美国妇产科医师学会、母胎医学学会以及产科麻醉和围产期学会已经发布了孕妇护理和分娩指南。

大流行早期阶段的数据表明，儿童仅占确诊病例的一小部分，大多数儿童 COVID-19 病例是轻症和自限性的。随后的数据表明，一定比例的儿科患者是无症状的。有症状的患者有发热和咳嗽；较低比例的患儿有典型的病毒性呼吸道症状，包括鼻塞、肌痛、疲劳和咽痛。不到 10% 表现为胃肠道症状。儿童病死率低于 0.5%，低于季节性流感。患有呼吸/心脏基础疾病的儿童面临的风险最大。

儿童多系统炎症综合征（MIS-C）最初在英国被描述为一种具有某些川崎病（川崎病是一种罕见的儿童血管炎，可导致冠状动脉瘤）特征的疾病，随后在世界范围内被报道。截至 2020 年 7 月中旬，已报告约 1000 例病例。目前该病的发病机制仍在定义中，但大多数定义都认为这是一种炎症性疾病，伴有发热和炎症标志物升高，涉及胃肠道、心血管、血液学、皮肤和呼吸系统等器官系统中的至少四个，大多数患者有 COVID-19 感染的证据。

这种疾病通常在 COVID-19 症状出现 2～4 周后。它发生在既往体健的 5 岁以上儿童中，包括青少年，而川崎病患者通常小于 5 岁。相对较高的比例（10%～20%）患儿有累及心血管和冠状动脉瘤的证据。治疗方法是使用抗炎药物。大多数患者康复，但死亡率可达 2%。关于这种罕见疾病的流行病学、临床特征和治疗的仍需进一步数据。

预防

本附录不再赘述复杂的流行病学及为预防和减轻 COVID-19 大流行采取的公共卫生工作。从武汉的经验可以清楚地看出，政府采取的严格措施，包括禁止进出武汉、严格隔离、佩戴口罩、关闭公共交通和公共集会、关闭企业、增加医疗服务能力等，在几个月内遏制了疫情。欧洲、美国和世界其他地区制定了稍逊严格的措施，限制的程度各不相同。在韩国等一些国家，接触者追踪已得到有效实施，但缺乏充分的检测和无症状患者的高比例使得这在许多情况下不切实际。

measures include face masks, social distancing, and restricting social gatherings.

Many countries have seen a marked reduction in cases due to initial public health measures and have begun loosening restrictions with a resultant increase in the number of cases. Early data on resurgent COVID-19 indicate that younger age groups are more affected and that the severity and mortality are less. It is possible, however, that the infection will spread to vulnerable populations, resulting in additional waves of the pandemic that need to be addressed and controlled. Mitigation efforts do not eliminate the virus and until herd immunity is widespread (presumably higher than 40%) and effective vaccines are available, viral transmission and infection will continue.

The downside of public health restrictions has included major negative effects on people. There has been an increase in stress, mental health issues such as depression and anxiety, and unfortunately increases in drug use including alcohol. In one survey, frequency of alcohol use increased 14% overall in 2020 compared to 2019 and affected women more than men. Many patients have avoided the medical care system for acute and routine care out of fear of catching COVID-19. According to a CDC survey early in June 2020, 41% of the US population had delayed or avoided medical care during the pandemic. Care for conditions such as acute infection, acute cardiac disease, and injuries has often not been readily accessible in many locations and as a result mortality has increased for some of these conditions. Routine care including elective surgery, vaccinations, and regular medical visits have been put on hold. Economic disruption with unprecedented economic contraction, massive worldwide unemployment, supply chain disruption, business failures, and food insecurity has wreaked havoc on all countries but has disproportionally affected the poorest and most vulnerable populations. One estimate of the total cost for the United States is $16 trillion resulting from economic disruption and medical costs. School closings and reopenings have been an extremely important issue that continues to be debated, but the downside of school closings has been enormous, particularly for children in minority populations. The balance between restrictions for the pandemic and opening society will be an ongoing issue for the foreseeable future.

SUGGESTED READINGS

Brooks JT, Butler JC, Redfield RR: Universal masking to prevent SARS-CoV-2 transmission—the time is now, JAMA 324(7):635–637, 2020.

Chou R, Dana T, Jungbauer R, Weeks C, McDonagh MS: Masks for prevention of respiratory virus infections, including SARS-CoV-2, in health care and community settings—a living rapid review, Annal Int Med 173(7):542–555, 2020.

Fineberg HV: The toll of COVID-19, JAMA 324(15):1502–1503, 2020.

Fontanet A, Couchemez S: COVID-19 herd immunity: Where are we? Nature Reviews 20(10):583–584, 2020.

Gupta A, Madhavan MV, Sehgal K, et al: Extrapulmonary manifestations of COVID 19, Nat Med 26:1017–1032, 2020.

MMWR, CDC, March 27, 2020 Severe Outcomes among Patients with Coronavirus Disease 2019 (COVID 19)—United States, February 12-March 16, 2020 page 343.

MMWR, CDC, October 2, 2020 Changing Age Distribution of the COVID-19 Pandemic—United States, May-August 2020, page 1404.

MMWR, CDC, October 23, 2020 Mortality due to COVID-19, page 1522.

Oran DP, Topol EJ: Prevalence of asymptomatic SARS-CoV-2 infection—a narrative review, Annal Int Med 173:362–367, 2020.

Sethuraman N, Jeremiah SS, Ryo A: Interpreting diagnostic tests for SARS-CoV-2, JAMA 323(22):2249–2251, 2020.

The WHO Rapid Evidence Appraisal for COVID-19 Therapies (REACT) Working Group: Association between administration of systemic corticosteroids and mortality among critically Ill patients with COVID-19 a meta-analysis, JAMA 324(13):1330–1341, 2020.

Wiersinga WJ, Rhodes A, Cheng AC, Peacock SJ, Prescott HC: Pathophysiology, transmission, diagnosis, and treatment of coronavirus disease 2019 (COVID 19) a review, JAMA 324(8):782–793, 2020.

戴口罩、保持社交距离、限制社交聚会等已被普遍接受为有效措施。

由于采取了初步的公共卫生措施，许多国家的病例已显著减少，并已开始放松限制，病例数又由此增加。关于COVID-19死灰复燃的早期数据表明，年轻年龄组受影响更大，严重程度和死亡率也更低。然而，这种感染有可能蔓延到脆弱人群，导致需要处理和控制的另一波大流行。缓解的措施并不能消除病毒，在群体免疫力普及（估计高于40%）和有效疫苗可用之前，病毒传播和感染将继续下去。

公共卫生限制的不利方面包括对人们的重大负面影响。压力、抑郁和焦虑等心理健康问题有所增加，不幸的是，包括酒精在内的化学品和毒品使用也增加。在一项调查中，与2019年相比，2020年饮酒频率总体上增加了14%，对女性的影响大于男性。由于害怕感染COVID-19，许多患者回避前往医疗系统进行急诊和常规诊疗。根据美国CDC 2020年6月初的一项调查，41%的美国人在疫情期间推迟或避免就医。在许多地方，对急性感染、急性心脏病和外伤等疾病往往得不到及时治疗，因此其中一些疾病的死亡率有所增加。包括择期手术、疫苗接种和定期随诊在内的常规照护被搁置。前所未有的经济萎缩、大规模的全球失业、供应链中断、企业倒闭和粮食安全问题给所有国家造成了严重破坏，但对最贫困和脆弱人口的影响尤为严重。据估计，美国因经济混乱和医疗费用而付出的总代价高达16万亿美元。学校的关闭和重新开放是一个非常重要的问题，人们一直在争论，但学校关闭的负面影响是巨大的，特别对少数族裔的孩子。在可预见的未来，限制疫情与开放社会之间的平衡将是一个持续的问题。

推荐阅读

Brooks JT, Butler JC, Redfield RR: Universal masking to prevent SARS-CoV-2 transmission—the time is now, JAMA 324(7):635–637, 2020.

Chou R, Dana T, Jungbauer R, Weeks C, McDonagh MS: Masks for prevention of respiratory virus infections, including SARS-CoV-2, in health care and community settings—a living rapid review, Annal Int Med 173(7):542–555, 2020.

Fineberg HV: The toll of COVID-19, JAMA 324(15):1502–1503, 2020.

Fontanet A, Couchemez S: COVID-19 herd immunity: Where are we? Nature Reviews 20(10):583–584, 2020.

Gupta A, Madhavan MV, Sehgal K, et al: Extrapulmonary manifestations of COVID 19, Nat Med 26:1017–1032, 2020.

MMWR, CDC, March 27, 2020 Severe Outcomes among Patients with Coronavirus Disease 2019 (COVID 19)—United States, February 12-March 16, 2020 page 343.

MMWR, CDC, October 2, 2020 Changing Age Distribution of the COVID-19 Pandemic—United States, May-August 2020, page 1404.

MMWR, CDC, October 23, 2020 Mortality due to COVID-19, page 1522.

Oran DP, Topol EJ: Prevalence of asymptomatic SARS-CoV-2 infection—a narrative review, Annal Int Med 173:362–367, 2020.

Sethuraman N, Jeremiah SS, Ryo A: Interpreting diagnostic tests for SARS-CoV-2, JAMA 323(22):2249–2251, 2020.

The WHO Rapid Evidence Appraisal for COVID-19 Therapies (REACT) Working Group: Association between administration of systemic corticosteroids and mortality among critically Ill patients with COVID-19 a meta-analysis, JAMA 324(13):1330–1341, 2020.

Wiersinga WJ, Rhodes A, Cheng AC, Peacock SJ, Prescott HC: Pathophysiology, transmission, diagnosis, and treatment of coronavirus disease 2019 (COVID 19) a review, JAMA 324(8):782–793, 2020.

索引 Index

A

Abscess (es)
   brain, 94-98, 96f, 96t-98t
      infectious endocarditis with, 102-104
      subdural empyema leading to, 98-100
   fever of unknown origin and, 44-46
   hepatic, 52, 172
   infectious endocarditis with, 102-104
   intra-abdominal, 56
   solid organ, 172
   spinal epidural, 100, 102f
   splenic, 172
Acquired immunodeficiency syndrome (AIDS)
   travel by patients with, 294
Acute bacterial endocarditis (ABE), 134, 142t
Acute bacterialotitis externa, 114-116
Acute bacterialotitis media, 116
Acute bacterial rhinosinusitis, 108-110
   clinical presentation of, 108
   complications of, 108-110, 110f
   definition and epidemiology of, 108
   pathogenesis and microbiology of, 108
   treatment for, 108
Acute HIV infection, 238
Acute kidney injury (AKI)
   in septic shock, 64
Acute respiratory distress syndrome (ARDS)
   in sepsis, 68
Acute retroviral syndrome, 240
   symptoms and signs of, 242t
Acute tubular necrosis (ATN)
   in septic shock, 64
Adaptive immunity, 6-8, 6f, 16-24, 16f
Aeromonas hydrophila, skin and soft tissue infection from, 152
Aeromonas schubertii, skin and soft tissue infection from, 152
Aeromonas veronii, skin and soft tissue infection from, 152
African tick-bite fever, 54
African trypanosomiasis, 296
Aging
   HIV infection and, 256-258
Alveolar cyst disease, 300
Alveolar macrophages, 16
Amebiasis, 296
American trypanosomiasis, 296-298
Amoxicillin, for acute bacterialotitis media, 116
Amphotericin B, for cryptococcal meningitis, 86
Anal cancer
   screening for, 262
Anaplasmosis, human granulocytic, 54
Anergy, in HIV infection, 238
Aneurysm (s)
   intracranial, in infectious endocarditis, 104
   mycotic, 104
Angular cheilosis, 242
Animal bites, 158
   treatment for, 160
Animal exposure, febrile syndromes associated with, 44t, 50-52
Antibiotic prophylaxis, for infective endocarditis, 144
Antibiotics
   for acute bacterialotitis media, 116
   for acute bacterial rhinosinusitis, 108

A

脓肿
   脑脓肿，95-99，97f，97t-99t
      感染性心内膜炎，103-105
      硬膜下积脓，99-101
   不明原因发热，45-47
   肝脓肿，53，173
   感染性心内膜炎，103-105
   腹腔内脓肿，57
   实质器官脓肿，173
   硬脊膜外脓肿，101，103f
   脾脓肿，173
获得性免疫缺陷综合征（AIDS）
   患者旅行，295
急性细菌性心内膜炎（ABE），135，143t
急性细菌性外耳炎，115-117
急性细菌性中耳炎，117
急性细菌性鼻窦炎，109-111
   临床表现，109
   并发症，109-111，111f
   定义和流行病学，109
   发病机制和微生物学，109
   治疗，109
急性 HIV 感染，239
急性肾损伤（AKI）
   感染中毒性休克，65
急性呼吸窘迫综合征（ARDS）
   感染中毒症，69
急性逆转录病毒综合征，241
   症状和体征，243t
急性肾小管坏死（ATN）
   感染中毒性休克，65
适应性免疫，7-9，7f，17-25，17f
嗜水气单胞菌，皮肤和软组织感染，153
舒伯特气单胞菌，皮肤和软组织感染，153
维氏气单胞菌，皮肤和软组织感染，153
非洲蜱咬热，55
非洲锥虫病，297
老化
   HIV 感染，257-259
泡型棘球蚴病，301
肺泡巨噬细胞，17
阿米巴病，297
美洲锥虫病，297-299
阿莫西林，治疗急性细菌性中耳炎，117
两性霉素 B，治疗隐球菌性脑膜炎，87
肛门癌
   筛查，263
人嗜粒细胞无形体病，55
无反应性，见于 HIV 感染，239
动脉瘤
   颅内动脉瘤，见于感染性心内膜炎，105
   真菌性动脉瘤，105
口角干裂，243
动物咬伤，159
   治疗，161
动物暴露，相关发热性综合征，45t，51-53
抗生素预防，治疗感染性心内膜炎，145
抗生素
   急性细菌性中耳炎，117
   急性细菌性鼻窦炎，109

Page numbers followed by "f" indicate figures, "t" indicate tables, and "b" indicate boxes.

页码数字中，"f"代表"图"，"t"代表"表格"，"b"代表"框"。

in bone and joint infections, 188
for peritonitis, 164
for pneumonia, 122
source control and timing of, 164
Antibodies, 16-20
major isotypes of, 18f
structure of, 20, 20f
Antigen-presenting cells, 16, 22, 22f
Antimalarial chemoprophylaxis, 294
Antimicrobial prophylaxis, immunocompromised host and, 282
Antimicrobial regimen, empirical, in septic patients, 70, 70t
Antimicrobial stewardship, importance of, 210
Antimicrobial therapy
for diarrhea, 180t, 186
for meningitis, 84-86, 88t-90t
Appendectomy, 164-166
Appendicitis, 164-166, 166f
Arcanobacterium haemolyticum, skin and soft tissue infection from, 152
Artemisinin, 294
Ascaris lumbricoides, 298
Aseptic meningitis, 252
Aseptic meningitis syndrome, 76
Aspergillosis
invasive pulmonary, 280f, 284f
Aspergillus
immunocompromised host and, 284, 286f
infection with, pneumonia in, 120
pulmonary infiltrates caused by, 272
Asplenia, in immunocompromised host, 270
Asymptomatic bacteriuria, 194
Atovaquone-proguanil, for malaria, 292-294
Atrial myxomas, mimicking subacute bacterial endocarditis, 140
Avian influenza, 42
Azithromycin
for chlamydia, 216
for granuloma inguinale, 228

B

B cells, 20
B lymphocytes, 16-20, 22f
Babesia microti, 296t
Bacillus anthracis, skin and soft tissue infection from, 152-154, 154f
Bacillus cereus, food poisoning from, 178
Bacteremia, 60-72
in fever of unknown origin, 50
Bacterial epiglottitis, 112-114
Bacterial food poisoning, 178
Bacterial infections, 42
Bartonella henselae, 56
skin and soft tissue infection from, 154
Basal ganglia
Toxoplasma abscesses in, 94-96
Basophils, 8-16
Biliary infection, 170-172
Bismuth subsalicylate, for diarrhea, 186
Blood cultures
in fever of unknown origin, 46
in osteomyelitis, 188-190
in pneumonia, 122
Body temperature, thermoregulation of, 40
Bone diseases
in HIV infection, 254-256
Borrelia burgdorferi, 54
infection with, 190
Bovine spongiform encephalopathy, 104
Breast cancer
in HIV infection, 250
Bronchopneumonia, 118

骨与关节感染，189
腹膜炎，165
肺炎，123
感染源控制和用药时机，165
抗体，17-21
主要类型，19f
结构，21,21f
抗原提呈细胞，17,23,23f
抗疟化学预防，295
预防性抗菌治疗，免疫妥协宿主，283
经验性抗菌治疗方案，感染中毒症患者，71,71t
抗菌药物管理，重要性，211
抗菌治疗
腹泻，181t,187
脑膜炎，85-87,89t-91t
阑尾切除术，165-167
阑尾炎，165-167,167f
溶血性隐秘杆菌，皮肤和软组织感染，153

青蒿素，295
蛔虫，299
无菌性脑膜炎，253
无菌性脑膜炎综合征，77
曲霉病
侵袭性肺曲霉病，281f,285f
曲霉菌
免疫妥协宿主，285,287f
感染，肺炎，121
导致肺部浸润，273
无脾，免疫妥协宿主，271
无症状菌尿，195
阿托伐醌-氯胍，治疗疟疾，293-295
心房黏液瘤，与亚急性细菌性心内膜炎相似表现，141
禽流感，43
阿奇霉素
衣原体感染，217
腹股沟肉芽肿，229

B

B细胞，21
B淋巴细胞，17-21,23f
微小巴贝虫，297t
炭疽杆菌，皮肤和软组织感染，153-155,155f
蜡样芽孢杆菌，食物中毒，179
菌血症，61-73
不明原因发热，51
细菌性会厌炎，113-115
细菌性食物中毒，179
细菌感染，43
汉赛巴尔通体，57
皮肤和软组织感染，155
基底神经节
弓形虫脓肿，95-97
嗜碱性粒细胞，9-17
胆道感染，171-173
次水杨酸铋，治疗腹泻，187
血培养
不明原因发热，47
骨髓炎，189-191
肺炎，123
体温调节，41
骨病
HIV感染，255-257
伯氏疏螺旋体，55
感染，191
牛海绵状脑病，105
乳腺癌
HIV感染，251
支气管肺炎，119

Brucellosis, 52
Bubonic plague, 56
Burn wounds, 160
　　treatment for, 162

C

C3 convertase, 8
Calcofluor, fluorescent staining with, 30, 34f
Campylobacter jejuni
　　diarrhea from, 178t-180t, 180
Candida albicans, immunocompromised host and, 282-284, 284f
Candida infections, 242
　　vulvovaginitis, 242
Candida pharyngitis, 240
Capnocytophaga canimorsus, skin and soft tissue infection from, 154
Carbuncle, 150
Cardiomegaly, 138
Cardiovascular disease (CVD)
　　in HIV infection, 254
Cat-scratch disease, 56
Catheter, vascular, infections associated with, 204-208
Catheter-associated urinary tract infections (CAUTI), 194, 202-204, 206t, 208f
CAUTI. *See* Catheter-associated urinary tract infections
Cavernous sinus thrombosis, septic, 100-102
$CD4^+$ T cells, 22-24
　　in HIV infection
　　　　opportunistic infections and, 242
　　　　progressive, 242t
　　　　monitoring interval for, 258
$CD8^+$ T cells, 24
Ceftriaxone, for Lyme meningitis, 84
Cell-mediated immunity deficits
　　agents causing infection in, 270
　　conditions causing, 272t
Cell-mediated response, 26
Cellulitis, 150, 152f
Central line-associated bloodstream infection (CLABSI), 204-208, 208f
Central nervous system (CNS)
　　diseases, without prominent focal signs, 252
　　focal lesions of, 250-252, 252t
Central nervous system infection, 276
Central venous catheter-related bloodstream infections, 144
Cerebral edema
　　magnetic resonance imaging of, 96f
Cerebritis, 96
Cerebrospinal fluid (CSF)
　　Creutzfeldt-Jakob disease and, 104-106
　　diagnosis of infection in, with India ink examination, 82-84
　　in encephalitis, 86-88
　　in infectious endocarditis, 104
　　in meningitis
　　　　bacterial, 74
　　　　fungal, 82-84
　　　　spirochetal, 82
　　　　tuberculous, 82
Cervical cancer
　　screening for, 262
Cervicitis, 214-220
Chagas' disease, 296-298
Chancroid, 56, 228
Chemokine receptors CCR5, 236-238
Chemokines, 8
Chest radiography
　　in pneumonia, 122
Chickenpox, 54
Chills, 42
　　in sepsis, 66

C

C3 转化酶，9
荧光增白剂，荧光染色，31，35f
空肠弯曲菌
　　腹泻，179-181t，181
白念珠菌，免疫妥协宿主，283-285，285f
念珠菌感染，243
　　外阴阴道炎，243
念珠菌性咽炎，241
犬咬二氧化碳嗜纤维菌，皮肤和软组织感染，155
痈，151
心脏肥大，139
心血管疾病（CVD）
　　HIV 感染，255
猫抓病，57
导管，血管，相关感染，205-209
导管相关尿路感染（CAUTI），195，203-205，207t，209f
CAUTI 参见导管相关尿路感染
海绵窦血栓形成，感染中毒性，101-103
$CD4^+$ T 细胞，23-25
　　HIV 感染
　　　　机会性感染，243
　　　　进展期，243t
　　　　监测间隔，259
$CD8^+$ T 细胞，25
头孢曲松，治疗莱姆病脑膜炎，85
细胞介导免疫缺陷
　　诱发感染物，271
　　导致细胞介导免疫缺陷的情况，273t
细胞免疫应答，27
蜂窝织炎，151，153f
中心静脉导管相关感染（CLABSI），205-209，209f
中枢神经系统（CNS）
　　疾病，无明显的局灶性体征，253
　　局灶性病变，251-253，253t
中枢神经系统感染，277
中心静脉导管相关血流感染，145
脑水肿
　　磁共振成像，97f
脑炎，97
脑脊液（CSF）
　　克-雅病，105-107
　　诊断脑脊液感染，墨汁染色检查，83-85
　　脑炎，87-89
　　感染性心内膜炎，105
　　脑膜炎
　　　　细菌性脑膜炎，75
　　　　真菌性脑膜炎，83-85
　　　　螺旋体脑膜炎，83
　　　　结核性脑膜炎，83
宫颈癌
　　筛查，263
宫颈炎，215-221
美洲锥虫病，297-299
软下疳，57，229
趋化因子受体 CCR5，237-239
趋化因子，9
胸部 X 线检查
　　肺炎，123
水痘，55
寒战，43
　　感染中毒症，67

Chinese liver fluke, 300
Chlamydia, 214-216
    clinical presentation of, 216
    definition of, 214
    diagnosis and differential diagnosis of, 216
    epidemiology of, 214
    pathology of, 214-216
    prognosis of, 216
    treatment of, 216
Chlamydia trachomatis, 214-216
    urethritis and, 214
Chlamydophila pneumoniae, infection with, pneumonia in, 120
Chloroquine, for malaria, 292-294
Cholangitis, 170-172
Cholecystitis, 170
    acalculous, 170
Chronic meningitis, 252
Chronic osteomyelitis, 188
Clonorchiasis, 300
Clonorchis sinensis, 300
Clostridioides difficile
    colitis, with fever, 46
    diarrhea from, 178t-180t, 182
Clostridioides difficile colitis, 168-170
Clostridioides difficile infection (CDI)
    infection, 210
Clostridioides perfringens
    food poisoning from, 178
    skin and soft tissue infection from, 154
Coagulopathy
    in sepsis, 68
Coccidioides immitis infection, meningitis in, 78
Colonoscopy
    in diverticulitis, 166
Colorectal cancer
    in HIV infection, 250
Common cold, 108
Compartment syndrome, 160
Complement deficits, in immunocompromised host, 270
Complement factors, 8, 18f
Connective tissue diseases
    fever of unknown origin and, 46
Cortical abscess (renal carbuncle), in urinary tract infections, 198t-200t
Cortical ribboning, 104-106
Cortical venous thrombosis, 98-100
Cortico-medullary abscess, in urinary tract infections, 198t-200t
Corticosteroids
    for meningitis, tuberculous, 86
COVID-19. *See* Coronavirus disease 2019
Coxiella burnetii infection, 44t, 50-52
Creutzfeldt-Jakob disease (CJD)
    sporadic, 104-106
Cryptococcal disease, 244-246
Cryptococcal meningitis, clinical presentation of, 80
Cryptococcus, immunocompromised host and, 284
Cryptococcus neoformans, 244-246
    infection, meningitis in, 78
Cryptosporidium, 178t-180t, 296t
Culture, 30-32, 36t
Culture-negative endocarditis
    diagnostic approach to, 142t
    infectious, 136
CURB-65 score, for pneumonia, 122
Cutibacterium acnes, 190
Cyclospora, 178t-180t
Cysticercosis, 300
Cytokines, 8, 10t-14t
    as endogenous pyrogens, 40
    skin and soft tissue infections and, 150

中国肝吸虫，301
衣原体，215-217
    临床表现，217
    定义，215
    诊断和鉴别诊断，217
    流行病学，215
    病理学，215-217
    预后，217
    治疗，217
沙眼衣原体，215-217
    尿道炎，215
肺炎衣原体，感染，肺炎，121
氯喹，治疗疟疾，293-295
胆管炎，171-173
胆囊炎，171
    无结石胆囊炎，171
慢性脑膜炎，253
慢性骨髓炎，189
华支睾吸虫病，301
华支睾吸虫，301
艰难梭菌
    结肠炎，发热，47
    腹泻，179t-181t，183
艰难梭菌结肠炎，169-171
艰难梭菌感染（CDI）
    感染，211
产气荚膜梭菌
    食物中毒，179
    皮肤和软组织感染，155
凝血功能障碍
    感染中毒症，69
粗球孢子菌感染，脑膜炎，79
结肠镜
    憩室炎，167
结直肠癌
    HIV 感染，251
普通感冒，109
间隔综合征，161
补体缺陷，见于免疫妥协宿主，271
补体因子，9，19f
结缔组织病
    不明原因发热，47
皮质脓肿（肾痈），见于尿路感染，199t-201t
皮质带，105-107
皮质静脉血栓形成，99-101
皮质-髓质脓肿，见于尿路感染，199t-201t
皮质类固醇
    结核性脑膜炎，87
COVID-19 参见 2019 冠状病毒病
贝纳柯克斯体感染，45t，51-53
克-雅病（CJD）
    散发性 CJD，105-107
隐球菌病，245-247
隐球菌性脑膜炎，临床表现，81
隐球菌，免疫妥协宿主，285
新型隐球菌，245-247
    感染，脑膜炎，79
隐孢子虫，179t-181t，297t
培养，31-33，37t
培养阴性的心内膜炎
    诊断方法，143t
    感染性，137
CURB-65 评分，针对肺炎，123
痤疮丙酸杆菌，191
环孢子虫，179t-181t
囊尾蚴病，301
细胞因子，9，11t-15t
    内源性致热原，41
    皮肤和软组织感染，151

Cytomegalovirus (CMV), 246
    immunocompromised host and, 282-288
    infection
        fever in, 54-56
        mononucleosis syndrome in, 42, 56
    retinitis, in HIV-infected patients, 242, 246
Cytomegalovirus colitis, 168
Cytomegalovirus disease, 246

D

Dementia
    in Creutzfeldt-Jakob disease, 104
Dendritic cells, 16
    immature, 24
Dexamethasone
    for bacterial meningitis, 86
    for cerebral edema, with brain abscess, 98
Diabetes mellitus
    in HIV infection, 256
Diabetic foot infections, 160, 160f
    treatment for, 162
Diarrhea, 276
    infectious, 176-186
        from bacterial food poisoning, 178
        clinical presentation of, 182-184
        cytotoxin-induced, 176
        definition and epidemiology of, 176
        diagnosis and differential diagnosis, 184, 184f
        enterotoxin-induced, 176
        invasive, 178
        pathology of, 176-178
        prognosis of, 186
        specific pathogens in, 178-182, 178t-180t
        treatment of, 184-186
    invasive, 178
    protozoan causes of, 182
    viral causes of, 182
Direct fluorescent antibody (DFA) staining, 30
Direct smear interpretation, 30, 34f
Disseminated intravascular coagulation (DIC)
    in sepsis, 68
Distal symmetrical peripheral neuropathy (PN), 252
Diverticulitis, 166, 168f
    Hinchey classification of, 170t
Doxycycline
    for chlamydia, 216
    for granuloma inguinale, 228
Drug-drug interactions, of immunocompromised host, 282
Drugs
    fever induced by, 42
Duke criteria, modified, for infective endocarditis diagnosis, 140t

E

Ear infections, subdural empyema and, 98-100
Echinococcus, 300
Echocardiography
    for infective endocarditis, 136
Ecthyma, 150
Ecthyma gangrenosum, 66
Edwardsiella tarda, skin and soft tissue infection from, 154
Ehrlichiosis, 54
Eikenella corrodens, skin and soft tissue infection from, 154
Elephantiasis, 298
Emphysematouspyelonephritis, in urinary tract infections, 198t-200t
Empyema
    subdural, 98-100
Encephalitis, 86-94
    Japanese, 290
    Toxoplasma, in HIV-infected patients, 246

D

痴呆
    克-雅病, 105
树突状细胞, 17
    未成熟树突状细胞, 25
地塞米松
    细菌性脑膜炎, 87
    脑水肿伴脑脓肿, 99
糖尿病
    HIV 感染, 257
糖尿病足感染, 161, 161f
    治疗, 163
腹泻, 277
    感染性腹泻, 177-187
        细菌性食物中毒, 179
        临床表现, 183-185
        细胞毒素诱导, 177
        定义和流行病学, 177
        诊断和鉴别诊断, 185, 185f
        肠毒素诱导, 177
        侵袭性腹泻, 179
        病理学, 177-179
        预后, 187
        特异性病原体, 179-183, 179t-181t
        治疗, 185-187
    侵袭性腹泻, 179
    原生动物病因, 183
    病毒性病因, 183
直接荧光抗体（DFA）染色, 31
直接涂片, 31, 35f
弥散性血管内凝血（DIC）
    感染中毒症, 69
远端对称性周围神经病变（PN）, 253
憩室炎, 167, 169f
    Hinchey 分类, 171t
多西环素
    衣原体感染, 217
    腹股沟肉芽肿, 229
药物相互作用, 免疫妥协宿主, 283
药物
    引起发热, 43
杜克标准修订版, 诊断感染性心内膜炎, 141t

E

耳部感染, 硬膜下积脓, 99-101
棘球蚴, 301
超声心动图
    感染性心内膜炎, 137
臁疮, 151
坏疽性深脓疱, 67
迟钝爱德华菌, 皮肤和软组织感染, 155
埃立克体病, 55
啮蚀艾肯菌, 皮肤和软组织感染, 155
象皮肿, 299
气性肾盂肾炎, 见于尿路感染, 199t-201t
积脓
    硬膜下积脓, 99-101
脑炎, 87-95
    乙型脑炎（日本脑炎）, 291
    弓形虫脑炎, 见于 HIV 感染者, 247

巨细胞病毒（CMV）, 247
    免疫妥协宿主, 283-289
    感染
        发热, 57
        单核细胞增多症综合征, 43, 57
        视网膜炎, HIV 感染者, 243, 247
巨细胞病毒结肠炎, 169
巨细胞病毒病, 247

Endarteritis, 144
Endocrine disorders
 in HIV infection, 256
Endoscopic retrograde cholangiopancreatography (ERCP), 164
Entamoeba histolytica, 178t-180t
 infections, 296, 296t
Enteric fever, 42
Enterobiasis, 298
Enteroviral infections, 42, 44t
Enteroviruses, in aseptic meningitis syndrome, 76
Entry inhibitors, for HIV infection, 262
Eosinophils, 8
Epidural abscess
 spinal, 100, 102f
 subdural empyema with, 98-100
Epstein-Barr virus (EBV)
 infection
  fever in, 54
  infectious mononucleosis in, 54
  mononucleosis syndrome in, 42
Erysipelas, 150, 152f
Erysipelothrix rhusiopathiae, skin and soft tissue infection from, 154
Escherichia coli, 292
 diarrhea-causing, 182
 enterotoxigenic, 176, 178t-180t
 P-fimbriated, 196
 Shiga toxin-producing, 176
 in urinary tract infections, 196
Eustachian tubes, 116

F

Familial fatal insomnia, 104
Febrile neutropenia, 50
Febrile syndromes, 40-58
Fever, 40-58
 acutely ill patient with, diagnostic approach to, 42-44
 after animal exposures, 44t, 50-52
 clinical findings and associated infections in, 50t
 deleterious effects of, 40
 factitious, self-induced illness and, 56
 vs. hyperthermia, 40
 infective endocarditis and, 136
 during inflammation and infection, 16
 with localized symptoms and signs, 42-44
 with lymphadenopathy, 54-56
 pathogenesis of, 40
 patterns of, 42
 rash and, 44, 44t-48t, 52-54
 in returning traveler, 294
  syndromes and diseases associated with, 48t
 in sepsis, 66
 of unknown origin, 44-50, 50t-52t
Fever of unknown origin, 276-278
Filariasis, lymphatic, 298
Fluid resuscitation
 in sepsis, 70
Fluid therapy, oral, for diarrhea, 186
Fluorescent in situ hybridization (FISH), 32-34
Fluorescent treponemal antibody absorption (FTA-ABS) test, for syphilis, 224
Folliculitis, 150
Food poisoning, bacterial, 178
Fosfomycintrometamol, for urinary tract infections, 196
Fournier gangrene, 150
Fracture, osteomyelitis from, 188
Francisella tularensis, skin and soft tissue infection from, 154, 154f
Fungal infections, in immunocompromised patients, 270
Fungal meningitis
 clinical presentation of, 80
 diagnosis of, 82-84

动脉内膜炎，145
内分泌疾病
 HIV 感染，257
内镜逆行胰胆管造影（ERCP），165
溶组织内阿米巴，179t-181t
 感染，297，297t
肠热症，43
蛲虫病，299
肠道病毒感染，43，45t
肠道病毒，见于无菌性脑膜炎综合征，77
HIV 进入抑制剂，263
嗜酸性粒细胞，9
硬膜外脓肿
 硬脊膜外脓肿，101，103f
 硬膜下积脓，99-101
EB 病毒（EBV）
 感染
  发热，55
  传染性单核细胞增多症，55
  单核细胞增多症综合征，43
丹毒，151，153f
猪红斑丹毒丝菌，皮肤和软组织感染，155
大肠埃希菌，293
 引起腹泻，183
 肠产毒性大肠埃希菌，177，179t-181t
 P 菌毛，197
 产志贺毒素大肠埃希菌，177
 尿路感染，197
咽鼓管，117

F

家族性致死性失眠，105
发热性中性粒细胞减少，51
发热性综合征，41-59
发热，41-59
 急性发热患者，诊断流程，43-45
 动物暴露后发热，45t，51-53
 临床表现和相关感染，51t
 有害作用，41
 伪热，人为性发热，57
 vs. 过热，41
 感染性心内膜炎，137
 炎症和感染期间，17
 局部症状和体征，43-45
 淋巴结肿大，55-57
 发病机制，41
 热型，43
 皮疹，45，45t-49t，53-55
 旅行者发热，295
  症状和疾病，49t
 感染中毒症，67
 不明原因，45-51，51t-53t
不明原因发热，277-279
丝虫病，淋巴系统，299
液体复苏
 感染中毒症，71
液体疗法，口服，治疗腹泻，187
荧光原位杂交（FISH），33-35
荧光密螺旋体抗体吸收（FTA-ABS）试验，梅毒，225
毛囊炎，151
食物中毒，细菌性，179
磷霉素氨丁三醇，治疗尿路感染，197
富尼埃坏疽，151
骨折，骨髓炎，189
土拉热弗朗西丝菌，皮肤和软组织感染，155，155f
真菌感染，免疫妥协宿主，271
真菌性脑膜炎
 临床表现，81
 诊断，83-85

epidemiology and etiology of, 78
Fungi
  in bone and joint infections, 190
  pneumonia and, 120
Furuncles, 150

G

Gardnerella vaginalis, in vaginitis, 218
Gastric acidity, 6
Gastrointestinal disease
  in HIV infection, 252-254
    large and small intestines, 252-254
    mouth and esophagus, 252
Genital ulcers, 220-228, 222t
  causes of, 228
Gerstmann-Sträussler-Scheinker syndrome, 104
Ghon complex, 126, 128f
Giardia lamblia, 178t-180t
  infections, 296t
  in returning traveler, 294
Giardiasis, in returning travelers, 294-296
Glucose
  cerebrospinal fluid, infection and, 82t, 92
Gonorrhea, 216-218
  clinical presentation of, 218
  definition of, 216
  diagnosis and differential diagnosis of, 218
  epidemiology of, 216
  pathology of, 216-218
  prognosis of, 218
  treatment of, 218
Granulocyte colony-stimulating factor (G-CSF)
  for neutropenia, 280
Granuloma, formation of, macrophages in, 16
Granuloma inguinale, 228
Group A streptococcal infections, lymphadenitis in, acute suppurative, 56
Group A streptococci, pharyngitis and, 110
Gummas, 224

H

Haemophilus influenzae infection
  meningitis in, 76
  pneumonia in, 118-120, 122f
Head and neck infections, 108-116
  acute bacterialotitis externa, 114-116
  acute bacterialotitis media, 116
  acute bacterial rhinosinusitis, 108-110
  common cold, 108
  deep neck space infections, 112-116, 114f
  pharyngitis and tonsillitis, 110-112
Heart
  acute congestive, infective endocarditis and, 142
  and bloodvessels, infections of, 134-148
    central venous catheter-related bloodstream infections, 144
    endarteritis, 144
    infective endocarditis, 134-144
    suppurative phlebitis, 144
Heart murmurs, in infective endocarditis, 136
Heatstroke, 40
Helminthic infections, 290-302, 300t
  common in travelers and immigrants, 298-300
  common in United States, 298
Hematogenousosteomyelitis, 188
Hematologic malignancies, in immunocompromised host, 272
Hematopoietic cell transplantation, 274, 276t
Hemorrhagic fevers, 54
Hepatitis A

G

阴道加德纳菌，见于阴道炎，219
胃液酸度，7
消化道疾病
  HIV 感染，253-255
    大肠和小肠，253-255
    口腔和食管，253
生殖器溃疡，221-229，223t
  病因，229
格斯特劳斯特斯勒尔-沙因克尔综合征，105
冈氏综合征，127，129f
蓝氏贾第鞭毛虫，179t-181t
  感染，297t
  返程旅行者，295
贾第虫病，见于返程旅行者，295-297
葡萄糖
  脑脊液，感染，83t，93
淋病，217-219
  临床表现，219
  定义，217
  诊断和鉴别诊断，219
  流行病学，217
  病理学，217-219
  预后，219
  治疗，219
粒细胞集落刺激因子（G-CSF）
  中性粒细胞减少，281
肉芽肿形成，巨噬细胞，17
腹股沟肉芽肿，229
A 组链球菌感染，急性化脓性淋巴结炎，57
A 组链球菌，咽炎，111
树胶肿，225

H

流感嗜血杆菌感染
  脑膜炎，77
  肺炎，119-121，123f
头颈部感染，109-117
  急性细菌性外耳炎，115-117
  急性细菌性中耳炎，117
  急性细菌性鼻窦炎，109-111
  普通感冒，109
  颈深间隙感染，113-117，115f
  咽炎和扁桃体炎，111-113
心脏
  急性充血，感染性心内膜炎，143
  血管，感染，135-149
    中心静脉导管相关血流感染，145
    动脉内膜炎，145
    感染性心内膜炎，135-145
    化脓性血栓性静脉炎，145
心脏杂音，感染性心内膜炎，137
热射病，41
蠕虫感染，291-303，301t
  常见于旅行者和移民，299-301
  常见于美国，299
血源性骨髓炎，189
恶性血液病
  免疫妥协宿主，273
造血细胞移植，275，277t
出血热，55
甲型肝炎

immunization for, 262
   in infectious diseases of travelers, 290
Hepatitis B
   immunization for, 262
Hepatobiliary disease, in HIV infection, 254
Herpes simplex virus (HSV), 226-228
   clinical presentation of, 226-228
   definition of, 226
   diagnosis and differential diagnosis of, 228
   epidemiology of, 226
   genital, 242
   immunocompromised host and, 282
   inguinal lymphadenopathy and, 56
   pathology of, 226
   prognosis of, 228
   skin and soft tissue infection from, 156
   treatment of, 228
Herpes simplex virus infection
   encephalitis in, 88-90
   meningitis in, 76-78
Herpes zoster, 54
Histamine, 8-16
Hookworm infections, 298
Hospital-acquired pneumonia, 204, 208t
HPV. See Human papillomavirus
HPV-associated cancers, 248
Human bites, 160
   treatment for, 162
Human immunodeficiency virus (HIV) infection, 232-268
   acute, 238
   aging and, 256-258
   antiretroviral treatment for, 262-266, 264t
   clinical diagnosis of, 238-240, 240f
   co-occurring disease and multimorbidity with, 250-258
   cure research, 266
   epidemiology of, 232-234, 234f
   fever of unknown origin in, 50
   history of, 232
   immunization for, 260-262, 260t
   immunology and inflammation in, 238
   infections in, CD4 counts and, 242
   malignancy and, 248-250
   management and treatment of, 258-262
      initial counseling and ambulatory evaluation, 258
      laboratory monitoring, 258-260
      screening for associated, 260
   natural progression of, 240-250
      acute retroviral syndrome, 240, 242t
      opportunistic infections, 242-248
      untreated disease, 240-242, 242t
   prevention of, 266-268
   primary, 56
   progression of, 238
   transmission of, 232
   viral load in, 238
   virology of, 234-238, 236f-238f
Human papillomavirus (HPV), 228
   immunization for, 260
Humoral response, 24-26
Hydatid disease, 300
Hyperglycemia
   in sepsis, 68
Hyperpyrexia, 40
Hyperthermia, 40
Hypoglycemia
   in sepsis, 68
Hypogonadism, 256
Hypotension, in sepsis, 68
Hypothermia, in sepsis, 66

免疫接种，263
   旅行者感染性疾病，291
乙型肝炎
   免疫接种，263
肝胆疾病，HIV 感染，255
单纯疱疹病毒（HSV），227-229
   临床表现，229
   定义，227
   诊断和鉴别诊断，229
   流行病学，227
   生殖器 HSV，243
   免疫妥协宿主，283
   腹股沟淋巴结肿大，57
   病理学，227
   预后，229
   皮肤和软组织感染，157
   治疗，229
单纯疱疹病毒感染
   脑炎，89-91
   脑膜炎，77-79
带状疱疹，55
组胺，9-17
钩虫感染，299
医院获得性肺炎，205，209t
HPV 参见人乳头瘤病毒
HPV 相关癌症，249
人咬伤，161
   处理，163
人类免疫缺陷病毒（HIV）感染，233-269
   急性感染，239
   老化，257-259
   抗逆转录病毒治疗，263-267，265t
   临床诊断，239-241，241f
   并发症与合并疾病，251-259
   治愈研究，267
   流行病学，233-235，235f
   不明原因发热，51
   历史，233
   免疫接种，261-263，261t
   免疫学和炎症，239
   感染，CD4$^+$ T 细胞计数，243
   恶性肿瘤，249-251
   管理和治疗，259-263
      初次咨询和门诊评估，259
      实验室监测，259-261
      相关筛查，261
   自然病程，241-251
      急性逆转录病毒综合征，241，243t
      机会性感染，243-249
      未经治疗的疾病，241-243，243t
   预防，267-269
   急性感染，57
   进展，239
   传播，233
   病毒载量，239
   病毒学，235-239，237f-239f
人乳头瘤病毒（HPV），229
   免疫接种，261
体液免疫应答，25-27
棘球蚴病，301
高血糖
   感染中毒症，69
超高热，41
过热，41
低血糖
   感染中毒症，69
性腺功能减退症，257
低血压，感染中毒症，69
体温过低，感染中毒症，67

I

Immune reconstitution inflammatory syndrome (IRIS), 250
Immunizations
    of immunocompromised host, 282
    travel-related illness, 290-292
Immunocompromised host
    cell-mediated immunity deficits, 270
    clinical presentation of, 276-278
    diagnosis of, 278-280, 278f
    diagnostic imaging for, 280
    epidemiology of, 270
    host considerations for, 278-280
    humoral immune deficits, 270
    infections in, 270-288, 272f
    neutropenia and, 270
    novel immunomodulatory medications for, 274-276
    pathogenesis of, 270-276
    prevention of infection, 282-288
    syndrome considerations of, 280
    treatment of, 280-282
Immunodeficiency syndromes, primary, 272t
Immunoglobulin(s)
    congenital deficiency of, 4
Immunology, in HIV, 238
Immunosuppressive therapy
    for immunocompromised host, 274t
Impetigo, 150
India ink examination, 84
Infections
    healthcare-associated, 202-212
        catheter-associated urinary tract infections, 202-204, 206t, 208f
        from *Clostridioides difficile*, 210
        definition of, 202
        epidemiology of, 202
        hospital-acquired pneumonia, 204, 208t
        multidrug-resistant pathogens in, 210-212, 210t
        prevention of, 202, 206t
        from vascular catheters, 204-208
    host defenses against, 4-26
        categories of, 4-24
        host *vs.* pathogen, 4
        nonimmunologic, 4-6
        response to pathogens, 24-26
    involving bones and joints, 188-192
        clinical presentation of, 188-190
        definitions of, 188
        diagnosis of, 188-190
        differential diagnosis of, 190
        pathophysiology of, 188
        prognosis of, 192
        treatment of, 190-192
    laboratory diagnosis of, 28-38
        culture with boost, 30-32, 36t
        diagnostic stewardship, 28, 30b
        direct smear interpretation in, 30, 34f
        metagenomic next-generation sequencing for pathogen detection, 34-36
        point-of-care or near-patient testing in, 36-38
        rapid diagnostic methods in, 28-30, 32t
        specimen collection and processing in, 28
        syndromic assay panels, 34
        trends in, 38, 38b
    pyogenic, 56
    reactivation, in tuberculosis, 130
    severe, definition of, 60
    tuberculosis and, 126-130
Infectious bowel disease, 166-170
Infectious colitis, 166-168
Infectious mononucleosis, 54

I

免疫重建炎症综合征（IRIS），251
免疫接种
    免疫妥协宿主，283
    旅行相关疾病，291-293
免疫妥协宿主
    细胞介导的免疫缺陷，271
    临床表现，277-279
    诊断，279-281，279f
    诊断性影像学检查，281
    流行病学，271
    宿主注意事项，279-281
    体液免疫缺陷，271
    感染，271-289，273f
    中性粒细胞减少症，271
    新型免疫调节剂，275-277
    发病机制，271-277
    预防感染，283-289
    综合征注意事项，281
    治疗，281-283
原发性免疫缺陷综合征，273t
免疫球蛋白
    先天性缺乏免疫球蛋白，5
免疫学（HIV），239
免疫抑制治疗
    免疫妥协宿主，275t
脓疱病，151
墨汁染色，85
感染
    医疗照护相关感染，203-213
        导管相关尿路感染，203-205，207t，209f
        艰难梭菌，211
        定义，203
        流行病学，203
        医院获得性肺炎，205，209t
        多重耐药病原体，211-213，211t
        预防，203，207t
        血管导管，205-209
    宿主防御，5-27
        分类，5-25
        宿主 *vs.* 病原体，5
        非免疫性宿主防御，5-7
        对病原体的防御反应，25-27
    累及骨和关节，189-193
        临床表现，189-191
        定义，189
        诊断，189-191
        鉴别诊断，191
        病理生理学，189
        预后，193
        治疗，191-193
    实验室诊断，29-39
        强化培养，31-33，37t
        诊断管理，29，31b
        直接涂片，31，35f
        用于病原体检测的宏基因组二代测序，35-37
        即时检测或近患者检测，37-39
        快速诊断方法，29-31，33t
        样本采集和处理，29
        综合征检测试剂盒，35
        趋势，39，39b
    化脓性感染，57
    再激活，见于结核，131
    严重感染，定义，61
    结核和感染，127-131
感染性肠病，167-171
感染性结肠炎，167-169
传染性单核细胞增多症，55

Infective endocarditis, 134-144
    blood cultures in, 42-44
    complications of, 142
    definition of, 134
    diagnosis of, 136-140, 138t-140t
        clinical features of, 136
        differential diagnosis and mimics, 138-140
        imaging studies of, 136-138
        laboratory findings in, 136, 142t
        modified Duke criteria for, 140t
    embolization in, 102-104
    epidemiology of, 134
    likely pathogen in, 138t
    neurologic complications of, 102-104
    pathogenesis of, 134-136
    prognosis of, 144
    prophylaxis for, 144
    prosthetic valve, 134
    treatment of, 140-142, 144t-146t
        antimicrobial, 146t
        surgical intervention in, echocardiographic indications for, 148t
Inflammation, 8
    in HIV, 238
Influenza, 42
    avian, 42
    travel-related illness, 290
Influenza vaccine, 124
Influenzavirus, immunization for, 260
Inguinal lymphadenopathy, 56
Innate immunity, 6-16, 6f
Integrase inhibitors, for HIV infection, 262
Integrasestrand transfer inhibitors (InSTIs), for HIV infection, 262
Integrins, 8
Interferon(s), antiviral action of, 8
Interferon-γ, 16
Intraabdominal abscess, 172
Intraabdominal infections, 164-174
    acalculouscholecystitis, 170
    appendicitis, 164-166, 166f
    cholecystitis, 170
    diverticulitis, 166, 168f
    infectious bowel disease, 166-170
    peritonitis, 164
Intrapelvic abscess, 172
Intravenous fluid therapy, for diarrhea, 186
Isospora, 180t

J

Janeway's lesions, infective endocarditis and, 136
Japanese encephalitis, 290

K

Kaposi's sarcoma, 248
Klebsiella pneumoniae, infection with, pneumonia in, 118-120

L

Lactate, serum, in sepsis, 68
Laparoscopiccholecystectomy, for cholecystitis, 170
Lateral pharyngeal space infection, 112
Lateral sinus thrombosis, septic, 102
Latex agglutination test, in cryptococcal meningitis, 84
Legionellapneumophila, infection with, pneumonia in, 118-120
Legionnaires' disease, infective endocarditis and, 136
Leishmania donovani, 296t
Leishmaniasis, 296
Lemierre syndrome, pharyngitis and, 112
Leptospirosis, 52
    meningitis in, 52

感染性心内膜炎，135-145
    血培养，43-45
    并发症，143
    定义，135
    诊断，137-141，139t-141t
        临床特征，137
        鉴别诊断与容易混淆的情况，139-141
        影像学研究，137-139
        实验室检查，137，143t
        改良杜克标准，141t
    栓塞，103-105
    流行病学，135
    可能的病原体，139t
    神经系统并发症，103-105
    发病机制，135-137
    预后，145
    预防，145
    人工瓣膜心内膜炎，135
    治疗，141-143，145t-147t
        抗菌治疗，147t
        手术干预，超声心动图指征，149t
炎症，9
    HIV 感染，239
流感，43
    禽流感，43
    旅行相关疾病，291
流感疫苗，125
流感病毒，免疫接种，261
腹股沟淋巴结肿大，57
先天免疫，7-17，7f
整合酶抑制剂，治疗 HIV 感染，263
整合酶链转移抑制剂（InSTI），治疗 HIV 感染，263
整合素，9
干扰素，抗病毒作用，9
干扰素 γ，17
腹腔内脓肿，173
腹腔内感染，165-175
    无结石胆囊炎，171
    阑尾炎，165-167，167f
    胆囊炎，171
    憩室炎，167，169f
    感染性肠病，167-171
    腹膜炎，165
盆腔内脓肿，173
静脉输液，治疗腹泻，187
等孢球虫属，181t

J

詹韦损害，感染性心内膜炎，137
乙型脑炎，291

K

卡波西肉瘤，249
肺炎克雷伯菌感染，119-121

L

血清乳酸，感染中毒症，69
腹腔镜胆囊切除术，治疗胆囊炎，171
咽旁间隙感染，113
侧窦血栓形成，感染中毒性，103
乳胶凝集试验，见于隐球菌性脑膜炎，85
军团菌肺炎，119-121
军团病，感染性心内膜炎，137
杜氏利什曼原虫，297t
利什曼病，297
Lemierre 综合征，咽炎，113
钩端螺旋体病，53
    脑膜炎，53

Lifestyle modifications
    of immunocompromised host, 282
Lipopolysaccharide (LPS), 64
Listeria monocytogenes infection
    bacteremia in, 42, 44t
    diarrhea from, 180-182
    meningitis caused by, 76
Liver
    abscess, 46
Liver cancer, in HIV infection, 250
Liver disease. See also Cirrhosis; Hepatitis
    sepsis in, 68
Loa loa (eyeworm), 300
Loperamide, for diarrhea, 186
Lower respiratory tract, infections of, 118-132
    clinical presentation of, 120
    definition of, 118
    diagnosis of, 120-122
    differential diagnosis of, 122
    epidemiology of, 118
    etiologic agents of, 118-120
    pathology of, 118-120
    pathophysiology of, 118
    prevention of, 124, 124f
    prognosis of, 124, 124f
    respiratory pathogens, transmission of, 118
    treatment for, 122-124, 124t
Ludwig angina, 112, 116f
Lumbar puncture, 80
Lung cancer
    in HIV infection, 248-250
Lyme disease, 54
    meningitis and, 80
Lymph node enlargement, in HIV infection, 242
Lymphadenopathy
    fever with, 54-56
    regional, infections causing, 56
Lymphatic filariasis (elephantiasis), 298
Lymphogranuloma venereum, 56

M

Macrophages
    fever and, 40
    properties and function of, 16
Magnetic resonance imaging (MRI)
    of brain abscess, 96, 96f
    in Creutzfeldt-Jakob disease, 104-106
    for infective endocarditis, 136-138, 164
    of spinal epidural abscess, 100, 102f
    of subdural empyema, 100
Malaria
    fever of unknown origin and, 46
    prophylaxis, 292
Malignancy
    HIV and, 248-250
Marantic endocarditis, 140
Marine lacerations and punctures, treatment for, 162
Matrix-assisted laser desorption ionization-time of flight mass spectrometry (MALDI-TOF MS), 30, 34f
Measles, 290
Men who have sex with men (MSM)
    chlamydia screening for, 214
    giardiasis in, 294-296
Meningeal coccidioidomycosis, 80
Meningismus, 78
Meningitis, 74-86
    bacterial, 52
        adjunctive therapy for, 86
        antimicrobial therapy for, 84-86, 88t-90t

生活方式修改
    免疫妥协宿主，283
脂多糖（LPS），65
单核细胞增生李斯特菌感染
    菌血症，43，45t
    腹泻，181-183
    脑膜炎，77
肝
    肝脓肿，47
肝癌，见于HIV感染，251
肝病 参见肝硬化；肝炎
    感染中毒症，69
罗阿丝虫（眼丝虫），301
洛哌丁胺，治疗腹泻，187
下呼吸道感染，119-133
    临床表现，121
    定义，119
    诊断，121-123
    鉴别诊断，123
    流行病学，119
    病原体，119-121
    病理学，119-121
    病理生理学，119
    预防，125，125f
    预后，125，125f
    呼吸道病原体，传播，119
    治疗，123-125，125t
脓性颌下炎，113，117f
腰椎穿刺，81
肺癌
    HIV感染，249-251
莱姆病，55
    脑膜炎，81
淋巴结肿大，见于HIV感染，243
淋巴结肿大
    发热，55-57
    局部淋巴结肿大，感染导致，57
淋巴性丝虫病（象皮肿），299
性病性淋巴肉芽肿，57

M

巨噬细胞
    发热，41
    特性和功能，17
磁共振成像（MRI）
    脑脓肿，97，97f
    克-雅病，105-107
    感染性心内膜炎，137-139，165
    硬脊膜外脓肿，101，103f
    硬膜下积脓，101
疟疾
    不明原因发热，47
    预防，293
恶性肿瘤
    HIV，249-251
非细菌性栓塞性心内膜炎，141
海洋割伤和穿刺伤，治疗，163
基质辅助激光解吸电离飞行时间质谱法（MALDI-TOF MS），31，35f
麻疹，291
男男性行为（MSM）
    衣原体筛查，215
    贾第虫病，295-297
脑膜球孢子菌病，81
脑膜刺激征，79
脑膜炎，75-87
    细菌性脑膜炎，53
        辅助治疗，87
        抗菌疗法，85-87，89t-91t

clinical presentation of, 78
diagnosis of, 80-82
differentiation from viral meningitis, 82
epidemiology and etiology of, 74-76
initial treatment of, 84, 84f, 86t
pathogens in, 74, 76t
clinical presentation of, 78-80
in cryptococcal disease, 244-246
definition of, 74
diagnosis of, 80-84
epidemiology and etiology of, 74-78
fungal, cryptococcal, 82-84
subacute or chronic, clinical presentation of, 78-80
symptoms of, 42
treatment of, 84-86
Meningococcal meningitis, 290-292
Meningococcemia, fever and rash in, 52
Meningoencephalitis, 252
Mental health
HIV infection and, 258
Metabolic syndrome
in HIV infection, 256
Methicillin-resistant *Staphylococcus aureus* (MRSA), 210-212
community-associated, skin and soft tissue infections, 150
Metronidazole, for vaginitis, 220
Microbiologic flora, normal, 6
Middle East respiratory syndrome (MERS), 42
Molecular assays, 32
Molecular diagnostics, 32-34
Monocytes
blood, 16
fever and, 40
Mononucleosis syndromes, 42
Monospot test, 54
Moraxella catarrhalis, infection with, pneumonia in, 118-120, 122f
Mucorales
invasive pulmonary, 286
pulmonary infiltrates caused by, 272
Multidrug-resistant pathogens, 210-212, 210t
Multiorgan failure, in severe sepsis, 60, 62f
Murine typhus, 54
Mycobacteria, invasive pulmonary, 286
Mycobacterium avium complex (MAC) infection, 242
regional lymphadenopathy caused by, 56
Mycobacterium leprae, skin and soft tissue infection from, 154
Mycobacterium marinum, skin and soft tissue infection from, 154
Mycobacterium scrofulaceum, regional lymphadenopathy caused by, 56
Mycobacterium tuberculosis, 120, 246
Mycotic aneurysms, 104

N

Native valve endocarditis (NVE), 134
Natural killer (NK) cells, 16
Near-patient testing, 36-38
Neck space infections, 112-116, 114f
Necrotizing fasciitis, 150, 152f
Neisseria gonorrhoeae, 216
Neisseria meningitidis, 290-292
in humoral immunity, 270
immunization for, 262
Neisseria meningitidis infection
bacteremia in, 66-68
meningitis in, 74-76
Nematodes, intestinal, 298
Nervous system infections, 74-106
brain abscess, 94-98, 96f, 96t-98t
subdural empyema leading to, 98-100
clinical presentation of, 78-80
diagnosis of, 80-84, 80t-82t

临床表现，79
诊断，81-83
与病毒性脑膜炎鉴别，83
流行病学和病因学，75-77
初始治疗，85, 85f, 87t
病原体，75, 77t
临床表现，79-81
隐球菌病，245-247
定义，75
诊断，81-85
流行病学和病因，75-79
真菌性脑膜炎和隐球菌性脑膜炎，83-85
亚急性或慢性脑膜炎，临床表现，79-81
症状，43
治疗，85-87
脑膜炎球菌性脑膜炎，291-293
脑膜炎球菌血症，发热和皮疹，53
脑膜脑炎，253
心理健康
HIV 感染，259
代谢综合征
HIV 感染，257
耐甲氧西林金黄色葡萄球菌（MRSA），211-213
社区相关感染，皮肤和软组织感染，151
甲硝唑，治疗阴道炎，221
正常微生物群，7
中东呼吸综合征（MERS），43
分子检测，33
分子诊断，33-35
单核细胞
血液单核细胞，17
发热，41
单核细胞增多症综合征，43
单斑试验，55
卡他莫拉菌，感染，肺炎，119-121, 123f
毛霉目真菌
侵袭性肺毛霉菌病，287
引起肺浸润，273
耐多药病原体，211-213, 211t
多器官功能衰竭，见于严重感染中毒症，61, 63f
鼠型斑疹伤寒，55
分枝杆菌，侵袭性肺分枝杆菌感染，287
鸟分枝杆菌复合群（MAC）感染，243
引起局部淋巴结肿大，57
麻风分枝杆菌，皮肤和软组织感染，155
海分枝杆菌，皮肤和软组织感染，155
瘰疬分枝杆菌，引起区域淋巴结肿大，57
结核分枝杆菌，121, 247
真菌性动脉瘤，105

N

自体瓣膜心内膜炎（NVE），135
自然杀伤（NK）细胞，17
近患者检测，37-39
颈深间隙感染，113-117, 115f
坏死性筋膜炎，151, 153f
淋病奈瑟球菌，217
脑膜炎奈瑟球菌，291-293
体液免疫，271
免疫接种，263
脑膜炎奈瑟球菌感染
菌血症，67-69
脑膜炎，75-77
线虫，肠，299
神经系统感染，75-107
脑脓肿，95-99, 97f, 97t-99t
硬膜下积脓导致的脑脓肿，99-101
临床表现，79-81
诊断，81-85, 81t-83t

parameningeal, 98-100
prion diseases, 104-106
sinus thrombosis, 100-102
spinal epidural abscess, 100, 102f
subdural empyema, 98-100
Neurologic disease
in HIV infection, 250-252
Neurosyphilis, 224
Neutropenia, 270
febrile, 46-50
in sepsis, 68
Neutrophilic dermatosis, febrile, 276
Neutrophils, 8
Nitric oxide
in sepsis, 64-66, 66f
skin and soft tissue infection and, 150
Nitrofurantoin
for urinary tract infections, 196
Nocardia, 286
Non-AIDS-defining cancers (NADC), 248-250
Nonalcoholic fatty liver disease (NAFLD)
in HIV infection, 256
Non-Hodgkin's lymphomas, 248
Nonimmunologic host defenses, 4-6
Non-nucleotide reverse transcription inhibitors (NNRTIs), for HIV infection, 262
Nontreponemal test, for syphilis, 224
Nontuberculous mycobacterial disease, 246
Nontyphoidal salmonellosis, 178-180
Norovirus, diarrhea from, 178t, 182
Nosocomial infective endocarditis, 136
Nucleic acid amplification, 158
Nucleic acid amplification testing (NAAT), 216
Nucleotide/nucleoside reverse transcriptase inhibitors (NRTIs), for HIV infection, 262

O

Obesity
in HIV infection, 256
Onchocerca volvulus infection, 300
Opportunistic infections, 272-274
Oral fluid therapy, for diarrhea, 186
Osler node, in infective endocarditis, 136
Osteomyelitis, 188
fever and, 42
Osteoporosis
in HIV infection, 254-256
Otitis externa, malignant, 116

P

Pancreatic infection, 172
Papanicolaou (Pap) smear, in HIV-infected women, 242
Papillary necrosis, in urinary tract infections, 198t-200t
Parameningeal infections, 98-100
Parasites, invasive pulmonary, 286-288
Paratyphoid fever, 42, 48t
Pasteurella multocida, skin and soft tissue infection from, 154
Pelvic inflammatory disease (PID), chlamydia and, 214
Penicillin, for syphilis, 226
Penicillin G, for CNS syphilis, 84
Penicillin therapy, for bacteremicpneumococcal pneumonia, 122
Perinephric abscess, in urinary tract infections, 198t-200t
Peritonitis
primary, 164
secondary, 164
Peritonsillar abscess, pharyngitis and, 112
Persistent chronic inflammation, in HIV infection, 238
Persistent diarrhea, 176

脑膜周围感染，99-101
朊病毒病，105-107
窦血栓形成，101-103
硬脊膜外脓肿，101, 103f
硬膜下积脓，99-101
神经系统疾病
HIV 感染，251-253
神经梅毒，225
中性粒细胞减少症，271
发热性中性粒细胞减少症，47-51
感染中毒症，69
发热性嗜中性细胞皮肤病，277
中性粒细胞，9
一氧化氮
感染中毒症，65-67, 67f
皮肤和软组织感染，151
呋喃妥因
尿路感染，197
诺卡菌，287
非艾滋病标志性癌症（NADC），249-251
非酒精性脂肪性肝病（NAFLD）
HIV 感染，257
非霍奇金淋巴瘤，249
非免疫宿主防御，5-7
非核苷类反转录酶抑制剂（NNRTI），治疗 HIV 感染，263
非梅毒螺旋体试验，针对梅毒，225
非结核分枝杆菌病，247
非伤寒沙门菌病，179-181
诺如病毒，腹泻，179t, 183
医院获得性心内膜炎，137
核酸扩增，159
核酸扩增试验（NAAT），217
核苷类反转录酶抑制剂（NRTI），治疗 HIV 感染，263

O

肥胖症
HIV 感染，257
旋盘尾丝虫感染，301
机会性感染，273-275
口服液体疗法，治疗腹泻，187
奥斯勒结节，见于感染性心内膜炎，137
骨髓炎，189
发热，43
骨质疏松症
HIV 感染，255-257
恶性外耳炎，117

P

胰腺感染，173
巴氏（Pap）涂片，用于 HIV 感染女性，243
乳头坏死，见于尿路感染，199t-201t
脑膜周围感染，99-101
寄生虫，侵袭肺部，287-289
副伤寒，43, 49t
多杀巴斯德菌，皮肤和软组织感染，155
盆腔炎（PID），衣原体，215
青霉素，治疗梅毒，227
青霉素 G，治疗 CNS 梅毒，85
青霉素治疗，治疗菌血症性肺炎球菌性肺炎，123
肾周脓肿，见于尿路感染，199t-201t
腹膜炎
原发性腹膜炎，165
继发性腹膜炎，165
扁桃体周脓肿，咽炎，113
持续性慢性炎症，见于 HIV 感染，239
持续性腹泻，177

Phagocytic cells, 16
Phagocytosis
 of *Mycobacterium tuberculosis*, 24
 by neutrophils, 16
Pharyngitis, 110-112
Phlebitis, suppurative, 144
Pinworm, 298
Plague, 56
Plasmodium falciparum, 292
Plasmodium species, 296t
Pneumococcallobar pneumonia, 118
Pneumocystis jirovecii pneumonia, 232, 244, 244t
Pneumonia, 232, 276
 bacterial, 118-120
  Chlamydophila pneumoniae, 120
  Klebsiella pneumoniae, 118-120
  Legionellapneumophila, 120
  S.pneumoniae, 120, 122f
  Staphylococcus aureus, 120, 122f
  Streptococcus pyogenes, 118-120
 clinical presentation of, 120
 definition of, 118
 diagnosis of, 120-122
 differential diagnosis of, 122
 epidemiology of, 118, 120f
 fungi, 120
 healthcare-associated, 208t
 hospital-acquired, 204, 208t
 pathology of, 118-120
 pathophysiology of, 118
 prevention of, 124, 124f
 prognosis of, 124, 124f
 treatment for, 122-124, 124t
 viruses and, 118-120
Pneumonia severity index (PSI), 122
Point-of-care testing, 36-38
Poisoning
 bacterial food, 178
Polio, 292
Polymerase chain reaction (PCR)
 in enteroviral meningitis diagnosis, 82
 real-time, 34
Polymyalgia rheumatica (PMR)
 fever in, 46
 with temporal arteritis, 46
Polyomaviruses, immunocompromised host and, 282
Postangina septicemia, 112
Pregnancy
 travel during, 294
Primaquine, for malaria, 292
Primary CNS lymphoma, 248
Prion diseases, 104-106
Progressive multifocal encephalopathy (PML), 278f
Progressive multifocal leukoencephalopathy (PML), 246
Prostaglandin E_2, fever and, 40
Prostaglandins (PGs)
 skin and soft tissue infection and, 150
Prostate cancer
 in HIV infection, 250
Prosthetic joint infections (PJI), 190
Prosthetic valve endocarditis (PVE), 134
 late, 136
Protease inhibitors (PIs), for HIV infection, 262
Protozoal infections, 294-298, 296t
 common in travelers and immigrants, 296-298
 in United States, 294-296
Pseudomonas aeruginosa, skin and soft tissue infection from, 154
Pubic lice, 228-230
Pyomyositis, 150

吞噬细胞，17
吞噬作用
　结核分枝杆菌，25
　中性粒细胞，17
咽炎，111-113
化脓性血栓性静脉炎，145
蛲虫，299
鼠疫，57
恶性疟原虫，293
疟原虫，297t
肺炎球菌性大叶性肺炎，119
耶氏肺孢子虫肺炎，233，245，245t
肺炎，233，277
　细菌性肺炎，119-121
　　肺炎衣原体，121
　　肺炎克雷伯菌，119-121
　　嗜肺军团菌，121
　　肺炎链球菌，121，123f
　　金黄色葡萄球菌，121，123f
　　化脓性链球菌，119-121
　临床表现，121
　定义，119
　诊断，121-123
　鉴别诊断，123
　流行病学，119，121f
　真菌性肺炎，121
　医疗相关肺炎，209t
　医院获得性肺炎，205，209t
　病理学，119-121
　病理生理学，119
　预防，125，125f
　预后，125，125f
　治疗，123-125，125t
　病毒性肺炎，119-121
肺炎严重程度指数（PSI），123
即时检测，37-39
中毒
　细菌性食物中毒，179
脊髓灰质炎，293
聚合酶链反应（PCR）
　肠病毒性脑炎诊断，83
　实时聚合酶链反应，35
风湿性多肌痛（PMR）
　发热，47
　颞动脉炎，47
多瘤病毒，免疫妥协宿主，283
咽峡炎后感染中毒症，113
妊娠
　妊娠期间旅行，295
伯氨喹，治疗疟疾，293
原发性中枢神经系统淋巴瘤，249
朊病毒病，105-107
进行性多灶性脑病（PML），279f
进行性多灶性白质脑病（PML），247
前列腺素 E_2，发热，41
前列腺素（PG）
　皮肤软组织感染，151
前列腺癌
　HIV 感染，251
假体关节感染（PJI），191
人工瓣膜心内膜炎（PVE），135
　晚期，137
蛋白酶抑制剂（PI），治疗 HIV 感染，263
原虫感染，295-299，297t
　旅行者和移民中常见的原虫感染，297-299
　美国原虫感染，295-297
铜绿假单胞菌，皮肤和软组织感染，155
阴虱，229-231
化脓性肌炎，151

Q

Q fever, 44t, 50-52
    infective endocarditis and, 136
Quinidine
    for malaria, 294

R

Rabies, encephalitis and, 92
Ramsay Hunt syndrome, 156
Rash
    fever and, 44, 44t-48t, 52-54
    from syphilis, 224
    viral infections associated with, 54
Renal disease
    in HIV infection, 254
Renal injury, in sepsis, 68
Resistance testing, for HIV infection, 262-264
Respiratory pathogens, transmission of, 118
Respiratory syncytial virus (RSV), 120
Retropharyngeal infection, 112
Reynolds pentad, 170
Rheumatoid arthritis
    juvenile, fever in, 46
Rhinoviruses, common cold and, 108
Rickettsial infections, 54
Rigors, 42
Rituximab
    in humoral immunity, 274-276
River blindness, 300
Rocky Mountain spotted fever (RMSF), 44
Roth spots, 136
Roundworm, 298

S

Sagittal sinus thrombosis, septic, 102
Salmonella, diarrhea due to, 178-180, 178t-180t
Salmonella paratyphi, 44t
Salmonella typhi, 44t
Scabies, 230
Schistosomiasis, 298
Scrofula, 56
Seizures
    brain abscess causing, 94-96
    in cysticercosis, 300
Sepsis, 60-72
    clinical presentation of, 66-68
    definition of, 60, 62f
    diagnosis of, 68
    diagnostic criteria for, 62t
    epidemiology of, 60
    immunopathogenesis of, 62-64, 66f
    microorganisms associated with, 60, 64t
    pathology of, 62-64
    prognosis of, 72
    treatment of, 70-72, 70t
Sepsis syndrome
    pathophysiology of, 60
    systemic inflammatory response syndrome and, 60
Septic arthritis, 188
    treatment of, 190-192
Septic shock
    clinical presentation of, 66-68
    definition of, 60, 62f
    epidemiology of, 60
    pathophysiology of, 64-66
    treatment of, 70-72, 70t
    in urinary tract infections, 198t-200t
Serotonin syndrome, 40

Q

Q 热，45t，51-53
    感染性心内膜炎，137
奎尼丁
    疟疾，295

R

狂犬病，脑炎，93
拉姆齐·亨特综合征，157
皮疹
    发热，45，45t-49t，53-55
    梅毒疹，225
    病毒感染，55
肾病
    HIV 感染，255
肾损伤，见于感染中毒症，69
耐药检测，HIV 感染，265
呼吸道病原体传播，119
呼吸道合胞病毒（RSV），121
咽后感染，113
雷诺五联征，171
类风湿关节炎
    幼年型类风湿关节炎，发热，47
鼻病毒，普通感冒，109
立克次体感染，55
寒战，43
利妥昔单抗
    体液免疫，275-277
河盲，301
落基山斑点热（RMSF），45
罗特斑，137
蛔虫，299

S

矢状窦血栓形成，感染中毒性，103
沙门菌属，引起腹泻，179-181，179t-181t
副伤寒沙门菌，45t
伤寒沙门菌，45t
疥疮，231
血吸虫病，299
瘰疬，57
癫痫发作
    脑脓肿导致的癫痫发作，95-97
    猪囊尾蚴病，301
感染中毒症，61-73
    临床表现，67-69
    定义，61，63f
    诊断，69
    诊断标准，63t
    流行病学，61
    免疫发病机制，63-65，67f
    相关微生物，61，65t
    病理学，63-65
    预后，73
    治疗，71-73，71t
感染中毒症综合征
    病理生理学，61
    系统性炎症反应综合征，61
化脓性关节炎，189
    治疗，191-193
感染中毒性休克
    临床表现，67-69
    定义，61，63f
    流行病学，61
    病理生理学，65-67
    治疗，71-73，71t
    尿路感染，199t-201t
5-羟色胺综合征，41

Sexually transmitted diseases, 56
Sexually transmitted infections (STIs), 214-230
    genital ulcer disease in, 220-228, 222t
    HIV infection and, 258-260
    urethritis and cervicitis in, 214-220
Shiga toxin-producing *Escherichia coli* (STEC)
    diarrhea from, 178t-180t
Shigella
    diarrhea due to, 178, 178t-180t
Sigmoidresection, for diverticulitis, 166
Significant bacteriuria, defined, 194
Sinus thrombosis, 100-102
Skin and soft tissue infections
    acute bacterial, 150-162
    causative organisms of, 152
    classification of bacterial and mycotic, 156t-158t
    definition of, 150
    diagnosis for, 158-160
    differential diagnosis for, 160
    epidemiology of, 150
    fungi and viruses, 154-156
    infectious mechanism of, 150
    manifestations of, 150
    pathology of, 150
    prognosis of, 162
    special considerations in, 158-160, 160f
    treatment for, 160-162
Skin cancer, in HIV infection, 250
Skin lesions
    biopsy of, 276
    of returning traveler, 294
Skin manifestations, 276
Solid organ abscess, 172
Solid organ transplantation (SOT), 272-274, 274t
Specialty staining, 30
Specimen(s), collection and processing of, 28
Spinal epidural abscess, 100, 102f
Spirochetal meningitis
    diagnosis of, 82
    epidemiology and etiology of, 78
Sporothrix schenckii, skin and soft tissue infection from, 156
Sputum
    Gram stain, 120, 122f
Staphylococcal toxic shock syndrome, 52-54, 152
Staphylococcus aureus
    skin and soft tissue infection from, 152
    urinary tract infections from, 196
Staphylococcus aureus infection
    in bone, 188
    infective endocarditis in, 134
    lymphadenitis in, acutesuppurative, 56
    pneumonia in, 120, 122f
    sepsis in, 42, 44t
    toxic shock syndrome in, 52-54
Streptococcal toxic shock syndrome, 152
Streptococcus agalactiae, skin and soft tissue infection from, 152
Streptococcus pneumoniae infection
    immunization for, 260
    meningitis in, 74, 82
    pneumonia in, 120, 122f
Streptococcus pyogenes infection
    pneumonia in, 118-120
    skin and soft tissue, 152
Strongyloides hyperinfection, 286
Strongyloidosis, 298
Subacute bacterial endocarditis (SBE), 134, 142t
    diagnosis of, 136-140
Subdural empyema, 98-100
Submandibular space infection, 112

性传播疾病，57
性传播感染（STI），215-231
    生殖器溃疡性疾病，221-229，223t
    HIV 感染，259-261
    尿道炎和宫颈炎，215-221
产志贺氏毒素大肠埃希菌（STEC）
    腹泻，179t-181t
志贺菌
    志贺菌引起的腹泻，179，179t-181t
乙状结肠切除术，治疗憩室炎，167
显性菌尿，定义，195
窦血栓形成，101-103
皮肤和软组织感染
    急性细菌性感染，151-163
    致病微生物，153
    细菌和真菌分类，157t-159t
    定义，151
    诊断，159-161
    鉴别诊断，161
    流行病学，151
    真菌和病毒，155-157
    感染机制，151
    临床表现，151
    病理学，151
    预后，163
    特殊诊断注意事项，159-161，161f
    治疗，161-163
皮肤癌，HIV 感染，251
皮病变
    活体组织检查，277
    返程旅客，295
皮肤表现，277
实质器官脓肿，173
实质器官移植（SOT），273-275，275t
特殊染色，31
样本，采集和处理，29
硬脊膜外脓肿，101，103f
螺旋体脑膜炎
    诊断，83
    流行病学和病因，79
申克孢子丝菌，皮肤和软组织感染，157
痰
    革兰氏染色，121，123f
葡萄球菌中毒性休克综合征，53-55，153
金黄色葡萄球菌
    皮肤和软组织感染，153
    尿路感染，197
金黄色葡萄球菌感染
    骨骼感染，189
    感染性心内膜炎，135
    急性化脓性淋巴结炎，57
    肺炎，121，123f
    感染中毒症，43，45t
    中毒休克综合征，53-55
链球菌中毒性休克综合征，153
无乳链球菌，皮肤和软组织感染，153
肺炎链球菌感染
    免疫接种，261
    脑膜炎，75，83
    肺炎，121，123f
化脓性链球菌感染
    肺炎，119-121
    皮肤和软组织，153
类圆线虫超感染，287
类圆线虫病，299
亚急性细菌性心内膜炎（SBE），135，143t
    诊断，137-141
硬膜下积脓，99-101
下颌下间隙感染，113

Substance use disorder, HIV infection and, 258
Surgical site infections, 206t, 208-210
Swimmer's ear, 114-116
Symptomatic therapy, for diarrhea, 186
Syndromic assay panels, 34, 36f
Syphilis, 220-226
    clinical presentation of, 220-224
    definition of, 220
    diagnosis and differential diagnosis of, 224
    epidemiology of, 220
    inguinal lymphadenopathyin, 56
    pathology of, 220
    prognosis of, 226
    serologic testing for, 224t
    treatment of, 226, 226t
Syphilitic meningitis, clinical presentation of, 78-80
Systemic inflammatory response syndrome (SIRS), 60
Systemic lupus erythematosus (SLE)
    fever in, 46
    subacute bacterial endocarditis and, 138

T

T lymphocytes, 20-24
Taenia solium, 300
Tamm-Horsfall proteins, 204
Tapeworms, 300
    intestinal, 300
T-cell receptors, 16
Temperature, thermoregulation of, 40
Tetralogy ofFallot
    infective endocarditis and, 134
Thrombocytopenia
    in sepsis, 68
Toll-like receptors (TLRs), 8, 10t-14t, 64
Tonsillitis, 110-112
Toxoplasma encephalitis, 246
Toxoplasma gondii infections, 246, 296t
Toxoplasmosis, 56
    in HIV-infected patients, cerebral, 98
    mononucleosis syndrome in, 42
Transesophageal echocardiography (TEE)
    in infective endocarditis, 136
Trauma
    osteomyelitis from, 188
Traumatic wounds, 160
Travelers, preparation of, 290-294
Traveler's diarrhea, 182
Traveler's infection
    AIDS and, 294
    diarrhea, 292-294
    helminth, 298-300
    pregnant women and, 294
    protozoal, 294-298
    in returning traveler, 294
Treponema pallidum, 220
    infection, meningitis in, 78
Trichomonas vaginalis, 296t
Trichomoniasis, 218
Trichuris trichiura, 298
Trimethoprim-sulfamethoxazole (TMP-SMX), for urinary tract infections, 196
Trypanosoma species, 296t
Trypanosomiasis
    African, 296
    American, 296-298
Tuberculosis, 124-130
    clinical manifestation of, 126-130
    definition of, 124
    diagnosis of, 126

药物滥用，HIV 感染，259
手术部位感染，207t，209-211
游泳耳，115-117
对症治疗，腹泻，187
综合征检测试剂盒，35，37f
梅毒，221-227
    临床表现，221-225
    定义，221
    诊断和鉴别诊断，225
    流行病学，221
    腹股沟淋巴结肿大，57
    病理学，221
    预后，227
    血清学检测，225t
    治疗，227，227t
梅毒性脑膜炎，临床表现，79-81
系统性炎症反应综合征（SIRS），61
系统性红斑狼疮（SLE）
    发热，47
    亚急性细菌性心内膜炎，139

T

T 淋巴细胞，21-25
猪带绦虫，301
T-H 蛋白，205
绦虫，301
    肠道绦虫，301
T 细胞受体，17
体温，体温调节，41
法洛四联症
    感染性心内膜炎，135
血小板减少症
    感染中毒症，69
Toll 样受体（TLR），9，11t-15t，65
扁桃体炎，111-113
弓形虫脑炎，247
刚地弓形虫感染，247，297t
弓形虫病，57
    HIV 感染患者，脑弓形虫病，99
    单核细胞增多症综合征，43
经食管超声心动图（TEE）
    感染性心内膜炎，137
创伤
    骨髓炎，189
外伤，161
旅行前准备，291-295
旅行者腹泻，183
旅行者感染
    AIDS，295
    腹泻，293-295
    蠕虫，299-301
    妊娠女性，295
    原虫，295-299
    返程旅行者，295
梅毒螺旋体，221
    感染，脑膜炎，79
阴道毛滴虫，297t
滴虫病，219
毛首鞭形线虫，299
甲氧苄啶-磺胺甲噁唑（TMP-SMX），治疗尿路感染，197

锥虫属，297t
锥虫病
    非洲锥虫病，297
    美洲锥虫病，297-299
结核病，125-131
    临床表现，127-131
    定义，125
    诊断，127

epidemiology of, 124-126
extrapulmonary, 130
fever of unknown origin and, 46
HIV infection screening of, 260
lymphadenopathyin, 54
microbiology of, 126
pathobiology of, 126, 128f
prognosis of, 130
treatment and prevention for, 130
Tuberculous meningitis
clinical presentation of, 80
diagnosis of, 82
epidemiology and etiology of, 78
23-valent pneumococcal polysaccharide vaccine, 124
Typhoid, 292
Typhoid fever, 42, 48t
Typhus, murine, 54

U

Ultrasonography
for appendicitis, 164
for cholecystitis, 170
Uncomplicated urinary tract infections, therapy for, 198t
Upper respiratory tract infections, viral, 42, 44t
Urethritis, 214-220
nongonococcal, 214
causes of, 220
Urinary tract, protection of, 6
Urinary tract infections (UTI), 194-200
catheter-associated, 202-204, 206t, 208f
complications of, 198, 198t-200t
definition of, 194
diagnosis of, 194
epidemiology of, 196
fever in, 46
laboratory findings of, 194-196
pathogenesis of, 196
treatment of, 196-198

V

Vaccination human papillomavirus, 228
Vaginitis, 218-220
clinical presentation of, 220
definition of, 218
diagnosis and differential diagnosis of, 220
epidemiology of, 218
pathology of, 218
prognosis of, 220
treatment of, 220
Vancomycin-resistant *Enterococcus* (VRE), 210-212
Varicella-zoster disease, 248
Varicella-zoster virus (VZV)
immunocompromised host and, 282
infection, 54
skin and soft tissue infection from, 156
Ventilator-associated pneumonia (VAP), 204
Vibrio cholerae, diarrhea from, 178t-180t, 180
Vibrio vulnificus, skin and soft tissue infection from, 154
Viral hepatitides, 254
Viral hepatitis, HIV infection screening of, 260
Viral infection, 42
Viral meningitis
clinical presentation of, 78
differentiation from bacterial meningitis, 82
epidemiology and etiology of, 76-78
Viridans streptococci, subacute bacterial infective endocarditis and, 134-136
Virology, of human immunodeficiency virus, 234-238, 236f-238f

流行病学，125-127
肺外结核，131
不明原因发热，47
HIV 感染筛查，261
淋巴结肿大，55
微生物学，127
病理生物学，127，129f
预后，131
治疗和预防，131
结核性脑膜炎
临床表现，81
诊断，83
流行病学和病因，79
23 价肺炎球菌多糖疫苗，125
伤寒，293
伤寒发热，43，49t
鼠型斑疹伤寒，55

U

超声检查
阑尾炎，165
胆囊炎，171
非复杂性尿路感染，治疗，199t
上呼吸道病毒性感染，43，45t
尿道炎，215-221
非淋菌性尿道炎，215
病因，221
尿路保护，7
尿路感染（UTI），195-201
导管相关 UTI，203-205，207t，209f
并发症，199，199t-201t
定义，195
诊断，195
流行病学，197
发热，47
实验室检查，195-197
发病机制，197
治疗，197-199

V

人乳头瘤病毒疫苗接种，231
阴道炎，219-221
临床表现，221
定义，219
诊断和鉴别诊断，221
流行病学，219
病理学，219
预后，221
治疗，221
万古霉素耐药肠球菌（VRE），211-213
水痘-带状疱疹病，249
水痘-带状疱疹病毒（VZV）
免疫妥协宿主，283
感染，55
皮肤和软组织感染，157
呼吸机相关肺炎（VAP），205
霍乱弧菌，腹泻，179t-181t，181
创伤弧菌，皮肤和软组织感染，155
病毒性肝炎，255
病毒性肝炎，HIV 感染筛查，261
病毒感染，43
病毒性脑膜炎
临床表现，79
与细菌性脑膜炎的鉴别诊断，83
流行病学和病因学，77-79
草绿色链球菌，亚急性细菌性心内膜炎，135-137
病毒学，人类免疫缺陷病毒，235-239，237f-239f

Viruses
    arthropod-borne, 42
    pneumonia and, 118-120

W

Warts, genital, 228
Whipworm, 298

X

Xanthogranulomatouspyelonephritis, in urinary tract infections, 198t-200t

Y

Yellow fever, 292
Yersinia enterocolitica
    diarrhea from, 178t-180t, 182
Yersinia pestis, 56

病毒
    虫媒病毒，43
    肺炎，119-121

W

生殖器疣，229
鞭虫，299

X

黄色肉芽肿性肾盂肾炎，见于尿路感染，199t-201t

Y

黄热病，293
小肠结肠炎耶尔森菌
    腹泻，179t-181t，183
鼠疫耶尔森菌，57